AF881028

Lung Cancer: Clinical and Surgical Specifications

Edited By

Akın Eraslan Balcı

Department of Thoracic Surgery
Euphrates University School of Medicine
Elazig
Turkey

CONTENTS

CHAPTER

FOREWORD

Carcinoma of the lung is the leading cause of cancer deaths. The management of lung cancer involved a questionnaire prior to treatment. It contains questions asked when taking a medical history, when forming a differential diagnosis, when choosing treatment, when performing an operation and when planning a postoperative treatment. Physicians who worked on lung cancer, regardless of speciality, are constantly confronted with questions posed from patients, from their collegues and, most importantly, from within themselves.

These considerations are behind developing a new textbook of this nature and caused the motivation. The book edited by Prof. Balci provides a broad overview of the lung cancer surgery, clinical and molecular aspects and pathology of it.

This textbook is a good resource to pulmonary and critical care specialist and their trainees, as well as thoracic surgeons, oncologists, and pulmonary pathologists. Major objectives are to present a summation of the current knowledge and clinical concepts of the surgical management of lung cancer. The pathophysiological alterations produced and the correction of these by appropriate intervention are emphasized throughout. Clinical features, pathological changes, surgical management, operative results and prognosis are included as integral part of the book.

We are most grateful to the numerous authors who put so many times into writing otustanding chapters. This book includes all the relevant and current information on lung cancer. Much information is completely updated. Although we believe that this book will provide a clear understanding of these manifestations, we invite our readers to inform us about differences of opinion they may have with its contents and areas that need improvment.

Yavuz Selim Ilhan

Euphrates University Hospital
Head of General Surgery Department
Elazig
Turkey

PREFACE

This book focuses on the lung cancer, which is the mostly encountered, and one of the most challenging malignant disease of the world. Worldwide, the annual number of new cases of lung cancer is estimated at more than one million and is expected to increase to ten million in 2025. Fortunately, the political efforts to reduce the use of tobacco are getting increasing attention in many countries and the statistics are now showing the first positive results.

Over the last decade there have been several improvements and changes in the lung cancer management. Among the epidemiologic changes we see a change in the histopathologic pattern, with a relative decrease in squamous cell carcinoma and a rise in adenocarcinoma. Much research is attempting to identify biomarkers to predict a high risk for developing lung cancer. This will be important for implementing screening and prevention strategies. There is a steady improvement of the overall management of lung cancer based on an increasing use of combined modality therapy, consisting of surgery, chemotherapy, and radiotherapy applied concurrently or sequentially in early stage disease. Furthermore, new techniques are gaining ground, both within surgery and radiotherapy, and targeted medical therapy is being offered to more and more patients.

This book is not intended as a comprehensive textbook, but as a concise summary of advances in lung cancer clinical research and treatment for the clinician. The textbook brings up-to-date information about lung cancer, based on worldwide experience, for the use of the many physicians involved in this field.

All of the authors have been selected for their expertise and proven achievement in these challenging fields; I would like to sincerely thank all of them for participating with enthusiasm in this project. I hope that the different contributions will help the readers to fill in the gaps and stimulate them for future developments.

Akın Eraslan Balcı

Euphrates University
School of Medicine
Department of Thoracic Surgery
Elazig
Turkey

List of Contributors

Abdurrahman Y.E. Oğur

Euphrates University, School of Medicine, Department of Radiology, Elazig, Turkey

Ozgur Ozyilkan

Division of Medical Oncology, Baskent University, Research and Treatment Center, Adana, Turkey

Akif Turna

Istanbul University Cerrahpasa Medical Faculty, Department of Thoracic Surgery, Kocamustafapasa/Fatih Istanbul, Turkey

Akın E. Balcı

Euphrates University School of Medicine, Department of Thoracic Surgery, Elazig, Turkey

Bülent Arman

Maltepe University School of Medicine, Department of Thoracic Surgery, İstanbul, Turkey

Mehmet A. Bedirhan

Yedikule Hospital for Chest Disease, Chief of Surgery, İstanbul, Turkey

Cem Onal

Baskent University, Faculty of Medicine, Adana Research and Treatment Center, Deparment of Radiation Oncology, Yuregir/ Adana, Turkey

Ahmet Hatipoğlu

Department of Thoracic Surgery, Baskent University Faculty of Medicine, Ankara Teaching and Medical Research Center, Bahcelievler/Ankara, Turkey

Ebru Ö. Etem

Department of Medical Biology, Firat University, Faculty of Medicine, Elazig, Turkey

Fulya Ilhan

Department of Immunology, Euphrates University, Faculty of Medicine, Elazığ, Turkey

Gamze Kirkil

Department of Respiratory Diseases, Euphrates University, Elazığ, Turkey

Günay Aydin

Department of Respiratory Diseases, İstanbul University, Cerrahpasa Medical School, Turkey

Ibrahim H. Ozercan

Department of Pathology, Euphrates University, School of Medicine, Elazig, Turkey

Kamil Kaynak

Department of Thoracic Surgery, Istanbul University Cerrahpasa Medical Faculty, Kocamustafapasa/Fatih Istanbul, Turkey

Mehmet O. Özyurtkan

Department of Thoracic Surgery, Firat University, Faculty of Medicine, Elazığ, Turkey

Selami A. Önal

Department of Pain, Euphrates University, Elazig, Turkey

Süleyman Özyalçın

Depratment of Algology, Istanbul University, Istanbul Faculty of Medicine, Monoblok, Capa, Istanbul, Turkey

Tansel A. Balci

Department of Nuclear Medicine, Firat Euphrates University School of Medicine, Elazig, Turkey

Tulin Cagatay

Istanbul University, Istanbul Medical Faculty, Department of Pulmonary diseases, CAPA, Istanbul, Turkey

Murat Kara

Department of Medical Genetics School of Medicine, Euphrates University, Elazig-Turkey

Semen Onder

Department of Pathology, Euphrates University, School of Medicine, Elazig, Turkey

Gulfer Okumus

Department of Pulmonary Diseases, Istanbul University, Istanbul Medical Faculty, CAPA, Istanbul, Turkey

Serdar Erturan

Department of Respiratory Diseases, İstanbul University, Cerrahpasa Medical School, Turkey

Dalokay Kiliç

Department of Thoracic Surgery, Baskent University Faculty of Medicine, Ankara Teaching and Medical Research Center, Bahcelievler, Ankara, Turkey

Alper Findikçioğlu

Department of Thoracic Surgery, Baskent University Faculty of Medicine, Adana Teaching and Medical Research Center, Adana, Turkey

Ahmet K. Poyraz

Department of Radiology, Euphrates University, School of Medicine, Elazig, Turkey

Ahmet Demirkaya

Department of Thoracic Surgery, Istanbul University, Cerrahpasa Medical Faculty, Kocamustafapasa/Fatih Istanbul, Turkey

Ezel Ersen

Department of Thoracic Surgery, State Hospital, Kocaeli, Turkey

Hassan V. Kara

Marmara University, School of Medicine, Department of Thoracic Surgery, İstanbul, Turkey

Alpay Orki

Department of Thoracic Surgery, Maltepe University School of Medicine, İstanbul, Turkey

Altuğ Koşar

Thoracic Surgery Department, Lutfi Kirdar Research and Training Hospital, Istanbul, Turkey

Burcu Kilic

Department of Thoracic Surgery, Istanbul University, Cerrahpasa Medical Faculty, Turkey

Fatih Kose

Division of Medical Oncology, Baskent University, Research Center, Adana, Turkey

Ahmet T. Sumbul

Division of Medical Oncology, Baskent University, Research Center, Adana, Turkey

Ayşegül A. Yücel

Department of Immunology, Gazi University, Faculty of Medicine, Beşevler, Ankara, Turkey

Selçuk Dinçer

Depratment of Algology, Istanbul University, Istanbul Faculty of Medicine, Monoblok, CAPA, Istanbul, Turkey

Sedat Altin

Yedikule Chest Disease Hospital, İstanbul, Turkey

Send Orders of Reprints at reprints@benthamscience.net
Lung Cancer: Clinical and Surgical Specifications, **2013, 3-12** **3**

CHAPTER 1

Epidemiology and Carciongenesis of Lung Cancer

Part A: Factors Related with Lung Cancer Epidemiology

Gamze Kirkil*

Firat University, Department of Chest Diseases, Elazig, Turkey

Abstract: Pulmonary carcinoma is the most commonly diagnosed cancer in worldwide, and it is the most common cause of cancer death. A variety of factors, such as ethnicity, age, gender, geographic location, and socioeconomic status, influence the rate in spesific groups. The known behavioral and environmental causes--cigarette smoking, diet, asbestos and other occupational carcinogens, radon, and environmental tobacco smoke--are responsible for the majority of cases. Passive smoking, the involuntary inhalation of tobacco smoke by nonsmokers, has also been found to cause lung cancer. Moreover familial aggregation and increased familial risk for lung cancer have been reported.

Keywords: Lung carcinoma, smoking, occupational carcinogens, familial aggregation.

INTRODUCTION

Pulmonary carcinoma is the most commonly diagnosed cancer in worldwide (1.61 million, 12.7% of the total), and it is the most common cause of cancer death (1.38 million, 18.2% of the total) [1]. At the end of the 20th century, lung cancer had become one of the leading causes of preventable death [2]. Routine mortality statistics confirmed the clinical impression that the lung cancer became more frequent across the first half of the 20th century. Where as lung cancer accounted for only 3% of all cancer deaths in women in 1950, in the year 2000, it accounted for an estimated 25% of all cancer deaths [3]. Because many of cancer individuals are between 50 and 70 years of age at the time of death, the neoplasm is responsible for the most years of life lost of any cancer.

A variety of factors, such as ethnicity, age, gender, geographic location, and socioeconomic status, influence the rate in specific groups. Rates in man exceed those in women, and rates in African American men exceed those in white men

***Address correspondence to Gamze Kirkil:** Firat University, Department of Chest Diseases, Elazig, Turkey; Tel: +90 535 2991523; Fax: 90 424 2388096; E-mail: gamkirkil@yahoo.com

[4]. In the United States, rates in men are currently in decline, however rates in white and African American women, also women in Japan, Norway, Poland, Sweden, United Kingdom, Australia, Denmark, New Zeland, Canada have continued to rise [5-8]. These rates are related to parallel trends in smoking prevalance.

The known behavioral and environmental causes--cigarette smoking, asbestos and other occupational carcinogens, radon, and environmental tobacco smoke--are responsible for the majority of cases [9]. Worldwide, tobacco smoking is associated with more of 90% of cases of lung cancer [10]. The vast majority of lung cancer deaths are attributable to cigarette smoking. The risk of dying from lung cancer is associated with age of initiation and duration of cigarette smoking. In countries where smoking has been a widespread habit, it is responsible for 80-90% of lung cancer deaths [11]. By the early 1950s, epidemiologic studies in Britain and the United States using the case-control method had shown that cigarettes were strongly associated with the risk for lung cancer [12-14]. As Wingo *et al.* have continued to follow lung cancer incidence and mortality rates, they have readily shown that their rise and decline parallel past trends of cigarette smoking [15]. In more developed countries, the incidence and mortality rates are generally declining, reflecting previous trends in smoking prevalence. However, in less developed countries lung cancer rates are predicted to continue to increase due to endemic tobacco use [16].

Lung cancer is also a leading cause of morbidity and mortality in patients with COPD as 33% of patients died of lung cancer over a 14.5-year follow-up [17]. In most cases this reflects cigarette smoke exposure which is able to induce an inflammatory response in the airways of smokers. Cigarette smoke induces the release of many inflammatory mediators and growth factors including TGF-β, EGFR, IL-1, IL-8 and G-CSF through oxidative stress pathways and this inflammation may persist for decades after smoking cessation. Mucus production is also increased by these inflammatory mediators, further linking airway inflammation to an important mechanism of lung cancer [18]. Smokers with silicosis are also at increased risk of lung cancer [19]. In a meta-analysis the relative risks of lung cancer due to silica and silicosis is estimated. The pooled relative risks were 1.32 (95% confidence interval (CI), 1.23-1.41) for silica, 2.37

(95% CI, 1.98-2.84) for silicosis and 0.96 (95% CI, 0.81-1.15) for non-silicosis with exposure to silica. They concluded that it was less possible that silica exposure directly increases lung cancer risk. On the other hand, the relative risk, 2.37 for silicosis suggested that silicosis increases lung cancer risk. Meta-analysis also revealed that cigarette smoking strongly increased the lung cancer risk in silicotic patients (relative risk, 4.47; 95% CI, 3.17-6.30) [20].

Passive smoking, the involuntary inhalation of tobacco smoke by nonsmokers, has also been found to cause lung cancer [21]. It has been reported that there was a close relationship between lung cancer risk and environmental tobacco smoke at workplace among non-smoking subjects. Especially for non-smoking women who expose to workplace environment tobacco smoke have a close relationship with lung cancer [22].

Although its predominant cause is now widely known (tobacco smoking), there are other causes as well, some acting in concert with smoking to synergistically increase risk. Radon is the first occupational respiratory carcinogen to be identified [23]. Radioactive radon is an inert gas that can migrate from soils and rocks and accumulate in enclosed areas, such as homes and underground mines. Studies of miners show that exposure to radon decay products causes lung cancer. In the miners, about 40% of all lung cancer deaths may be due to radon progeny exposure, in the United States, 10% of all lung cancer deaths might be due to indoor radon exposure [24]. Krewski *et al.* [25] conducted a study to evaluate the risk associated with prolonged residential radon exposure, a combined analysis of the primary data from seven large scale case-control studies of residential radon and lung cancer risk. The combined data set included a total of 4081 cases and 5281 controls, representing the largest aggregation of data on residential radon and lung cancer conducted to date. Residential radon concentrations were determined primarily by a-track detectors placed in the living areas of homes of the study subjects in order to obtain an integrated 1-yr average radon concentration in indoor air. Conditional likelihood regression was used to estimate the excess risk of lung cancer due to residential radon exposure, with adjustment for attained age, sex, study, smoking factors, residential mobility, and completeness of radon measurements. The estimated odds ratio (OR) of lung cancer generally increased with radon concentration. The OR trend was consistent with linearity (p =.10), and the excess OR (EOR) was 0.10 per Bq/m3 with 95% confidence limits (-0.01, 0.26). They concluded that these results provide direct evidence of an association between residential radon and lung cancer risk, a finding predicted by extrapolation of results from occupational studies of radon-exposed underground miners. A case-control study of residential radon and lung cancer was conducted in five countries in New Jersey and involved 561 cases and 740 controls. The authors concluded that while the odds ratios (ORs) for whole data were suggestive of an increased risk for exposures >75 Bq m(-3), these associations were not statistically significant. The adjusted excess OR (EOR) per 100 Bq m(-3) was -0.13 (95% CI: -0.30 to 0.44) for males, 0.29 (95% CI: -0.12 to 1.70) for females and 0.05 (95% CI: -0.14 to 0.56) for all subjects combined. An analysis of radon effects by histological type of lung cancer showed that the OR was strongest for small/oat cell carcinomas in both males and females. They found no statistical heterogeneity of radon effects by demographic factors (age at disease occurrence, education level and type of respondent). Analysis by categories of smoking status, frequency or duration did not modify the risk estimates of radon on lung cancer [26].

The list of human occupational causes of lung cancer also includes arsenic, asbestos, chromates, chloromethyl ethers, nickel, polycyclic aromatic hydrocarbons, radon progeny, and other agents [27]. Outdoor air pollution, which includes combustion-generated carcinogens, is also considered to contribute to the lung cancer burden in urban dwellers. In some developing countries, exposure to fumes from cooking stoves and fires is associated with lung cancer risk. Associations of diet with lung cancer risk have been vigorously investigated with the anticipation that dietary micronutrients that modify the high lung cancer risk in smokers might be found [28].

Epidemiologic studies showed that asbestos cumulative exposures increase the risk of lung cancer to a variable extent, depending on the manufacturing process and the specific job. The risk appears relatively small and is detectable after massive exposures only. Clinical diagnosis of asbestos-related lung cancer is based upon medical history, possible lung fibrosis and counts of asbestos bodies and fibers in bronchoalveolar lavage and lung tissues. The multiplicative interaction between smoke and asbestos is only detectable when the risk associated with asbestos exposure is increased, *i.e.* after high exposures [29].

Although it is known that smoking is a predominant cause of lung cancer, 15% of lung cancer patients are never-smoked, more often women and adenocarcinoma. Primary factors closely tied to lung cancer in never smokers include exposure to known and suspected carcinogens including radon, second-hand tobacco smoke, and other indoor air pollutants. Several other exposures have been implicated. However, a large fraction of lung cancers occurring in never smokers cannot be definitively associated with established environmental risk factors, highlighting the need for additional epidemiologic research in this area. Lung cancer in never-smoker appears to be a distinct entity from lung cancer in smoker, with specific molecular characteristics such as frequent EGFR mutations. Limited research has been conducted evaluating familial aggregation and genetic linkage of lung cancer, particularly among never smokers in whom such associations might be expected to be strongest. Data emerging over the past several years show that lung cancers in never smokers are much more likely to carry activating mutations of the epidermal growth factor receptor (EGFR), a key oncogenic factor and direct therapeutic target of several newer anticancer drugs. EGFR mutant lung cancers may represent a distinct class of lung cancers, enriched in the never-smoking population, and less clearly linked to direct tobacco carcinogenesis [30]. Epidermal growth factor receptor gene mutations, which are correlated with sensitivity to EGFR-tyrosine kinase inhibitors (EGFR-TKIs), are more frequent in never-smoker lung cancers. In a study, microRNA (miRNA) expression profiling of 28 cases of never-smoker lung cancer identified aberrantly expressed miRNAs, which were much fewer than in lung cancers of smokers and included miRNAs previously identified (*e.g.*, up-regulated miR-21) and unidentified (*e.g.*, down-regulated miR-138) in those smoker cases. The changes in expression of some of these miRNAs, including miR-21, were more remarkable in cases with EGFR mutations than in those without these mutations. A significant correlation between phosphorylated-EGFR (p-EGFR) and miR-21 levels in lung carcinoma cell lines and the suppression of miR-21 by an EGFR-TKI, AG1478, suggest that the EGFR signaling is a pathway positively regulating miR-21 expression. In the never-smoker-derived lung adenocarcinoma cell line H3255 with mutant EGFR and high levels of p-EGFR and miR-21, antisense inhibition of miR-21 enhanced AG1478-induced apoptosis. In a never-smoker-derived adenocarcinoma cell line H441 with wild-type EGFR, the antisense miR-21 not only showed the additive effect with AG1478 but also induced apoptosis by itself. These results suggest that aberrantly increased expression of miR-21, which is enhanced further by the activated EGFR signaling pathway, plays a significant role in lung carcinogenesis in never-smokers, as well as in smokers, and is a potential therapeutic target in both EGFR-mutant and wild-type cases [31].

New molecular targets are on investigation, such as EML4-ALK translocation [32]. In Shaw *et al.* study [33] it is shown that patients with EML4-ALK-positive tumours, like patients who harbored EGFR mutations, also were more likely to be never/light smokers compared with patients in the wild type (WT)/WT cohort.

Familial aggregation and increased familial risk for lung cancer have been reported in several studies, subsequently [34-36]. Gu *et al.* [37] explored the relationship between family history of lung cancer and lung cancer risk by searching PubMed, CENTRAL, CBM, CNKI and VIP, they collected both domestic and overseas published documents before November, 2009 on family history of lung cancer and lung cancer risk. In this study, twenty-eight publications were included into the combined analysis, which indicated that the lung cancer risk of the probands' first-degree relatives was 1.88 times higher than that of their controls'. Moreover, in the sub-study, compared with the controls' father mother and siblings, the OR of the probands' father mother and siblings was 1.62 ($p<0.001$), 1.96 ($p<0.001$) and 1.92 ($p<0.001$), respectively. For gender categories, lung cancer risk in first-degree relatives of female probands was 1.89 ($p<0.001$) times higher than that of their corresponding controls'. And for male subjects, the lung cancer risk was 1.99 ($p<0.001$) times higher in proboands' first-degree relatives.

A critical review of epidemiological studies on diet and lung cancer over the last 20+ years has not provided overwhelming evidence that higher consumption of vegetables, fruit, low-fat/low-cholesterol foods or such micronutrients as carotenoids, selenium and vitamins A, C or E is associated with reduced lung cancer risk. Results from case-control studies have been more positive, with about one half showing fruit and vegetables or their associated micronutrients to be associated with reduced risk. However, most results from cohort and serum micronutrient studies, which avoid the problems of inaccurate accounting of diet and recall bias, were statistically insignificant. Moreover, although most studies were conducted on white male smokers in North America and Europe, the few studies which found significant contrary trends were among subjects of different backgrounds, *i.e.*, black American males and Chinese women in China. Since male smokers *vs.* nonsmokers in Europe, North America and Japan have been shown in other studies to be lower consumers of fruit/vegetables, and less likely to pursue "perceived healthier lifestyles," the possibility that some of the epidemiological findings on diet and lung cancer are artifactually due to inadequate adjustment for behavioral correlates of smoking and health seekers in a particular society must be considered [38].

A case-control study was conducted in Uruguay to estimate the odds ratios associated with lung cancer risk. They showed that fried meat, barbecued meat, and salted meat were positively associated with risk (OR of the highest quartile of salted meat *versus* the lowest, 2.90, 95 % CI 1.99-4.25, p-value for trend<0.0001), boiled red meat was mainly protective. They conclude that salted meat was the main risk factor [39]. In an other study it is concluded that consumption of red meat, was associated with an increased risk of lung cancer even after controlling for total fat, saturated fat, cholesterol, fruit, yellow-green vegetable consumption and smoking history, while yellow-green vegetables are associated with a decreased risk of lung cancer [40].

Case-control studies of newly diagnosed lung cancer have shown that HDL-cholesterol levels are reduced in lung cancer cases relative to levels observed in the control groups [41-44]. Kucharska-Newton *et al.* [45] examined prospectively the association of baseline plasma HDL-cholesterol levels with incidence of lung cancer in subject of the Atherosclerosis Risk in Communities (ARIC) cohort. They found relatively weak inverse association of HDL-cholesterol with lung cancer that was dependent on smoking status, even after exclusion of cases diagnosed within 5 years of baseline. Biological mechanisms that might link low plasma levels of HDL-cholesterol with cancer are not well understood. HDL regulation of cell cycle entry through a mitogen activated protein kinase-dependent pathway [46] and apoptosis [47] modulation of cytokine production, and antioxidative function [48] has been considered and is biologically plausible.

A consideration of the epidemiology of lung cancer consistently reinforces one major theme: the pandemic of lung cancer is a consequence of the tragic and widespread addiction to cigarettes throughout the world. Curtailing the pandemic of lung cancer will require preventing youths from starting to smoke cigarettes and effectively promoting smoking cessation among addicted smokers. There are other causes that also need control, but fortunately there have been successes in reducing exposures to occupational carcinogens in countries of the developed world.

ACKNOWLEDGEMENTS

Declared none.

CONFLICT OF INTEREST

The author confirms that this article content has no conflict of interest.

REFERENCES

[1] Ferlay J, Shin HR, Bray F, *et al.* Estimates of worldwide burden of cancer in 2008: GLOBOCAN 2008. Int J Cancer 2010Jun 17. [Epub ahead of print].
[2] Rosen G. A history of public health: expanded edition. Baltimore, MD: The Johns Hopkins University Press, 1993.
[3] Jemal A, Chu KC, Tarone RE. Recent trends in lung cancer mortality in the United States. J Natl Cancer Inst 2001; 93: 277-83.
[4] Schwartz AG, Swanson GM. Lung carcinoma in African Americans and whites: A population-based study in metropolitan Detroit, Michigan. Cancer 1997; 79: 45-52.
[5] Travis WD, Lubin J, Ries L, Devesa S. United States lung carcinoma incidence trends-declining for most histologic types among males, increasing among females. Cancer 1996; 77: 2464-70.
[6] Fry WA, Menck HR, Winchester DP. The National Cancer Data base report on lung cancer. Cancer 1996; 77: 1947-55.
[7] Stanley K, Stjernsward J. Lung cancer-a worldwide health problem. Chest 1989; 96: 1-5.
[8] Lopez-Abente G, Pollan M, de la Iglesia P, Ruiz M. Characterization of the lung cancer epidemic in the European Union (1970-1990). Cancer Epidemiol Biomarkers Prev 1995; 4: 813-20.
[9] Beckett WS. Epidemiology and etiology of lung cancer. Clin Chest Med 1993; 14: 1-15.
[10] Jemal A, Siegel R, Ward E, *et al.* Cancer statistics, 2009. CA Cancer J Clin 2009; 59: 225–49.
[11] US Department of Health and Human Services. The Health Consequences of Smoking. Cancer: a report of the Surgeon General. US Department of Health and Human Services, Office on Smoking and Health. DHHS publication No. (PHS) 82-50179, 1982.

[12] Doll R, Hill AB. Smoking and carcinoma of the lung; preliminary report. BMJ 1950; 2: 739-48.
[13] Levin ML, Goldstein H, Gerhardt PR. Cancer and tobacco smoking; a preliminary report. J Am Med Assoc 1950; 143: 336-8.
[14] Wynder EL, Graham EA. Tobacco smoking as a possible etiologic factor in bronchiogenic carcinoma; a study of 684 proved cases. J Am Med Assoc 1950; 143: 329-36.
[15] Wingo PA, Ries LA, Giovino GA, *et al.* Annual report to the nation on the status of cancer, 1973–1996, with a special section on lung cancer and tobacco smoking. J Natl Cancer Inst 1999; 91: 675-90.
[16] Youlden DR, Cramb SM, Baade PD. The international epidemiology of lung cancer: geographical distribution and secular trends. J Thorac Oncol 2008; 3: 819-31.
[17] Anthonisen NR, Skeans MA, Wise RA, *et al.* The effects of a smoking cessation intervention on 14.5-year mortality: a randomized clinical trial. Ann Intern Med 2005; 142: 233-9.
[18] Adcock IM, Caramori G, Barnes PJ. Chronic obstructive pulmonary disease and lung cancer: new molecular insights. Respiration 2011; 81: 265-84.
[19] Lo AI, Huang Y, Lam SY, *et al.* Early detection of central airway lung cancer in smokers with silicosis. Int J Tuberc Lung Dis 2011; 15: 523-7.
[20] Kurihara N, Wada O. Silicosis and smoking strongly increase lung cancer risk in silica-exposed workers. Ind Health 2004; 42: 303-14.
[21] The health consequences of involuntary smoking: a report of the Surgeon General. Washington, DC: US Government Printing Office, US Department of Health and Human Services, 1986; publication 87–8398.
[22] Wang X, Qin Y, Gu J, *et al.* Systematic review of studies of workplace exposure to environmental tobacco smoke and lung cancer risk. Zhongguo Fei Ai Za Zhi 2011; 14: 345-50.
[23] Samet JM. Radon and lung cancer. J Natl Cancer Inst 1989; 81: 745-57.
[24] Lubin JH, Boice JD Jr, Edling C, *et al.* Lung cancer in radon-exposed miners and estimation of risk from indoor exposure. J Natl Cancer Inst 1995; 87: 817-27.
[25] Krewski D, Lubin JH, Zielinski JM, *et al.* A combined analysis of North American case-control studies of residential radon and lung cancer. J Toxicol Environ Health A 2006; 69: 533-97.
[26] Wilcox HB, Al-Zoughool M, Garner MJ, *et al.* Case-control study of radon and lung cancer in New Jersey. Radiat Prot Dosimetry 2008; 128: 169-79.
[27] Coultas DB, Samet JM. Occupational lung cancer. Clin Chest Med 1992; 13: 341-54.
[28] Alberg AJ, Ford JG, Samet JM. Epidemiology of lung cancer: ACCP Evidence-Based Clinical Practice Guidelines (2nd Edition). Chest 2007; 132: 29S-55S.
[29] Lotti M. Asbestos-related lung cancer. G Ital med Lav Ergon 2010; 32: 381-4.
[30] Rudin CM, Avila-Tang E, Harris CC. Lung cancer in never smokers: molecular profiles and therapeutic implications. Clin Cancer Res 2009; 15: 5646-61.
[31] Seike M, Goto A, Okano T, *et al.* MiR-21 is an EGFR-regulated anti-apoptotic factor in lung cancer in never-smokers. Proc Natl Acad Sci USA 2009; 106: 12085-90.
[32] Hadoux J, Besse B, Planchard D. Lung cancer in never smoker: Epidemiology, molecular profiles and treatment. Presse Med 2011; 40: 371-8.
[33] Shaw AT, Yeap BY, Mino-Keudson M, *et al.* Clinical features and outcome of patients with non-small-cell lung cancer who harbor EML4-ALK. J Clin Oncol 2009; 27: 4247-53.

[34] Jin YT, Xu YC, Yang RD, *et al.* Familial aggregation of lung cancer in a high incidence area in China. Br J Cancer 2005; 92: 1321-5.

[35] Jin Y, Xu Y, Xu M, Xue S. Increased risk of cancer among relatives of patients with lung cancer in China. BMC Cancer 2005; 5: 146.

[36] Sellers TA, Ooi WL, Elston RC, *et al.* Increased familial risk for non-lung cancer among relatives of lung cancer patients. Am J Epidemiol 1987;126: 237-46.

[37] Gu J, Hua F, Zhong D, *et al.* Systematic review of the relationship between family history of lung cancer and lung cancer risk. Zhongguo Fei Ai Za Zhi 2010; 13: 224-9.

[38] Koo LC. Diet and lung cancer 20+ years later: more questions than answers? Int J Cancer 1997; 10: 22-9.

[39] Stefani ED, Ronco AL, Boffetta P, *et al.* Meat consumption, meat cooking and risk of lung cancer among uruguayan men. Asian Pac J Cancer Prev 2010; 11: 1713-7.

[40] Alavanja MC, Field RW, Sinha R, *et al.* Lung cancer risk and red meat consumption among Iowa women. Lung Cancer 2001; 34: 37-46.

[41] Siemianowicz K, Gminski J, Stajszczyk M, *et al.* Serum HDL cholesterol concentration in patients with squamous cell and small cell lung cancer. International Journal of Molecular Medicine 2000; 6(3): 307-11.

[42] Umeki S. Decreases in serum cholesterol levels in advanced lung cancer. Respiration 1993; 60(3): 178-81.

[43] Dessi S, Batetta B, Pulisci D, *et al.* Altered pattern of lipid metabolism in patients with lung cancer. Oncology 1992; 49(6): 436-41.

[44] Fiorenza AM, Branchi A, Sommariva D. Serum lipoprotein profile in patients with cancer. A comparison with non-cancer subjects. International Journal of Clinical and Laboratory Research 2000; 30(3): 141-5.

[45] Kucharska-Newton AM, Rosamond WD, Schroeder JC, *et al.* HDL-cholesterol and the incidence of lung cancer in the Atherosclerosis Risk in Communities (ARIC) study. Lung Cancer 2008; 61(3): 292-300.

[46] Nofer JR, Junker R, Pulawski E, *et al.* High density lipoproteins induce cell cycle entry in vascular smooth muscle cells *via* mitogen activated protein kinase-dependent pathway. Thrombosis and Haemostasis 2001; 85(4): 730-5.

[47] Nofer JR, Levkau B, Wolinska I, *et al.* Suppression of endothelial cell apoptosis by high density lipoproteins (HDL) and HDL-associated lysosphingolipids. Journal of Biological Chemistry 2001; 276(37): 34480-5.

[48] Von Eckardstein A, Hersberger M, Rohrer L. Current understanding of the metabolism and biological actions of HDL. Current Opinion in Clinical Nutrition and Metabolic Care 2005; 8(2): 147-2.

Send Orders of Reprints at reprints@benthamscience.net
Lung Cancer: Clinical and Surgical Specifications, 2013, 13-20

CHAPTER 1

Part B: Lung Cancer Cancerogenesis

Murat Kara*

Department of Medical Genetics School of Medicine, Mugla Sitki Kocman University, Mugla, Turkey

Abstract: Lung cancer is one of the most common cancers and is the leading cause of cancer mortality worldwide. The development of lung cancer is a multifactorial process that involves a series of genetic and epigenetic changes. Smoking tobacco is an important etiologic risk factor for lung cancer. Other risk factors include occupational and environmental long-term exposure, diet, familial aggregation, and genetic factors. Lung carcinogenesis involves identified genetic alterations, namely oncogenes, tumour suppressor genes, epigenetic alterations, and chromosomal abnormalities. New diagnostic and therapeutic approaches to lung cancer are urgently needed. Molecular genetic studies have focused on oncogenes, tumour suppressor genes, and chromosomal abnormalities.

Keywords: Lung cancer, chromosomal aberrations, smoking, oncogenes, tumour suppressor genes.

LUNG CANCER CANCEROGENESIS

Cancer is a considerable health issue around the world. Lung cancer is the most common cause of cancer death in both sexes in the United States, with an estimated 180,000 new cases and 150,000 deaths expected annually in the United States [1].

In human beings, carcinogenesis generally has multifactorial and complex mechanisms. Tumour development is affected by different factors and different mechanisms at different stages. Carcinogenesis is usually initiated by mutagens, which are classified as either endogenous or exogenous factors. Both endogenous and exogenous mutagens may cause human cancers. The exogenous carcinogens, which are chemical, physical, or biological agents, are the main causes of cancer.

***Address correspondence to Murat Kara:** Department of Medical Genetics, School of Medicine, Mugla Sitki Kocman University, Mugla, Turkey; Tel: 0-252-2115151; E-mail: dr.muratkara@gmail.com

Nickel, cadmium, arsenic, nitrosamines, trichloroethylene, arylamines, benzopyrene, aflatoxins, and reactive oxygen species are examples of chemical carcinogens. Examples of physical carcinogens are UV with irradiation and ionizing radiation. Human papilloma virus (*e.g.* strain 16), Epstein-Barr virus, Hepatitis virus B, Schistosoma mansoni, and Helicobacter pylori are among the biological carcinogens. Some of the endogenous carcinogens are DNA replication, metabolic reactions generating reactive oxygen species, and chronic inflammation [2, 3].

Failures of the mechanisms that usually control the growth and proliferation of cells lead to cancer. Cancer arises from the occurrence of abnormal gene expressions. Gene expression changes as a result of some DNA damage, such as a point mutation in the gene, translocation, amplification, deletion, and loss of heterozygosity (LOH) [2]. Mutations on proto-oncogenes and tumour suppressor genes have been implicated in the onset of cancer. Mutations leading to the over-expression of a proto-oncogene or the silencing of a tumour suppressor gene may lead to tumour formation.

Lung cancer may develop as a result of the accumulation of multiple molecular abnormalities that lead to genomic instability. The levels at which the alterations can take place are gene silencing through DNA sequence changes, methylation, DNA segment amplification or deletion, and whole-chromosome gains or losses [4, 5]. Accumulation of multiple genetic changes, including chromosome deletions, oncogene mutations, and methylation of tumour-suppressor gene promoters, is the main cause of lung cancer. The activation of mutations in oncogenes and the inactivation of mutations in tumour-suppressor genes are key genetic changes and are among the most common factors leading to cancer [6]. The current research on carcinogenesis of non-small-cell-lung cancer (NSCLC) has shown that the accumulation of multiple genetic and epigenetic alterations should occur in a cell prior to (malignant) transformation.

Epigenetic alterations occur as heritable changes in gene expression and do not lead to changes in DNA sequence. The effects of epigenetic mechanisms occur mostly in the early stages of tumour development. Epigenetic changes are aberrant DNA methylation and histone modification in chromatin. Both genomic

DNA hypomethylation leading to genomic instability and aberrant promoter hypermethylation leading to inactivation of tumour suppressor genes have been observed in human cancers; they resulted in oncogene over-expression and therefore cancer development and progression. Promoter hypermethylation has been detected in bronchial lavage fluid and pleural fluid of lung cancer patients. Recent studies have reported that histone deacetylase inhibitors had antitumour activity against NSCLC. Epigenetic changes are reversible modifications of histone proteins and CpG islands of gene promoters, and they exist nearly in 40% of mammalian genes [7, 8]. Deletion and epigenetic silencing of LRP1B have been observed in lung cancer cell lines [9].

Lung Cancer and Tobacco Smoke

Smoking constitutes the major risk for lung cancers for smokers or ex-smokers. Risk factors for lung cancer stemming from smoking are total consumption, initiation age, and years of smoking. Tobacco smoke contains more than 20 carcinogens, including polycyclic aromatic hydrocarbons and the tobacco-specific nitrosamine 4-(methylnitrsosamino)- 1-(3-pyridyl)-1-butanone, aromatic amines that are strongly associated with lung cancer development [10]. Other risk factors are occupational and environmental exposure (radiation, asbestos, uranium), diet (cholesterol, vitamin A, vitamin E), and host (familial aggregation) and genetic factors. Tobacco smoke contains a variety of carcinogens initiating and/or promoting. Tobacco smoke induces oxidative DNA lesions, such as 8-oxoguanine, which causes G-to-T transversion [11]. Lung inflammation and lung carcinogenesis are highly correlated. Cigarette smoke in particular is a considerable cause of lung inflammation, which plays a key role in lung carcinogenesis [12, 13].

Oncogenes and Tumour Suppressor Genes in Lung Cancer Carcinogenesis

Molecular genetic studies have investigated the contribution of multiple genetic loci to sporadic lung cancers as a result of the molecular abnormalities in growth-promoting oncogenes and growth-suppressing tumour suppressor genes. The tumour suppressor genes p16, p53, RB, PTEN, and FHIT have been associated with the lung cancer. These gene mutations lead to the initiation or progression of the disease. Abnormal transcription of the FHIT gene, the function of which is related to proapoptotic signaling, was defined in 40% of NSCLC [7]. Methylation of numerous tumour suppressor genes, including DAPK1, CDKN2A, RARβ, RASSF1A, MLH1, APC, CDH13, GSTP1, and MSH2, has been implicated in lung cancer pathogenesis [14].

The p53 gene, a nuclear transcription factor which is located at the short arm of chromosome 17 (17p13), is a key regulator in cellular growth control. It is involved in many biological processes, including DNA repair, cell-cycle arrest, autophagy, apoptosis, metabolism, senescence, and aging [15, 16]. It is also the most mutated gene in human cancer and is inactive due to the mutation in over 50% of human tumours [16]. Single base substitutions in p53 mutations frequently occur in exons 5-8. It is necessary to note that there is a sex-related difference in the incidence of p53 mutations, which are more frequent in females than in males [17]. These mutations are more common in small cell and squamous cell cancers [18].

Phosphatase and tensin homolog (PTEN), also known as mutated in multiple advanced cancers (MMA-1 C) and TGF beta regulated and epithelial cell enriched phosphatase (TEP-1), is a tumour suppressor gene located on chromosome 10q23.3 that is highly susceptible to mutation in many tumour types [19, 20]. PTEN is a member of the protein tyrosine phosphatase family that encodes a 403 amino acid protein. It has important roles in controlling cell growth, cellular transformation, promoting apoptosis, down-regulating adhesion, and inducing cell cycle arrest. Mutations of the PTEN gene have been reported in a number of human malignancies, such as endometrial carcinoma, glioblastoma, breast, colon, and prostate cancers, and lung carcinoma [21, 22].

The inactivation of p53 and PTEN tumour suppressor genes has been observed to be a widespread genetic event in lung cancer. PTEN and p53 tumour suppressors are two frequently altered genes in lung and other human cancers. Around 50% of all NSCLCs have mutations in one allele of p53. PTEN inactivation in lung cancer takes place as a result of mutations and homozygous deletions. However, these genetic events are relatively rare in NSCLCs. Promoter hypermethylation and LOH are the predominant cause for the reduction or loss of PTEN expression in NSCLC tumours [23, 24]. A tumour suppressor gene and critical member of the

Rb pathway, p16 is inactivated in more than 40% of NSCLCs. Loss of heterozygosity on 9p21 and point mutations provide alternative mechanisms for inactivation in 30–50% of NSCLCs [4].

The mutation is about 30% for the oncogene KRAS in lung adenocarcinomas. The mutations in KRAS can transform airway epithelial cells into cancer cells by activating the ERK-MAP kinase pathway. KRAS mutations that are mostly G-T transversions (a glycine → valine amino acid) have been positively correlated with the use of tobacco [25]. Activating point mutations at KRAS codon 12, 13, and 61 have been observed in NSCLC [17].

The epidermal growth factor receptor (EGFR) family is a member of the transmembrane receptor tyrosine kinase superfamily, which consists of EGFR (HER1 or ERBB1), HER2 (EGFR2 or ERBB2/NEU), HER3 (EGFR3 or ERBB3), and HER4 (EGFR4 or ERBB4) [26]. EGFR gene mutations have been discovered associated with lung cancer. This discovery has emphasized that lung cancer has multiple unique phenotypes reflecting different pathways and etiologies of carcinogenesis. Most of the EGFR mutations are point mutations in exon 21 or exon 19 deletions. Oncogenic transformation can be caused by mutations in EGFR tyrosine kinase in NSCLC, and this may lead to sensitivity to inhibitors of the enzyme. Frequent over-expression of EGFR has been observed in NSCLC (50–90%), particularly in SCCs [27].

Some of the genes in NSCLC, namely MYC, Cyclin D1, and EGFR15, are amplified and over-expressed by about 2.5–10%, 5%, and 6%, respectively. Over-expression of C-erbB2 (Her-2/neu) is involved in about 25% of cases. Novel mutations in BRAF have been observed in about 3% of adenocarcinoma patients [28]. It is possible to observe the deregulated expression of MYC genes in many forms of human cancer, including lung cancer. Amplification or transcriptional dysregulation activate the MYC gene in almost all SCLC and almost 50% of the NSCLC and its precursor lesion [29].

Chromosomal Aberrations in Lung Cancer Pathogenesis

Gene mutations and a series of chromosomal aberrations such as translocations, inversions, internal deletions and amplifications lead to cancer cells. The regions codin genes for essential tumour suppressor and DNA repair involved in the pathogenesis of several tumour types are subjected to frequent losses. The genome of lung cancer commonly has large areas of deletions (*e.g.* chromosome 3p, 9p) or amplifications (*e.g.* 1q, 3q). Squamous cell cancers have more chromosomal changes determined by LOH and comparative genomic hybridization (CGH) than adenocarcinoma of the lung. The most commonly seen alterations are the allelic loss of chromosomes 3p21.3 and 9p21, deletions of the chromosomal arm on 5q21, and mutations of p53 associated with LOH on 17p. Loss of chromosomes 3p and 9p and deletions of the chromosomal arm on 5p are the most common genetic alterations in NSCLC. According to the analysis of allelic losses in NSCLC, there has been 70–100% LOH of 3p [11, 17, 30]. The chromosomal aberrations in 3p, 6q, 9p (p16), 16p, 17p (p53), and 19p were more frequent in smokers than in those who had never smoked [14, 31]. The linkage analysis of high risk pedigrees showed that the 6q23-25 region, which includes LATS1, IGF2R, PARK2, SASH1, and TCF21, is the susceptibility locus for lung cancer [32].

Research on lung cancer has concentrated on the role of specific genetic modifications related to chromosomal abnormalities, the inactivation of specific tumour suppressor genes, the activation of specific oncogenes, the expression of hormone receptors, and growth factor production.

ACKNOWLEDGEMENTS

Declared none.

CONFLICT OF INTEREST

The author confirms that this article content has no conflict of interest.

REFERENCES

[1] V.A. Joshi, R. Kucherlapati, Lung cancer genetics and pharmacogenomics. Cytogenet Genome Res 115 (2006) 298-302.
[2] R.W. Ruddon, Cancer Biology. fourth edition (2007) 7-8.
[3] J.S. Bertram, The molecular biology of cancer. Mol Aspects Med 21 (2000) 167-223.
[4] P.P. Massion, D.P. Carbone, The molecular basis of lung cancer: molecular abnormalities and therapeutic implications. Respir Res 4 (2003) 12.

[5] M.R. Stratton, P.J. Campbell, P.A. Futreal, The cancer genome. Nature 458 (2009) 719-724.

[6] X. Xue, Y.M. Zhu, P.J. Woll, Circulating DNA and lung cancer. Ann N Y Acad Sci 1075 (2006) 154-164.

[7] A. Risch, C. Plass, Lung cancer epigenetics and genetics. Int J Cancer 123 (2008) 1-7.

[8] W.B. Liu, L. Ao, Z.Y. Zhou, Z.H. Cui, Y.H. Zhou, X.Y. Yuan, Y.L. Xiang, J. Cao, J.Y. Liu, CpG island hypermethylation of multiple tumour suppressor genes associated with loss of their protein expression during rat lung carcinogenesis induced by 3-methylcholanthrene and diethylnitrosamine. Biochem Biophys Res Commun 402 (2010) 507-514.

[9] C.X. Liu, S. Musco, N.M. Lisitsina, E. Forgacs, J.D. Minna, N.A. Lisitsyn, LRP-DIT, a putative endocytic receptor gene, is frequently inactivated in non-small cell lung cancer cell lines. Cancer Res 60 (2000) 1961-1967.

[10] S.S. Hecht, Tobacco smoke carcinogens and lung cancer. J Natl Cancer Inst 91 (1999) 1194-1210.

[11] M. Sato, D.S. Shames, A.F. Gazdar, J.D. Minna, A translational view of the molecular pathogenesis of lung cancer. J Thorac Oncol 2 (2007) 327-343.

[12] J.L. Pauly, G. Paszkiewicz, Cigarette smoke, bacteria, mold, microbial toxins, and chronic lung inflammation. J Oncol 2011 (2011) 819129.

[13] G. Lee, T.C. Walser, S.M. Dubinett, Chronic inflammation, chronic obstructive pulmonary disease, and lung cancer. Curr Opin Pulm Med 15 (2009) 303-307.

[14] J. Subramanian, R. Govindan, Molecular genetics of lung cancer in people who have never smoked. Lancet Oncol 9 (2008) 676-682.

[15] A. Mogi, H. Kuwano, TP53 mutations in nonsmall cell lung cancer. J Biomed Biotechnol 2011 (2011) 583929.

[16] E.C. Pietsch, O. Humbey, M.E. Murphy, Polymorphisms in the p53 pathway. Oncogene 25 (2006) 1602-1611.

[17] R.H. Breuer, P.E. Postmus, E.F. Smit, Molecular pathology of non-small-cell lung cancer. Respiration 72 (2005) 313-330.

[18] E. Gabrielson, Worldwide trends in lung cancer pathology. Respirology 11 (2006) 533-538.

[19] L.M. Chow, S.J. Baker, PTEN function in normal and neoplastic growth. Cancer Lett 241 (2006) 184-196.

[20] M.J. Wishart, J.E. Dixon, PTEN and myotubularin phosphatases: from 3-phosphoinositide dephosphorylation to disease. Trends Cell Biol 12 (2002) 579-585.

[21] M.M. Rizvi, M.S. Alam, A. Ali, S.J. Mehdi, S. Batra, A.K. Mandal, Aberrant promoter methylation and inactivation of PTEN gene in cervical carcinoma from Indian population. J Cancer Res Clin Oncol 137 (2011) 1255-1262.

[22] T.H. Cheung, K.W. Lo, S.F. Yim, L.K. Chan, M.S. Heung, C.S. Chan, A.Y. Cheung, T.K. Chung, Y.F. Wong, Epigenetic and genetic alternation of PTEN in cervical neoplasm. Gynecol Oncol 93 (2004) 621-627.

[23] T. Andjelkovic, J. Bankovic, J. Stojsic, V. Milinkovic, A. Podolski-Renic, S. Ruzdijic, N. Tanic, Coalterations of p53 and PTEN tumour suppressor genes in non-small cell lung carcinoma patients. Transl Res 157 (2011) 19-28.

[24] G. Jin, M.J. Kim, H.S. Jeon, J.E. Choi, D.S. Kim, E.B. Lee, S.I. Cha, G.S. Yoon, C.H. Kim, T.H. Jung, J.Y. Park, PTEN mutations and relationship to EGFR, ERBB2, KRAS, and TP53 mutations in non-small cell lung cancers. Lung Cancer 69 (2010) 279-283.

[25] G.J. Riely, J. Marks, W. Pao, KRAS mutations in non-small cell lung cancer. Proc Am Thorac Soc 6 (2009) 201-205.

[26] Z. Zhang, A.L. Stiegler, T.J. Boggon, S. Kobayashi, B. Halmos, EGFR-mutated lung cancer: a paradigm of molecular oncology. Oncotarget 1 (2010) 497-514.

[27] P.A. Janne, B.E. Johnson, Effect of epidermal growth factor receptor tyrosine kinase domain mutations on the outcome of patients with non-small cell lung cancer treated with epidermal growth factor receptor tyrosine kinase inhibitors. Clin Cancer Res 12 (2006) 4416s-4420s.

[28] P.K. Paik, M.E. Arcila, M. Fara, C.S. Sima, V.A. Miller, M.G. Kris, M. Ladanyi, G.J. Riely, Clinical characteristics of patients with lung adenocarcinomas harboring BRAF mutations. J Clin Oncol 29 (2011) 2046-2051.

[29] N. Shivapurkar, J. Reddy, P.M. Chaudhary, A.F. Gazdar, Apoptosis and lung cancer: a review. J Cell Biochem 88 (2003) 885-898.

[30] W. Digel, M. Lubbert, DNA methylation disturbances as novel therapeutic target in lung cancer: preclinical and clinical results. Crit Rev Oncol Hematol 55 (2005) 1-11.

[31] J. Wen, J. Fu, W. Zhang, M. Guo, Genetic and epigenetic changes in lung carcinoma and their clinical implications. Mod Pathol 24 (2011) 932-943.

[32] J.E. Bailey-Wilson, C.I. Amos, S.M. Pinney, G.M. Petersen, M. de Andrade, J.S. Wiest, P. Fain, A.G. Schwartz, M. You, W. Franklin, C. Klein, A. Gazdar, H. Rothschild, D. Mandal, T. Coons, J. Slusser, J. Lee, C. Gaba, E. Kupert, A. Perez, X. Zhou, D. Zeng, Q. Liu, Q. Zhang, D. Seminara, J. Minna, M.W. Anderson, A major lung cancer susceptibility locus maps to chromosome 6q23-25. Am J Hum Genet 75 (2004) 460-474.

Send Orders of Reprints at reprints@benthamscience.net
Lung Cancer: Clinical and Surgical Specifications, **2013, 21-48**

CHAPTER 2

Histopathologic Features of the Lung Cancer

Semen Onder* and Ibrahim Hanifi Ozercan

Department of Pathology, Euphrates University School of Medicine, Elazig, Turkey

Abstract: Lung cancer is one of the leading cause of cancer death in the world today. The predominant cause of the lung cancer is tobacco smoking. The other main causative agents are asbestos, silica, radon and heavy metals. Histologically carcinomas comprise nearly 99% of lung cancers. Lung carcinomas have two major groups in the classification of the World Health Organization [WHO]. There is a new multidisciplinary classification of lung adenocarcinomas published by the International Association for the Study of Lung Cancer, American Thoracic Society and European Respiratory Society. With the improvements in the knowledge of the lung cancer biology, there may be more changes in the histological classification and the treatment.

Keywords: Lung cancer, histology, classification, adenocarcinoma.

INTRODUCTION

Lung cancer is the third common cancer in the United States and Europe [1-4]. It is the leading cause of cancer mortality in both sexes. The majority of the patients are men [Male to female ratio is 2.7]. Lung cancer is very related to tobacco smoking [1, 5]. There is a strong relation between cancer death and smoking indicated by the large groups of studies. The other risk factors can be summarized as occupational exposures to carcinogens and air pollution. Asbest, silica, radon and heavy metals are regarded as the most important lung carcinogens [1-3].

Lung cancers have two major histological groups in the classification of the World Health Organization [WHO]: Small cell lung carcinoma and non-small cell lung carcinoma (Table **1**). This seperation has also clinical importance. Small cell carcinomas have special clinical, biological and histological features which will be considered below. Non small cell carcinomas represent approximately 80% of

***Address correspondence to Semen Onder:** Department of Pathology, Euphrates University School of Medicine, Elazig, Turkey; Tel: +90 2333555/2181; Fax: +90 424 2388096; E-mail: semen_yesil@yahoo.com.tr

Akın Eraslan Balcı (Ed)

all lung cancers and have 3 main subtypes including: adenocarcinoma, squamous cell carcinoma and large cell carcinoma. It is very common to see the mixture of these types in majority of the cases.

Recently, a new multidisciplinary classification of lung adenocarcinomas was published by the International Association for the Study of Lung Cancer, American Thoracic Society and European Respiratory Society. This classification is intended to support clinical practice, research investigation and clinical trials [6].

Table 1: WHO Classification of Tumours of the Lung [1]

Malignant Epithelial Tumours
• Squamous cell carcinoma
• Papillary
• Clear cell
• Small cell
• Basaloid
• Small cell carcinoma
• Combined small cell carcinoma
• Adenocarcinoma
• Adenocarcinoma, mixed subtype
• Acinar adenocarcinoma
• Papillary adenocarcinoma
• Bronchioloalveolar carcinoma
o Nonmucinous
o Mucinous
o Mixed nonmucinous and mucinous or indeterminate
• Solid adenocarcinoma with mucin production
o Fetal adenocarcinoma
o Mucinous adenocarcinoma
o Mucinous cystadenocarcinoma
o Signet ring adenocarcinoma
o Clear cell adenocarcinoma
• Large cell carcinoma
• Large cell neuroendocrine carcinoma
o Combined large cell neuroendocrine carcinoma
• Basaloid carcinoma

Table 1: contd...

• Lymphoepithelioma-like carcinoma
• Clear cell carcinoma
• Large cell carcinoma with rhabdoid phenotype
• Adenosquamous carcinoma
• Sarcomatoid carcinoma
• Pleomorphic carcinoma
• Spindle cell carcinoma
• Giant cell carcinoma
• Carcinosarcoma
• Pulmonary blastoma
• Carcinoid tumour
• Typical carcinoid
• Atypical carcinoid
• Salivary gland tumours
• Mucoepidermoid carcinoma
• Adenoid cystic carcinoma
• Epithelial-myoepithelial carcinoma
Mesenchymal Tumours
• Epitheloid haemangioendothelioma
• Angiosarcoma
• Pleuropulmonary blastoma
• Chondroma
• Congenital peribronchial myofibroblastic tumour
• Diffuse pulmonary lymphangiomatosis
• Inflammatory myofibroblastic tumour
• Lymphangioleiomyomatosis
• Synovial sarcoma
o Monophasic
o Biphasic
• Pulmonary artery sarcoma
• Pulmonary vein sarcoma
Lymphoproliferative Tumours

SQUAMOUS CELL CARCINOMA

Definition

Squamous cell carcinoma [SCC] is a malignant epithelial tumour that displays keratinization, keratin pearls and/or intercellular bridges [1, 2]. It is also called as 'epidermoid carcinoma'.

Gross Findings

Tumour masses have typically white-greyish colour and the texture can be firm with focal carbon pigment deposits in the center and gritty. Cavitation and necrosis are the common findings. At least 50% of all squamous cell carcinomas arise centrally from the first to third order bronchi [3]. Generally central tumours are seen as polypoid masses. They can give rise to atelectasis, obstructive pneumonia or bronchopneumonia as a result of infiltration of the bronchial wall [1-3]. Tumours of peripheral origin usually have nodular growth form with well-defined borders. Extensive coagulation necrosis and cavitation are the common features of peripheral origin [3, 7]. Peripheral squamous cell carcinoma can be divided into two groups macroscopically: 1). Tumour with central or subpleural fibrosis with anthracosis 2). Tumour without scar having no anthracotic pigments on the cut surfaces [3, 8]. Early squamous cell carcinoma is defined as a tumour confined to the wall of a bronchus. There should be no lymph node metastasis to use this term [1, 3, 9]. There are two known patterns of early squamous cell carcinoma: In 'creeping type' the tumour replaces the surface epithelium and also invades submucosal glandular ducts. The second pattern is known as 'penetrating type' which forms small polypoid mucosal lesions [1, 3, 10].

Microscopical Findings

Squamous cell carcinoma displays keratinization, intercellular bridges and keratin pearl due to the degree of differentiation (Fig. **1**) [1-3, 11]. If these features are present, the tumour is graded as well differentiated. However, most of the squamous cell carcinomas of the lung appear to be moderately to poorly differentiated [2]. Adjacent to the invasive tumour *in situ* component can be seen in airway mucosa [2]. As it is pointed out earlier, squamous cell carcinoma has an intraepithelial *in situ* like extension. As adenocarcinoma and small cell carcinomas of the lung tend to grow beneath the epithelial surface, they do not replace the bronchial epithelium. This feature is a good indicator for deciding the histologic type of tumour in cases of small biopsy specimens [3].

Histological variants of squamous cell carcinoma include papillary, clear cell, small cell, space filling type and basaloid subtypes. Papillary variant of squamous cell carcinoma usually form exophytic growth. Most of the lesions are well differentiated and invasion is frequently observed. The clear cell variant is composed of cells having clear cytoplasm. It must be distinguished from lung adenocarcinoma with clear cell change and metastatic renal clear cell carcinoma. Tumour cells of small cell variant show morphologic features of a non-small cell carcinoma. Focal squamous differentiation is present but this variant must be described as a poorly differentiated squamous cell carcinoma with small tumour cells [1-3, 12]. These small tumour cells do not show the characteristic nuclear features of small cell carcinoma and usually have more cytoplasm [1, 2]. Basaloid variant has nuclei with peripheral palisading of nuclei and shows squamous differentiation [1, 2]. Alveolar space-filling type consists nearly 5% of total peripheral squamous cell carcinomas and does not destroy alveolar structure [1].

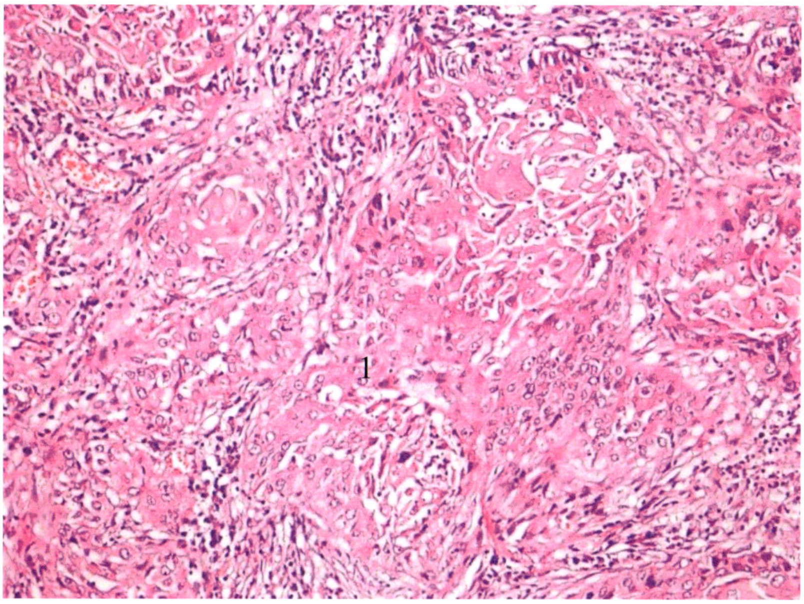

Figure 1: Squamous Cell Carcinoma. Keratin pearl formation and intercellular bridges are present in the tumour.

Immunohistochemistry

Most of the squamous cell carcinomas express predominantly high molecular weight keratin [34βE12], cytokeratins 5/6 and carcinoembryonic antigen [CEA]. Some of these carcinomas express low molecular weight keratin [35βH11] and very small proportion of them express thyroid transcription factor-1 [TTF-1], p63 or cytokeratin 7 [CK7] [1, 2].

Differential Diagnosis

Squamous papilloma can easily be misdiagnosed as carcinoma on small biopsies. The distinction is based on the presence of sufficient cytological atypia even though invasive growth is not clear. Large cell carcinoma can be diagnosed with the presence of squamous differentiation [1]. Small cell variant of squamous cell carcinoma shares the same features of small cell carcinoma except for the nuclear features such as fine chromatin and nuclear molding. Squamous cell carcinoma can entrap alveolar pneumocytes and resemble adenosquamous carcinoma [1, 13].

Diffuse alveolar damage may also mimic carcinoma as well as it shows squamous metaplasia with cytologic atypia. The typical changes that favor a metaplastic change are hyaline membranes and pneumocytic hyperplasia in addition to diffuse proliferation of alveolar connective tissue [1].

SMALL CELL CARCINOMA

Definition

Small cell carcinoma of the lung is a malignant epithelial tumour that is composed of small cells with special features. These cells do not have clear cell borders and fine nucleoli, and typically do have granular nuclear chromatin [1].

Gross Findings

Generally this tumour originates from major bronchi and the masses are white and soft [1, 2]. Perihilar tumoural masses display extensive necrosis and nodal involvement is so common. Only 5% of them appear as peripheral masses [1-3, 14]. Lymphatic involvement is present within bronchovascular bundles and interlobular septa. Central fibrosis may be present with anthracosis. Small cell carcinoma usually disseminates widespread, so these carcinomas are staged as limited or extensive disease [1, 15].

Microscopical Findings

Tumour cells have a size of less than three lymphocytic diameter. They have round, ovoid or sometimes spindle shaped nuclei and finely granular nuclear chromatin with a 'salt and pepper' appearance (Fig. **2**) [1-3]. Nuclei are absent or inconspicuous and there is a thin nuclear membrane. The nuclear to cytoplasmic ratio is very high and nuclear molding is common. The most frequent presentation of this tumour is sheet-like growth without a neuroendocrine morphologic pattern [1-3]. Sometimes they show these neuroendocrine morphologic features such as nesting, trabeculae, peripheral palisading and rosette formation [1-3]. The mitotic rate is usually very high, mean value is like 60 mitoses per 10 high-power fields/2 mm^2 [1, 2]. As the stroma is delicate and vascular, the crush artefact is frequently detected. There is no *in situ* phase of this tumour [1]. Sometimes, tumour cells may be larger in size, more pleomorphic and show extensive necrosis. These findings are more frequent in larger specimens. Basophilic nuclear DNA deposits can be found around the blood vessel walls and this phenomenon is called 'Azzopardi's sign'. However this finding is not regarded as pathognomonic for small cell carcinoma.

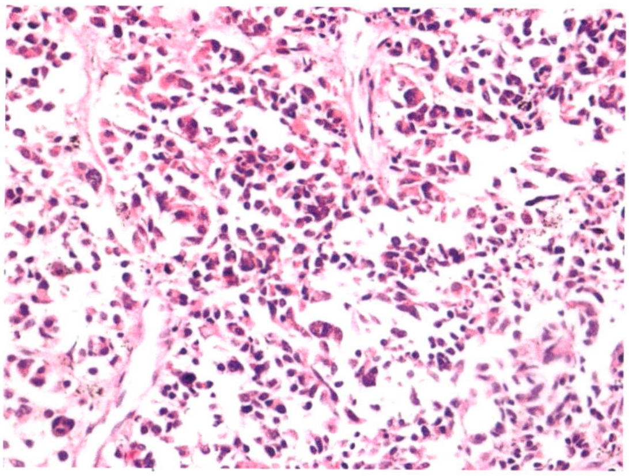

Figure 2: Small Cell Carcinoma. There are sheets of small tumour cells with granular nuclear chromatin.

If there is non-small cell carcinoma elements such as squamous, glandular or large cells in the tumour, then the neoplasm is designated as 'combined small cell carcinoma'. There must be at least 10% of each small cell carcinoma and non-small cell component [1-3, 16].

Immunohistochemistry

Most of the cases are positive for at least one of the neuroendocrine markers including CD56, synaptophysin and chromogranin [1-3]. All these neuroendocrine markers are negative in less than 10% of small cell lung carcinoma [1]. Eighty five percent of small cell lung carcinomas express TTF-1 with a nuclear pattern of staining [1, 2, 17, 18]. Beside these markers, tumour cells are often stained positively with antibodies to enzymes such as aromatic l-amino acid decarboxylase [AADC], neuron specific enolase [NSE] and creatin kinase BB [CK-BB]; to peptide hormones, such as gastrin-releasing peptide [GRP], calcitonin and various pituitary and brain-gut peptide hormones [3, 19-21]. In literature c-kit [CD117] expression has also been reported in some cases [2].

Differential Diagnosis

The differential diagnosis must be included the other neuroendocrine tumours, other 'small round blue cell tumours' and primary or metastatic non-small carcinomas [1-3, 22]. Especially when crush artifact is present, the distinction can sometimes be more difficult. It is widely accepted that crush artifact is not specific for small cell carcinoma, it can also be seen with poorly differentiated non-small cell carcinomas, carcinoids and lymphomas [1]. To make the right diagnosis we should observe some preserved tumour cells in these crushed specimens.

Carcinoid tumours and tumourlets might be misdiagnosed as small cell carcinomas and can be differentiated owing to their extensive areas of necrosis and frequent mitotic activity [more than 20 per 10 high-power fields] like small cell carcinoma [1-3]. They do not stain with TTF-1, but small cell carcinomas show diffuse positivity.

Primitive neuroectodermal tumours [PNET] which are one of the small round blue cell tumours generally show less mitotic activity when compared to small cell carcinomas. The tumour cells of PNET also stain with MIC-2 [CD99], but not for TTF-1 and cytokeratins [1, 23].

Merkel cell carcinoma can be differentiated from small cell carcinoma by using immunohistochemistry. The tumour cells of this entity show positivity for Cytokeratin 20 but not for Cytokeratin 7 and TTF-1.

It is sometimes very hard to differentiate small carcinoma from non-small cell carcinoma when there is marked crush artefact especially in suboptimal preserved tissue preparations [2]. Large cell neuroendocrine carcinoma is the most differential diagnosis with small cell carcinoma and can be separated from small cell carcinoma with architectural criteria such as large cell size, vesicular nuclei with conspicuous nucleoli. These two tumours both show large areas of necrosis, high mitotic count and TTF-1 positivity [2]. Small cell variants of squamous cell carcinoma, some solid adenocarcinomas can be defined as other non-small cell carcinomas that are present in differential diagnosis. These tumours do not show positive staining with neuroendocrine markers and especially squamous cell carcinomas of small cell type are usually negative for TTF-1, but are stained with Cytokeratin 1, 5, 10 and 14 [1, 2, 24].

ADENOCARCINOMA

Definition

Adenocarcinoma of the lung is defined as a malignant tumour that shows papillary, acinary, bronchiolealveolar or solid growth pattern with mucin production [1]. It is the most frequent histologic type seen in women and non-smokers among all lung carcinomas.

Gross Findings

Pulmonary adenocarcinomas have 6 different macroscopic patterns. Peripheral type is the most frequent pattern. They usually have grey-white cut surfaces and include anthracotic pigment. Due to anthracotic pigment, desmoplastic fibrosis can be seen in the central region. Some peripheral adenocarcinomas may have gelatinous appearance associated with mucin production [1, 25]. The tumour may have ill-defined borders or may be lobulated. The other type is known as endobronchial or central tumour which is very rare [1]. This type may cause obstructive lipoid pneumonia with bronchial luminal collapse. Another pattern is composed of lobar consolidation like a diffuse pneumonia that we usually see in mucinous bronchioloalveolar carcinoma [1, 2]. Diffuse and bilateral lung involvement can also be seen as another pattern like an interstitial pneumonia. The fifth macroscopic form has a mesothelioma-like appearance due to the thickening visceral pleura [1, 2].

Adenocarcinoma generally disseminates by hematogenous, lymphatic and aerogenous routes. Aerogenous spreading culminates in separate lesions from the main mass and is commonly seen in bronchoalveolar carcinoma [1].

Microscopic Findings

Adenocarcinoma of the lung generally shows six cytologic types: Bronchial surface cell type, goblet cell type, bronchial gland cell type, type II alveolar epithelial cell type and mixed cell type. Most of the adenocarcinomas appear as clara cell or type II alveolar epithelial cell type. Clara cells are columnar cells with apical nuclei and eosinophilic cytoplasm. Type II cells are recognized as cuboidal cells (Fig. **3**) with cytoplasmic vacuoles or intranuclear eosinophilic inclusions [1, 2]. The main histologic subtypes of adenocarcinoma are papillary, acinary, solid and bronchioloalveolar and mixed subtype. The most frequent pattern is the mixed type which includes different histologic subtypes and differention degrees. Papillary structures with fibrovascular cores replacing the underlying lung represent the papillary type. Lung invasion and necrosis can be seen in this type. Acinary pattern shows tubules and acini that are made of columnar or cuboidal cells (Fig. **3**). The appearence looks like bronchial gland. Due to the degree of gland, tubule or papillary formation, histologic grade for papillary and acinary pattern can be well, moderate or poorly differentiated (Fig. **4**). Solid adenocarcinoma consists of large polygonal cells without acini, papillar or tubular formation and mucin is present in at least 5 tumour cells in two high power fields. Bronchoalveolar carcinoma [BAC] is a special entity that has a favourable prognosis [1, 2, 26, 27]. There must be no stromal, vascular or pleural invasion for this diagnosis. BAC shows lepidic, aerogenous growth or septal widening with sclerosis (Fig. **5**). Lepidic growth is defined as dissemination of tumour cells along alveolar septa and is not accepted as an invasion pattern [1, 28, 29]. The variants of BAC are mucinous, non-mucinous and mixed or indeterminate type. Mucinous BAC is composed of tall columnar cells that contain mucin like goblet cells and typically has satellite nodules around the main mass. Clara cells and/or type II cells are usually seen in non-mucinous BAC which comprises the majority of the cases especially the solitary ones.

Noguchi *et al.* published a classification for adenocarcinomas that are smaller than 2 cm in diameter to their growth pattern [30]. There are two main groups which are believed to have different prognosis and clinical findings. For example Type A and Type B tumours show similar histology and have favorable prognosis. When compared with first group, Type D-E and Type F tumours have poor prognosis and similar to the third WHO classification by definition (Table **2**).

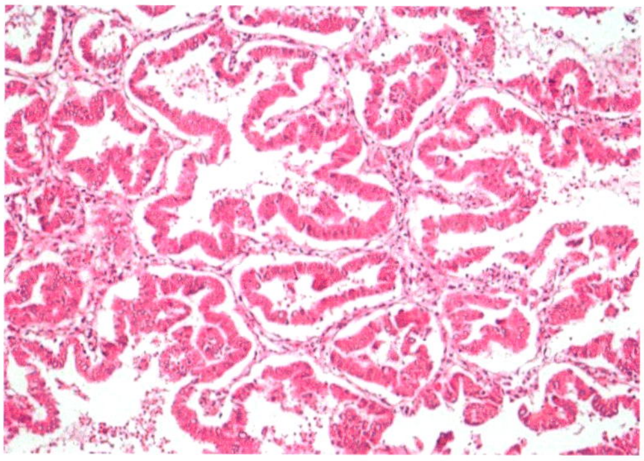

Figure 3: Acinar Adenocarcinoma. There are irregular shaped glands with malignant cells.

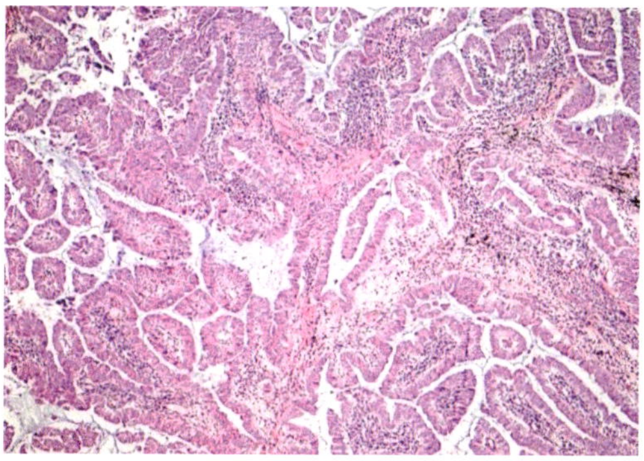

Figure 4: Adenocarcinoma. The tumour cells show glandular proliferation with mucin.

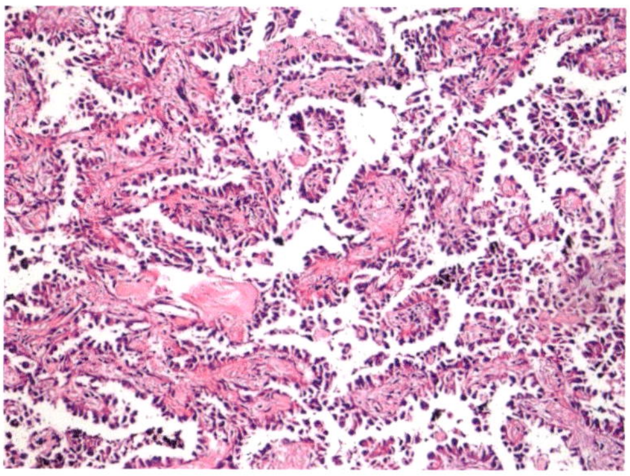

Figure 5: Bronchioloalveolar Carcinoma. Columnar cell shaped cells infiltrate alveolar walls.

The variants of adenocarcinoma are fetal, mucinous, signet ring and clear cell adenocarcinoma. Mucinous cystadenocarcinoma is the fifth variant. Fetal adenocarcinoma is a different tumour resembling fetal lung and is rarely seen with the other histologic types of adenocarcinomas. Clear cell variant is usually seen focally with the other patterns of adenocarcinoma. The other variants are identical to the gastrointestinal tumours with the same name.

Table 2: Noguchi's Classification for Small-Sized Adenocarcinoma

⇒ **Replacement type [lepidic type] adenocarcinoma**
Type A: Localized bronchioloalveolar carcinoma [LBAC]
Type B: LBAC with focal collapse of the alveolar structure
Type C: LBAC with focus of fibroblastic proliferation
⇒ **Nonreplacement type [nonlepidic type] adenocarcinoma**
Type D: Poorly differentiated adenocarcinoma
Type E: Tubular or acinar adenocarcinoma
Type F: True papillary adenocarcinoma

Nowadays with the improvement in radiological and surgical technics, adenocarcinomas are began to studied particularly. New mutations and amplifications are found in adenocarcinomas such as HER2, PIK3CA, BRAF, EML4-ALK mutations. EGFR and K-ras mutations are detected in 30-50% of the cases [1, 2, 31, 32]. As standard treatment many drugs targeting on this mutations are commonly used. So with the increasing knowledge about adenocarcinomas a new international classification of lung adenocarcinoma came from the International Association for the Study of Lung Cancer [IASLC], the American Thoracic Society [ATS], and the European Respiratory Society [6] (Table **3**). They recommend discontinuing the use of the term 'BAC.' There are three types of adenocarcinoma in this new classification used instead of BAC: *in situ* adenocarcinoma, minimal invasive adenocarcinoma and adenocarcinoma with lepidic pattern. Clear cell and signet ring cell variants are not considered to be specific histologic subtypes and are removed from this new classification. It is recommended to use of the term 'lepidic predominant adenocarcinoma' and discontinuing the term 'mixed subtype'. The suggestion is to give the proportions of different patterns or variants in pathology reports. There is also a new variant which is called 'enteric type' in the new classification. This variant is like colonic adenocarcinoma with its morphological and phenotypic aspects.

Table 3: IASLC/ATS/ERS Classification of Lung Adenocarcinoma in Resection Specimens

Preinvasive Lesions • Atypical adenomatous hyperplasia • Adenocarcinoma *in situ* [≤3 cm formerly BAC] 1. Nonmucinous 2. Mucinous 3. Mixed mucinous/nonmucinous
Minimally Invasive Adenocarcinoma [≤ 3 cm lepidic predominant tumour with ≤ 5 mm invasion] • Nonmucinous • Mucinous • Mixed mucinous/nonmucinous
Invasive Adenocarcinoma • Lepidic predominant [formerly nonmucinous BAC pattern, with ≥ 5 mm invasion] • Acinar predominant • Micropapillary predominant • Solid predominant with mucin production.
Variants of Invasive Adenocarcinoma • Invasive mucinous adenocarcinoma [formerly mucinous BAC] • Colloid • Fetal [low and high grade] • Enteric BAC: Bronchioloalveolar carcinoma; IASLC: International Association for the Study of Lung Cancer; ATS: American Thoracic Society; ERS: European Respiratory Society.

Immunohistochemistry

Adenocarcinomas typically express epithelial markers which are epithelial membrane antigen, carcinoembryonic antigen, AE1/AE3 and CAM5.2. Thyroid transcription factor 1 [TTF-1] is expressed in 75% of the adenocarcinomas [1, 33]. Cytokeratin 7 is positive, Cytokeratin 20 is less positive or negative [1, 2]. There is an exception in mucinous tumours which express both CK7 and CK20, also do not express TTF-1 [1, 33-35]. Adenocarcinomas also display CEA, MOC31, BerEP4 and leu M1 [1].

Differential Diagnosis

The differential diagnosis comprises malign mesothelioma and metastatic adenocarcinoma. Peripheral type adenocarcinomas especially if the tumour cells do not produce mucin are easily misdiagnosed as mesothelioma [1-3]. In this cases, it must be used clinical, macroscopical, immunohistochemical or electron microscopical analysis for the differentiation. Mesothelioma cases usually express thrombomodulin, calretinin and WT1. On the other side the expression of TTF-1, CEA and surfactan protein is absent or weaker as compared to adenocarcinomas.

Metastatic lesions are generally multiple. When the lesion is solitary, it must be considered for other histological features and immunohistochemistry results. Cytokeratin 7 [CK7], CK20 and TTF-1 antibodies are useful to separate primary adenocarcinomas. To differentiate metastatic thyroid carcinoma, thyroglobulin must be used. If there is both positive staining for TTF-1 and thyroglobulin, this favours metastatic thyroid carcinoma over a primary adenocarcinoma of the lung.

ADENOSQUAMOUS CARCINOMA

Definition

Adenosquamous carcinoma is defined by WHO as a carcinoma displaying features of both adenocarcinoma and squamous cell carcinoma. Each component consists at least 10% of the tumour. It occurs especially in smokers.

Gross Findings

They generally form tan peripheral masses that may have a central scar [1, 2]. These tumours have poor prognosis due to their tendency to show early metastasis.

Microscopical Findings

Adenocarcinoma component usually show acinary, papillary or bronchioloalveolar pattern. If there is a solid pattern with mucin production, then we have to search for more than five mucin droplets per high power field to diagnose as an adenocarcinoma. Squamous component can sometimes show focal mucin. The two component may be seen in equal proportion or one of them may be predominant. The criteria for the diagnosis is to include each of two components at least 10% of the tumour. Large cell carcinoma can be seen as a minor component of the tumour. Occasionally adenosquamous carcinoma can have an amyloid-like stroma [1, 36].

Immunohistochemistry

They usually express CK7, AE1/AE3, CAM 5.2. The tumour cells generally do not stain with CK20. Adenocarcinoma component show immunoreactivity for TTF-1 by contrast with squamous component.

Differential Diagnosis

The differential diagnosis includes squamous cell carcinoma containing normal alveolar structures, mucoepidermoid carcinoma and adenocarcinoma with squamous metaplasia [1-3]. Mucoepidermoid carcinomas show squamous and glandular differention like their salivary gland complement. They usually arise from central locations in contrast to peripherally located adenosquamous carcinoma. If a tumour does not contain squamous pearls, keratinization, *in situ* squamous cell carcinoma or tubular, acinary and papillary pattern, it is probably a mucoepidermoid carcinoma rather than an adenosquamous carcinoma [1, 2]. But it is not always possible to separate this antity reliably from mucoepidermoid carcinoma especially if it is high grade [1, 37].

LARGE CELL CARCINOMA

Definition

Large cell carcinoma is a malignant tumour that does not show glandular or squamous differentiation. All types are usually seen in older patients [average age is 60] that are predominantly smokers and male. Lymphoepithelioma-like carcinoma is an exceptional type occuring in younger patients [mean age 57] mostly female and non-smoker patients [1, 2].

Gross Findings

We usually see large [>4 cm] and peripheral masses with frequent necrosis. Only basaloid carcinomas present as exophytic bronchial masses. Chest wall involvement can be detected in case of delayed therapy recieved patients [1-3].

Metastases are usually seen in hilar or mediastinal nodes followed by pleural metastasis. The pattern of dissemination is like other non-small cell carcinomas.

Microscopic Findings

Large cell carcinoma cells usually have large vesicular nuclei, prominent nucleoli and abundant cytoplasm. These large sized polygonal cells typically form solid nests or sheets [1-3]. Generally the diagnosis is made when other possibilities like squamous cell carcinoma, adenocarcinoma or small cell carcinoma are excluded. It is logical to entitle the tumour as a poorly differentiated non-small cell carcinoma in small biopsies. There are five histologic variants defined by the WHO: large cell neuroendocrine carcinoma, basaloid carcinoma, lymphoepithelioma-like carcinoma, clear cell carcinoma and large cell carcinoma with rhabdoid phenotype.

Large cell neuroendocrine carcinoma displays typical neuroendocrine features like trabecular growth, organoid pattern, rosettes or perilobular palisading. Tumour cells are large and polygonal with vesicular chromatin and low nuclear cytoplasmic ratio. The mitotic rate is relatively high like 11 or more per 10 high power fields [1-3]. For the diagnosis we have to show strong immunoreactivity for at least one of the neuroendocrine markers which are chromogranin, synaptophysin and CD56. Extensive necrosis is a common feature. If a large cell neuroendocrine carcinoma includes other non-small cell carcinoma component then it is called as 'combined large cell neuroendocrine carcinoma'. Basaloid carcinoma is another histologic variant of large cell carcinoma which has small, monomorphic cells with granular chromatin and hyperchromatic nuclei. The mitotic activity is very high like 15-50 mitoses per 10 high power fields. There is no squamous differention and nuclear molding, however rosettes can be present. Similar to its nasopharyngeal or timic component, pulmonary lymphoepithelioma-like carcinoma usually displays syncytial growth pattern with prominent lymphocytic infiltration. Amyloid may be present within the tumour. Another variant is clear cell carcinoma which has large cells containing clear or foamy cytoplasm. Large cell carcinoma with rhabdoid phenotype is a tumour consisting of rhabdoid cells in at least 10% proportion. Rhabdoid cells having typically eosinophilic globules in cytoplasm are stained with vimentin and cytokeratin [1, 38]. Pure form is very rare.

Immunohistochemistry

Each histologic variant of large cell carcinoma shows different staining pattern. Large cell neuroendocrine carcinoma always express strong reactivity for one neuroendocrine marker [chromogranin, synaptophysin CD56]. Tumour cells sometimes show reactivity for TTF-1, but generally do not have the expression of cytokeratin 1, 5, 10, 14, 20 [34β12]. Basaloid carcinoma usually stain with cytokeratin 1, 5, 10, 14, 20 [34β12] but not TTF-1. There is generally no reactivity for neuroendocrine markers, might be a weak reactivity in less than 20% of all the tumour cells [1, 2, 39]. Staining with EBER-1 RNA is a feature of lymphoepithelioma-like carcinoma. Large cell carcinoma with rhabdoid phenotype shows positive reactivity for vimentin and cytokeratin [1, 38].

Differential Diagnosis

Large cell carcinoma with classical features [NOS] must be separated from other poorly differentiated non-small cell carcinomas like solid type adenocarcinoma and poorly differentiated squamous cell carcinoma. If there is a foci of keratinization, intracellular bridges or a minimum of 5 mucinous droplets in at least 2 high power fields then it must be excluded the possibility of large cell carcinoma. If we handle large cell neuroendocrine carcinoma, differential diagnosis will be included basaloid carcinoma, atypical carcinoid, large cell carcinoma [NOS] and small cell carcinoma. Basaloid carcinoma is known to share similar histologic features, so immunohistochemical analysis is essential for the seperation. Cytokeratin coctail [34β12] is positive and TTF-1 is typically negative for basaloid carcinoma. In contrast large cell neuroendocrine carcinoma shows immunoreactivity for TTF-1 but not for 34β12. Differentiation from large cell carcinoma [NOS] depends on showing neuroendocrine features. When compared to atypical carcinoid, large cell neuroendocrine carcinoma has a higher mitotic rate [11 or more per 10 high power fields] and more extensive necrosis [1, 2]. Small cell carcinoma has smaller sized cells with higher nuclear to cytoplasmic ratio and have granular nuclear chromatin instead of vesicular chromatin when compared to large cell neuroendocrine carcinoma. But two types of neoplasm sometimes show similar nuclear features, it is impossible to separate them. We use the term 'combined small cell carcinoma' as a final diagnosis, if there is a recognisable foci of small cell carcinoma [2]. It is necessary to differentitate the basaloid from poorly differentiated squamous cell carcinoma and small cell carcinoma. The presence of squamous cell differentiation is necessary to use the term 'basaloid variant of squamous cell carcinoma'. Nuclear features of small cell carcinoma as we described before, are used in seperation from basaloid carcinomas. The differential diagnosis for lymphoepithelioma-like carcinoma contains malignant lymphoma, İnflammatory pseudotumour and primary lymphoid hyperplasia. Showing the mixed population in tumour by immunohistochemistry is helpful in differentiation from malignant lymphoma. And before diagnosing a lung tumour as a clear cell carcinoma, metastatic clear cell carcinomas from various origin like kidney, thyroid or salivary gland must be excluded first.

SARCOMATOID CARCINOMA

Definition

Sarcomatoid carcinomas belong to non-small cell lung carcinomas which exceptionally show sarcoma-like features [1]. These carcinomas are usually seen in elder population [mean age is 60 year] with male dominance. But pulmonary blastoma is an exception which effects younger people with no gender selection.

Gross Findings

They usually form larger masses especially in the upper lung lobes. Peripheral tumours generally show inclination to have large and well-circumscribed masses when compared to centrally located ones which are smaller and more infiltrable tumours [1, 40, 41]. Necrosis can be detected in the specimens. Sarcomatoid carcinomas have the agressive behaviour with metastasis like other non small cell lung carcinomas.

Microscopical Findings

Sarcomatoid carcinomas include different histologic and morphological patterns. The 5 histologic subgroups defined by the WHO are: pleomorphic carcinoma, spindle cell carcinoma, giant cell carcinoma, carcinosarcoma and pulmonary blastoma. Pleomorphic carcinomas are usually poor-differentiated non-small cell carcinomas including at least 10% malignant giant and/or spindle cells [1-3]. Spindle cells can show epitheloid, mesenchymal or smooth muscle features and can form fascicules while giant cells. These tumours can have myxoid or fibrous stroma. Spindle cell carcinoma do not show any other non-small cell lung carcinoma pattern and only consists of malignant spindle cells which are described in pleomorphic carcinomas by description. They sometimes inlude lymphoplasmacytic infiltration. The third subgroup is called as giant cell carcinoma which is composed of purely large and multinucleated cells and does not show other morphologic patterns like spindle cell carcinoma [1-3]. If the tumour shows the features of adenocarcinoma, it is better to use the term 'pleomorphic adenocarcinoma with giant cells' for this situation [3]. The tumour also includes neutrophil predominant inflamatory infiltration most of the time [1, 42, 43]. Another histologic variant of sarcomatoid carcinomas are known as carcinosarcomas. These tumours are biphasic malignant tumours which have both the carcinomatous and the sarcomatous components. Squamous cell carcinoma is the most frequent type seen as the carcinomatous component [1-3]. The second component of the tumour has spindle shaped cells resembling fibrosarcoma, and it is usually a poorly differentiated spindle cell sarcoma. Pulmonary blastoma is a dual tumour comprising the both primitive epithelial and mesenchymal components [1]. The epithelial component is composed of glycogen rich tubules lined by non-ciliated columnar cells with clear cytoplasms. This appearance is similar to well-differentiated fetal adenocarcinoma. The cytoplasmic vacuoles usually show PAS-positive staining. Stromal component has a blastamel-like appearance like *Wilms*' tumour of the kidney [1]. Pulmonary blastoma can sometimes include foci of spindle cell carcinoma, rhabdomyosarcoma or osteosarcoma.

Immunohistochemistry

The tumour cells of pleomorphic, spindle or giant cell carcinoma show immunoreactivity for cytokeratin, vimentin, carcinoembryonic antigen [CEA] and smooth muscle antigens [1, 44, 45]. In pulmonary blastoma reactivity with epithelial markers [EMA, keratin, CEA] and sometimes neuroendocrine markers are seen in epithelial component. Similar to developing fetal lung tubules epithelial cells also express *Clara* cell antigen and surfactan apoprotein [46]. Stromal component of blastomas contains vimentin, smooth muscle actin, desmin or S-100 protein.

Differential Diagnosis

Primary/metastatic carcinomas, other carcinomas of the same group and reactive processes constitute the differential diagnosis group of pleomorphic carcinoma. A detailed macroscopic examination and sampling [at least one section per centimeter of tumour diameter] will be adequate for the identification of epithelial component [1]. Spindle cell carcinomas have to be distinguished from synovial sarcomas, inflammatory myofibroblastic tumour. Synovial sarcoma is stained focally positive for keratin but show X:18 translocation. Carcinosarcomas are sometimes confused with other tumours in this group and metastatic lesions like teratomas of the female or male genital tract. It must be distunguished pulmonary blastoma from fetal adenocarcinoma, pleuropulmonary blastoma and primary or metastatic sarcomas. Fetal adenocarcinomas do not include malignant mesenchymal component and similarly pleuropulmonary blastoma and metastatic sarcomas do not have malignant epithelial component while pulmonary blastomas consist of both malignant mesenchymal and glandular elements [2]. Finally; the differential diagnosis of giant cell carcinoma includes sarcomas [primary or metastatic] like pleomorphic rhabdomyosarcoma, metastatic choriocarcinoma and other pleomorphic sarcomas [1, 47].

CARCINOID TUMOUR

Definition

Carcinoid tumours are one of the neuroendocrine tumours of the lung which show organoid, insular, trabecular, ribbon and rosette-like growth pattern [1]. The main age at diagnosis is 47 years old usually with no cigarette smoking.

They share common morphological, ultrastructural and immunohistochemical features with small cell carcinoma and large cell neuroendocrine carcinoma, however they are different in respect to their prognosis and clinical findings. Neuroendocrine tumours may be a component of MEN1 syndrome which is related with inactivation of the gene locus at 11p13.

Gross Findings

They are usually well circumscribed and yellowish tumours. Some carcinoids grow as polypoid endrobronchial masses while others present as peripheral tumours with invading more extensively in the adjacent lung tissue [1, 2, 48]. Squamous metaplasia can be found.

Microscopic Findings

There are two main subgroups of carcinoid tumours including typical and atypical carcinoids. Typical carcinoid was called also as a well differentiated neuroendocrine carcinoma. Nowadays WHO defined this tumour as a 'carcinoid tumour that show fewer than 2 mitoses per 2 mm^2 and lack necrosis. These tumours usually present as endobronchial masses. Atypical carcinoids which were known as moderately differentiated neuroendocrine carcinomas, are accepted as 'carcinoid tumours with 2-10 mitoses per 2 mm^2 and/or foci of necrosis' due to the WHO definition [1]. Generally they usually form peripheral masses and effects elder people with cigarette smoking as a risk factor. It is hard to separate these two subgroups in a bronchial biopsy, a resection specimen is needed for the final diagnosis. They do not combine with other lung tumours but they can be multiple.

Carcinoid tumours generally consist of polygonal uniform cells with inconspicuous nucleoli, finely granular chromatin and eosinophilic cytoplasm (Fig. **6**). Different growth patterns are recognised especially organoid and trabecular pattern. The stroma is commonly vascularized but sometimes hyalinized. There may be neuroendocrine cell hyperplasia in the adjacent epithelium.

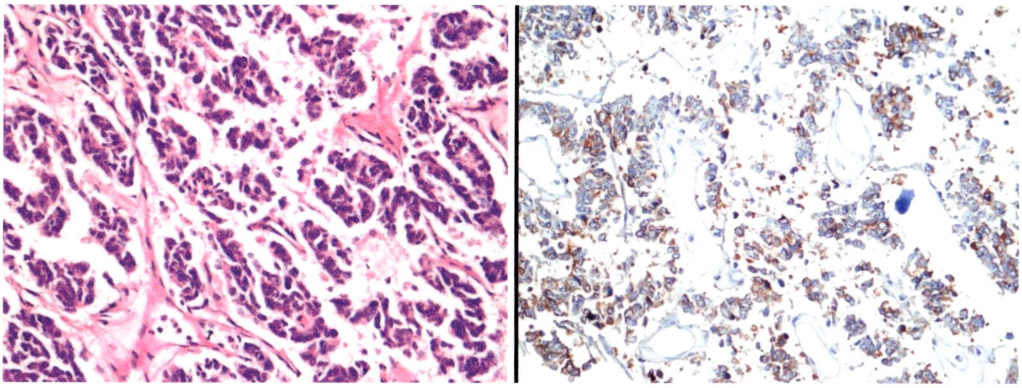

Figure 6 and 7: Carcinoid Tumour. Polygonal uniform cells with organoid pattern. H&E. Tumour cells stain with Chromogranin A.

Immunohistochemistry

They usually show positive reactivity to neuroendocrine markers including (Fig. **7**) chromogranin, synaptophysin, CD57 and CD56. The staining pattern may be focal or patchy in atypical carcinoids. Most of the carcinoid tumours are immunoreactive for cytokeratins [cytokeratin 8, 18 and 19] [49, 50]. But cytokeratins 1, 5, 10 and 14 [34β12] are not typically positive in carcinoids. Different staining patterns with TTF-

1 have been reported in the literature [1, 51]. Ki67 is believed to be more positive in atypical carcinoids. Carcinoids sometimes are stained with CD99 [1, 52, 53].

Differential Diagnosis

Carcinoid tumours especially typical ones are usually confused with carcinoid tumourlets [1, 54]. Tumourlets are typically less than 5 mm in diameter unlike carcinoid tumours. The differential diagnosis includes other neuroendocrine tumours which are small cell carcinoma and large call neuroendocrine carcinoma. These are high grade carcinomas with a mitotic rate more than 10 per 2 mm^2 and differ easily from carcinoids. Some carcinoid tumours resemble adenocarcinomas if they show gland like patterns. Adenocarcinomas usually have more mucin but show less staining with neuroendocrine markers. The other entities in the differential diagnosis are paraganglioma, glomus tumour and sclerosing hemangioma [55]. Paragangliomas do not stain with cytokeratins and similarly glomus tumours and hemangiomas are not reactive for neuroendocrine markers.

2. SALIVARY GLAND TUMOURS

These tumours share the similar histologic features of their salivary gland counterparts but originate from the tracheal and bronchial seromucous glands. The subgroups seen in the tracheabronchial tree are mucoepidermoid carcinoma, adenoid cystic carcinoma and epithelial-myoepithelial carcinoma, acinic cell carcinoma, carcinoma ex-pleomorphic adenoma and malignant endobronchial myxoid tumour [1, 2].

MUCOEPIDERMOID CARCINOMA

Definition

Mucoepidermoid carcinoma is defined as a rare malignant epithelial tumour that consists of mucinous, intermediate and squamoid type cells. This uncommon tumour effects a wide range of people with 3-78 years [1-3].

Gross Findings

They generally present as polypoid endobronchial masses with mucoid or cystic appearence. Especially in high grade tumours infiltration of lung parenchyma and metastasis to adjacent organs are more common [1, 2, 56].

Microscopic Findings

According to their cytologic and morphologic features, mucoepidermoid carcinomas are examined in two groups: high and low grade types. Low grade tumours generally form cystic masses that contain mucin and comprised of columnar epithelium and eosinophilic round-oval, mucin rich cells. The stroma usually has an amyloid like appearence. High grade tumours resemble adenosquamous carcinomas and include mostly solid areas of intermediate and squamoid cells. Nuclear atypia, hyperchromasia, high mitotic accounts and necrosis are commonly found in high grade mucoepidermoid carcinomas [57, 58].

Immunohistochemistry

The tumours cells stain with pancytokeratins and cytokeratin 7. They do not show immunoreactivity for TTF-1 and cytokeratin 20 [2].

Differential Diagnosis

Mucous gland adenomas can be confused with low grade tumours and separated by comprising squamous differentiation and intermediate cells. The differential diagnosis of high grade type includes squamous cell carcinoma and especially adenosquamous carcinoma. The features favoring the diagnosis of high grade mucoepidermoid carcinoma are the absence of *in situ* carcinoma, squamous pearl formation with showing low grade mucoepidermoid carcinoma like areas or keratinization [1-3].

ADENOID CYSTIC CARCINOMA

Definition

Adenoid cystic carcinoma is a malignant tumour that consists of cribriform, glandular and tubular patterns of cells scattered in hyalinized and mucinous matrix [1]. It effect people in the fourth and fifth decades without gender selection.

Gross Findings

This tumour can form polypoid lesions or diffuse infiltrating plaques but has always infiltrative margins. It is the most common tumour arising from the tracheabronchial glands while it comprises less than 1% of all lung tumours originating from mainstem or lobar bronchi [2].

Microscopic Findings

The tumour cells are typically small with dark hyperchromatic nuclei and scanty cytoplasm. These cells commonly make cribriform pattern which has a'Swiss cheese' appearance with the nests of cells around spaces filled with PAS positive basophilic mucoid material [2]. Mitotic figures are rare, but perineural invasion and extention to the bronchial wall are nearly common [1-3].

Immunohistochemistry

The luminal cells stain with cytokeratins, CEA, EMA while the cells around pseudocysts show immunoreactivity for vimentin, smooth muscle actin, S100 protein and p63 indicating myoepithelial origin.

Differential Diagnosis

Basaloid carcinomas, small cell carcinomas and usual adenocarcinomas of the lung with trabecular or cribriform patterns are usually separated from adenoid cystic carcinomas by using immunohistochemistry. It is hard to distinguish from metastatic adenoid cystic carcinoma without clinical findings.

EPITHELIAL MYOEPITHELIAL CARCINOMA

Definition

Epithelial myoepithelial carcinoma is a tumour composed of myoepithelial cells and ductal epithelial cells with various patterns [1]. The synonyms of this tumour are assumed as adenomyoepithelioma, myoepithelioma and epithelial-myoepithelial tumour. It is a rare tumour that usually effects middle-aged patients (mean age is 50).

Gross Findings

They usually form well-demarcated endobronchial lesions with white-grey coloured cut surface.

Microscopic Findings

Myoepithelial component is composed of spindle or round shaped cells with eosinophilic or abundant cytoplasms. There is variable amount of ducts composed of dual layer of cells in the tumour.

Immunohistochemistry

The myoepithelial cells stain with S100, Smooth muscle actin, CD10, Calponin and p63. Inner layer of ducts is positive for EMA and keratins.

Differential Diagnosis

The differential diagnosis of this entity includes other biphasic tumours like pleomorphic adenoma, adenoid cystic carcinoma, metastatic epithelial-myoepithelial carcinoma and clear cell tumours [pulmonary or metastatic] when clear cell are predominate [2, 59, 60].

ACKNOWLEDGEMENTS

Declared none.

CONFLICT OF INTEREST

The authors confirm that this article content has no conflict of interest.

REFERENCES

[1] Travis WD, Brambilla E, Muller-Hermelink HK, *et al.* Pathology and Genetics. Tumours of the Lung, Pleura, Thymus and Heart. Lyon, France: IARC Press, 2004.

[2] Zander DS, Farver CF, *et al.* Pulmonary Pathology. A volume in the series foundations in diagnostic pathology. Philadephia, Pennsylvania: Churchill Livingstone, Elsevier, 2008.

[3] Mills SE, Carter D, Greenson JK, Reuter VE, Stoler MH, *et al.* Sternberg's Diagnostic Surgical Pathology, Volume I. Philadelphia: Lippincott Williams& Wilkins, 2010.

[4] Ferlay J, Parkin DM, Steliarova-Foucher E [2010]. Estimates of cancer incidence and mortality in Europe in 2008. European Journal of Cancer 46: 765-781.

[5] Doll R, Peto R. The causes of cancer: quantative estimates of avoidable risks of cancer in the United States today. J Natl Cancer Inst 66: 1191-1308.

[6] Travis WD, Brambilla E, Noguchi M, Nicholson AG, *et al.* International Association for the Study of Lung Cancer/American Thoracic Society/European Respiratory Society International Multidisciplinary Classification of Lung Adenocarcinoma. Journal of Thoracic Oncology; 6[2]: 244-285.

[7] Funai K, Yokose T, Ishii G, Araki K, Yoshida J, Nishimura M, Nagai K, Nishiwaki Y, Ochiai A [2003]. Clinicopathologic characteristics of peripheral squamous cell carcinoma of the lung. Am J Surg Pathol 27: 978-984.

[8] Mackay B, Lukeman JM, Ordonez NG [1991]. Tumours of the Lung. WB Saunders: Philadelphia.

[9] Shimosato Y, Amemiya R. Pathology of early stage squamous cell carcinoma of the hilar type. In Ikeda M, Oho K, Oshibe M, *et al*, eds. Atlas of Early Cancer of Major Bronchi. Tokyo: Igaku-Shoin, 1976: 29-37.

[10] Nagamoto N, Saito Y, Suda H, Imai T, Sato M, Ohta S, Kanma K, Sagawa M, Takahashi S, Usuda K [1989]. Relationship between length of longitudinal extension and maximal depth of transmural invasion in roentgenographically occult squamous cell carcinoma of the bronchus [nonpolypoid type]. Am J Surg Pathol 13: 11-20.

[11] Dulmet-Brender E, Jaubert F, Huchon G [1986]. Exophytic endobronchial epidermoid carcinoma. Cancer 57: 1358-1364.

[12] Brambilla E, Lantuejoul S, Sturm N [2000]. Divergent differentiation in neuroendocrine lung tumours. Semin Diagn Pathol 17: 138-148.

[13] Colby TV, Koss M, Travis WD [1995]. Tumours of the Lower Respiratory Tract. 3rd ed. Armed Forces Institute of Pathology: Washington DC.

[14] Curan WJJr [2001]. Therapy of limited stage small cell cancer. Cancer Treat Res 105: 229-252.

[15] Lally BE, Urbanic JJ, Blackstock AW, Miller AA, Perry MC. Small cell lung cancer: Have we made any progress over the last 25 years? Oncologist. 2007; 12[9]: 1096-1104.

[16] Nicholson SA, Beasley MB, Brambilla E, Hasleton PS, Colby TV, Sheppard MN, Falk R, Travis WD [2002]. Small cell lung carcinoma: a clinicopathologic study of 100 cases with surgical specimens. Am J Surg Pathol 26: 1184-1197.

[17] Folpe AL, Gown AM, Lamps LW, Garcia R, Dail DH, Zarbo RJ, Schmidt RA [1999]. Thyroid transcription factor-1: immunohistochemical evaluation in pulmonary neuroendocrine tumours. Mod Pathol 12: 5-8.

[18] Kaufmann O, Dietel M [2000]. Expression of thyroid transcription factor-1 in pulmonary and extrapulmonary small cell carcinomas and other neuroendocrine carcinomas of various primary sites. Histopathology 36: 415-420.

[19] Nomori H, Shimosato Y, Kodama T, *et al.* [1986]. Subytpes of small cell carcinoma of the lung: morphometric, ultrastructural and immunohistochemical analyses. Hum Pathol 17: 604-613.

[20] Shimosato Y, Nakajima T, Hirohashi S, *et al.* [1986]. Biological, pathological and clinical features of small lung cancer. Cancer Lett; 33: 241-258.

[21] Minna JD [1986]. Genetic events in the pathogenesis of lung cancer. Chest; 96: 178-238.

[22] Sattler M, Salgia R [2003]. Molecular and cellular biology of small cell lung cancer. Semin Oncol; 30: 57-71.

[23] Lumadue JA, Askin FB, Perlman EJ. MIC2 analysis of small cell carcinoma. Am J Clin Pathol. 1994; 102: 692-694.

[24] Hirsch FR, Matthews MJ, Yesner R [1982]. Histopathologic classification of small cell carcinoma of the lung: comments based on an interobserver examination. Cancer 50: 1360-1366.

[25] Shimosato Y, Suzuki A, Hashimoto T, Nishiwaki Y, Kodama T, Yoneyama T, Kameya T [1980]. Prognostic implications of fibrotic focus in small peripheral lung cancers. Am J Surg Pathol 4: 365-373.

[26] Sica G, Yoshizawa A, Sima CS, *et al.* [2010]. A grading system of lung adenocarcinomas based on histologic pattern is predictive of disease recurrence in stage I tumours. Am J Surg Pathol; 34: 1155-1162.

[27] Motoi N, Szoke J, Riely GJ, *et al.* [2008]. Lung adenocarcinoma: modification of the 2004 WHO mixed subtype to include the major histologic subtype suggests correlations between papillary and micropapillary adenocarcinoma subtypes, EGFR mutations and gene expression analysis. Am J Surg Pathol; 32: 810-827.

[28] Borczuk AC, Qian F, Kazeros A, *et al.* [2009]. Invasive size is an independent predictor of survival in pulmonary adenocarcinoma. Am J Surg Pathol; 33: 462-469.

[29] Yim J, Zhu LC, Chiriboga L, *et al.* [2007]. Histologic features are important prognostic indicators in early stages lung adenocarcinomas. Mod Pathol; 20: 233-241.

[30] Noguchi M, Morikawa A, Kawasaki M, *et al.* [1995]. Small adenocarcinoma of the lung. Histologic characteristics and prognosis. Cancer; 75: 2844-2852.

[31] Chiosea S, Shuai Y, Cieply K, Nikiforova MN, Dacic S [2010]. EGFR fluorescence *in situ* hybridization-positive lung adenocarcinoma: incidence of coexisting KRAS and BRAF mutations. Hum Pathol, in press.

[32] Okada A, Shimmyo T, Hashimoto T, Kobayashi Y, Miyagi Y, Ishikawa Y, Nakagawa K, Hayashi J, Tsuchiya E. Predictive advantage of a cell type classification for pulmonary adenocarcinoma coupled with data for p53, K-ras and EGFR alterations. Cancer Science; 3; 27-30.

[33] Zamecnik J, Kodet R [2002]. Value of thyroid transcription factor-1 and surfactan apoprotein A in the differential diagnosis of pulmonary carcinomas.: a study of 109 cases. Virchows Arch 440: 353-361.

[34] Lau SK, Desrochers MJ, Luthringer DJ [2002]. Expression of thyroid transcription factor-1, cytokeratin 7 and cytokeratin 20 in bronchioloalveolar carcinomas: an immunohistochemical evaluation of 67 cases. Mod Pathol 15: 538-542.

[35] Shah RN, Badve S, Papreddy K, Schindler S, Laskin WB, Yeldandi AV [2002]. Expression of cytokeratin 20 im mucinous bronchioloalveolar carcinoma. Hum Pathol 33: 915-920.

[36] Lynch TJ, Bell DW, Sordella R, Grubhagavatula S, Okimoto RA, Brannigan BW, Haris PL, Haserlat SM, Supko JG, Haluska FG, Louis DN, Christiani DC, Settleman J, Haber DA [2004]. Activating mutations in the Epidermal Growth Factor Receptor Underlying Responsiveness of Non-Small Cell Lung Cancer to Gefitinib. N Engl J Med 10: 133-138.

[37] Mooi WJ [1996]. Common lung cancers. In: Spencer's Pathology of the Lung, Hasleton PS, ed., 5th ed. McGraw-Hill: New York, pp. 1009-1064.

[38] Cavazza A, Colby TV, Tsokos M, Rush W, Travis WD [1996]. Lung tumours with a rhabdoid phenotype. Am J Clin Pathol 105: 182-188.

[39] Sturm N, Lantuejoul S, Laverriere MH, Papotti M, Brichon PY, Brambilla C, Brambilla E [2001]. Thyroid transcription factor 1 and cytokeratins 1, 5, 10, 14 [34 beta 12] expression in basaloid and large cell neuroendocrine carcinomas of the lung. Hum Pathol 32: 918-925.

[40] Cabarcos A, Gomez Dorronsoro M, Lobo Beristain JL [1965]. Pulmonary carcinosarcoma. A case study and review of the literature. Br J Dis Chest 79: 83-94.

[41] Fischer DR, Beerman LB, Park SC, Bahnson HT, Fricker FJ, Mathews RA [1984]. Diagnosis of intracardiac rhabdomyoma by two dimensional echocardiography. Am J Cardiol 53: 978-979.

[42] Johnson RL, Donnell RM [1979]. Diffuse granulocytic infiltration of giant cell carcinoma of the lung: a distinctive histologic finding with clinical significance. Lab Invest 40: 262.

[43] Travis WD, Colby TV, Corrin B, Shimosato Y, Brambilla E [1999]. WHO Histologic Classification of Tumours. Histologic Typing of Lung and Pleural Tumours. 3rd ed. Springer-Verlag: Berlin.

[44] Addis BJ, Dewar A, Thurlow NP [1988]. Giant cell carcinoma of the lung-immunohistochemical and ultrastructural evidence of dedifferentiation. J Pathol 155: 231-240.

[45] Attanoos RL, Papagiannis A, Suttinont P, Goddard H, Papotti M, Gibbs AR [1998]. Pulmonary giant cell carcinoma: pathological entity or morphological phenotype? Histopathology 32: 225-231.

[46] Yousem SA, Wick MR, Randhawa P, Manivel JC [1990]. Pulmonary blastoma. An immunohistochemical analysis with comparison with fetal lung in its pseudoglandular stage. Am J Clin Pathol 93: 167-175.

[47] Boucher LD, Yoneda K [1995]. The expression of trophoblastic cell markers by lung carcinomas. Hum Pathol 26: 1201-1206.

[48] Colby TV, Koss M, Travis WD [1995]. Tumours of the Lower Respiratory Tract. 3rd ed. Armed Forces Institute of Pathology: Washington, DC.

[49] Travis WD, Linnoila RI, Tsokos MG, Hitchcock CL, Cutler GBJr, Nieman L, Chrousos G, Pass H, Doppman J [1991]. Neuroendocrine tumours of the lung with proposed criteria for large cell neuroendocrine carcinoma. An ultrastructural, immunohistochemical and flow cytometric study of 35 cases. Am J Surg Pathol15: 529-553.

[50] Travis WD, Rush W, Flieder DB, Falk R, Fleming MW, Gal AA, Koss MN [1998]. Survival analysis of 200 pulmonary neuroendocrine tumours with clarification of criteria for atypical carcinoid and its seperation from typical carcinoid. Am J Surg Pathol 22: 934-944.

[51] Sturm N, Rossi G, Lantuejoul S, Papotti M, Frachon S, Claraz C, Brichon PY, Brambilla C, Brambilla E [2002]. Expression of thyroid transcription factor-1 in the spectrum of neuroendocrine cell lung proliferations with special interest in carcinoids. Hum Pathol 33: 175-182.

[52] Wick MR [2000]. Immunohistology of neuroendocrine and neuroectodermal tumours. Semin Diagn Pathol 17: 194-203.

[53] Pelosi G, Fraggetta F, Sonzogni A, Fazio N, Cavallon A, Viale G [2000]. CD99 immunoreactivity in gastrointestinal and pulmonary neuroendocrine tumours. Virchows Arch 437: 270-274.

[54] Churg A, Warnock ML [1976]. Pulmonary tumourlet. A form of peripheral carcinoid. Cancer 37: 1469-1477.

[55] Barbareschi M, Ferrero S, Frigo B, Mariscotti C, Mosca L [1988]. Bronchial carcinoid with S-100 positive sustentacular cells. Tumouri 74: 705-711.

[56] Hussain SP, Hofseth LJ, Harris CC [2001]. Tumour suppressor genes: at the crossroads of molecular carcinogenesis, molecular epidemiology and human risk assessment. Lung Cancer 34 Suppl 2: 7-15.

[57] Heitmiller RF, Mathisen DJ, Ferry JA, Mark EJ, Grillo HC [1989]. Mucoepidermoid lung tumours. Ann Thorac Surg 47: 394-399.

[58] Naunheim KS, Taylor JR, Skosey C, Hoffman PC, Ferguson MK, Golomb HM, Little AG [1987]. Adenosquamous lung carcinoma: clinical characteristics, treatment, and prognosis. Ann Thorac Surg 44: 462-466.

[59] Doganay L, Bilgi S, Ozdil A, Yoruk Y, Altaner S, Kutlu K [2003]. Epithelial-myoepithelial carcinoma of the lung. A case report and review of the literature. Arch Pathol Lab Med 127: 177-180.

[60] Fulford LG, Kamata Y, Okudera K, *et al.* [2001]. Epithelial-myoepithelial carcinomas of the bronchus. Am J Surg Pathol 25: 1508-1514.

CHAPTER 3

Genetics of Lung Cancer

Ebru Önalan Etem*

Firat University, Faculty of Medicine, Department of Medical Biology, 23119, Elazig, Turkey

Abstract: Lung cancer is developed through the accumulation of genetic alterations. The number of potential lung cancer-related genes have been enlightened over the last 20 years. Several molecular genetic abnormalities have been described in the pathogenesis of lung cancer, including the mutational activations of oncogenes, the inactivation of tumour suppressor genes and the alterations in the genes responsible for cell cycle regulation and DNA repair. Lung cancer progression is characterised by cumulative alterations in key molecules involved in the cell cycle, signaling and angiogenesis pathways. The identification of developmentally regulated pathways active in tumourigenesis provides insights into lung carcinogenesis and suggests early steps may differ according to the eventual tumour morphology. Developing novel biological agents to target lung cancer, and new microarray-based technologies provide new methods for predicting prognosis and response to treatment. In this chapter, particulars that have been focus on major recent advances in the molecular study of the origins and biology of lung cancer.

Keywords: Lung cancer, cytogenetic, molecular genetic, signaling mechanism, oncogene, tumour suppressor gene.

INTRODUCTION

Despite new developments in molecular techniques and better knowledge on lung cancer tumour biology, many genetic alterations associated with the development and progression of lung carcinogenesis still remain unclear. Lung tumourigenesis is a complex and heterogeneous process that might result from several clonal molecular genetic alterations including, but not limited to, gains and losses in the genome and silencing or deletion of tumour suppressor genes, among others. By identifying "repetitive" chromosomal changes th, there is a chance of discovering a

***Address correspondence to Ebru Önalan Etem:** Firat University, Faculty of Medicine, Department of Medical Biology, 23119, Elazig, Turkey; Tel: +(90) 0424 2370000/ 4656; Fax: +(90) 0424 2379138; E-mail: ebruetem@gmail.com tumour-specific gene signature associated with lung tumour development and progression [1].

CYTOGENETIC OF LUNG CANCER

Cytogenetic abnormalities in lung cancer are very complex. However, a number of recurrent cytogenetic abnormalities have been identified. Many of these changes are common in both major histological groups of lung cancer while certain chromosomal abnormalities have been correlated with the stage or the grade of the tumours [2,3].

Chromosomal Changes in Primary Lung Adenocarcinoma (AC)

The most frequently altered locus was gain of 16p followed by gain of 20q, with the minimal overlapping regions at 16p13.1-p13.2 and 20q13.2, respectively. Other over-represented loci with > 30% frequency were observed at 5p, 7p, 8q, 17q, and 19q; and high-level DNA amplifications were detected at 1q, 7p, 12q, 19q, and 20q. DNA under-representation was observed less commonly and included 8p, 9p, 13q and 18q [4].

Chromosomal Changes in Non-Small Cell Lung Cancer (NSCLC)

In NSCLCs, karyotypic changes typically are extensive, with multiple numerical and structural changes, and the karyotypes are often near-triploid The chromosome arm most frequently contributing to losses was 9p (~84%). Other chromosome arms lost in at least 60% of cases included 3p, 6q, 8p, 9q, 13q, 17p, 18q, 19p, 21q, 22q and the short arms of each of the acrocentric chromosomes. The chromosome arms most frequently involved in gains were 7p and 7q, each observed in 60% of cases. Extra copies of chromosome arms 1q, 3q, 5p, 11q and 12q were also common [5]. Masuda et al reported that chromosomal gains are frequent in 5p, the long arm of chromosome 8 (8q), 17q and 19q in NSCLC and whereas chromosome losses are frequent in 1p, 4q, 5q, 6q, 8p, 9p, 13q and 17p in NSCLC [6].

Genomic Inbalanced in NSCLC

Comparative genomic hybridisation (CGH) revealed regions on 5p, 3q, 8q, 11q, 2q, 12p and 12q to be commonly over-represented and regions on 9p, 3p, 6q, 17p,

22q, 8p, 10p, 10q and 19p to be commonly under-represented in NSCLC. Translocations between chromosomes 5 and 14, 5 and 11 and 1 and 6, loss of the Y chromosome and gains of chromosomes 20 and 5p were also frequent. Chromosomes 4, 5, 8, 11, 12 and 19 were most frequently involved in interchromosomal translocations [7].

Chromosomal Changes in Small Cell Lung Cancer SCLC

Chromosomal gains are frequent 3q, 5p, 8p and Xq in SCLC, whereas chromosome losses are frequent in 5q, 13q and 17p in SCLC [6]. Cytogenetic losses of chromosome 5q13–2, including the gene encoding the p85α regulatory unit of phosphatidylinositol-3 kinase and *APC* are freguent in SCLC. The p53 gene, *TP53*, is located at band 17p13.1 and has been shown to be a frequent target for molecular alteration in lung cancer [5].

Genomic Inbalanced in SCLC

The most frequent sites of chromosome loss are 3p, 5q and 13q, each observed in 90% of cases according to CGH result, including loss of 4q, 10q and 16q, and gains of 3q and 5p, were each identified in 60-70% of cases. Gains of 8q and 19q were also observed in ~40% of the tumours. Amplification at chromosome bands 1p32, 2p23 and 8q24.1, sites of *MYCL, MYCN* and *MYC*, respectively, were also observed Several candidate genes in deleted regions of 3p have been identified, including the β-retinoic acid receptor gene, the protein-tyrosine phosphatase-γ gene, the semaphorin IV and A(V) genes, the von Hippel Lindau tumour suppressor gene, *VHL*, and the fragile histidine triad gene, *FHIT* [5].

Ploidy

DNA content is the most significant cellular parameter able to monitor the cell proliferation and the neoplastic transformation [8]. Nuclear DNA content analysis has been assigned some prognostic significance in SCLC, but some studies failed to confirm any prognostic value of the ploidy in SCLCs. Aneuploid tumours seem to carry a poorer prognosis, with this finding being independent of tumour stage. Aneuploidy correlates with postoperative chemosensitivity of SCLC; the less aneuploid tumours are more chemoresistant. ACs are more frequently aneuploid than typical carcinoids (TCs) [9].

LUNG CANCER TUMOURIGENESIS

Cancer is driven by the activation/inactivation of key genes that are essential point controllers in regulatory pathways, such as signal transduction, cell cycles, DNA repair, and apoptosis. Global gene mutational profiles have identified recurrent nonsystemic mutations in many putative oncogenes and tumour suppressor genes [10]. Similarly, comparative genomic hybridisation and single nucleotide polymorphism studies have led to the identification of several sites of recurrent amplicons in lung cancers, and have resulted in the identification of putative oncogenes [11]. In the case of lung cancer, several gene alterations are known to contribute to its development, including activating mutations or gene amplification of the oncogenes; inactivating point mutations; homozygous deletions; and promoter hypermethylation of the tumour suppressor genes [10].

Molecular Alterations of Genes

Overexpression of oncogenes, loss of tumour suppressor genes and amplification of chromosome copy number have all been associated with lung carcinogenesis. Hundreds of studies have demonstrated increases in chromosomal copy numbers of 1p, 1q, 3q, 5p, 6p, 8q, 12, 17q, 19p, 19q, 20p, 20q, and X chromosome regions, implying that direct-acting oncogenes relevant to the tumourigenic process reside in these chromosomal regions [12].

Oncogenes

In the particular case of lung cancer, several gene alterations are known to contribute to its development, including activating mutations and gene amplification at the oncogenes [13]. Some important oncogenes in lung cancer tumourigenesis were given in Table **1**.

B-related factor 2 (BRF2): Genetic activation of BRF2, which encodes a RNA polymerase III (Pol III) transcription initiation factor, was found to be associated with increased expression of small nuclear RNAs (snRNAs) that are involved in processes essential for cell growth, such as RNA splicing. Ectopic expression of BRF2 in human bronchial epithelial cells induced a transformed phenotype and demonstrates downstream oncogenic effects. Genetic activation of BRF2 represents a unique mechanism of SCLC lung tumourigenesis through the increase of Pol III-mediated transcription. Focal amplification of a BRF2 may plays a key role in squamous cell lineage specificity of the lung cancer [12].

Myelocytomatosis oncogenes (MYC family): The MYC gene family encodes nuclear phospho-proteins (C-MYC, N-MYC, L-MYC) that control cellular growth, proliferation, differantiation and apoptosis [9, 13]. Their amplification and/or overexpression is very frequent in SCLCs [15].

N-MYC is frequently activated in SCLC by gene amplification. Several studies demonstrated that *N-MYC* is required for lung development. Embryos homozygous for a hypomorphic mutation of *N-MYC* die at birth with lungs half of the normal size. *N-MYC* RNA expression is highest in embryonic lung and is very low in the adult lung. Thus, the role of *N-MYC* in lung organogenesis appears to be centered on maintaining a population of undifferentiated, proliferating progenitor cells in the developing lung tissue. L-and N-MYC amplification is specific for neuroendocrine lung tumours, including SCLC and large cell neuroendocrine carcinoma (LCNEC) [16].

Table 1: Chromosomal location and functions of some oncogenes found to be altered in lung cancer

Localization	Related Gene/Genes	Functions	The Role of Lung Cancer
3q26.3-q27	SRY (sex determining region Y)-box 2 (SOX2)	A transcription factor Controlling pluripotency	Low-level gains in about 80% of the tumours and high-level amplifications in 20% of lung SCC are found [17].
3q26.3	Phosphoinositide-3-kinase, catalytic, alpha polypeptide (PIK3CA)	p110-alpha subunit of phosphoinositide-3-kinase	*Amplification* is found infrequently in lung cancer [10].
4q11-q12	Mast/stem cell growth factor receptor (c-kit)	A tyrosine kinase receptor A chemotactic factor for SCLC	The stem cell factor (SCF)/kit autocrine loop is functional in the majority of SCLCs [9].
6p12.3	G protein-coupled receptor (GPR110)	G protein-coupled receptor A known function	Greatly overexpressed in human lung adenocarcinoma tissue [18]. (Lum).
8p11.23	B-related factor 2 subunit of RNA polymerase III (BRF2)	Transcription initiation factor	Focal amplification of a BRF2 may plays a key role in squamous cell lineage specificity of the lung cancer [12].

Table 1: contd….

8q24.21	v-myc myelocytomatosis viral oncogene homolog (MYC)	A transcription factor, Regulating cellular growth, differentiation and apoptosis	Activated by increased expression or amplification. Altered expression of *c-myc* is often correlated with adverse prognosis in SCLCs [11].
11q13	Cyclin D1 (CCND1)	Cyclin D1 encoded by the *CCND1* gene The member of the G1 cyclin family Controlling cell cycle, G1/S transition	Recurrent numeric gene aberrations, particularly high-level amplifications, of cyclin D1 were obvious in lung cancers [19].
11q23.3	v-ets erythroblastosis virus E26 oncogene homolog 1 (c-ets-1)	A transcription factor	Expressed in Neuroendocrin) NE tumours of advanced stages—SCLCs and LCNECs—suggesting a potential role in tumour invasion[9].
12p12.1	Kirsten rat sarcoma viral oncogene homolog (Ras Family)	Signal transduction p21 membrane-associated protein proliferation, differentiation and survival	K-ras mutated in 30% of adenocarcinomas Not in SCLC [20].
17q21.1	Erythroblastic leukemia viral oncogene homolog 2 (ERBB2)	Membran receptor Transmembrane glycoprotein Structural homology to epidermal growth factor receptor Intracellular tyrosine kinase domain Receptor function? Activated by amplification and overexpression	EGFR overexpression is often associated with adverse prognosis. Amplification rare SCLC, rare overexpression NSCLC, overexpressed in 35% of cases [20].
8q24	Myelocytomatosis oncogenes (MYC family)	Nuclear phosphoproteins Regulation of gene transcription c-myc expression coupled to cell cycle Can cooperate with ras in transforming	SCLC, amplified in 30-50% of cell lines and 11-24% of tumours; overexpressed in 89% of cell lines and 83% of tumours NSCLC, amplified in 8% of tumours [20].

Table 1: contd....

		primary cells Activated by increased expression or amplification	

More frequently than amplification, a high level of transcription leads to over expression of MYC proteins [11]. Myc amplification has been reported that *c-myc* overexpression occurs in classic SCLC, whereas *L-myc* and *N-myc* overexpression is likely to lead to the variant phenotype of SCLC. Gains on *8q*, the region harboring *c-myc*, are frequently observed in SCLC [9]. (koumatsu). Activated by increased expression or amplification, amplified in 11-24% of SCLC; overexpressed in 83% of NSCLC, amplified in 8% of tumours. Altered expression of *c-myc* is often correlated with adverse prognosis in SCLCs [13].

Tumour Supressor Genes (TSG)

A tumour suppressor may possess multiple mechanisms to suppress cancer cell growth four major mechanisms have been revealed for tumour suppressors: suppression of cell division, induction of apoptosis, DNA damage repair and inhibition of metastasis [21]. TSGs are rendered inactive by chromosomal loss of one allele (loss of heterozygosity (LOH)) and damage to the other by genetic mutation or the epigenetic hypermethylation of its promoter [13].

Suppression of Cell Division

The tumour suppressors that adopt suppression of cell division include retinoblastoma protein (Rb), adenomatosis polyposis coli (APC), alternate reading frame (ARF), RIZ1, p15, p16, p18, p19, p21, p27, and p53.

Tumour Protein (p53)

p53 is a nuclear phosphoprotein, have multiple cellular activities, such as G1 and G2 checkpoint control, maintenance of genomic integrity, DNA repair, replication, transcription, apoptosis, and differentiation. *17p* losses seem to be absent in TCs and rare in ACs. Absence of p53 mutations in TCs might be responsible for their benign clinical course, and their presence in some ACs could explain their higher aggressiveness [9]. Allelic losses and/or p53 mutations detected in the majority of SCLCs are likely to be related with smoking and the carcinogens found in tobacco and seem to be correlated with poorer prognosis in lung tumours. Approximately 90% of SCLCs and 50% of NSCLCs have mutated p53. Inactivation occurs in >75% of SCLCs and about 50% of NSCLCs with mutations correlating with cigarette smoking [22].

Retinoblastoma (Rb) Gene

RB is a key component of the cell-cycle regulatory machinery, which normally inhibits G1/S transition by sequestering the E2F-1 transcription factor [16]. Loss of heterozygosity at *Rb* gene is significantly more frequent in SCLCs (67%) than in NSCLCs (31%) [9]. RB is mutated in more than 90% of SCLCs but in only a small fraction of NSCLCs [20]. Functional loss of the RB gene can include deletions, nonsense mutations, or splicing abnormalities leading to protein abnormalities in most SCLCs and 15–30% of NSCLCs [22]. E2F-1, a member of the E2F family of transcriptional modulators, plays a key regulatory role in cell-cycle progression, apoptosis, and differentiation. E2F-1 is overexpressed in both SCLCs and LCNECs and is accompanied by increased Ki-67 index and a Bcl-2:Bax ratio >1, suggesting a strong implication of E2F-1 deregulation in SCLC and NSCLCs tumourigenesis [9].

p27KIP1 protein is a cyclin-dependent kinase (CDK) inhibitor, acting as a negative regulator of the cell cycle. Recent evidence however, suggests that p27 may function as an oncogene rather than a tumour suppressor gene [23]. Interestingly, and in contrast to NSCLCs, expression of p27 is elevated in SCLCs *in vivo* [9]. p27 may not appear to be an independent prognostic factor in patients with NSCLC [19,23].

p15INK4B is a cell-cycle inhibitor that belongs to the INK4 family, are highly expressed in normal lung tissue [9]. The *p16INK4A* is part of the p16-cyclin D1-CDK4,6-RB pathway that is central to controlling the G1–S transition of the cell cycle by inbiting CDK4,6. This critical cell cycle regulatory pathway is functionally altered or mutated in many cancers including those of lung origin [22]. Homozygous alterations (*i.e.*, deletions, point mutations, aberrant methylation) of this gene ocur more frequently in NSCLCs than in SCLCs. *p16* aberrant methylation has been considered to be an early event in NSCL carcinogenesis [9]. The p16INK4 gene has been inactivated by hypermethylation of the promoter region could have an advantage in progression and metastasis in non-small cell lung cancers, especially in the tumours with normal p53, and that the frequency of p16INK4 gene inactivation by hypermethylation could vary in clinical course [24]. p16INK4 and p15INK4B gene mutations are associated with tumour progression of a subset of NSCLC, but not of SCLC, and that p15INK4B mutations might also be an early event in the molecular pathogenesis of a subset of NSCLC [25].

Induction of Apoptosis (Programmed Cell Death)

Examples of this group of tumour suppressors are p53, APC, cluster of differentiation 95 (CD95), bridging integrator 1 (Bin1) and phosphatase and tensin homolog (PTEN) [21, 26]. p53 mediates apoptosis through two major pathways, the extrinsic pathway, which activates a caspase cascade including caspase-9,-3,-6 and-7, and the intrinsic pathway, which promotes the apoptosome formation *via* the Bcl-2 family [21]. The family of apoptotic regulators also includes BCL-XL, BCL-XS, Bax, Bad, Bak, MCL-1, *etc.* Specifically, Bax and Bak induce apoptosis, and myeloid cell leukemia-1(MCL-1) prevents cell death. The majority of SCLCs overexpress the Bcl-2 protein, thus resisting the apoptotic process. In metastatic SCLCs both *Bcl-2* and *Bax* expression are decreased, may be indicative of development of metastatic clones that are resistant to apoptosis [9].

DNA Damage Repair

The tumour suppressors that can help in DNA damage repair, include mutS homolog 2 (MSH2), mutL homolog 1 (MLH1), Ataxia-telangiectasia mutated gene product (ATM), breast cancer protein (BRCA), p53, *etc.* ATM is a general sensor to DNA damage. BRCA and p53 work together in nucleotide excision repair of DNA adducts [21].

Inhibition of Metastasis

Tumour suppressors that can inhibit metastasis consist of metastin, breast cancer metastasis suppressor 1 (BRMS1), tissue inhibitor of metalloproteinase (TIMP), cofactor required for specificity protein 1 activation (CRSP), and KAL1/CD82. The binding of metastin to the metastin receptor (orphan G protein-coupled receptor GPR54) increases the expression and activity of focal adhesion kinase (FAK) and inhibits the metastasis of melanoma cells. BRMS1 regulates gene transcription through interaction with the mSin3 histone deacetylase (HDAC) complex. TIMPs can bind not only all matrix metalloproteinases (MMPs) in their active forms but also MMP-2 and MMP-9 in their latent forms. TIMPs reduce cancer metastasis by inhibiting the cancer cell-released MMPs, maintaining the integrity of extracellular matrices, and preventing the penetration of cancer cells through the base membrane of blood vessels. CRSP can up-regulate the expression of metastin. CD82 is a cell surface glycoprotein activated by p53. The expression levels of CD82 and p53 are strongly correlated. The exact mechanism for CD82 to inhibit cancer metastasis is still unclear; however, it may inhibit cancer cell migration/invasion through the FAK-Lyn-p130CAS-CrkII pathway [21].

LOH Studies in Lung Cancers

A genome wide search for LOH in 36 lung cancer cell lines using, 400 high resolution polymorphic markers showed that tumours had a mean of 17–22 "hot spots" of chromosomal loss. There were 22 different regions with more than 60% LOH, 13 with a preference for SCLC, seven for NSCLC, and two affecting both histological types. The sharing of some LOH regions and the specificity of others may provide an insight into the genes common to lung cancer development and others specific to subtype differentiation. The chromosomal arms with the most frequent LOH were 1p, 3p, 4p, 4q, 5q, 8p, 9p (p16 TSG locus), 9q, 10p, 10q, 13q (RB-retinoblastoma TSG locus), 15q, 17p (p53 TSG locus), 18q, 19p, Xp, and Xq [22].

FHIT at the 3p14.2 region; lung cancer cells frequently express abnormal mRNA transcripts of FHIT apart from normal wild type transcripts. Homozygous deletions and loss of heterozygosity (LOH) at the *FHIT* locus have been frequently reported in lung cancer cell lines and primary tumours; aberrant *FHIT* mRNA transcripts have been detected in 40 to 80% of tumour samples, whereas mutations are rare. Loss of FHIT protein expression is observed in almost 70% of primary tumours, mainly in those arising in smokers, and in 90% of preinvasive lesions. The promoter region around exon 1/intron 1 of the *FHIT* gene contains CpG islands that have been shown to be hypermethylated in lung cancer and methylation was associated with loss of *FHIT* mRNA and protein expression [27].

Brahma/SWI2-related gene 1(BRG1, SMARCA4): BRG1, a central component of the SWI/SNF chromatin-remodeling complex. Depending on the cellular context, the complex can regulate transcriptional transactivation or repression by remodeling the chromatin structure, upon disturbing DNA–histone interactions at the nucleosomes in an ATP-dependent manner. The SWI/SNF complex functions, including regulation of gene transcription, occur through the remodeling of the chromatin structure. Direct interaction of BRG1, or other components of the complex, with different proteins such as retinoblastoma (RB), BRCA1, nuclear receptors and transcription factors play a role in orchestrating different biological pathways including arrest of the cell cycle, DNA repair, as well as cell differentiation and regulation of apoptosis. BRG1 is somatically inactivated by point mutations or large deletions in lung tumours featuring LOH of chromosome 19p [28].

Semaphorin 3 B and F (SEMA3F): 3p23 undergoes frequent loss of heterozygosity (LOH) and both *SEMA3F* and *SEMA3B* transcripts are underrepresented in squamous cell carcinomas. SEMA3B induces apoptosis of lung and the target of the tumour suppressor p53. SEMA3F is abundantly expressed in normal lung and cultured bronchial epithelial cells. In contrast, it is markedly down-regulated in most human lung cancers and loss of SEMA3F protein staining is significantly correlated with advanced stage of disease and vascular endothelial growth factor-165 (VEGF165) overexpression SEMA3F blocked tumour formation by H157 lung cancer cells in a rat orthotopic model. This was associated with loss of activated AVB3 integrin, impaired cell adhesion to extracellular matrix components, and down-regulation of phospho-extracellular signal-regulated kinase 1/2 (ERK1/2). SEMA3F inhibited the activity of integrin-linked kinase (ILK) although this appeared to account only for the loss of phospho-ERK1/2. Thus, SEMA3F has emerged as a potent tumour suppressor and antagonist of VEGF-driven tumour neovascularization [29].

Table 2: Chromosomal location and functions of some tumour suppressor genes found to be altered in lung cancer

Localization	Related Gene	Functions	The Roles of Lung Cancer
3p25.3	Von Hippel-Lindau (VHL)	An E3 ubiquitin ligase the regulation of gene expression by hypoxia.	An important biological markers for lung carcinogenesis [30]. (Neal).
5q22.2	Adenomatous polyposis coli (APC)	Modulate the base excision repair (BER) pathway.	Hypermethylation of the APC gene promoter in plasma is a potential diagnostic marker for lung cancer diagnosis [31,32,33]. (Jaiswall). Hawes). (pan XY).
10q23.2	Phosphatase and tensin homolog (PTEN)	Acts as a phosphatase to dephosphorylate phosphatidylinositol (3,4,5)-trisphosphate (PtdIns (3,4,5)P_3 or PIP_3).	The expression level of PTEN may predict the effect of radiotherapy, chemotherapy and prognosis of NSCLC [26]. (Zhang H).
11p15.1	HIV-1 Tat interactive protein 2 (CC3)	A small protein (also known as TIP30) with metastasis suppressor properties.	*CC3* expression is absent in the highly aggressive variant SCLCs, but it is detected in the less metastatic classic type of SCLCs, in other tumours, and in normal tissue [9].
11q13.1	Multiple endocrine neoplasia type 1 (MEN1)	Menin encoded by the MEN1 gene is associated with chromatin and the nuclear matrix.	Reduction of menin is closely correlated with increased lung cancer metastasis to lymph nodes [34].
17q11.2	Neurofibromatosis type 1 (NF1)	Encodes for the protein a regulator of ras guanosine triphosphatase activity (GTPase-activating protein, GAP).	NF1 gene mutation could imply a poor prognosis [35,36].
18q21.2	Deleted in pancreatic carcinoma, locus 4 (Smad4 DPC4)	The key intracellular mediators of transcriptional responses to TGF-β.	Importance for the initiation and development of NSCLC. It can be used as prognostic factors of NSCLC [37,38].

Table 2: contd....

18q21.3	Serpin peptidase inhibitor, clade B (ovalbumin), member 5 (Maspin, SERPINB5)	The serpin protease inhibitor family.	The expression of maspin is frequently lost in human lung cancer [39].
19p13.3	Serine/threonine kinase 11 (STK11, LKB1)	The regulation of the cell energetic checkpoint through the phosphorylation and activation of adenosine monophosphate-dependent kinase (AMPK).	Mutated in 30% of NSCLC tumours, and recent evidence points to a prominent role in NSCLC metastasis [28].
19p13.2	SWI/SNF related, matrix associated, actin dependent regulator of chromatin, subfamily a, member 4 (BRG1)	A central component of the SWI/SNF chromatin-remodeling complex.	The presence of BRG1 alterations was significantly more frequent in the NSCLC-type cell lines [28].
22q12.2	Ras association (RalGDS/AF-6) domain family member 1 (RASSF1A)	Downregulate the expression of cyclin D1. Induces apoptoisis.	Promoter acquired hypermethylation in 90% of SCLCs and 30–40% of NSCLCs [40].

Familial Lung Cancer

Recent genome-wide association studies have identified multiple genetic loci and single nucleotide polymorphisms (SNPs) associated with either increased or decreased risk of lung cancer. A genome-wide screen for lung cancer loci identified strong evidence for linkage to 6q23-25 and suggestive evidence for linkage to 12q24 and 12p12-12q12 [41]. Allelic loss in 6q23–25 (146–164 cM) has been reported in a number of tumour types. The region identified is large, encompassing 74 known genes and 41 unknown genes, including four putative tumour suppressor genes (*SASH1*, *LATS1*, *IGF2R*, and *PARK2*), as well as genes involved in regulating cellular proliferation and preventing DNA damage [42]. In the human, Kras2 and Krag have been mapped to 12p12.1 and 12p11.2. One potential candidate gene for lung function is microsomal *GSTM1*, located on 12p, which is involved in detoxification of oxygen radicals and matrix Gla protein, a lung extracellular matrix component (Ann). Other chromosomes also suggestive for linkages, including 5p15.33, 5q31-q33, 6p21.33,12p11.2, 13q31.3, 14q11, 15q25.1, 16q24, and 19q13.2–3 [42-45]. Candidate genes that suggests possible overlap between genes predicting lung function, COPD, and lung cancer are presented in Table **3**.

A significant association was also seen at 19q13.3. *ERCC1* and *XPD*, DNA repair genes, are located in this region at 19q13.2–3. There is evidence that some polymorphisms in DNA repair genes play a role in carcinogenesis, most notably the ERCC2 Lys751Gln and XPA G23A polymorphisms. The variant allele of each of the three polymorphisms was associated with about a 30% decrease or increase in lung cancer risk. The XPA G23A polymorphism itself may alter the transcription and/or translation of the gene. The nearby proximal nucleotides to the AUG initiation codon are important for the initiation of translation because the 40S ribosomal subunit binds initially at the 5′-end of the mRNA. A functional association between the G23A polymorphism and DRC was reported, which showed significantly higher repair efficiency in healthy subjects with at least one G allele. The Gln allele of the ERCC2 Lys751Gln polymorphism is associated with a higher DNA adduct level or lower DNA repair efficiency. The meta-analysis by Hu *et al.*, showed that the Gln/Gln genotype had a significant 23% increased risk of lung cancer compared with individuals with the Lys/Lys genotype among Caucasians [41, 46].

Neutrophil elastase (NE), a member of the serine protease family, synthesized at the promyelocyte stage of granulocyte differentiation. Mutations in the gene encoding neutrophil elastase have been associated with cyclic and severe congenital neutropenia, a hematologic disorder characterized by early-stage maturation arrest of myelopoiesis [47]. IL-4 is structurally related to IL-13, which has been attributed mainly to a shared use of the receptor complex for the IL-4 type II receptor, predominantly composed of the IL-4Rα and IL-13Rα1. IL-4 acts as a survival factor on epithelial cells by increasing the expression of antiapoptotic molecules rendering them resistant to the induction of apoptosis. One of the main physiological functions of IL-4 is to influence the immune system toward the production of T_H2 cells and suppression of the production of IFN-γ-producing T_H1 cells, the latter being important in efficient tumour immunity [48].

Associations between markers on chromosome 6q to both lung cancer and lung function, and on 12 to lung cancer, chronic obstructive pulmonary disease

(COPD), and lung function, together with overlap in candidate genes for these outcomes, suggest that future research into underlying genetic mechanisms of lung disease would benefit from broadening the collection of family history and lung function data [42].

Table 3: Candidate genes in familial lung cancer

Chromosomal Region	Related Gene/Genes	Functions
1q42.1	Microsomal epoxide hydrolase (*EPHX*) Low-activity haplotype (His113–His139)	An enzyme associated with the metabolism and detoxification of xenobiotic chemicals [49].
2q	Interleukin-8 receptor-α gene (*IL8RA*)	A cytokine involved in neutrophil recruitment to the lung [50].
5q31	Interleukin-8 receptor- α (*IL4RA)* Q551R genotype	An autocrine survival factor in epithelial cells [51].
6q	*SMOC2* (secreted modular calcium-binding protein 2)	The encoded protein contains a serine protease inhibitor domain [52].
11q22.3	Matrix metalloproteinases (*MMP1)* 2G/2G genotype	Extracellular matrix (ECM) degradation, invasion, and cytokine mobilization [53].
12p	Microsomal *GSTM1*	Detoxification of oxygen radicals and matrix Gla protein, a lung extracellular matrix component [50].
19p13.3	Neutrophil elastase (*ELA2*) T-903G [REP-a] TT genotype G-741A [REP-b] GG genotype	Granulocyte differentiation [47].

Lung Cancer in Never-Smokers: A Different Disease

Lung cancer in never-smokers demonstrates a marked sex bias worldwide, occurring more frequently among females, and especially in Asiatic countries. Although smoking-related carcinogens act on both proximal and distal airways, inducing all the major forms of lung cancer, cancers arising in never-smokers target the distal airways and favour ADC histology. While the conventional thought is that lung cancer in never-smokers is due to environmental tobacco smoke, this is a relatively weak carcinogen and can only account for a minority of lung cancers arising in neversmokers. The cause of lung cancer in never-smokers remains controversial, but no conclusive cause for most cases has been identified. Molecular epidemiology studies, in particular of the TP53, KRAS and EGFR genes, demonstrate strikingly different mutation patterns and frequencies between lung cancers in never-smokers and smokers [11]. *TP53, KRAS and STK11* (*LBK1*) mutations are lower in non-smokers than smokers. *EGFR, HER2*mutations, *EML4-ALK* transloations and N-tyr expression are higher frequency in non-smokers than smokers [54]. In addition, there are major clinical differences between lung cancers arising in neversmokers and smokers, and their response to targeted therapies. These facts strongly suggest that lung cancer arising in neversmokers is a disease distinct from the more common tobaccorelated forms of lung cancer. Clearly, further efforts are needed to identify the major causes of lung cancers arising in neversmokers and the reasons for its marked pathological, geographical and sex differences [11].

SOME IMPORTANT PATHWAYS IN LUNG CANCER TUMOURIGENESIS

Integrated approaches to whole genome analyses are likely to be of greater benefit than individual platforms, and have already led to the identification of cancer-related abnormalities in signaling pathways [11].

1. Ras/Raf/MEK/ERK and Lung Cancer

In humans three Ras proto-oncogenes encode four isoforms (H-Ras, K-Ras4A, K-Ras4B and N-Ras) that function as molecular switches. Ras proteins predominantly sit on the inner leaflet of the plasma membrane and switched on when a wide range of cell surface receptors become activated. Oncogenic Ras mutations interfere with the ability of GAPs to interact with Ras producing constitutively active Ras proteins Ras activation promotes cell proliferation, differentiation and survival amongst many other cell regulatory functions. These proteins have transforming potential in humans. Signal transduction was activated by point mutation. K-ras mutated in 30% of adenocarcinomas, not in SCLC [55, 56].

Raf and phosphatidylinositol 3-kinase (PI3K) were the first two Ras effectors. Raf promotes cell proliferation and differentiation through the MAP kinase (MAPK) pathway whilst PI3K generates antiapoptotic signaling. At least 20 effectors links to pathways regulating cytoskeletal organisation, membrane trafficking, cell migration, cell cycling and transcription [56]. (Jasminka). The phosphoinositide-3-kinase

(PI3K)/PTEN/AKT signaling pathway is frequently deregulated in human lung cancers. PI3K/Akt activation was demonstrated to be involved in the regulation of several cellular functions like cell survival, cell growth and angiogenesis stimulation, inhibition of apoptosis, translation of several proteins and hence, in the development of lung cancer [57]. PIK3CA is a gene that encodes for the p110-alpha subunit of PI3K. PIK3CA amplification is found infrequently in lung cancer, and thus, gene amplification may constitute a mechanism for oncogenic activation of *PIK3CA*, especially in lung squamous cell carcinomas, offering a candidate marker that is sensitive to therapy with inhibitors of PI3K activity [10].

Raf is a serine/threonine protein kinase that participates in the mitogen-activated protein kinase/extracellular signal-regulated kinase (MAPK/ERK) signal transduction pathways [9]. Ras proteins show varying abilities to activate the Raf/MEK/ERK and PI3K/Akt cascades. K-Ras is a stronger induce of Raf/MEK/ERK than H-Ras. In contrast, Ha-Ras may be a stronger inducer of PI3K/Akt than Raf/MEK/ERK [56]. The raf–MEK–MAPK pathway has been shown to relate with Notch signaling. The effect of Notch activation seems to be the suppression of SCLC growth. However, the Notch signaling pathway has to be further analyzed, not only in SCLCs but also in the rest of the NE lung tumours [9].

ErbB, Ras, Src, Abl, Raf, PI3K, Akt, Jun, Fos, Ets and NF-κB (Rel) oncogenes are connected to the Ras/Raf/MEK/ERK and PI3K/PTEN/PDK/Akt pathways and either feed into this pathway (*e.g.,* BCR-ABL, ErbB) or are downstream targets, which regulate gene expression (*e.g.,* Jun, Fos, Ets, and NF-κB) [55].

The Ras/Raf/MEK/ERK pathway has what often appears to be conflicting roles in cellular proliferation, differentiation, and the prevention of apoptosis. Classical studies have indicated that Ras/Raf/MEK/ERK can promote proliferation and malignant transformation in part due to the stimulation of cell growth and at the same time the prevention of apoptosis. Furthermore, an often overlooked aspect of Raf/MEK/ERK is the production of growth factors which can stimulate growth. The latest "hot" area of the Ras/Raf/MEK/ERK pathway is the discovery of mutation of the B-Raf gene in human cancer, which can promote proliferation and transformation. The Raf/MEK/ERK pathway is intimately linked with the PI3K/PTEN/Akt pathway. Ras can regulate both pathways. Furthermore, in some cell types, Raf activity is negatively regulated by Akt indicating a cross-talk between the two pathways. Both pathways may result in the phosphorylation of many downstream targets and impose a role in the regulation of cell survival and proliferation [56].

2. PI3K/Akt/mTOR Signaling Pathway

mTOR plays a critical role in transducing proliferative signals mediated through the PI3K and Akt signaling pathways, principally activating downstream protein kinases that are required for both ribosomal biosynthesis and translation of mRNAs of proteins that are essential for G_1 to S phase traverse. It has been reported that constitutive activation of the PI3K/Akt/mTOR signaling network is a common feature of lung cancer.

PI3K—The family of PI3K enzymes is characterized by the ability to phosphorylate the 3'-OH group in inositol lipids and comprises three different classes, I, II, and III. Class I PI3K is divided further into A and B subtype. Class IA PI3Ks are heterodimeric enzymes composed of a regulatory (p85α, p85β, p55α, p55γ, p50α) and of catalytic (p110α, p110β, p110δ) subunits. Class IB PI3K comprises a p101 regulatory and a p110γ catalytic subunit. p110γ and p110δ PI3Ks are mostly related to the immune system functions. Activating mutations in the gene coding for p110α (PIK3CA) have been found in lung cancer subtypes.

Akt—Akt (the cellular homolog of the *v-akt) is* a 57-kDa serine/threonine protein kinase. The Akt interacts with PtdIns (3,4,5)P3. Once Akt is recruited at the plasma membrane, its activation loop is phosphorylated by PDK1 while the mTOR complex 2 (mTORC2) phosphorylates in the Akt. Active Akt migrates to both the cytosol and the nucleus. Nuclear Akt may fulfil important anti-apoptotic roles. Akt substrates (over 100 Akt) include Bad, caspase-9, murine double minute 2 (MDM2), IκB kinase (IKK) α, proline-rich Akt substrate 40-kDa (PRAS40), the FOXO family of Forkhead transcription factors, apoptosis signal-regulated kinase 1 [ASK1, a negative regulator of pro-apoptotic c-Jun N-terminal kinase (JNK)], Raf, p27Kip1, p21Cip1, glycogen synthase kinase 3β (GSK3β). Each of these substrates has a key role in the regulation of cell survival and proliferation. Phosphorylated-Akt is a reliable prognostic factor in patients with small cell carcinoma of the lung [58,59].

mTOR—mTOR is an atypical 289-kDa serine/threonine kinase, belongs to the PI3K-related kinase family. mTOR exists as two complexes, referred to as mTOR complex 1 (mTORC1) and mTORC2 (Fig. **1**) [60].

mTORC1 signaling integrates environmental clues (growth factors, hormones, nutrients, stressors) and information from the cell metabolic status. Thus, mTORC1 controls anabolic processes for promoting protein synthesis and cell growth. mTORC1 regulates translation in response to nutrients/growth factors by phosphorylating components of the protein synthesis machinery, including p70S6 kinase (p70S6K) and eukaryotic initiation factor 4E-binding protein 1 (4E-BP1). eIF4E is a key component for translation of genes encoding growth promoting molecules, such as c-Myc, cyclin D1, Cdk 2, RB, p27Kip1, vascular endothelial growth factor (VEGF), and signal activator and transducer of transcription 3 (STAT3). Furthermore, mTORC1 negatively regulates autophagy, a non-apoptotic form of cell death Akt also phosphorylates PRAS40, an inhibitor of the interactions between mTORC1 and its substrates, and by doing so, prevents PRAS40 ability to suppress mTORC1 signaling. Moreover, mTORC1 signal transduction is inhibited by the master metabolic regulator, energy-sensing AMP-dependent protein kinase (AMPK), given that AMPK phosphorylates and activates TSC2 [58].

mTORC2 activation requires PI3K and the TSC1/TSC2 complex. mTORC2 phosphorylates Akt which enhances subsequent Akt phosphorylation by PDK1 and plays a role in cytoskeleton organization by controlling actin polymerization and phosphorylates protein kinase C (PKC) α. Another downstream target of mTORC2 is serum-and glucocorticoid-induced protein kinase 1 (SGK1).

Akt and mTORC1/2 are linked to each other *via* positive and negative regulatory feedback Circuits. Assuming that an equilibrium exists between mTORC1 and mTORC2, when mTORC1 is formed, it antagonizes the formation of mTORC2 and reduces Akt activity. Indeed, once mTORC1 is activated through Akt, the former elicits a negative feedback loop for inhibiting Akt activity. This negative regulation of Akt activity by mTORC1 is a consequence of p70S6K-mediated phosphorylation of insulin receptor substrate (IRS) 1 adapter protein, downstream of insulin receptor and/or Insulin-like Growth Factor-1 Receptor (IGF-1R). mTORC1 is capable of downregulating also IRS2 expression by enhancing its proteosomal degradation [58].

The mammalian target of rapamycin (mTOR) acts as a downstream effector for Akt. Activation of the Akt/mTOR signal is a contributing factor to decreased radiation sensitivity. Rapamycin can enhance the effect of radiation through the repression of pro-survival signals and the reduction in the apoptotic threshold. Taken together, inhibition of the mTOR signal may be a promising strategy for radiosensitization with no relevance to p53 gene status from the aspects of cell lethality and cell growth depression [61].

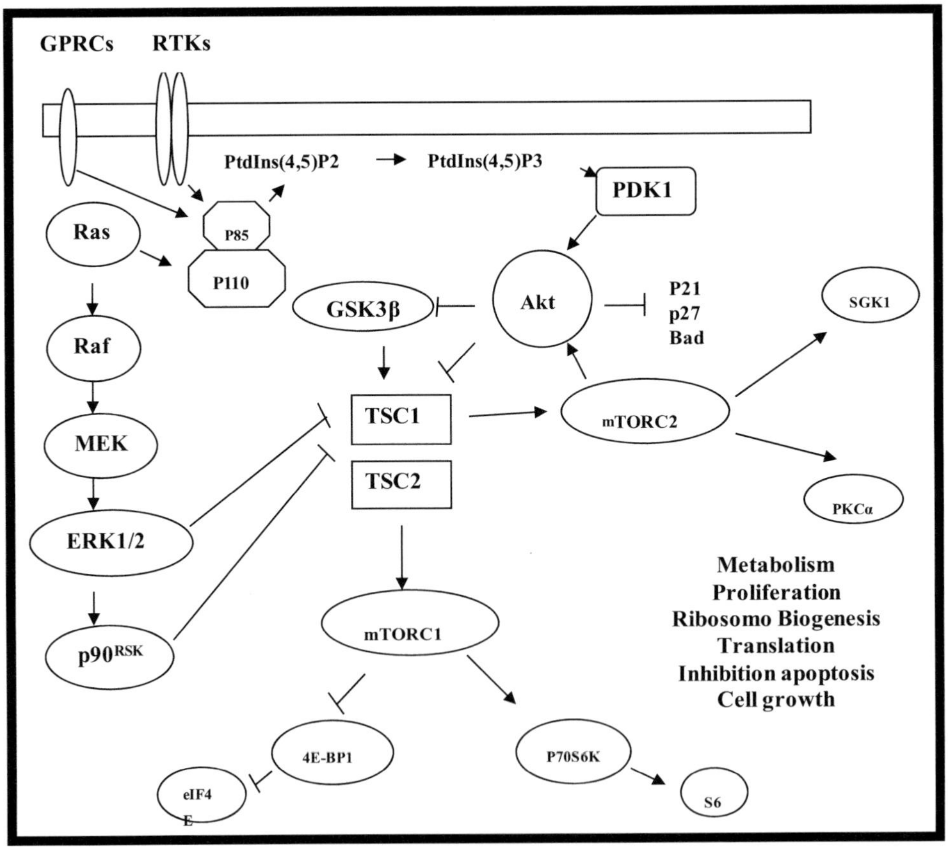

Figure 1: The PI3K/Akt/mTOR signaling pathway.

G protein coupled receptors (GPCRs), receptor tyrosine kinases (RTKs), and Ras activate PI3K. PI3K generates phosphatidylinositol 3,4,5 trisphosphate [PtdIns (3,4,5)P3] from phosphatidylinositol 4,5 bisphosphate [PtdIns (4,5) P2]. PtdIns (3,4,5) P3 attracts to the plasma membrane phosphoinositide-dependent protein kinase 1 (PDK1) which phosphorylates Akt. Most of the Akt substrates are inactivated by phosphorylation. Active Akt inhibits Tuberous Sclerosis 2 or hamartin (TSC2) activity through direct phosphorylation. Akt-driven Tuberous Sclerosis 1 or tuberin (TSC1)/TSC2 complex inactivation allows Ras homolog enriched in brain (Rheb) to accumulate in a GTP bound state. Rheb-GTP then activates the protein kinase activity of mTORC1. mTORC1 targets p70S6 kinase (p70S6K) and eukaryotic initiation factor 4E-binding protein (4E-BP1) which are critical for translation. 4E-BP1 phosphorylation by mTORC1 results in the release of eIF4E, while p70S6K phosphorylates ribosomal S6 protein. The TSC1/2 complex is required to activate also mTORC2. Ras/Raf/MEK/ERK 1/2 signaling positively regulates mTORC1 activity, as both ERK 1/2 and p90 ribosomal S6 kinase (p90RSK) phosphorylate TSC2, thus suppressing its inhibitory function on Rheb.

3. Sonic Hedgehog Signaling (SHH) and GLI Gene Family

The Hedgehog signaling pathway is a major regulator of cell differentiation, tissue polarity and cell proliferation. The Hh family consists of three secreted proteins including Sonic Hedgehog (Shh), Desert Hedgehog (Dhh), and Indian Hedgehog (Ihh). The receptor of Hh ligands is Patched (Ptc), which is located on membrane. In the absence of Hh, Ptc catalytically inhibits the activity of Smoothened (Smo) which is the seven-transmembranespan receptor-like protein. Binding of Hh to Ptc leads to the loss of Ptc activity, and consequent activation of Smo, which transduces the Hh signal to the cytoplasm. Subsequently, the activated Smo causes the activation of Gli (glioma-associated oncogene family zinc finger) family of transcriptional effectors through complex interactions with Costal2 (Cos2), Fused (Fu) and Suppressor of fu (Sufu), leading to the up-regulation of Ptc, Wnt, BMP, *etc.* Therefore, the Hh ligands, Sonic Hedgehog, Desert Hedgehog, and Indian Hedgehog stimulate Gli transcription factors which constitute the final effectors of the Hh signaling pathway (Fig. **2**) [62]. c-Jun and JunB known as transcription factors are final effectors in the Hh signaling pathway, have antagonistic activities of in the transcription of genes coding for major cell cycle regulators such as CyclinD and p16INK4A [63].

Somatic mutations which activate Hh pathway have been linked to a variety of human cancers. Emerging evidence clearly suggesting the activation of Hh signaling in lung cancer. Hh plays a central role in the control of proliferation and differentiation of stem cells, the aberrant activation of Hh signaling could lead to the generation of cancer stem cell (CSCs) and the development of cancer. Recent studies also showed that activation of Hedgehog signaling is critically related to CSCs and acquisition of epithelial to mesenchymal transition (EMT), EMT features in many types of cancers [62]. The signaling cascade reaches the *GLI* oncogenes (*GLI1*,*GLI2* and *GLI3*) which activate or repress gene transcription. All three GLI genes are expressed in the mesoderm around the developing trachea and primary bronchi. Animals with targeted disruption of *SHH* or *GLI3* eventually developed several lung anomalies. Both SCLC and NSCLC have been shown to require an active hedgehog signaling pathway. An antagonist of the hedgehog pathway inhibited proliferation of NSCLC cell lines containing a hedgehog autocrine loop [16] The expression levels of several important components of the Hh pathway in lung cancers such as Smoothened (SMO), Rab23, the downstream target platelet-derived growth factor receptor alpha (PDGFRalpha), hedgehog interacting protein (HIP) and hepatocyte nuclear factor 3-beta (HNF3beta) was determined [64]. It was repoted that a significant correlation of lymph node metastases with expression of SMO in all NSCLC histological types and with nuclear GLI1 immunolocalization only in adenocarcinomas. HH-signaling pathway is activated in NSCLC and correlates with histological type, prognostic parameters of the tumours as well as with the increased expression of FOXM1 [65].

Hedgehog (Hh) signals by binding to Patched (PTC), a protein with 12 transmembrane domains. In the absence of Hh, Patched represses the activity of the G-protcin-coupled receptor Smoothened (SMO). Repression is associated with reduced Smoothened stability. Gli forms a complex with COS2, Fu, and Su (Fu) (suppressor of Fu), by which it associates with microtubules. In the absence of Smoothened signaling, GLI family transcription factors are multiply phosphorylated by protein kinase A (PKA), glycogen synthase kinase (GSK) and casein kinase (CSK). Phosphorylation targets GLI for processing by the proteasome, converting the full-length transcriptional activator (GliAct) to a shorter transcriptional repressor (GliR). When hh (SHH, IHH, DHH) binds to Ptc, the inhibitory effect upon SMO is suppressed, followed by the activation of SMO signal pathway. Activated Smoothened then inhibits phosphorylation of GLI (Ci) proteins, thereby preventing degradation of the repressor form. The COS2-Fu-Su(Fu) complex dissociates from microtubules, and an active form of Gli translocates to the nucleus where it switches on transcription of the target genes.

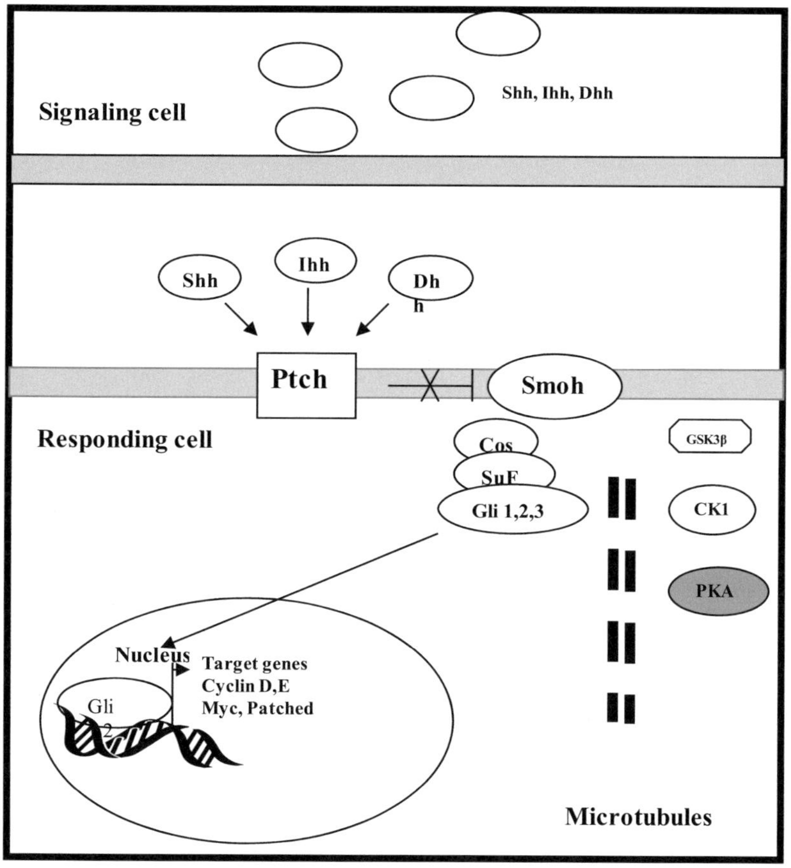

Figure 2: Hedgehog signaling.

4. Wingless-Type MMTV Integration Site Family (WNT)/β-Catenin Pathway

At the cellular level WNT and β-catenin pathway regulates a variety of cellular processes such as epithelial-mesenchymal interactions, cell fate, proliferation *versus* differentiation, survival *versus* apoptosis, and migration during morphogenesis. Using a conditional strategy to specifically inactivate β-catenin in lung cells, ablation of β-catenin interferes with peripheral airway formation without major impact on the proximal airway. Of all the 19 WNT genes, WNT5a has been shown to be critical to the distal lung morhphogenesis and WNT7b is essential to mesenchymal proliferation and vascular development in the lung. Also during tumourigenesis the Wnt signaling pathway has a central role and inappropriate activation of this pathway are observed in human lung cancers. In NSCLC, activation of WNT/β-catenin pathway has been reported in 75% of all cases tested [16].

Canonical Wnt signals are transduced through membrane Frizzled (FZD) receptors and low density lipoprotein receptor-related protein (LRP) to the β-catenin signaling cascade (Fig. **3**). Wnt signaling target genes are implicated in the cytoskeletal reorganization during invasion and metastasis, suggesting the importance of noncanonical Wnt signaling in cancer invasion and metastasis. The aberrant activation of the canonical Wnt/β-catenin signaling is one of the most frequent signaling abnormalities known in human cancers. During the development of human cancer, activated Wnt signal promotes β-catenin accumulation in the nucleus, resulting in the consequent transcriptional activation of specific target genes. The inappropriate expression of the Wnt ligand and Wnt binding proteins and the inappropriate activation of the Wnt signaling have been found in a variety of human cancers. Mutations in APC and other components of the β-catenin destruction complex promote the activation of Wnt signaling. In addition, loss or reduction of E-cadherin together with abnormal expression of Wnt ligands, receptors, inhibitors, and other co-regulators could also contribute to the activation of Wnt signaling in cancers with the acquisition of EMT phenotype of cancer cells [62].

In the absence of active WNT (a), The β-catenin degradation complex is assembled by Axin, and contains β-catenin, APC, GSK3 and CK1. PP1 and WTX may also associate with the Axin complex. β-catenin phosphorylation by CK1 and GSK3 results in β-catenin recognition by β-Trcp, thereby triggering its degradation. β-catenin is degraded, and prospective target genes are in a repressed state.

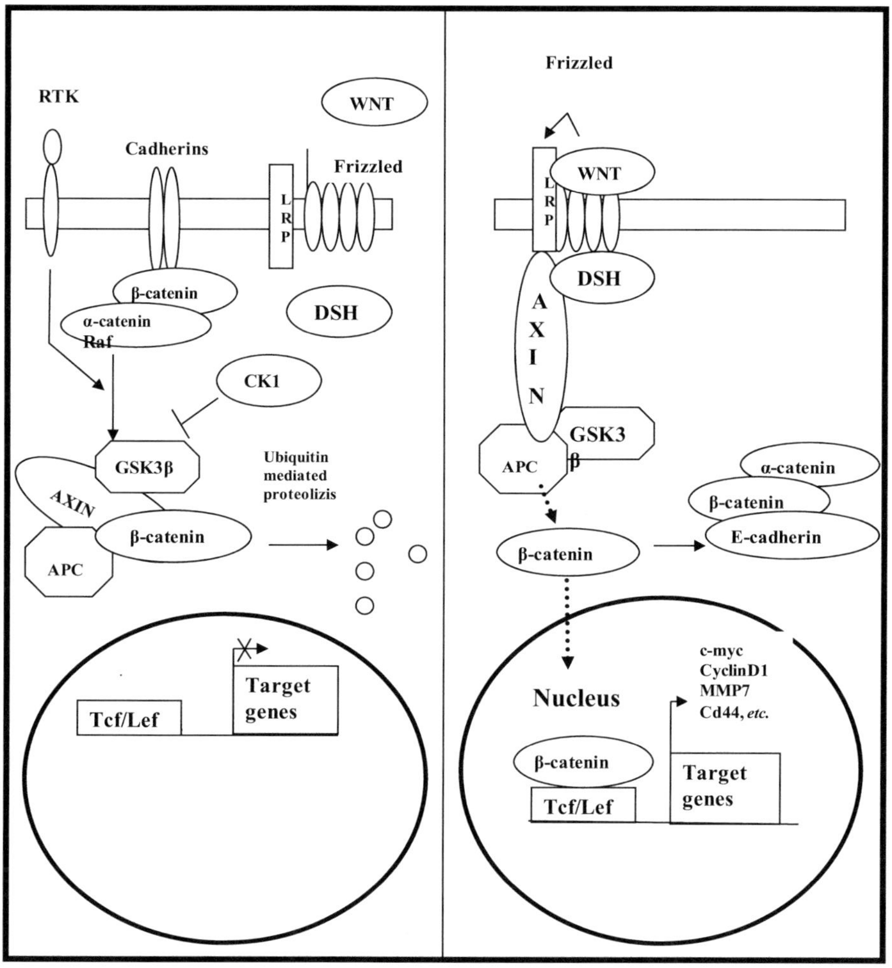

Figure 3: Wnt/β-catenin pathway.

If WNT signaling (b) is active, β-catenin degradation is reduced. As β-catenin accumulates, it enters the nucleus, binds to T cell factor/lymphoid enhancer factor (TCF/LEF) transcription factors and Legless family docking proteins (BCL9 and BCL9L) associated with PYGO family coactivators. The TCF/LEF-β-catenin complex then activates the transcription of Wnt signaling target genes such as FGF20, DKK1, Myc, cyclin D1, *etc.*

The components shown are described in more detail in the text. APC, adenomatous polyposis coli; β-cat, β-catenin; CBP, CREB-binding protein; CK, casein kinase; DSH, Dishevelled; GBP, GSK3-binding protein; GSK, glycogen synthase kinase; LRP, LDL-receptor-related protein; P, phosphorylation; sFRP, secreted Frizzled-related protein; TCF, T-cell factor.

5. Epidermal Growth Factor Receptor Signaling Pathway

Of the 90 known tyrosine kinases (TKs), the receptor TKs (RTKs) form a group of 58 cell-surface growth factor receptors with ligand-mediated TK activity. Whereas RTK activity in normal resting cells is tightly regulated, mutations or deregulated expression might cause them to function as potent oncogenes. Epidermal growth factor receptor is the prototypical member of a family of four RTKs, EGFR (ERBB1, HER1), ERBB2 (HER2, Neu), ERBB3 (HER3) and ERBB4 (HER4). Multiple ligands activate the different family members; those for EGFR include epidermal growth factor (EGF), transforming growth factor-α (TGF-α) and amphiregulin (AR). EGFR, the product of the *HER-1* oncogene, is a 170-kD TM glycoprotein with intracellular tyrosine kinase activity. Ligand binding enables the formation of homo or heterodimer complexes and results in TK activation and receptor transphosphorylation. This results in the activation of pathways including Ras, phosphatidylinositol-3-kinase (PI3K) (Fig. **4**). EGFR deregulation has been observed in multiple tumour types, including NSCLCs. Intracellular tyrosine kinase domain activated by amplification and overexpression [20]. EGFR overexpression is often associated with adverse prognosis. It was identified frequent EGFR protein overexpression (62%) in NSCLCs of squamous cell and ADC subtypes. EGFR amplification rare SCLC, rare overexpression NSCLC. EGFR expression correlates with poor prognosis in extensive disease or advanced stage of SCLCs [9].

The Ras/mitogen-activated protein kinase and PI3K/Akt pathways are major signaling networks linking EGFR activation to cell proliferation and survival. EGFR signaling pathway genes have been found to be mutated in NSCLC (and very rarely in other tumours). Depending on the geographical location, EGFR and KRAS mutations have been identified in 10–30% of NSCLCs. EGFR mutations are independently associated with ADC histology, East Asian ethnicity, never-smoking status and female sex. Mutations of KRAS also target ADC histology, but otherwise differ from EGFR mutations because they are relatively rare in East Asians and occur more frequently in males and smokers. Less commonly, somatic mutations have also been found in other EGFR pathway genes, including HER2 (2%), HER4 (2%), BRAF (2%) and PIK3CA (4%). The mutations target critical regions of the TK domain associated with downstream signaling (exons 18–21) and are of several types, including deletions, insertions and activating point mutations. However, two major types account for 85% of mutations: deletions in exon 19 and point mutation L858R in exon 21.

As a consequence of the frequent deregulation of EGFR pathway genes in NSCLC, EGFR became one of the first rationally selected molecules for targeted therapy. While initial targeted approaches utilised monoclonal antibodies, which block the ligand–receptor interaction, newer approaches have utilised small molecule reversible TK inhibitors (TKIs). The TK activity of EGFR is required for the biochemical responses induced by this receptor. Two TKIs, gefitinib and erlotinib have been widely used in the treatment of advanced or recurrent NSCLC. Responses were noted in subsets, notably East Asian ethnicity, female sex, never-smoking status and ADC histology. Subsequently, EGFR mutations in the TK domain were found to predict response to TKI in the same subset of patients. According to a meta-analysis of 1,170 patients,.70% of NSCLCs with EGFR mutations responded to TKIs, whereas 10% of tumours without EGFR mutation responded. However, not all activating mutations are associated with response to TKIs, and a point mutation T790M is associated with secondary resistance. In addition, insertion mutations in exon 20 are also associated with primary resistance. Further studies indicated that factors other than EGFR mutations may play a role in determining response and survival after TKI therapy. EGFR gene copy number gain was associated with significantly improved TKI sensitivity and survival in a large unselected study with appropriate controls. In addition, other members of the EGFR family, *i.e.* HER2 and EGFR3 may be important factors involved in TKI sensitivity. A further complexity is the clinical observation that somatic mutations of KRAS confer intrinsic resistance to TKIs [11].

Ligands, such as epidermal growth factor (EGF), transforming growth factor (TGF)-a, or others, bind to the specific receptors, resulting in activation and receptor transphosphorylation. This creates docking sites for the adaptor proteins, Grb2 and Sos, which recruit Ras and phosphatidylinositol 3-kinase (PI3K), leading to the formation of three major signaling pathway branches, Ras/MAPK, PI3K/Akt and

JAK/Stat. These networks result in, amongst others, proliferation, evasion of apoptosis and angiogenesis. MAPK: mitogen-activated kinase-like protein.

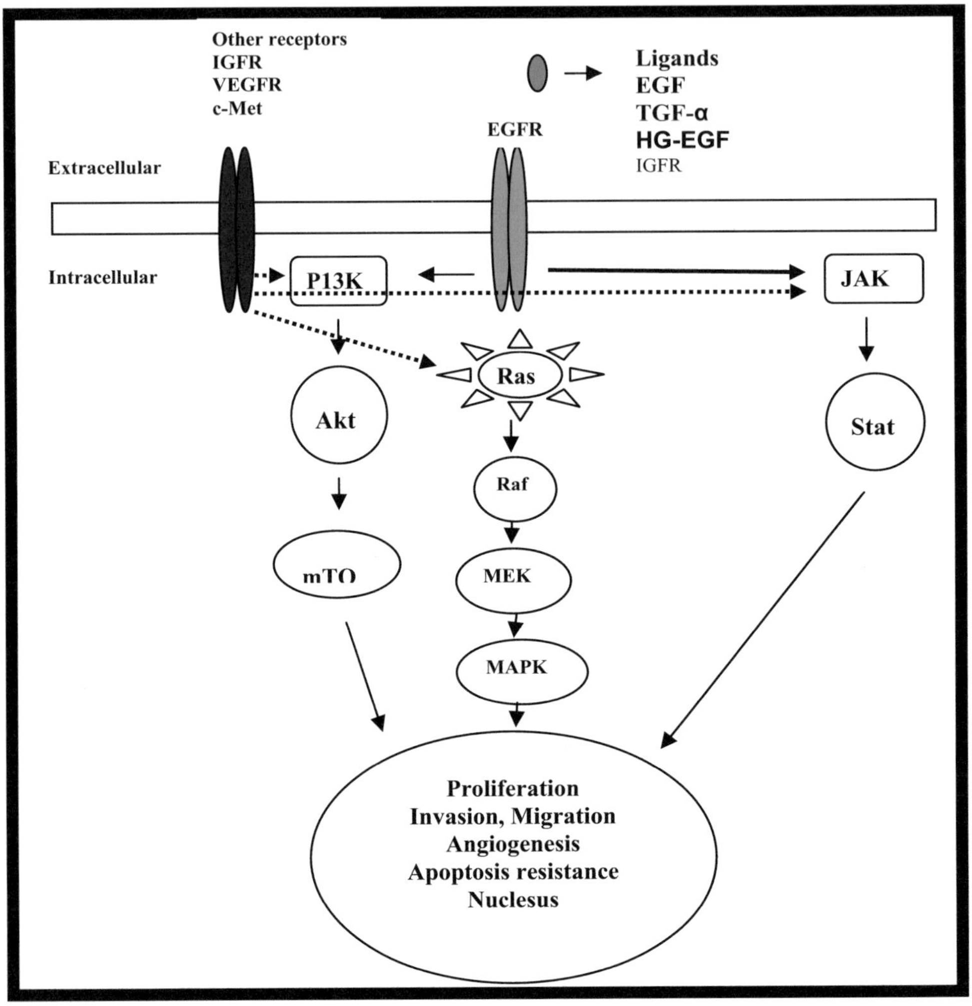

Figure 4: Epidermal growth factor receptor (EGFR) pathway.

6. The Insulin-Like Growth Factor (IGF)

The insulin-like growth factor (IGF) family consists of IGF-I, IGF-II, and relaxin. They bind to IGF-I and-II receptors, which bear tyrosine kinase activity. IGFs participate in mitogenesis, transformation, and survival of cells through endocrine, autocrine, and paracrine stimulation. Specifically, IGF-I mediates proliferation of the SCLC tumour cells *via* an autocrine feedback loop [9].

7. Notch Signaling

Notch signaling is activated upon binding of Notch receptors (Notch 1-4) with their ligands (Delta-like1, 3 and 4 and Jagged1 and 2) expressed on adjacent cells. The binding of Notch with its ligands triggers a series of proteolytic cleavages resulting in the release of the Notch intracellular domain (NICD) capable of binding to the CSL (*C*BF1/RBPjk). In the absence of NICD, CSL inhibits transcription by associating with co-repressor proteins. NICD activates transcription by competing with these repressor proteins and facilitating the binding of activator complexes to CSL (Fig. **5**). This activating complex is then capable of transcribing target genes including Hes and Hey, and genes implicated in cancer development, such as c-myc, cyclin D1 and p21/Waf1.

Notch signaling has also been associated with a number of human cancers and altered in approximately one third of non–small-cell lung carcinomas (NSCLCs), which are the leading cause of cancer-related deaths: in ≈30% of NSCLCs, loss of Numb expression leads to increased Notch activity, while in a smaller fraction of cases (around 10%), gain-of-function mutations of the NOTCH-1 gene are present. Activation of Notch correlates with poor clinical outcomes in NSCLC patients without TP53 mutations [66, 67]. Delta-like ligand 4 and Notch-1 are independent prognostic factors in NSCLC, but have diverse impacts in SCC and AC. The coexpression of tumour cell Notch-1/VEGF-A has a major impact on survival [68, 69].

Target sites of MicroRNA-430 (miR-430) are detected in the mammalian *Nodal* gene suggesting that miRNA-dependent regulation of Nodal could occur in humans. In fact, web based analyses of potential miRNA targets predict that members of the miR-302 cluster, the human homolog of miR-430, may regulate Nodal expression. Notch signaling is also regulated by miRNAs in mammalian cells. Specifically,miR-1 negatively affects Notch signaling by repressing the expression of the Notch ligand, Delta-like1 [70].

Binding of Notch receptors to ligands expressed on adjacent cells leads to enzymatic cleavage by gamma-secretase (γ-SC) and intracytoplasmic release of the active Notch intracellular domain (NICD). The CSL DNA binding protein can function as a transcriptional repressor. When NCID binds to CSL it forms an activator complex leading to target gene transcription.

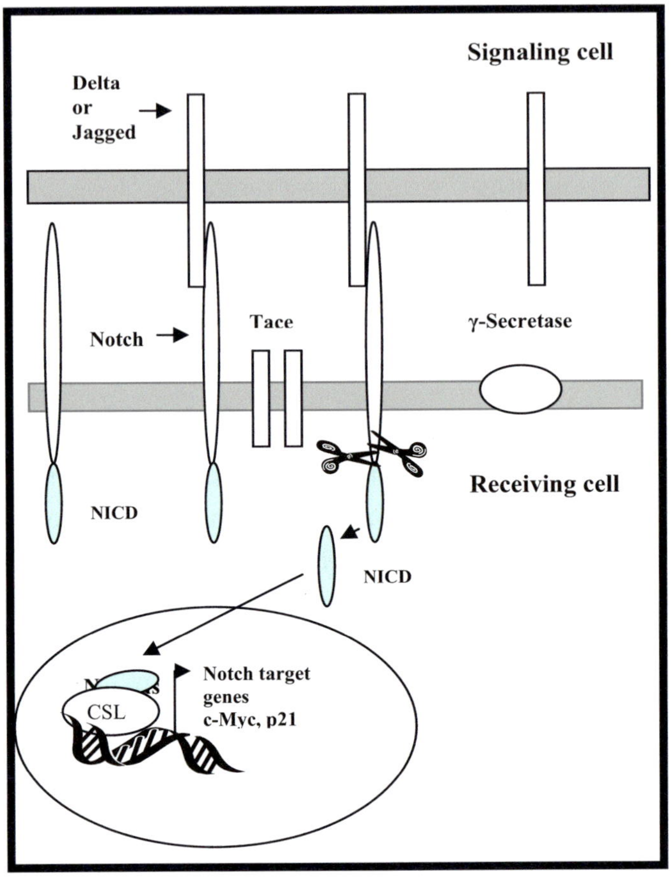

Figure 5: Notch signaling.

8. Anaplastic Lymphoma Kinase Fusion Proteins

A recurrent gene fusion between echinoderm microtubule associated protein-like 4 (EML4; and, occasionally, of other fusion partners) and the anaplastic lymphoma kinase (ALK) gene occurs in 7% of NSCLCs, resulting in activation of a potent ALK fusion protein. ALK fusion protein is usually found in never-smoker subjects. Although relatively rare, the relative paucity of fusion proteins known to contribute to lung cancer pathogenesis makes this a finding of biological interest. Although present understanding of the ALK fusion protein is limited, it may play a role in activating RAS. Thus it is negatively associated with the presence of KRAS or EGFR mutations, and may favour ADC histology and never-smoker status [11].

EPIGENETIC CHANGES IN LUNG CANCER

Epigenetics may be defined as heritable changes in gene expression that are not due to any alteration in the DNA sequence. Epigenetic modifications refer to a number of molecular mechanisms that regulate gene expression without changing the DNA sequence. These include the following: 1) alteration of the methylation status of DNA within CpG islands, with hypermethylation of CpG island promoters of tumour suppressor genes leading to their silencing; 2) covalent modification of histone tails; and 3) gene regulation by micro-RNA (miRNA) [11].

DNA Methylation and Lung Cancer

The epigenome of cancer cells has been most commonly studied at the level of DNA CpG methylation [40]. The best-known epigenetic marker is DNA methylation, occurs as one part of a complex chromatin network that is influenced by modifications in histone structure. Methylation is a normal physiological function and essential for the development and regulation of gene expression. In postnatal life, it controls expression of oncofetal genes, imprinted genes and tissue-specific gene expression. Three forms of abnormal methylation may play roles in tumour pathogenesis, including global hypomethylation, hypermethylation of tumour-suppressor genes and the recent finding that methylation may regulate expression of some miRNAs. DNA methylation is restricted to cytosines that are upstream of guanines (CpG sites). In the human genome, the promoter of 50% of genes are rich in CpG sites (CpG islands). In expressed genes, CpG islands are usually unmethylated, while in other regions of the genome, most of the CpG sites are methylated. Loss of methylation at the latter sites (usually in noncoding regions of the genome) is common in tumours and leads to genomic instability. In contrast, methylation occurs at multiple CpG islands in tumours, resulting in loss of expression of tumour suppressor genes. Altered CpG methylation patterns discriminate tumour tissue from its nonmalignant counterpart tissue or normal adjacent tissue [40].

The importance of CpG island methylation in functional inactivation of lung cancer suppressor genes is becoming increasingly recognized. For example, *RASSF1A* is inactivated by promoter methylation in about 30–40% of non-small cell lung cancers (37% of squamous cell carcinomas) and in close to 80% of small cell lung cancers. In lung cancer, many genes (perhaps hundreds) have been found to be silenced by promoter methylation. The most well-studied genes include RARB, CDKN2A, TIMP3, MGMT, DAPK, CDH1, CDH13 and RASSF1A, *p16*, *RARbeta*, *MGMT*, *GSTP1*, *CDH13*, *APC*, *DAPK*, *RASSF1A*, *GSTP1* and *APC*. Methylation begins early during lung cancer pathogenesis. In squamous cell carcinomas of the lung, CpG methylation patterns undergo substantial changes relative to normal lung epithelium [40]. Multiple genes often intensively methylated in SCLC are *RASSF1A*, *hsRBC*, *CAV1* and *RARB*. In contrast, the frequencies of methylation of *MGMT*, *PAX5-alpha, PAX5-beta*, *TSLC1*, *hMLH1, hMLH2*, *DAPK*, *P14IRF*, *FHIT, beta-Catenin* are remarkably higher in NSCLC than SCLC. The *P16* gene is more frequently methylated in SCC than AC, but the *APC*, *CDH13* [71]. DNA methylation may predict for early recurrence in stage I NSCLC. Restoration of expression of epigenetically silenced genes is a new targeted therapeutic approach, and histone deacetylase inhibitors are being investigated for the treatment of lung cancer [11].

Epigenetic Modifications of Histones: The Histone Code of Lung Cancer

Human cancers undergo a massive overall loss of DNA methylation, although they acquire specific patterns of hypermethylation of certain promoters. DNA methylation occurs in the context of other epigenetic modifications. Methyl-CpG binding proteins and DNA methyltransferase are associated with histone deacetylases and histone methyltransferases. The status of acetylation and methylation of specific lysine residues within the tail of nucleosomal core histones play a crucial role in regulating chromatin packaging, nuclear architecture, gene expression and genomic stability. In cancer cells, including lung cancer, hypermethylation of promoter CpG islands of transcriptionally repressed tumour suppressor genes are associated with a particular combination of histone markers, such as deacetylation of histones H3 and H4, loss of histone H3 lysine 4 trimethylation, and gain of H3K9 and H3K27 trimethylation. The impact of histone code changes in lung cancer progression in tumourigenesis and prognosis has been shown by an epigenetic landscape of cancer cells that are profoundly distorted in appearance compared with normal candidate stem cells. Excessive acetylation of H4K5/H4K8 and loss of trimethylation of H4K20 was shown in NSCLC and pre-invasive bronchial dysplastic lesions. H4K20 loss of trimethylation was shown to identify a subpopulation of early stage (I) ADC with shorter survival. In addition, histone H2 and H3 modifications in acetylation and trimethylation status were also detected in NSCLC and SCLC, allowing detection of subpopulations with differential prognosis, and suggesting that histone code epigenetic changes play an important role in lung cancer tumourigenesis. Recent technologies using genome-wide, cancer epigenetics approaches showed that global alterations of histone modifications patterns are linked to DNA methylation and are causal in lung cancer [11].

miRNA in Lung Cancer

MicroRNAs play a key role in diverse biological processes, including cell development, proliferation, differentiation, and apoptosis. miRNAs are a class of short, 19-to 25-nucleotide-long RNAs that regulate gene expression by binding to sequences in the 3′ untranslated region (3′UTR) of an expressed mRNA, resulting in either modulation of translation efficiency or degradation of the mRNA. that form short stem-loop structures when transcribed and produce either one or two mature miRNAs. Mature miRNAs are typically only partially complementary to their target mRNAs, meaning that each miRNA can regulate a broad set of targets [72]. Early *in vitro* studies investigating the function of miRNAs uncovered their critical role in regulating various cellular processes such as differentiation, cell growth, proliferation and apoptosis. Similarly, it was repeatedly observed that dysregulated miRNA expression underpinned a variety of pathological events, including carcinogenesis. Many miRNAs have tissue-specific expression patterns (miRNA fingerprints), and miRNA expression is commonly dysregulated in a variety of cancers, including lung cancer [11, 73]. The association of aberrant miRNA expression with cancer, and functional analyses of specific miRNAs which has established their roles as tumour suppressors or oncogenes. To date, there are ~700 annotated human miRNA loci. It is of interest that miRNAs may function both as oncogenes and as tumour suppressor genes, and thus may be either up-or downregulated in cancers. The gene target of only a minority of miRNAs is known with certainty, while several others have putative targets. However, miRNA genes are frequently located at fragile sites, as well as in minimal regions of loss of heterozygosity, minimal regions of amplification, or common breakpoint regions, indicating that they may play important roles in cancer pathogenesis. A unique miRNA molecular profile is characteristic of lung cancer and the miRNA signature of lung cancer differs from normal lung epithelial cells and in different tumour histology. As an example, six miRNA are expressed differently in ADC *versus* epidermoid carcinoma. miRNA expression profiles were correlated with survival of lung ADCs, including those classified as disease stage I, indicating that miRNA expression profiles are diagnostic and prognostic markers of lung cancer. The let-7 family of miRNAs inhibit Ras protein expression, which is mutated and overactive in many smoker-related ADCs. Let-7 shows a decreased expression in lung cancer as compared with surrounding normal lung tissue. Two species of Let-7 (Let-7a-1 and Let-7f-1) define two clusters of expression with low levels of expression correlating with shorter survival. Let-7 expression regulates cell cycle gene expression, such as cyclin E, E2F1, SKP2 and MCM, and cellular division, by regulating aurora A and B, and also regulates response-DNA damage response genes (BRCA1-2, RRM1-2, CHK1, HMGA2). As RAS mutations are rarely found in never-smoker tumours, expression of the let-7 family is predicted to show differences between smoker and never-smoker tumours. miRNAs are connected to the oncogenic pathway of Myc and E2F1: the cluster miR-17-92, contained in an amplicon at 13q31, is overexpressed in lung cancer and, typically, in SCLC. miR-34 reproduces almost all functions of p53, thereby completing the puzzle of the p53 network. Indeed, miR-34 recapitulates the main p53 activities towards cell cycle arrest and promotion of apoptosis. Deletions of miR-34 family miRNAs are reported in human cancer, as miR-34a is located within chromosome 1p36, a frequent region of heterozygous deletion. Minimal deletions and reduced expressions containing miR-34 are found in lung cancer and in lung cancer cell lines. Maturation enzymes of miRNA, such as DICER, are necessary for the bronchial branching in lung development. DICER expression decreases in a pre-invasive lesion from atypical alveolar hyperplasia to ADC *via* bronchioloalveolar carcinoma. Interestingly, the level of DICER is predictive of survival, with a low DICER level in ADC leading to shorter survival time [11, 73].

Upregulation of miR-21 (represses apoptosis, increases proliferation), miR-17-92 (induces angiogenesis, represses apoptosis) and miR-221/222 (represses apoptosis, induces proliferation, restricts angiogenesis) and down regulation of miR-34a-c (induces p53-dependent cellular stress responses), miR-29 (induces apoptosis, decreases tumourigenicity), let-7/miR-98 (decreases proliferation and apoptosis), miR-15/16 (induces Rb-dependent cell cycle arrest), miR-128b (reduces EGFR-mediated proliferation), miR-200/429 (increases E-cadherin expression, represses EMT, reduces metastasis), miR-197 (decreases proliferation), miR-93 (decreases proliferation) and miR-126 (reduces invasion, migration, and adhesion, decreases angiogenesis) have induced some important changes in lung tumourigenesis [72].

Mitochondrial Mutations

Somatic mitochondrial DNA (mtDNA) mutations have been increasingly observed in primary human cancers. The biological impact of a given mutation may vary, depending on the proportion of mutant mtDNAs carried by the cell. mtDNA mutations occur early during pre-neoplasia, and have great potential as cancer biomarkers. D-loop alterations are frequent in lung cancers and their cell lines, and these changes are weakly associated with certain clinical parameters [11].

Gene Expressing Profile

Multiple techniques technologies allow for simultaneous high-throughput measurement of expression of thousands of genes from several hundred samples. Gene expression microarrays is a technique that can be used to compare normal and cancerous tissues, serve to categorize tumours sharing common characteristics (eg, specific outcome, tumour histology) [12]. In lungs, expression profiling has been shown to discriminate between healthy lung tissue and lung tumours, as well as profiling distinct lung tumour histologies and clinical entities. In using expression profiles to discriminate lung cancer histologies, several studies agree that gene expression profiles clearly segregate lung adenocarcinoma from squamous cell carcinoma and from small cell lung cancer [10] (sanchez). Perhaps this could reach clinically significant relevance in the future, because we have recently learned that histology matters in lung cancer treatment decisions [10, 74]. Genomic technology has several potential applications to lung cancer research including a better understanding of the pathogenesis of lung cancer, facilitating early detection of cancer, improving pathological staging, defining prognosis, individualizing therapy and finding new targets of therapy [12].

METASTASIS STEPS OF LUNG CANCER

Invasion, Cell Adhesion and Matrix Molecules in Lung cancer

EGF, as well as TGF-α, AR, CRIPTO, heregulin, and heparin-binding EGF are members of the EGF family. The actions of EGF, TGF-α, and AR are mediated through the EGFR, which implies parallel functional roles in carcinogenesis. EGF signaling plays a modulatory role in tumour cell adhesion to extracellular matrix (ECM) proteins *via* integrins, either by inhibiting or by stimulating this process. A synergistic interaction has been observed between EGF and thrombospondin-1 (TSP-1), an adhesive protein, which leads to neurotypic differentiation and growth suppression of SCLCs *via* $\alpha3\beta1$ integrin-mediated adhesion of SCLC cells on TSP-1 [9].

Integrins are a group of TM glycoproteins with two subunits (α and β) that participate mainly in cell-to-matrix interactions. In comparison to NSCLC cells, integrins in SCLC cells are underexpressed and are composed of fewer types. Integrin $\alpha3\beta1$ is the predominant cell surface $\beta1$ integrin molecule in SCLCs. $\alpha3\beta1$ may be described as a multiple receptor: it interacts with laminin, collagen, entactin, and fibronectin at different receptor-binding domains in the presence of specific cations. It is considered to be the most important laminin-binding integrin for the anchorage of alveolar and bronchial epithelial cells to the basement membrane of human lung. It has been reported that SCLC cells expressing *c-myc* display decreased expression of $\alpha3\beta1$, an event that could explain the poor prognosis in SCLCs with *c-myc* overexpression [9].

Cadherins (CDHs) are TM glycoproteins containing dimeric, zipper-like adhesive structures that enable cellular interactions in the presence of calcium. SCLCs express several types of CDHs, including epithelial CDH (E-CDH). It has been suggested that CDH-mediated adhesion is regulated by the small GTP-binding protein Rho in SCLCs. E-CDH forms a structural complex with the cytoplasmic β-catenin molecule. Impairments in the E-CDH/catenin complex have been associated with tumour invasion and metastasis in lung cancer cells. (Koutsami). Tumours with an increased expression of dysadherin and a reduced expression of E-cadherin showed the worst prognosis [75].

Catenins are intracellular cytoplasmic proteins comprising β-and γ-catenin, which bind to E-CDH, and α-catenin, which mediates the linkage of this complex to the cytoskeleton. Tyrosine phosphorylation of α-catenin may lead to an enhanced migration capacity of lung cancer cells. α-catenin cytoplasmic overexpression is associated with poor prognosis in SCLCs [9]. δ-Catenin is the only member of the p120 catenin (p120ctn) subfamily that its primary expression is restricted to the brain. δ-catenin is upregulated in human lung cancer. Increased δ-catenin expression is critical for maintenance of the malignant phenotype of lung cancer [76].

CD99 is a TM glycoprotein encoded by *MIC2* located both on chromosomes X and Y. It acts as an adhesion molecule, as well as a modulator of the action of IGF-I, insulin, and growth hormone. CD99 is detected in TCs [9].

Dysregulation of transforming growth factor- β (TGF-β) signaling was identified as an important mediator of tumour invasion. The CC chemokine RANTES (Regulated on Activation, Normal T-cell Expressed, and presumably Secreted) was upregulated in invasive tumours and was required for invasion in cells with repressed levels of the TGF-β type II receptor. Transforming growth factor-β (TGF-β) type II receptor (TβRII*)*, TβRII repression was required for lung adenocarcinoma invasion, TGF-β, the ligand for the TGF-β type II receptor is a pleiotropic cytokine comprised of family members TGF-β 1, 2, 3 that regulate tissue homeostasis and prevent tumour initiation by inhibiting cellular proliferation, differentiation, and survival. It is secreted as a latent molecule and is activated by cleavage by proteases and other molecules. Signaling primarily occurs through SMAD protein dependent pathways whereby ligand binding to TBRII induces phosphorylation and activation of TGF-β type I receptor (TβRI*)*. Afterinteraction with TβRI, phosphorylated SMAD2 and SMAD3 dissociate to form a heterotrimeric complex with SMAD4 and translocate into the nucleus to regulate gene transcription. TGF-β signaling may also proceed *via* less well understood SMAD independent pathways. These "non-canonical" pathways involve various signaling cascades including Ras/ERK, Rho/ROCK, and

TAK1/MAPK, and are likely to have important roles in mediating the pro-tumourigenic effects of TGF-β. Depending upon context, TGF-β signaling may alternatively function to suppress tumour growth or to promote tumour cell invasion and metastasis [9].

TGF-β signaling occurs primarily *via* SMAD dependent pathways. A. Ligand binding to the TGF-β type II receptor (TβRII) induces phosphorylation and activation of type I receptor (TβRI), which phosphorylates and activates the receptor complex SMAD2 and SMAD3. Dissociated SMAD2/3 forms a heterotrimeric complex with SMAD4 that translocates into the nucleus to regulate gene transcription. TGF-β signaling may also proceed *via* SMAD-independent pathways that involve various signaling cascades including Ras/ERK, Rho/ROCK, and TAK1/MAPK. These "noncanonical" pathways are likely to have important roles in mediating the pro-tumourigenic effects of TGF-β. The histological distinction between bronchioloalveolar carcinoma (BAC) and other adenocarcinomas is tissue invasion. Invasion requires loss of cell-cell adhesion, migration, membrane degradation with vascular intravasation and extravasation and establishment of the metastatic niche angiogenesis and recruitment of stromal elements (top panel). Repression of TGF-β type II receptor in lung adenocarcinoma cells increases invasiveness and have used microarray analyses and inhibitor studies to identify the CC chemokine RANTES as an important mediator of lung adenocarcinoma invasion in TβRII deficient tumours [77].

Matrix metalloproteinases (MMPs) belong to a family of ECM-degrading enzymes, participating in tumour invasion, metastasis, and angiogenesis. To date, 16 MMPs have been identified, either in insoluble form or as TM proteins on the cell surface. It have observed elevated expression of MMP-3, MMP-11, and MMP-14 by SCLC cells, which was associated with adverse prognosis. The activities of MMPs are regulated by a class of proteins known as tissue inhibitors of MMPs (TIMPs) comprising TIMP-1,-2,-3, and-4 (184). TIMPs are widely expressed in SCLCs. However, only TIMP-1 underexpression in SCLCs was found to be statistically significant by multivariate analysis, being associated with better response to therapy [9].

The urokinase-type plasminogen activator (u-PA) is a serine protease that converts plasminogen into plasmin. This event leads to degradation of several components of the ECM. The plasminogen activator inhibitors PAI-1 and-2 control the activity of u-PA. Binding of u-PA to its receptor seems to enhance tumour-cell invasion. The u-PA system is implicated in the activation of several GFs, cell migration, and apoptosis. In SCLC and LCNEC both stromal and epithelial u-PA expression are observed, and the stromal expression is related to lymph node metastasis; u-PA is not detectable in TCs. PAI-1 and-2 are inversely expressed in the spectrum of NE tumours, with PAI-1 being highly expressed in SCLCs and LCNECs and PAI-2 being more elevated in TCs, thus implying a favorable prognostic value of the latter. A possible mechanism for this is the synergic activity of PAI-1 with u-PA in high-grade NE tumours, in contrast to PAI-2, which probably prevents tumour progression *via* the blockade of u-PA–mediated proteolysis [9].

CD44 is a TM glycoprotein that belongs to the immunoglobulin superfamily, acting as an ECM binding glycan as well as a hyaluronate receptor. It has a number of variant isoforms. These isoforms (CD44v1–v10) are the product of alternative splicing; the most abundant isoform is CD44 standard (CD44S). CD44S levels decrease in SCLCs and ACs, whereas it is overexpressed in TCs. Loss of CD44v6 is associated with more aggressive types of SCLCs and ACs, although it is probably related with nodal metastasis in TCs. The CD44v10 variant is mainly expressed in SCLCs, correlating with the expression of characteristic proteins of tumour growth and progression [9]. CD44s expression was associated with squamous cell carcinoma, a longer survival was observed in CD44-expressing adenocarcinomas [78].

CRMP-1 is a protein involved in mediating the effect of collapsins. Lung cancer specimens showed that reduced expression of CRMP-1 is associated with advanced disease, lymph node metastasis, early postoperative relapse, and shorter survival, indicating that CRMP-1 is involved in cancer invasion and metastasis. Collapsins are part of the semaphorin family, so CRMP-1 may provide another indication of the role of semaphorins and the pathways they mediate in the pathogenesis of lung cancer. Laminins and integrins are being intensively studied as key markers of tissue invasion through the basement membrane and subsequent development of metastases. The expression of laminin a chains (a3 and a5) is often reduced in lung cancer cells; this might contribute to basement membrane fragmentation and subsequent proliferation of stromal elements, as well as having a role in the process of cancer cell invasion.131 The LAMB3 gene (encoding the laminin b3 chain, a unique component of laminin-5) was expressed in NSCLC cells and not in SCLC cells. Laminin-5 is a heterotrimeric protein consisting of the a3, b3, and c2 chains, and another unique component of laminin-5, the c2 chain encoded by the LAMC2 gene. Since α6β4-integrin, the specific laminin-5 binding receptor, is known to be expressed only in NSCLCs and not in SCLCs, it appears that laminin-5 is a critical microenvironmental factor for the growth of NSCLC but not of SCLC cells. Survival analysis revealed that overexpression of laminin-5 was associated with shorter patient survival and was an independent prognostic factor in NSCLC [22].

Enzymes

Human telomeres consist of tandem repeats (TTAGGG), a number of which are lost by the end of each cell division cycle. Telomerase composed of 2 main components, the telomerase RNA component or hTR, the RNA template for telomere synthesis, and telomerase reverse transcriptase, the catalytic subunit, is reactivated in the majority of the lung cancer [79]. The ribonucleoprotein telomerase is capable of synthesizing such telomeric sequences, thus protecting chromosomal ends from mitotic senescence. The fraction of cells possessing telomerase activity is approximately 100% in SCLCs. Telomerase levels are regarded as an indicator of the mortal-to-immortal cell ratio in a tumour. This leads to the conclusion that SCLCs mainly consist of immortal cells. Besides, with the exception of TCs, all NE tumours display high telomerase expression, which seems to be associated with adverse prognosis [9].

Angiogenesis and Lymphangiogenesis

The majority of cancer death is caused by metastasis. The most common method involves development of metastases due to spread of neoplastic cells with the circulating blood and within lymphatic vessels [80]. During metastasis, tumour cells have signal interactions with endothelial cells to initiate angiogenesis and break down vascular walls. These actions promote their spread [21]. Angiogenesis, the formation of new blood vessels and assessed by tumour microvessel density, represents an essential process for tumour growth and metastasis [9].

It is not associated with metastatic status, tumour size, or prognosis in SCLCs. However, the prognostic role of the inducers and inhibitors that control the angiogenetic process appears to be very promising. Vascular endothelial growth factor (VEGF) is a potent inducer of angiogenesis that acts by forming heterodimeric complexes with two tyrosine kinase receptors: VEGF receptor 1 or Flt-1 (Fms-like tyrosine kinase), and VEGF receptor 2, also known as KDR/Flk-1 (kinase insert domain-containing receptor). VEGF has been shown to increase during lung cancer progression and this up-regulation is often associated with hypoxia. High serum levels of VEGF are correlated with short life expectancy and increased levels of VEGF detected before chemotherapy are correlated with chemoresistance and, therefore, with adverse prognosis in SCLC patients [9].

The FGF family members with heparin sulfate in the ECM, forming a reservoir of GFs that participate in development, hematopoiesis, angiogenesis, and wound repair. The best-characterized members are FGF-1 (acidic FGF) and FGF-2 (bFGF). Increased serum bFGF levels not only associate with favorable prognosis of SCLC patients [9].

TSP-1 is an ECM protein regulating growth, motility, and adhesion of cells, which can act as an angiogenetic inhibitor. TSP-1 induces $\alpha 3\beta 1$ integrin adhesion and neurite-like differentiation, and it prevents proliferation of SCLC cells [9].

There is growing evidence that the signal pathway between hepatocyte growth factor (HGF) and its receptor c-Met plays an important role in the development of lung cancer, although the specificity of such role is to be clarified. It seems clear that the HGF/c-Met signal contributes to the metastasis of cancer cells to the lung by stimulating the hyperproduction and overactivation of cytokines and enzymes, *e.g.* HGF, vascular endothelial growth factor and matrix metalloproteases [81].

Tumour lymphangiogenesis represents the principal factor in the process of metastases formation. Lymphangiogenesis involves a process of formation of new lymphatic vessels from already existing lymphatic capillaries and stimulated by vascular endothelial growth factors (VEGF) and other, recently reported factors, such as, *e.g.*, cyclooxygenase 2, fibroblast growth factor 2, angiopoetin-1 and the insulin-resembling growth factor. In lymphangiogenesis a key role is played by neutropilin 2 or podoplanin. Activation of VEGF-C/VEGF-D/VEGFR-3 axis increases motility and invasiveness of neoplastic cells, promotes development of metastases in several types of lung. In a positive correlation was detected between expressions of VEGF-C/D and VEGFR-3 in non-small cell lung cancer. In patients with lung cancer with high expression of VEGF-C a markedly abbreviated survival was noted. Positive correlation was detected between expression of VEGF-C and VEGF-D on one hand and expression of LYVE-1 on the other in sentinel lymph nodes with metastases of neoplastic cells in patients with non-small cell lung cancer. Also, high density of lymphatic vessels and high density of intraneoplastic microvessels proved to be independent poor prognostic indices in patients with non-small cell lung cancer [80].

Escape from Immune Surveillance in Lung Tumours

Tumour cells develop a variety of immune surveillance escaping mechanisms. The antigen-major histocompatibility complex (MHC) class I complex pathway represents a frequent target in lung cancer. It includes (i) MHC class I, which is responsible for the presentation of foreign antigenic peptides to cytotoxic T-lymphocytes; (ii) _2-microglobulin, which forms the light chain of class I molecules; (iii) LMP2 (latent membrane protein 2), which is a MHC-encoded proteasome subunit; and (iv) TAP (transporters associated with antigen presentation). After degradation of cytoplasmic proteins in proteasome, TAP convey intracellular peptides into the endoplasmic reticulum, so that a complex with MHC class I is created. This complex formation leads to recognition by cytotoxic T lymphocytes. Underexpression of *TAP-1* and *LMP2* genes has been observed in SCLC cell lines, providing a further explanation for the host immune surveillance escape. Host immune defense against lung cancer is reinforced by the presence of tumour-infiltrating lymphocytes (TILs). In human tumours, the majority are T cells. TILs secrete several cytokines that inhibit tumour progression, and it is through such mechanisms that the tumour-associated antitumour action of macrophages is regulated in lung cancer. Especially in SCLCs, T cells and macrophages are more abundant. It has been shown that a high proportion of intratumoural T cells, CD8 cells, and macrophages seem to improve prognosis in SCLCs, particularly in cases of low-grade tumours. Fas ligand (FasL) and its receptor Fas (also known as APO-1 or CD95) have a modulatory role in the apoptotic process of activated T cells. Both SCLC and NSCLC human cell lines express FasL, suggesting that the FasL–Fas interaction may be a possible mechanism for the peripheral deletion of tumour-reactive T-cell clones observed in these tumours.

The levels of the cytokines IFN-α, IFN-γ, TNF-α, and IL-2 are decreased in SCLCs. The factor behind this immunosuppressive effect seems to be TGF-α1. TNF-α is primarily produced by macrophages and monocytes. Its participation in pulmonary NE cell differentiation of SCLC cell lines has been suggested. Its 10.5/10.5-kb allele detection has been associated with favorable prognosis in patients with lung cancer. Decreased levels of IL-2 have been associated with adverse survival in SCLCs. Soluble IL-2 receptors are increased in this type of carcinoma and are correlated with poor prognosis, because IL-2 is unable to participate in cytotoxicity induced by lymphocytes [9].

Metastatic cancer cell in blood flow are sensitive to apoptosis and die. There is a tenfold decrease in the number of apoptotic cancer cells that are found at the secondary site 1 hour following the injection of cells rendered resistant to apoptosis *via* overexpression of Bcl2. Cancer cell death might occur as a result of two major mechanisms: cell destruction by mechanical stress and cell destruction by the immune system. Cancer cells circulating in the blood are submitted to strong mechanical forces caused by blood flow. This is especially important in narrow capillaries and within the microvasculature of contracting skeletal and heart muscle, in which sphere-to-cylinder shape transformation is lethal to most cancer cells NO and ROS are known to trigger apoptosis of cancer cells, and their production is activated by mechanical forces including shear and pulsatile stresses and contraction of the endothelium. Cancer cells have developed several ways to survive the mechanical stresses associated with circulation. Notably, they express high levels of stress proteins such as HSP70. Shear stress can induce pathways in the cancer cells that involve activation of integrins leading to adhesion of cancer cells to endothelial cells, thereby allowing them to escape anoikis. Nevertheless, these surviving processes are effective to only a small percentage of circulatory cancer cells since only 0.01% of these form metastases. In summary, the balanced response of tumour cells to mechanical destruction and adhesion initiation by

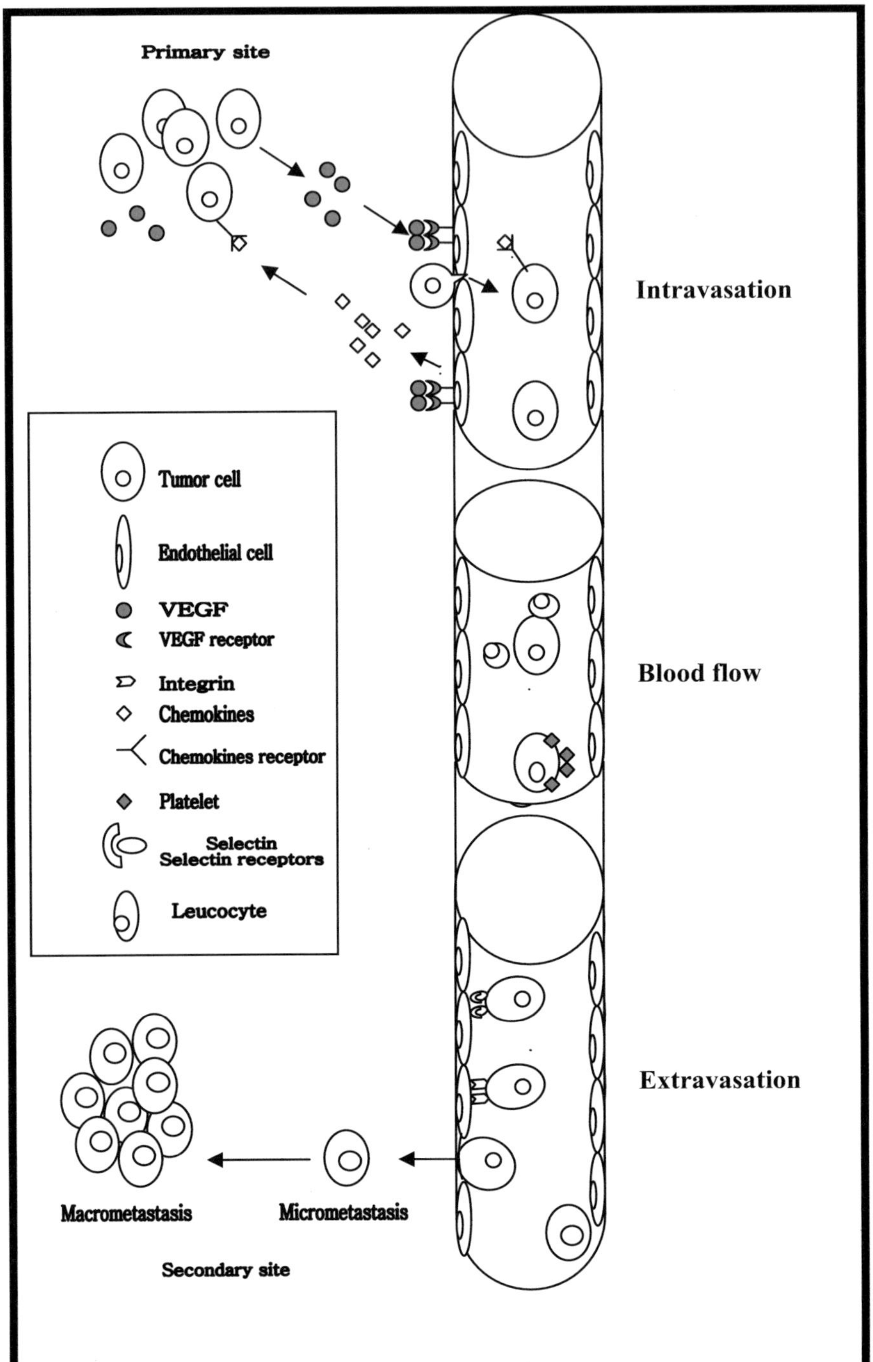

Figure 6: The journey of a metastatic cell: from the primary site to the secondary site. This journey comprises several steps that are summarized as follows.

circulating stress is an important mechanism that regulates the spread of hematogenous cancer. Circulating cancer cells have developed several mechanisms to escape immunosurveillance. In some cases, they can interact with platelets and fibrinogen to form clots that protect them against immune cells and facilitate their arrest and their adhesion on the endothelium. Furthermore, cancer cells may use inflammation-associated mechanisms to further protect themselves against apoptosis. For example acute-phase glycoproteins reach abnormally high levels in patients with cancer, which correlate with the extent of disease. It has been shown that these glycoproteins, synthesized by the liver in response to an inflammatory stimulus, may act as 'non-specific blocking factors' protecting tumours against the host's immunological attack [82].

1. **Intravasation:** Proliferation of primary tumour, local invasion of detached cells, intravasation in a capillary, and tumour cell survival in blood circulation. Mechanisms of VEGF-induced intravasation of cancer cells across blood vessels. Primary tumour cells secretes VEGF. VEGF activates blood endothelial cells that in turn may secrete chemotactic factors. This will contribute to attract cancer cells bearing appropriate chemokine receptors to the growing blood vessels, and enable their adhesion and their intra-vessel intravasation.

2. **Blood Flow in Tumour Cell:** Interaction with leukocytes that may be destructive or not; 2, aggregation with platelets, which protects cancer cells against mechanical stress and leukocytes. Tumour cell–cell aggregation, which protects against stress and formation of intra capillary thrombosis. d Arrest and extravasation in a target organ.

3. **Extravasation:** Extravasation of cancer cells is a multi-step process. The first step consists in the transient adhesion of cancer cells to the endothelium. It involves endothelial adhesion molecules such as E-selectin and P-selectin and their counter-receptors present on cancer cells. This step is associated with the rolling of the cancer cells on the endothelium. The second step consists in a firmer adhesion of cancer cells to endothelial cells. It is mediated through chemoattractants and cell adhesion molecules on the endothelium and integrins on the

cancer cells. The third step is characterized by the extravasation of cancer cells through endothelial cell–cell junctions. Metastatic growth in the new appropriate environment and formation of a secondary neoplasm.

Early and Late Molecular Events in Carcinogenesis of Lung Tumours

Somatic Mutations in Lung Cancer

There were five genes known to be mutated at high frequency in lung adenocarcinoma—*TP53, KRAS, STK11, EGFR* and *CDKN2A*— as well as several known genes with lower mutation frequencies— *PTEN, NRAS, ERBB2, BRAF* and *PIK3CA*. The newly identified genes that mutated in lung cancer include tumour suppressor genes (*NF1, RB1, ATM* and *APC*) along with tyrosine kinase genes (ephrin receptor genes, *ERBB4, KDR, FGFR4* and *NTRK* genes) that may function as protooncogenes. Many of these genes are also targeted by copy number alterations and/or gene expression changes. Additionally, there is a significant excess of mutations and copy number alterations in genes from the MAPK, p53, Wnt, cell cycle and mTOR signaling pathways, suggesting links to the disease.

The progression of epithelial tumours is accompanied by multiple genetic events. The increasing incidence of these events during the preneoplastic stage is not random, but it is mediated *via* specific steps. In epidemiologic, pathologic, and molecular terms, TCs and SCLCs are distinct, unrelated entities and ACs and LCNECs do not appear to represent intermediate stages between them, which may be indicative of a different process followed in their development. SCLCs are not accompanied by specific preneoplastic changes, whereas carcinoids are associated with inflammatory lesions in the airway.

Based on their profiles, it has been proposed that SCLCs may originate from either normal or hyperplastic epithelia, without passing through characteristic preneoplastic pathologic changes. The most characteristic early molecular events, occurring during the course of SCL carcinogenesis, are allele losses and microsatellite alterations. These aberrations, leading to inactivation of several growth-inhibitory pathways, are present both in normal bronchial epithelium associated with SCLC, as well as in hyperplasia and squamous metaplasia accompanying SCLCs. Simultaneous alterations of *FHIT* and *Rb*, as well as *Rb* and *p53*, which are located on the respective areas, are necessary for SCLC development. Furthermore, *3p* and *p16* are considered to be targets of aberrant methylation in SCLCs. Taking into account that hypermethylation is regarded as an early event in NSCL carcinogenesis, additional studies are needed to define its role in SCL carcinogenesis.

A number of molecular alterations are necessary for progression to the metastatic stage. Amplification of *c-myc* is considered to be a late event. This aberration is more frequently detected in SCLC cell lines derived from metastatic lesions than in primary tumours, in chemotherapy-treated patients, and in variant SCLCs. Overexpression of *c-myc* seems to down-regulate $\alpha 3\beta 1$ integrin. Impairments in E-CDH/catenin complex have also been associated with tumour invasion and metastasis. Moreover, it should be noted that the observed gradual increase of Bcl-2 in the clinical spectrum of NE tumours is not the case for metastatic SCLCs. In metastatic disease Bcl-2 is decreased, with a parallel decrease of Bax, which eventually leads to the attenuation of apoptosis. This may be attributed to the possible development of metastatic resistant-to-apoptosis clones. *c-erbB-2* and *c-ets* expression have been associated with extensive disease in SCLCs, and it is likely that their expressionmay enhance tumour invasion. Inactivation of *CC3* has been observed in the highly aggressive variant SCLCs; it is also expressed in the less metastatic classic type of SCLCs. Interestingly, telomerase activity becomes more apparent inextensive than in limited SCLCs. No specific genetic alteration is linked to metastatic carcinomas [9].

Organogenesis and Tumourigenesis of the Lung

Tumourigenesis and organogenesis share similar steps including rapid cell growth and vasculature restructuring. Kendall and co-workers investigated profiling DNA copy number alterations in 250 human lung cancer DNA. Five of the six most frequent amplicons harbored well-established oncogenes: *MYC*, *KRAS*, *EGFR*, *CCND1* and *L-MYC*. Intriguingly, the second most frequent amplicon did not contain an established oncogene. There were only three genes—*TTF1*, *NKX2-8* and *PAX9* (14q13). The RNAs of all three genes were overexpressed in amplified samples to varying degrees. *TTF1*, *NKX2-8* and *PAX9* synergistically stimulated proliferation of premalignant bronchial epithelial cells. Using RNAi to determine the tumour maintenance function, continuous expression of *NKX2-8* and *PAX9* was shown to be required to sustain tumourigenicity in an amplified squamous cell line that does not express *TTF1* (in general, squamous carcinomas do not in general expressed *TTF1*). It is very interesting that three functionally cooperating developmental transcription factors are coamplified by one specific amplicon to confer oncogenic advantage. In addition, it is clear that at least two of the three coamplified genes (*TTF1* and *NKX2-8*) mediate lung organogenesis [16].

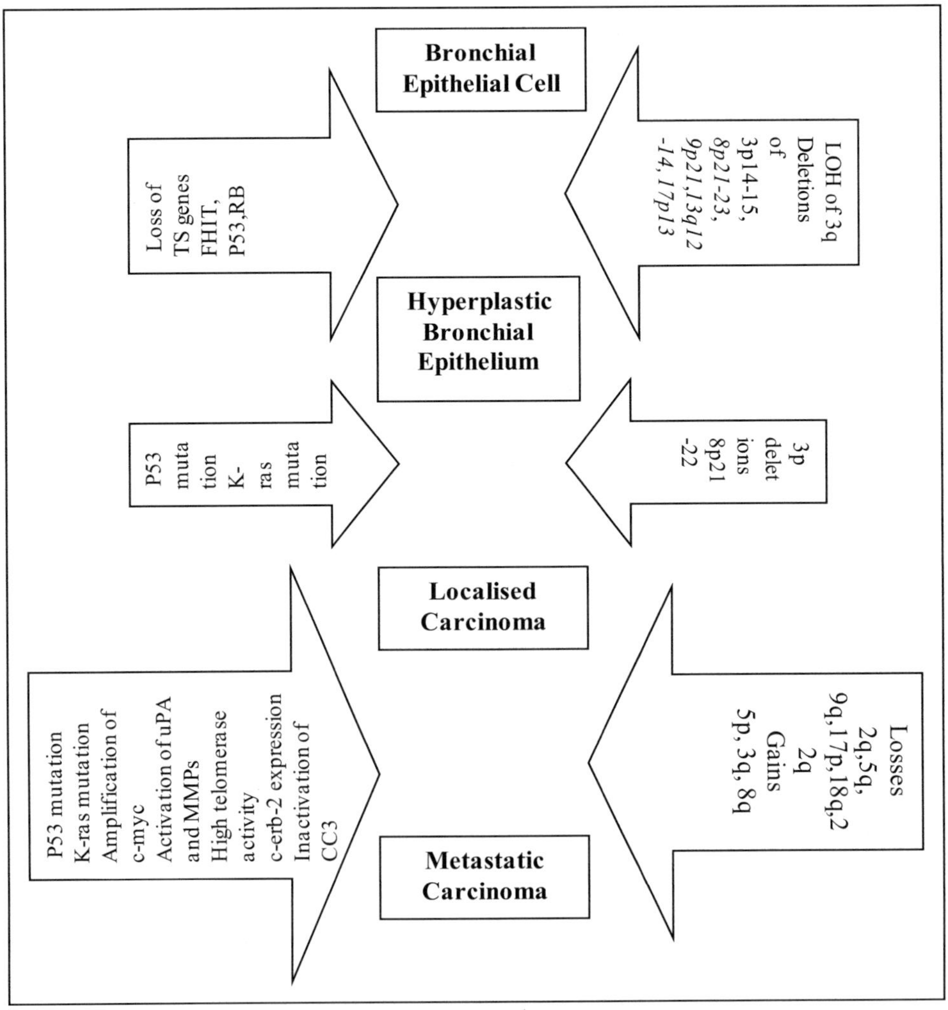

Figure7: Early and late molecular events in SCLC carcinogenesis.

Thyroid Transcription Factor 1 (TITF1)

Thyroid transcription factor 1 (TITF1; also known as NKX2-1) is a master transcription factor essential for the development of the peripheral airways, and is a lineage-specific marker for tumours developing from the terminal respiratory unit, *i.e.* peripheral ADCs. It is frequently overexpressed and occasionally amplified in these tumours. Inhibition of TITF1 by RNA interference induced growth inhibition and apoptosis in a subset of lung ADC cell lines expressing TTF1 (the protein product of TITF1); sustaining TTF1 expression is crucial for TTF1-expressing ADC. As most EGFR mutant ADCs arise from the terminal respiratory unit, they strongly express TITF1. In adult tissues, TITF1 has a very limited distribution, in only peripheral airway and thyroid epithelial cells. However, it is also expressed in the fetal forebrain, and perhaps that is the reason why it is also expressed in SCLCs [11].

Multidrug Resistance

The shield of tumour cells against chemotherapy is multidrug resistance (MDR). The fundamental mechanisms of MDR are either decrease of cellular drug levels or prevention of drug-induced apoptosis. Multidrug resistance-associated protein (MRP) is a TM 190-kDa glycoprotein, member of the ABC(ATP-binding cassette) superfamily. It functions as a TM transporter by keeping drug levels low *via* active efflux, thus offering MDR to tumour cells. MRP is present in normal lung tissue and is expressed in SCLC tumour cells, being the main mechanism of MDR in these tumours. P-glycoprotein, encoded by the *MDR1* gene, is another member of the ABC superfamily. Overexpression of P-glycoprotein causes active efflux of several drugs, leading to MDR. Interestingly, P-glycoprotein is rarely expressed in SCLCs. It was detected P-glycoprotein in clinical samples that it may be related to the clinically acquired MDR in SCLCs. Increased P-glycoprotein levels are associated with bad prognosis.

Another mechanism of MDR, which leads to increased drug detoxification, is that of glutathione (GSH) conjugation and transport of glutathione–drug conjugates out of the cell. This system consists of GSH, GSH-related enzymes, and glutathione-conjugate export pump (GS-X pump). The export of GSH conjugates of anticancer drugs is accomplished either by GS-X pump or by MRP. Each factor of this system is capable of rising independently or in conjunction with the other factors of the system in SCLCs. For instance, increase of GSH has been observed in drug-resistant human SCLC lines, without any alteration in the levels of GSH-related enzymes, and increased GSH may be accompanied by elevated activity of GS-X pump in human lung cancer cells.

Topoisomerase II (Topo II) participates in DNA replication, transcription, and recombination. There are two subtypes of this enzyme: Topo IIα (170 kDa) and Topo IIβ (180 kDa). Their expression is not correlated and this may be indicative of their different role in the progression of the cell cycle. Specifically, Topo IIα is produced during cell division, and Topo IIβ is expressed throughout the cell cycle, displaying higher levels in resting cells. It has been demonstrated that the expression of Topo IIα is higher in lung carcinomas than in normal lung tissue. Additionally, it is more elevated in SCLCs than NSCLCs. Topo IIβ levels exhibit no significant difference in these carcinomas. Topo II gene expression is associated with multidrug sensitivity, making it a possible chemosensitivity marker in lung cancer cell lines. Pretreatment Topo IIα levels are considered to reflect chemosensitivity of SCLC to Topo IIα-targeting drugs, such as etoposide, better than MRP and P-glycoprotein do. Furthermore, increased levels of Topo IIα correlate with adverse prognosis. In pulmonary carcinoid tumours, Topo IIα expression is more elevated in ACs than in TCs.

Metallothionein is a metal-binding protein rich in cysteine that has high affinity for Cd, Cu, and Zn. It has been suggested to correlate with resistance to cisplatin. overexpression of metallothionein is associated with adverse prognosis in SCLC patients receiving chemotherapy [9].

Diagnostic Biomarkers

Sensitive and specific biomarkers are critical tools for early detection and monitoring of cancer, in addition to representing potential therapeutic targets. The identification of novel molecular tumour markers remains a high priority in order to reduce cancer-associated morbidity and mortality, and provide clinicians with new strategies for targeted therapy of individual malignancies [73].

Kinetic Parameters—Proliferation Markers

Proliferating cell nuclear antigen (PCNA) is a 36-kDa non-histone nucleoprotein that binds to DNA polymerase and participates in DNA replication. PCNA labeling index can be a diagnostic tool for distinguishing between TCs and ACs. However, its role as a prognostic marker is very limited in patients with SCLC. The most reliable method for estimating the proliferating status is immunohistochemical analysis using the nuclear marker Ki-67, a monoclonal antibody assessing the growth fraction of human tumours. Increased proliferation is associated with poor survival in SCLCs and well differentiated NE carcinomas. Finally, proliferation rates are more elevated in ACs than in TCs, implying a higher risk for patients with ACs [9].

New Biomarkers and New Targets for Therapy

There are several distinct types of cancer biomarkers based on different areas: genetics, epigenetics, proteomics, metabolomics, imaging technology, and general physical techniques Genetics based cancer biomarkers utilize DNA arrays, polymerase chain reaction (PCR), reverse transcriptase polymerase chain reaction (RT-PCR), DNA sequencing, fluorescent *in situ* hybridization (FISH) *etc.* to detect the genetic alterations occurring in the cancerous state (Table **4**) [83].

Table 4: Genetic-based biomarkers

Groups	**Types of Genes**
Chromosomal changes	Deletion of chromosome 3p
Hypermethylation	P16, FHIT, Serine protease family member-trypsinogen VI(PRSS3) Tissue inhibitor of metalloproteinase (TIMP)-3 Death associated protein (DAP)-kinase
Genetic changes	K-ras P53 c-myc EGFR

The best example of genetic mutations discovered in lung cancer and subsequent development of biological agents is epidermal growth factor receptor (EGFR). Alterations in EGFR have been discovered in approximately 10% of patients with NSCLC. The treatment of these patients with tyrosine kinase inhibitors (ie. gefitinib, erlotinib) has been developed into a clinically useful therapy. Other single gene mutations that have been discovered in lung cancer include LKB1, EML4-ALK, p110, Kras, Her2 and BRAF. High-throughput methods to analyze effects of multiple biological agents on multiple genes simultaneously is being developed ("pharmacogenomics") [12].

ACKNOWLEDGEMENT

Declared none.

CONFLICT OF INTEREST

The author confirms that this article content has no conflict of interest.

REFERENCES

[1] Santos ES, Perez CA, Raez LE. How is gene-expression profiling going to challenge the future management of lung cancer? Future Oncol. 2009;5(6):827-35.

[2] Panani AD, Roussos C. Cytogenetic and molecular aspects of lung cancer. Cancer Lett. 2006; 28;239(1):1-9.

[3] Minna JD, Battey JF, Brooks BJ, Cuttitta F, Gazdar AF, Johnson BE, Ihde DC, Lebacq-Verheyden AM, Mulshine J, Nau MM, *et al.* Molecular genetic analysis reveals chromosomal deletion, gene amplification, and autocrine growth factor production in the pathogenesis of human lung cancer. Cold Spring Harb Symp Quant Biol. 1986;51 Pt 2:843-53

[4] Wang X, Li K, Chen H, Wang D, Zhang Y, Bai C.Does hepatocyte growth factor/c-Met signal play synergetic role in lung cancer? J Cell Mol Med. 2010 Apr;14(4):833-9. Epub 2010 Jan 30.

[5] Balsara BR, Testa JR. Chromosomal imbalances in human lung cancer. Oncogene. 2002 Oct 7;21(45):6877-83.

[6] Masuda A, Takahashi T. Chromosome instability in human lung cancers: possible underlying mechanisms and potential consequences in the pathogenesis. Oncogene. 2002 Oct 7;21(45):6884-97.

[7] Berrieman HK, Ashman JN, Cowen ME, Greenman J, Lind MJ, Cawkwell L. Chromosomal analysis of non-small-cell lung cancer by multicolour fluorescent *in situ* hybridisation. Br J Cancer. 2004 Feb 23;90(4):900-5.

[8] D'urso V, Collodoro A, Mattioli E, Giordano A, Bagella L. Cytometry and DNA Ploidy: Clinical Uses and Molecular Perspective in Gastric and Lung Cancer. J. Cell. Physiol. 222: 532–539, 2010.

[9] Koutsami MK, Anagnostopoulou ID, Papavassiliou AG, Gorgoulis VG. Genetic and Molecular Coordinates of Neuroendocrine Lung Tumours, with Emphasis on Small-cell Lung Carcinomas Molecular Medicine 8(8): 419–436,

[10] Sanchez MC. The Impact of Gene Expression Microarrays in the Evaluation of Lung Carcinoma Subtypes and DNA Copy Number. Archives of Pathology & Laboratory Medicine 2008; 32(10): 1562-1565.

[11] Brambilla E, Gazdar A. Pathogenesis of lung cancer signaling pathways: roadmap for therapies. Eur Respir J. 2009;33(6):1485-97.

[12] Singhal S, Miller D, Ramalingam S, Sun SY. Gene expression profiling of non-small cell lung cancer. Lung Cancer. 2008;60(3):313-24.

[13] Blanco R, Iwakawa R, Tang M, Kohno T, Angulo B, Pio R, Montuenga LM, Minna JD, Yokota J, Sanchez-Cespedes M. A gene-alteration profile of human lung cancer cell lines. Hum Mutat. 2009;30(8):1199-206.

[14] Lockwood WW, Chari R, Coe BP, Thu KL, Garnis C, Malloff CA, Campbell J, Williams AC, Hwang D, Zhu CQ, Buys TP, Yee J, English JC, Macaulay C, Tsao MS, Gazdar AF, Minna JD, Lam S, Lam WL. Integrative genomic analyses identify BRF2 as a novel lineage-specific oncogene in lung squamous cell carcinoma. PLoS Med. 2010: 27;7(7).

[15] Paulson KG, Lemos BD, Feng B, Jaimes N, Peñas PF, Bi X, Maher E, Cohen L, Leonard JH, Granter SR, Chin L, Nghiem P. Array-CGH reveals recurrent genomic changes in Merkel cell carcinoma including amplification of L-Myc. J Invest Dermatol. 2009;129(6):1547-55.

[16] Powers S, Mu D. Genetic similarities between organogenesis and tumourigenesis of the lung. Cell Cycle 2008;7:2, 200-204.

[17] Hussenet T, du Manoir S. SOX2 in squamous cell carcinoma: Amplifying a pleiotropic oncogene along carcinogenesis. Cell Cycle. 2010 Apr 13;9(8). [Epub ahead of print]

[18] Lum AM, Wang BB, Beck-Engeser GB, Li L, Channa N, Wabl M. Orphan receptor GPR110, an oncogene overexpressed in lung and prostate cancer. BMC Cancer. 2010 Feb 11;10:40.

[19] Sterlacci W, Fiegl M, Hilbe W, Jamnig H, Oberaigner W, Schmid T, Augustin F, Auberger J, Obermann EC, Tzankov A. Deregulation of p27 and cyclin D1/D3 control over mitosis is associated with unfavorable prognosis in non-small cell lung cancer, as determined in 405 operated patients. J Thorac Oncol. 2010 Sep;5(9):1325-36.

[20] Giuseppe Giaccone. Tumourigenesis Oncogenes and Antioncogenes in Lung. *Chest* 1996;109;130S-134S

[21] Wanpeng Sun and Jian Yang. Functional Mechanisms for Human Tumour Suppressors. *Journal of Cancer* 2010; 1:136-140

[22] Fong KM, Sekido Y, Gazdar AF, Minna JD. Lung cancer 9: Molecular biology of lung cancer: clinical implications. Thorax 2003;58:892-900

[23] Sion-Vardy N, Freedman J, Lazarov I, Bolotin A, Ariad S. p27kip1 Expression in non-small cell lung cancer is not an independent prognostic factor. Anticancer Res. 2010;30(9):3699-704.

[24] Seike M, Gemma A, Hosoya Y, Hemmi S, Taniguchi Y, Fukuda Y, Yamanaka N, Kudoh S. Increase in the frequency of p16INK4 gene inactivation by hypermethylation in lung cancer during the process of metastasis and its relation to the status of p53. Clin Cancer Res. 2000;6(11):4307-13.

[25] Okamoto A, Hussain SP, Hagiwara K, Spillare EA, Rusin MR, Demetrick DJ, Serrano M, Hannon GJ, Shiseki M, Zariwala M, *et al.* Mutations in the p16INK4/MTS1/CDKN2, p15INK4B/MTS2, and p18 genes in primary and metastatic lung cancer. Cancer Res. 1995; 1;55(7):1448-51.

[26] Zhang H, Shu H, Jiang W. Expression of PTEN, p53 and P-glycoprotein in Non-small cell Lung Cancer and Their Predictive Values. Zhongguo Fei Ai Za Zhi. 2009; 20;12(11):1213-6.

[27] Verri C, Roz L, Conte D, Liloglou T, Livio A, Vesin A, Fabbri A, Andriani F, Brambilla C, Tavecchio L, Calarco G, Calabrò E, Mancini A, Tosi D, Bossi P, Field JK, Brambilla E,

Sozzi G; EUELC Consortium. Fragile histidine triad gene inactivation in lung cancer: the European Early Lung Cancer project. Am J Respir Crit Care Med. 2009;1;179(5):396-401.

[28] Rodriguez-Nieto S, Sanchez-Cespedes M. BRG1 and LKB1: tales of two tumour suppressor genes on chromosome 19p and lung cancer. Carcinogenesis. 2009;30(4):547-54.

[29] Vincent A. Potiron1,2, Joëlle Roche2, and Harry A. Drabkin1 Semaphorins and their receptors in lung cancer. *Cancer Lett.* 2009; 8; 273(1): 1–14.

[29] Potiron VA, Sharma G, Nasarre P, Clarhaut JA, Augustin HG,Gemmill RM, Roche J, Drabkin HA. Semaphorin SEMA3F Affects Multiple Signaling Pathways in Lung Cancer Cells *Cancer Res* 2007;67:8708-8715.

[30] Neal CS, Michael MZ, Rawlings LH, Van der Hoek MB, Gleadle JM. The VHL-dependent regulation of microRNAs in renal cancer. BMC Med. 2010; 21;8:64.

[31] Jaiswal AS, Narayan S. A novel function of adenomatous polyposis coli (APC) in regulating DNA repair. Cancer Lett. 2008; 28;271(2):272-80.

[32] Hawes SE, Stern JE, Feng Q, Wiens LW, Rasey JS, Lu H, Kiviat NB, Vesselle H. DNA hypermethylation of tumours from non-small cell lung cancer (NSCLC) patients is associated with gender and histologic type. Lung Cancer. 2010;69(2):172-9.

[33] Pan SY, Xie EF, Shu YQ, Gao L, Zhang LX, Chen D, Chen JB, Zhao WJ, Mu Y, Zhang JN. [Methylation quantification of adenomatous polyposis coli (APC) gene promoter in plasma of lung cancer patients] Ai Zheng. 2009;28(4):384-9.

[34] Feng ZJ, Gao SB, Wu Y, Xu XF, Hua X, Jin GH. Lung cancer cell migration is regulated *via* repressing growth factor PTN/RPTP β/ζ signaling by menin. Oncogene. 2010; 30;29(39):5416-26.

[35] Boyd KP, Korf BR, Theos A. Neurofibromatosis type 1. J Am Acad Dermatol. 2009;61(1):1-14.

[36] Furukawa K, Yanai N, Fujita M, Harada Y. Novel mutations of neurofibromatosis type 1 gene in small cell lung cancers. Surg Today. 2003;33(5):323-7.

[37] Yang G, Yang X. Smad4-mediated TGF-beta signaling in tumourigenesis. Int J Biol Sci. 2010; 1;6(1):1-8.

[38] Tong XD, Liu HX, Zhao HR, Xu SG, Li Y, Han LB, Zhang L. [The role of Smad4 and MAPK proteins in signal transduction pathway in non-small cell lung cancer] Zhonghua Zhong Liu Za Zhi. 2006;28(10):741-5.

[39] Nam E, Park C. Maspin Suppresses Survival of Lung Cancer Cells through Modulation of Akt Pathway. Cancer Res Treat. 2010;42(1):42-7.

[40] Pfeifer GP, Rauch TA. DNA methylation patterns in lung carcinomas. Semin Cancer Biol. 2009;19(3):181-7.

[41] Yanagitani N, Kohno T, Kim J-G, Kunitoh H, Tamura T, Takei Y, Tsuchiya S, Saito R, Yokota J. Identification of *D19S246* as a novel lung adenocarcinoma susceptibility locus by genome survey with 10-cM resolution mircrosatellite markers. *Cancer Epidemiol Biomarkers Prev* 2003;12:366–371.

[42] Ann G. Schwartz and John C. Ruckdeschel Familial Lung Cancer American Journal of Respiratory and Critical Care Medicine 2006;173:16-22,

[43] Broderick P, Wang Y, Vijayakrishnan J, Matakidou A, Spitz MR, Eisen T, Amos CI, Houlston RS. Deciphering the impact of common genetic variation on lung cancer risk: A genome-wide association study. *Cancer Res*. 2009; 15; 69(16): 6633–6641

[44] Yokota J, Shiraishi K, Kohno T. Genetic basis for susceptibility to lung cancer recent progress and future directions. Adv Cancer Res. 2010;109:51-72.

[45] Fang S, Pinney SM, Bailey-Wilson JE, de Andrade M, Li Y, Kupert E, You M, Schwartz AG, Yang P, Anderson M, Amos CI. Ordered subset analysis identifies loci influencing lung cancer risk on chromosomes 6q and 12q. Cancer Epidemiol Biomarkers Prev. 2010 Oct 28. [Epub ahead of print]

[46] Kiyohara C, Takayama K, Nakanishi Y. Lung cancer risk and genetic polymorphisms in DNA repair pathways: a meta-analysis. J Nucleic Acids. 2010; 14;2010:701760.

[47] Horwitz M, Benson KF, Person RE, Aprikyan AG, Dale DC. Mutations in ELA2, encoding neutrophil elastase, define a 21-day biological clock in cyclic haematopoiesis. Nat Genet. 1999;23: 433-436.

[48] Todaro M, Lombardo Y, Francipane MG, Alea MP, Cammareri P, Iovino F, Di Stefano AB, Di Bernardo C, Agrusa A, Condorelli G, Walczak H, Stassi G.Apoptosis resistance in epithelial tumours is mediated by tumour-cell-derived interleukin-4. Cell Death Differ. 2008;15(4):762-72.

[49] Penyige A, Poliska S, Csanky E, Scholtz B, Dezso B, Schmelczer I, Kilty I, Takacs L, Nagy L. Analyses of association between PPAR gamma and EPHX1 polymorphisms and susceptibility to COPD in a Hungarian cohort, a case-control study. BMC Med Genet. 2010; 2;11:152.

[50] Palmer LJ, Celedon JC, Chapman HA, Speizer FE, Wiess ST, Sliverman EK. Genome-wide linkage analysis of bronchodilator responsiveness and post-bronchodilator spirometric phenotypes in chronic obstructive pulmonary disease. *Hum Mol Genet* 2003;12:1199–1210.[

[51] He JQ, Connett JE, Anthonisen NR, Sandford AJ. Polymorphisms in the *IL13, IL13RA1,* and *IL4RA* genes and the rate of decline in lung function in smokers. *Am J Respir Cell Mol Biol* 2003;28:379–385.

[52] Joost O, Wilk JB, Cupples A, Harmon M, Shearman AM, Baldwin CT, O'Conner GT, Myers RH, Gottlieb DJ. Genetic loci influencing lung function: a genomewide scan in the Framingham study. *Am J Respir Crit Care Med* 2002;165:795–799.

[53] Page-McCaw A, Ewald AJ, Werb Z. Matrix metalloproteinases and the regulation of tissue remodelling. Nat Rev Mol Cell Biol. 2007;8(3):221-33.

[54] Rudin CM, Avila-Tang E, Haris CC, Herman JG, Fred R. Hirsch3, William Pao4, Ann G. Schwartz5, Kirsi H. Vahakangas6, and Jonathan M. Samet. Lung cancer ın never smokers: molecular profiles and therapeutıc ımplıcatıons. *Clin Cancer Res*. 2009;15; 15(18): 5646–5661.

[55] Omerovic j, laude AJ, Prior IA. Ras proteins: paradigms for compartmentalised and isoform specific signaling. *Cell Mol Life Sci*. 2007;64(19-20): 2575–2589.

[56] McCubrey JA, Steelman LS, Chappell WH, Abrams SL, Wong EW, Chang F, Lehmann B, Terrian DM, Milella M, Tafuri A, Stivala F, Libra M, Basecke J, Evangelisti C, Martelli AM, Franklin RA. Roles of the Raf/MEK/ERK pathway in cell growth, malignant transformation and drug resistance. Biochim Biophys Acta. 2007 Aug;1773(8):1263-84.

[57] Barbi S, Cataldo I, De Manzoni G, Bersani S, Lamba S, Mattuzzi S, Bardelli A, Scarpa A. The analysis of PIK3CA mutations in gastric carcinoma and metanalysis of literature suggest that exon-selectivity is a signature of cancer type. J Exp Clin Cancer Res. 2010; 16;29:32.

[58] Qi H, Fan L. PI3K/Akt/mTOR Signaling Pathway and Non-small Cell Lung Cancer. Zhongguo Fei Ai Za Zhi. 2010; 20;13(12):1149-1154.

[59] Ikeda S, Takabe K, Inagaki M, Suzuki K. Expression of phosphorylated Akt in patients with small cell carcinoma of the lung indicates good prognosis. Pathol Int. 2010;60(11) Epub 2010 Oct 6.

[60] LoPiccolo J, Blumenthal GM, Bernstein WB, Dennis PA. Targeting the PI3K/Akt/mTOR pathway: effective combinations and clinical considerations. *Drug Resist Updat*. 2008; 11(1-2): 32–50.

[61] Nagata Y, Takahashi A, Ohnishi K, Ota I, Ohnishi T, Tojo T, Taniguchi S. Effect of rapamycin, an mTOR inhibitor, on radiation sensitivity of lung cancer cells having different p53 gene status. Int J Oncol. 2010;37(4):1001-10.

[62] Fazlul H. Sarkar, Yiwei Li, Zhiwei Wang, and Dejuan Kong. The role of nutraceuticals in the regulation of Wnt and Hedgehog signaling in cancer *Cancer Metastasis Rev*. 2010; 29(3): 383–394.

[63] Shaulian E. AP-1--The Jun proteins: Oncogenes or tumour suppressors in disguise? Cell Signal. 2010;22(6):894-9.

[64] Huang S, Yang L, An Y, Ma X, Zhang C, Xie G, Chen ZY, Xie J, Zhang H. Expression of hedgehog signaling molecules in lung cancer. Acta Histochem. 2010. [Epub ahead of print]

[65] Gialmanidis IP, Bravou V, Amanetopoulou SG, Varakis J, Kourea H, Papadaki H. Overexpression of hedgehog pathway molecules and FOXM1 in non-small cell lung carcinomas. Lung Cancer. 2009;66(1):64-74.

[66] Garnis C, Campbell J, Davies JJ, Macaulay C, Lam S, Lam WL. Involvement of multiple developmental genes on chromosome 1p in lung tumourigenesis. Hum Mol Genet 2005; 14:475-82.

[67] Westhoff B, Colaluca IN, D'Ario G, Donzelli M, Tosoni D, Volorio S, Pelosi G, Spaggiari L, Mazzarol G, Viale G, Pece S, Di Fiore PP. Alterations of the Notch pathway in lung cancer. Proc Natl Acad Sci U S A. 2009; 29;106(52):22293-8.

[68] Donnem T, Andersen S, Al-Shibli K, Al-Saad S, Busund LT, Bremnes RM. Prognostic impact of Notch ligands and receptors in nonsmall cell lung cancer: Coexpression of Notch-1 and vascular endothelial growth factor-A predicts poor survival. Cancer. 2010 15;116(24):5676-85.

[69] Donnem T, Andersen S, Al-Shibli K, Al-Saad S, Busund LT, Bremnes RM. Prognostic impact of Notch ligands and receptors in nonsmall cell lung cancer: coexpression of Notch-1 and vascular endothelial growth factor-A predicts poor survival. Cancer. 2010 15;116(24):5676-85.

[70] Strizzi L, Hardy KM, Seftor EA, Costa FF, Kirschmann DA, Seftor RE, Postovit LM, Hendrix MJ. Development and cancer: at the crossroads of Nodal and Notch signaling. Cancer Res. 2009;15;69(18):7131-4.

[71] Tang M, Xu W, Wang Q, Xiao W, Xu R.Potential of DNMT and its Epigenetic Regulation for Lung Cancer Therapy. Curr Genomics. 2009;10(5):336-52.

[72] Du D& Pertsemlidis A. microRNAs and lung cancer: tumours and 22-mers. Cancer Metastasis Rev 2010; 29:109–122.

[73] Heneghan HM, Miller N, Lowery AJ, Sweeney KJ, Kerin MJ. MicroRNAs as Novel Biomarkers for Breast Cancer. J Oncol. 2009;2009:950201.

[74] Mollberg N, Surati M, Demchuk C, Fathi R, Salama AK, Husain AN, Hensing T, Salgia R. Mind-mapping for lung cancer: Towards a personalized therapeutics approach. Adv Ther. 2011;28(3):173-94.

[75] Ono K, Uramoto H, Hanagiri T. Expression of dysadherin and cytokeratin as prognostic indicators of disease-free survival in patients with stage I NSCLC. Anticancer Res. 2010;30(9):3273-8.

[76] Dai SD, Wang Y, Zhang JY, Zhang D, Zhang PX, Jiang GY, Han Y, Zhang S, Cui QZ, Wang EH. Upregulation of δ-catenin is associated with poor prognosis and enhances transcriptional activity through Kaiso in non-small-cell lung cancer. Cancer Sci. 2010 [Epub ahead of print]

[78] Leung EL, Fiscus RR, Tung JW, Tin VP, Cheng LC, Sihoe AD, Fink LM, Ma Y, Wong MP. Non-Small Cell Lung Cancer Cells Expressing CD44 Are Enriched for Stem Cell-Like Properties. PLoS One. 2010 Nov 19;5(11):e14062.

[79] Lantuéjoul S, Salon C, Soria JC, Brambilla E. Telomerase expression in lung preneoplasia and neoplasia. Int J Cancer. 2007; 1;120(9):1835-41.

[77] Rebecca L. Toonkel, M.D.1, Alain C. Borczuk, M.D.2, and Charles A. Powell, M.D. TGF-ß Signaling Pathway in Lung Adenocarcinoma Invasion. J Thorac Oncol. 2010; 5(2): 153–157.

[80] Weryńska B, Dziegiel P, Jankowska R. Role of lymphangiogenesis in lung cancer. Folia Histochem Cytobiol. 2009;47(3):333-42.

[81] Wang X, Li K, Chen H, Wang D, Zhang Y, Bai C. Does hepatocyte growth factor/c-Met signal play synergetic role in lung cancer? Journal of Cellular and Molecular Medicine 2010; 14(4): 833–839.

[82] Stéphanie Gout & Jacques Huot Role of Cancer Microenvironment in Metastasis: Focus on Colon Cancer. Cancer Microenvironment 2008; 1:69–83

[83] Sung HJ & ChoJY Biomarkers for the lung cancer diagnosis and their advances in Proteomics. BMB reports 2008; 41(9): 615-625

Lung Cancer: Clinical and Surgical Specifications, **2013, 106-118**

CHAPTER 4

Symptoms, Clinical Findings and Paraneoplastic Syndromes in Lung Cancer

Tulin Cağatay* and Gulfer Okumus

Istanbul University, Istanbul Medical Faculty, Department of Pulmonary Diseases, CAPA, Istanbul, Turkey

Abstract: Signs and symptoms of lung tumours depend on tumour location and size, extent of the tumour or its stage and presence or absence of metastasis. Common symptoms are Cough (especially persistent cough), Hemoptysis, Dyspnea, Wheezing, Chest pain, and, Hoarseness. Less commonly, symptoms may arise due to introthoracic tissue and organ involvement, superior vena cava syndrome, Horner's syndrome or distance metastasis. Systemic effects like weight loss, anorexia, weakness may be seen and symptoms of paraneoplastic syndrome observed.

On physical examination, findings are due to the extent of the disease such as crackles, ronchi, and localised wheeze. If there is collapse of lung tissue or pleural effusions, dullness in precussion and decreased breath sounds will be found. Rarely, findings of paraneoplastic syndromes may dominate the picture. If there is respiratory failure its signs can be found on physical examination. The most important finding is finger clubbing.

Keywords: Lung Cancer, Symptoms, Clinical Findings, Paraneoplastic Syndrome.

INTRODUCTION

Signs and symptoms of lung tumours depend on tumour location and size, extent of the tumour or its stage and presence or absence of metastasis. However lung tumours are generally associated with a certain constellations of signs and symptoms which we grouped to facilitate understanding under four titles [1-4]. These are symptoms and signs arising:

***Address correspondence to Tulin Cağatay:** Istanbul University, Istanbul Medical Faculty, Department of Pulmonary Diseases, CAPA/Istanbul/Turkey; Tel: +90 212 4142000/31889; Fax +90 212 6352708; E-mail: tulcagat@istanbul.edu.tr

1. from the local spread of the tumour in thorax
2. from distant metastasis
3. due to systemic effects
4. due to paraneoplastic effects

1. SYMPTOMS AND SIGNS DUE TO LOCAL SPREAD OF THE PRIMARY TUMOUR

A. Symptoms Caused by Centrally Located Tumours

— **Cough** is the most common symptom of lung cancer. It is often present in endobronchial tumours located in the large airways. Cough that might be nonproductive or productive is present in 50% to 75% of lung cancer patients.

— **Hemoptysis**, a symptom more often seen in tuberculosis and bronchiectasia is present in 25 to 50% of patients with lung cancer [5-7].

— **Dyspnea** occurs in 25% of patients with lung cancer. Dyspnea may be due to airway obstruction, atelectasis, tumour emboli, lymphangitic spread, pleural and pericardal effusion, or pneumothorax [5, 6]. Dyspnea can also be due to diaphragmatic paralysis caused by phrenic nerve invasion.

— **Wheezing** especially localized to the affected lung area, can occur due to the obstruction caused by the tumour and postobstructive pneumonia.

B. Symptoms Due to Peripherally Located Tumours

— **Cough**

— **Dyspnea**

— **Chest** pain occurs due to parietal pleura and chest wall infiltration and vertebral and rib metastases. The chest pain is present 20% patients with lung cancer.

— **Hoarseness** arises due to tumoural involvement of recurrent laryngeal nerves. It mostly occurs in left upper lobe tumours due to the longer course of the left recurrent laryngeal nerve in thorax.

— **Dysphagia** may develop due to the tumour invasion of the esophagus, compression of the esophagus by the lymphatic glands and recurrent laryngeal nerve invasion by the tumour. Tracheal or broncooesophageal fistula may also cause dysphagia.

— **Pancoast syndrome** is a constellation of symptom and signs caused by local invasion of chest wall, satellite ganglion and lower brachial plexus by a tumour located in the apices of the lung. It is seen in less than 5% of the lung tumours [8].

— **Horner's syndrome** is caused by the compression of the cervical symphatetic nerve plexus by a superior sulcus lung tumour (Pancoast tumours). Findings of Horner's syndrome are ipsilateral ptosis, miosis, enophthalmos, and anhidrosis [9].

— **Pericardial or pleural effusions** are seen in 15% –50% of patients due to direct invasion of the visceral pleura by the tumour, or rarely due to mediastinal lymph invasion and the resulting lymphatic obstruction. Symptoms are vary according to the amount of pleural fluid accumulation, but chest pain, cough and dyspnea are common [10].

— **Superior vena cava syndrome** due to obstruction of superior vena cava by external compression, direct vessel invasion or vascular thrombosis. It mostly occurs in right lung tumours. Symptoms are dyspnea, cough, swelling of face and neck, cyanosis, headache, and dizziness. Signs are face, neck and arm edema, dusky skin coloration and possibly conjunctival edema, neck, upper extremity and thorax wall venous dilation and collateral vessel formation with retrograde flow [11].

C. Intrathoracic Extension of Lung Cancer

Lung tumours can extend to mediastinum and thoracic wall by direct expansion or by lymphatics. It can be seen in 10% of the patients. Mediastinum great vessels, esophagus, heart, pericardium, recurrent laryngeal nerve, phrenic nerve, brachial plexus can be involved.

Heart and pericardium are usually involved by direct lymphatic spread. The tumour most frequently implicated in pericardial spread (37%) is the tumour of the lung. If the mass is big enough, it may become noticable during the physical examination.

2. SYMPTOMS AND SIGNS DUE TO METASTASIS

The signs and symptoms are those of the organ that the tumour metastised. **Headache, mental status changes,** fits for **cranial metastasis, hepatomegaly** for hepatic metastasis, or **skin** or **soft tissue** masses for skim and soft tissue metastasis *etc.* **Extrapulmonary metastasis** is present in 60% and 30-40% of the patients with (SCLC) or without (NSCLC) small cell lung cancer respectively.

— **Bone**: All the bones in the body are involved of lung carcinomas. The bone metastasis can cause localised pain and local mass. Sometimes may also be painless [12]. Patients with lung carcinomas can be go to Doctor symptoms of bone metastasis.

— **Central nervous system** metastasis is present in 10% of the lung cancer patients. Symptoms are related to the region and the extend of the involved area but are generally nonspecific like headache, dizziness, mental status changes, focal and generalized fits.

— **Liver** metastases are more commonly seen in SCLC than in NSCLC (3.8%-17.5%) Generally it is symptomless rarely nonspecific findings such as emesis, loss of weight, fever may be seen.

— **Surrenal gland** involvement is an important signs during staging of lung cancer.

A. Subcutaneous Nodules

Lymphatic invasion, distant lymphatic involvement is less than 10%.

Lung parenchymal involvement can be seen and causes cough and dyspnea.

3. SYSTEMIC SYMPTOMS AND SIGNS

Patients may **lose weight** and may be in obvious **respiratory distress**. Lung cancer patients frequently present with weight loss in the context of the cachexia syndrome. Systemic symptoms and findings such as **malaise, fever** and anemia are seen in 55–88% of the lung cancer patients. **Anemia** is frequent in patients with lung cancer and can contribute to fatigue and dyspnea [13, 14].

On physical examination, the findings are due to the extent of the disease such as **crackles, ronchi** and localised **wheeze** besides the presence of **dullness** in percussion. If there are collapse and pleural effusions cause dullness and decreased breath sounds. If there is respiratory failure it's signs can be found on physical examination. The most important finding is **finger clubbing** [15].

4. PARANEOPLASTIC SYNDROMES

Paraneoplastic effects of a tumour are not related to the direct invasion, obstruction, or metastasis. Paraneoplastic syndromes (PS) are attributed to tumour secretion of functional peptides and hormones or immune cross-reactivity between tumour and normal host tissues. Thus, successful treatment of the underlying tumour often improves these conditions. Usually, PS is detected after a cancer diagnosis and the development of these disorders does not necessarily correlate with cancer stage. In some cases, PS is manifest before a cancer diagnosis. Therefore, their timely recognition may lead to detection of an otherwise clinically occult tumour at an early and highly treatable stage. Paraneoplastic syndromes related to bronchogenic carcinoma occur in 10-20% of patients (Table **1**) (Adapted from 16th literature).

A. Paraneoplastic Endocrine Syndromes

Hypercalcemia: Malignancy-associated hypercalcemia (MAH) is found in up to 10% of all patients with advanced cancer [17]. There are some mechanisms for hypercalcemia in cancer patients: Secretion of parathyroid hormone-related protein by tumour cells accounts for 80% of cases and occurs most commonly with squamous cell tumours. Another 20% of patients arise directly from osteolytic activity at sites of skeletal metastases [18]. Hypercalcemia in patients with lung

Table 1: Paraneoplastic syndromes associated with lung cancer

Endocrinologic Syndromes	**Neurologic Syndromes**	**Hematologic Syndromes**	**Cutaneous Syndromes**
Hypercalcemia SIADH Cushing's syndrome Carcinoid syndrome Hyper/hypo-glycemia Gynecomastia Galactorrhea	Lambert-Eaton syndrome Peripheral neuropathy Encephalopathy Myelopathy Cerebellar degeneration Psychosis	Leukemoid reaction Thrombocytosis Polycythemia Hypercoagulable state Eosinophilia Hemolytic anemia Thrombophlebitis	Clubbing Erythema multiforme Dermatomyositis Acanthosis nigricans Pruritus Hyperpigmentation Urticaria
GH excess Calcitonin secretion TSH	Dementia	Arterial thrombosis Nonbacterial thrombotic endocarditis Red cell aplasia Dysproteinemia Thrombocytopenic purpura	Scleroderma
Musculoskeletal syndromes	**Miscellaneous**		
Hypertrophic osteoarthropathy Polymyositis Osteomalacia Myopathy	Cachexia Hyperuricemia Nephrotic syndrome		

cancer may arise from a bony metastasis or less commonly tumour secretion of a parathyroid hormone-related protein, calcitriol or other cytokines, including osteoclast activating factors.

Hiraki *et al.* was found that, hypercalcemia is 6% in 1149 consecutive patients with lung cancer [19]. Among those with hypercalcemia, squamous cell carcinoma, adenocarcinoma, and SCLC were responsible in 51, 22, and 15% of cases, respectively. Most patients with hypercalcemia have advanced disease (stage III or IV) and a median survival of a few months [19].

The symptom severity of hypercalcemia depends on the degree of hypercalcemia (>14 mg/dL), the rapidity of onset baseline neurologic and renal function [18]. The symptoms of hypercalcemia include anorexia, nausea, vomiting, constipation, lethargy, polyuria, polydipsia, and dehydration. Confusion and coma are late manifestations, as are renal failure and nephrocalcinosis [17].

Symptomatic patients require treatment that includes hydration and intavenous bisphosphonate [20].

Syndrome of Inappropiate Antidiuretic Hormone (SIADH) Secretion: The syndrome of inappropriate antidiuretic hormone secretion (SIADH), which is charecterized by hypo-osmotic, euvolemic hyponatremia, frequently caused by small cell lung cancer (SCLC). SCLC accounts for approximately 75% of all malignancy-related of SIADH [21- 22].

The severity of symptoms is related to the degree of hyponatremia and the rapidity of the fall in serum sodium. Symptoms include anorexia, nausea, and vomiting. Cerebral edema can occur with the onset of hyponatremia is rapid. Symptoms caused by cerebral edema may include irritability, restlessness, personality changes, confusion, coma, seizures, and respiratory arrest.

The treatment of SIADH focuses on treating the malignancy. The hyponatremia will resolve within weeks of starting chemotherapy, in the most of the patients with SCLC. Chronic hyponatremia or that of unclear duration may be treated with normal saline infusion to euvolemia, fluid restriction and demeclocycline or a vasopressin-receptor antagonist [23].

Cushing Syndrome: Ectopic production of adrenal corticotropin can cause Cushing's syndrome. Approximately 5% to 10% of patients with Cushing syndrome are paraneoplastic and 50% of these patients had neuroendocrine lung tumours (SCLC and bronchial carcinoids) [24- 26]. Patients often present with symptoms of paraneoplastic Cushing syndrome before a cancer diagnosis is made. Also, relapse of paraneoplastic Cushing syndrome may show tumour recurrence [27-28].

Patients typically present with muscle weakness, weight loss, hypertension, hirsutism, and osteoporosis. Hypokalemic alkalosis and hyperglycemia are usually present. Weight gain with centripetal fat distiribution is more common in nonparaneoplastic than in paraneoplastic Cushing syndrome [28].

B. Paraneoplastic Neurologic Syndromes

The paraneoplastic neurologic syndromes associated with lung cancer; typically these are associated with SCLC. Paraneoplastic neurologic manifestations include

Lambert-Eaton myasthenic syndrome (LEMS), cerebellar ataxia, subacute sensory neuropathy, limbic encephalitis, encephalomyelitis, autonomic neuropathy, retinopathy, and opsomyoclonus [29]. The frequency of any of these neurologic syndromes in SCLC is about 5%, and neurologic symptoms may precede the diagnosis by months to years.

LEMS is which may be seen in 2-4% of patients with SCLC, the most common of paraneoplastic neurologic syndromes [30]. The neurologic symptoms of LEMS precede the diagnosis of SCLC in more than 80% of cases. Proximal muscle weakness, hyporeflexia and autonomic dysfunction characterize LEMS. Cranial nerve involvement may be present and does not differentiate LEMS from myasthenia gravis. Also, LEMS has been strongly associated with anticalcium channel binding antibodies of peripheral cholinergic nerve terminals. These antibodies have been identified in over 90% of patients with LEMS and block the normal release of acetylcholine at the neuromuscular junction. Calcium channel autoantibodies have been identified in 25% of SCLC patients who are not affected by neurologic problems. The diagnosis of LEMS is based on charecteristic electromyographic findings [16].

70% of the patients who have SCLC and an associated paraneoplastic neurologic syndrome have limited stage disease [31]. The finding of a paraneoplastic autoantibody in patients presenting with a neurologic syndrome should lead to an evaluation for malignancy.

Immune modulation is a key component of paraneoplastic neurologic syndromes therapy. Specific modalities include corticosteroids, corticosteroid-sparing agents (eg, azathioprine, cyclophosphamide), IVIG, rituximab and plasmapheresis. These syndromes generally do not improve with immunosuppressive treatment. Because paraneoplastic neurologic syndromes may cause irreversible pathologic changes to the nervous system, treatment often results in symptom stability rather than improvement [32].

C. Paraneoplastic Hematologic Syndromes

A number of hematologic abnormalities are seen in patients with lung cancer. Paraneoplastic hematologic syndromes are rarely symptomatic. These conditions are usually detected after a cancer diagnosis and these are seen in association advanced disease. Paraneoplastic hematologic syndromes may improve with successful therapy of the underlying malignancy [33-35].

Leukocytosis: Paraneoplastic leukocytosis is about in 15% of patients with lung cancer (particularly large cell lung cancer). The leucocyte count ranges from 12-30×10^9 but in some cases exceeds 50×10^9/L [36]. Nearly all had non-SCLC, and the leukocytosis was thought to be due to overproduction of granulocyte-colony stimulating factor [37]. Leukocytosis in association with lung cancer is associated with a poor prognosis and has also been associated with hypercalcemia [19, 37].

Anemia: Anemia is frequent in patients with lung cancer and can contribute to fatigue and dyspnea. In one series 40% of untreated patients had a hemoglobin $\leq$12 g/dL, while the incidence of anemia was 80% in those on chemotherapy [38].

Thrombocytosis: Thrombocytosis is common and may be present in as many as 14% of patients with lung cancer at presentation [25]. The platelet count is greater than 400×10^9/L in about 35% of patients with thrombocytosis. Paraneoplastic thrombocytosis is thought to occur from tumour production of cytokines such as IL-6 [19]. Thrombocytosis is usually associated with advanced disease and worse clinical outcomes [39].

Eosinophilia: Paraneoplastic eosinophilia appears due to tumour production of the eosinophil growth factors interleukin (IL)-3, IL-5, and GM-CSF (40). Paraneoplastic eosinophilia in tissue or blood is rare, but has been reported in patients with large cell carcinoma. It is usuallly asymptomatic, but in certain cases it can cause wheezing and dyspnea [35].

Hypercoagulable Disorders: A variety of hypercoagulable disorders have been associated with lung cancer and other malignancies [33-35, 41]. These hypercoagulable disorders include:

1. Trousseau's syndrome (migratory superficial thrombophlebitis).

2. Deep venous thrombosis and thromboembolism.

3. Disseminated intravascular coagulopathy.
4. Thrombotic microangiopathy.
5. Nonthrombotic microangiopathy.

D. Paraneoplastic Rheumatologic and Dermatologic Syndromes

Development of paraneoplastic rheumatologic and dermatologic syndromes often precedes a diagnosis of cancer or recurrence of a previously treated malignancy. Management of these disorders consist of cancer-directed treatment plus standard treatments of the nonparaneoplastic counterparts of these syndromes. Generally, these syndromes are less responsive to treatment than are the nonparaneoplastic equivalents [41, 42].

Hypertrophic Osteoarthropathy: Hypertrophic pulmonary osteoarthropathy (HPO) is defined by the presence of clubbing and periosteal proliferation of the tubular bones associated with lung cancer or other lung disease. HPO, particularly digital clubbing, is present in up to 10% of patients with lung cancer [41- 42]. Clinically, HPO is characterized by a symmetrical, painful arthropathy that usually involves the ankles, knees, wrists, and elbows. The metacarpal, metatarsal, and phalangeal bones may also be involved. A radiograph of the long bones (*i.e.*, tibia and fibula) shows characteristic periosteal new bone formation in patients with HPO. An isotope bone scan or PET typically demonstrates diffuse uptake by the long bones. The symptoms of HPO may resolve after tumour resection. For patients who are not operable, the usual treatment is with nonsteroidal antiinflammatory agents or a bisphosphonate [43].

Dermatomyositis: Dermatomyositis is inflammatory myopathy featuring multiple skin changes before the onset proximal muscle weakness. This inflammatory myopathy can be the presenting symptom in patients with lung cancer or can develop later in the course of disease. Dermatologic findings in dermatomyositis include heliotrop rash on the upper eyelids, an erythematous rash on the face, neck, back, chest and shoulders; and Gottron papules, a scaly eruption over the phalangeal joints that may mimic psoriasis. About 10%-to 25% of patients are paraneoplastic [42, 44].

ACKNOWLEDGEMENTS

Declared none.

CONFLICT OF INTEREST

The authors confirm that this article content has no conflict of interest.

REFERENCES

[1] Vaporciyan A, Kies MS, Stevens CW, Komaki R, Roth J. Cancer of the lung. In: Kufe DW, Pollock RE, Weichselbaum RR, Free III E, editors. Holland- Frei Cancer Medicine. 6th ed. London: BC Decker Inc; 2003. p. 1051-3.

[2] The American Thoracic Society and The European Respiratory Society. Pretreatment evaluation of non-small-cell lung cancer. Am J Respir Crit Care Med 1997; 156(1):320-32.

[3] Kraut M, Wozniak A. Lung cancer: Principles and Practice. In: Pass IH, Mitchell JB, Johnson DH, Turrisi AT, Minna JD, editors. Lung Cancer. 2nd ed. Philadelphia: Lippincott Williams□□Wilkins Publishers; 2000. p.35-73.

[4] Ginsberg JR, Vokes EE, Rozensweig K. Non-small cell lung cancer In: DeVita TV, Hellman S, Rosenberg SA. DeVita, editors. Cancer: Principles and Practice of Oncology. 6th ed. Philadelphia: Lippincott Williams & Wilkins Publishers; 2001. P.925-.

[5] Hyde L, Hyde CI.Clinical manifestations of lung cancer. Chest 1974; 65:299.

[6] Chuta CG, Greenberg ER, Baron J, *et al.* Presenting conditions of 1539 population based lung cancer patients by cell type and stage in New Hampshire and Vermont. Cancer 1985; 56 2107.

[7] Soares Pires F, Teixeira N, Coelho F, Damas C. Hemoptysis--etiology, evaluation and treatment in a university hospital. Rev Port Pneumol. 2011 Jan;17(1):7-14.

[8] Arcasoy SM, Jett JR. Superior Pulmonary Sulcus Tumours and Pancoast's Syndrome. N Engl J Med.1997; 337(19):1370-6.

[9] Kong YX, Wright G, Pesudovs K,†Day JO, Wainer Z, Weisinger H. Horner syndrome: Clin Exp Optom 2007; 90: 5: 336–344.

[10] Lim E, Ali A, Theodorou P, Nicholson AG, Ladas G, GoldstrawP. Intraoperative pleural lavage cytology is an independent prognostic indicator for staging non-small cell lung cancer. J Thorac Cardiovasc Surg 2004;127(4):1113-8.

[11] Pires NF, Morais A, Queiroga H. Superior vena cava syndrome as tumour presentation. Rev Port Pneumol. 2010 Jan-Feb;16(1):73-88.

[12] Vandecandelaere M, Flipo RM, Cortet B, Catanzariti L, DuquesnoyB, Delcambre B. Bone metastases revealing primary tumours. Comparison of two series separated by 30 years. Joint Bone Spine 2004;71(3):224-9.

[13] Beckles MA., Spiro SG, Colice GL, Rudd RM. Initial evaluation of the patient with lung cancer: symptoms, signs, laboratory tests, and paraneoplastic syndromes. Chest 2003;123(1 Suppl):97S- 104S.

[14] LGioulbasanis I, Georgoulias P, Vlachostergios PJ, Baracos V, Ghosh S, Giannousi Z, Papandreou CN, Mavroudis D, Georgoulias V. Mini Nutritional Assessment (MNA) and

biochemical markers of cachexia in metastatic lung cancer patients: Interrelations and associations with prognosis. Lung Cancer. 2011 May 30. [Epub ahead of print]abstract.

[15] Hamilton W, Peters TJ, Round A, Sharp. What are the clinical features of lung cancer before the diagnosis is made? A population based case-control study Thorax 2005;60: 1059-1065.

[16] Midhun DE, Jett JR. Lung Tumours. Section 8, Chapter 43.Comprehensive Respiratory Medicine Editors: Richard Albert, Stephen Spiro, James Jett MOSBY, Harcourt Brace and Company Limited 1999 ISBN: 0 7234 3118 3, p:8.43.1-8.43-24).

[17] Lumachi F,Brunello A, Roma A, Basso U. Medical treatment of malignancy-associated hypercalcemia. Curr Med Chem. 2008;15:415-421.

[18] Stewart AF. Hypercalcemia associated with cancer.N Engl J Med. 2005;15:415-421.

[19] Hiraki A, Ueoka H, Takata I, *et al.* Hypercalcemia- leukocytosis syndrome associated with lung cancer. Lung Cancer.2004;43:301.

[20] Thomas L, Kwok Y, Edelman MJ.Management of paraneoplastic syndromes in lung cancer. Curr Treat Options Oncol 2004;5:51.

[21] List AF, Hainstworth JD, Davis BW, *et al.* The syndrome of inappropriate secretion of antidiuretic hormone (SIADH) in small-cell lung cancer. J Clin Oncol 1986;4:1191.

[22] Hansen O, Sorensen P, Hansen KH. The occurrence of hyponatremia in SCLC and the influence on prognosis: A retrospective study of 453 patients treated in a single institution in a 10year period. Lung Cancer 2010;68:111.

[23] Ellison DH, Berl T. Clinical practice. The syndrome of inappropriate antidiuresis. N Engl J Med 2007;356:2064.

[24] Ilias I, Torpy DJ, Pacak K, *et al.* Cushing's syndrome due to ectopic corticotropin secretion: twenty years' experience at the National Institutes of Health. J Clin Endocrinol Metab 2005; 90:4955..

[25] Delisle L, Boyer MJ, Warr D, *et al.* Ectopic corticotropin syndrome and small-cell carcinoma of the lung. Clinical features, outcome, and complications. Arch Intern Med 1993; 153:746.

[26] Shepherd FA, Laskey J, Evans WK, *et al.* Cushing's syndrome associated with ectopic corticotropin production and small- cell lung cancer. J Clin Oncol 1992;10:21.

[27] Morandi U, Casali C, Rossi G. Bronchial typical carcinoid tumours. Semin Thorac cardiovasc Surg. 2006;18: 191-198.

[28] Teves DA. Clinical approach of Cushing syndrome resulting from ACTH- producing metastatic neuroendocrine tumour. Endocrinologist. 2005; 15:401-404.

[29] Honnorat J, Antoine JC. Paraneoplastic neurological syndromes. Orphanet J Rare Dis. 2007;2:27.

[30] Elrington GM, Murray NM, Spiro SG, Newsom-Davis J. Neurological paraneoplastic syndromes in patients with small cell lung cancer. A prospective survey of 150 patients. J Neurol Neurosurg Psychiatry 1991;54:764.

[31] Sillevis Smitt P, Grefkens J, de Leeuw B, *et al.* Survival and outcome in 73 anti-Hu positive patients with paraneoplastic encephalomyelitis/sensory neuronopathy. J Neurol 2002;249:745.

[32] De Beukelaar JW, Sillevis Smitt PA. Managing paraneoplastic neurological disorders. Oncologist.2006; 11:292-305.

[33] Kessler CM. The link between cancer and venous thromboembolism: a review. Am J Clin Onkol. 2009;32:3-7.

[34] Sierko E; Wojtukiewicz MZ. Platelets and angiogenesis in malignancy. Semin Thromb Hemost. 2004;30:95-108.

[35] Jameson JL, Johnson BE. Paraneoplastic syndromes: endocrinologic/hematologic. In:Fauci AS, Braunwald E, Kasper DL, Hauser SL, Longo DL, jameson JL, Loscalzo J,eds. Harrison's Principles of Internal Medicine. 17th ed. New York, NY: McGraw Hill Medical;2008:617-622.

[36] Shonfeld Y, Tal A, Berliner S, Pinkhas J. Leukocytosis in nonhematological malignancies- a possible tumour-associated marker. J cancer Res Clin Oncol. 1986; 111:54-58.

[37] Kasuga I, Makino S, Kiyokawa H, *et al.* Tumour-related leukocytosis is linked with poor prognosis in patients with lung carcinoma. Cancer 200192:2399.

[38] Kosmidis P, KrzakowskiM, ECAS Investigators. Anemia profiles in patients with lung cancer: what have we learned from the European Cancer Anemia Survey (ECAS)? Lung Cancer. 2005;50:401.

[39] Aoe K, Hiraki A, Ueoka H, *et al.* Thrombocytosis as a useful prognostic indicator in patients withlung cancer. Respiration 2004;71:170.

[40] Anagnostopoulus GK, sakorafas GH, Kostopoulos P, *et al.* Disseminated colon cancer with severe peripheral blood eosinophilia and elevated serum levels of interleukine-2, interleukine-3, interleukine-5, and GM-CSF. J Surg Onkol.2005;89:273-275.

[41] Pelosof LC, Gerber DE. Paraneoplastic syndromes: An approach to diagnosis and treatment. Mayo Clin Proc. 2010;85(9):838-854.

[42] Thiers BH, Sahn RE, Callen JP. Cutaneous manifestations of internal malignancy. CA cancer J Clin. 2009;59:73-98.

[43] Amital H, Applbaum YH, Vasiliev L, Rubinow A. Hypertrophic pumonary osteoarthropathy: control of pain and symptoms with pamidronate. Clin Rheumatol 2004;23:330.

[44] Dalakas MC, Hohlfeld R. Polymyositis and dermatomyositis. Lancet. 2003;362:971-982.

Lung Cancer: Clinical and Surgical Specifications, **2013, 119-128** **119**

CHAPTER 5

Radiological Evaluation of Lung Cancer

Ahmet Kürşad Poyraz and Abdurrahman Yasin Erkin Oğur*

Firat University, School of Medicine, Department of Radiology, Elazig, Turkey

Abstract: Chest radiography is often the first imaging study performed in patients with lung cancer. Average size at detection is approximately 2.5 cm by radiography. Multidetector computed tomography (CT) is widely available, fast, offers excellent spatial resolution and with current scanners is able to provide multiplanar reconstructions. Contrast enhanced computed tomography of the chest should be performed in patients who have known or suspected lung carcinoma who are eligible for treatment. A definitive surgical staging of lung cancer is possible with contrast enhanced computed tomography. Magnetic resonance imaging has no advantage over CT in staging of the mediastinum.

Adenocarcinoma is typically a peripheral nodule or mass of subpleural location and occurs primarily in the upper lobes. Squamous cell carcinomas usually manifests as a hilar or perihilar mass lesion with cavitation. Bronchial obstruction is common and may result in atelectasis or post-obstructive pneumonia. Large mediastinal mass extending to at least one hilum is characteristic of small-cell lung cancer on radiography. Computed tomography reveals bulky mediastinal mass, post-obstructive pneumonitis or collapse, bronchial encasement or obstruction, pleural effusion and pulmonary nodule.

Bronchial carcinoids are lobular central mass which may have an endobronchial component and may demonstrate intense contrast enhancement and variable patterns of calcification.

Keywords: Computed tomography, radiography, non-small cell cancer, small cell cancer.

INTRODUCTION

Lung cancers are divided into two main types called small cell lung cancer and non small cell lung cancer (NSCLC). Non-small cell lung cancers have 3

***Address correspondence to Abdurrahman Yasin Erkin Oğur:** Euphrates University, School of Medicine, Department of Radiology, Elazig, Turkey; Tel: +90 424 2333555/1397; Fax: +90 424 2388096; E-mail: erkinogur@yahoo.com subtypes: adenocarcinoma, squamous cell carcinoma and large cell carcinoma. The most common subtype of lung cancer is adenocarcinoma. Lung cancers which originate from neuroendocrine cells and infiltrate the bronchial submucosa called small cell lung cancers. Pulmonary nodule is a mass lesion smaller than 3 cm diameter with round or oval shape. The role of imaging is to separate benign from malignant nodules.

Lung cancers including non-small cell, small cell and carcinoids are classified using TNM staging system.

Table 1(a): TNM Classification of Malignant Tumours - 7th edition (International Union Against Cancer)

Tx	Primary tumour can not be assessed
T0	No evidence of primary tumour
Tis	Carcinoma *in situ*
T1 **T1a** **T1b**	<3 cm <2 cm >2 – 3 cm
T2 **T2a** **T2b**	Main bronchus >2 cm from carina, invades visceral pleura, partial atelectasis >3- 5 cm >5 cm -7 cm
T3	>7 cm; chest wall, diaphragm, pericardium, mediastinal pleura, main bronchus <2 cm from carina, total atelectasis, separate nodule(s) in same lobe
T4	Mediastinum, heart, great vessels, carina, trachea, esophagus, vertebra; separate tumour nodule(s) in a different ipsilateral lobe
Nx	Regional lymph nodes cannot be assessed
N0	No regional lymph node metastasis
N1	Ipsilateral peribronchial, ipsilateral hilar
N2	Ipsilateral mediastinal, subcarinal
N3	Contralateral mediastinal or hilar, scalene or supraclavicular
Mx	Distant metastasis cannot be assessed
M0	No distant metastasis
M1 **M1a** **M1b**	 Separate tumour nodule(s) in a contralateral lobe; pleural nodules or malignant pleural or pericardial effusion Distant metastasis

Table 1(b): TNM Classification of Malignant Tumours - 7th edition (International Union Against Cancer)

	T	N	M
Occult Carcinoma	Tx	N0	-
Stage 0	Tis	N0	-
Stage IA	T1a,b	N0	-
Stage IB	T2a	N0	-
Stage IIA	T2b T1a,b T2a	N0 N1 N1	-
Stage IIB	T2b T3	N1 N0	-
Stage IIIA	T1a,b – T2a,b T3 T4	N2 N1, N2 N0, N1	-
Stage IIIB	T4 Any T	N2 N3	-
Stage IV	Any T	Any N	M1

NON-SMALL CELL LUNG CANCER

NSCLC accounts for about 80% of lung cancers. Lung cancer is 1.5 times more likely to occur in the right lung than in the left lung [1]. Approximately half of primary pulmonary adenocarcinomas manifest as isolated peripheral solitary pulmonary nodule, while squamous cell carcinomas that manifest as solitary pulmonary nodule are more likely to be centrally located and associated with cavitation [2].

Nodule morphology is associated with mean survival time in NSCLC. Nodules with smooth and well defined edges are related with longer survival time than smooth and poor defined edges. The shortest survival time is related to tumours with spiculated edges. Patients, whose tumours with homogenous structure had the longest median survival time. Tumours with air bronchogram, cavitation and inhomogenous internal structure are related to shorter survival time, respectively. Tumours showing peripheral halo sign related to long median survival period however, bronchovascular bundle thickening around tumour related to shortest median survival [3].

Adenocarcinoma is typically a peripheral nodule or mass of subpleural location and occurs primarily in the upper lobes. The borders of the tumour may be lobulated and well defined or spiculated and ill defined. Pleural involvement may be extensive and circumferential and may mimic mesothelioma (Fig. **1**) [4].

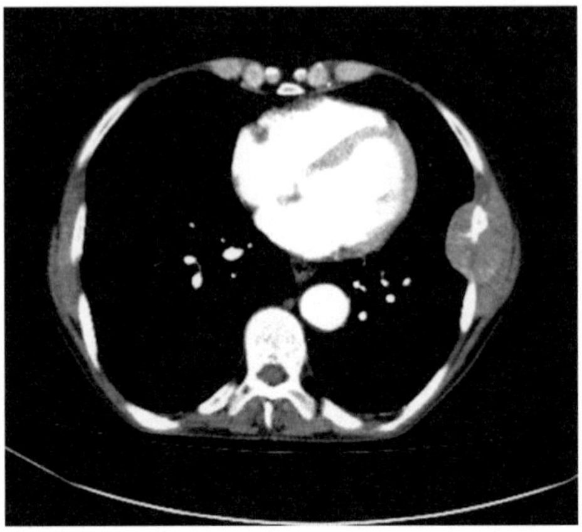

Figure 1: Axial CECT shows peripheral homogenous well defined mass lesion with osseous invasion. Found to be adenocarcinoma at histology. Circumferential pleural involvement mimics mesothelioma.

Squamous cell carcinomas usually manifests radiologically as a hilar or perihilar mass. Bronchial obstruction is common and may result in atelectasis or post-obstructive pneumonia (Figs. **2, 3**) [5].

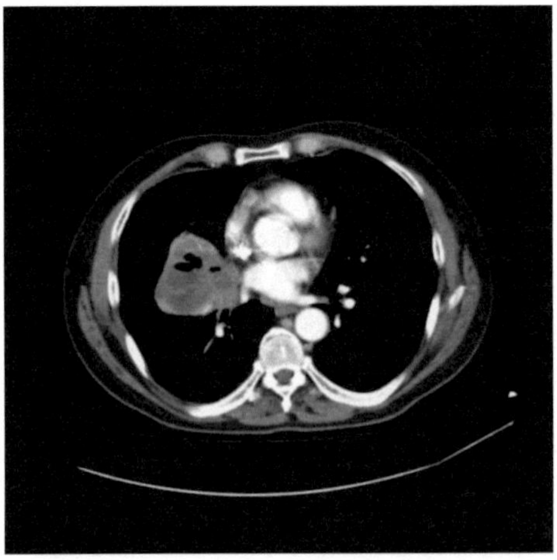

Figure 2: Axial CECT shows large necrotic mass in right lung with cavitation. Lesion diagnosed as squamous cell carcinoma at histology.

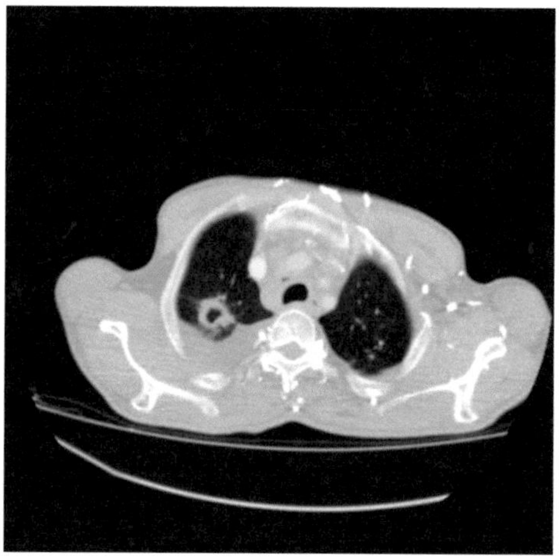

Figure 3: Axial CECT shows ill defined cavitary lesion in right upper lobe with ground glass opacity and pleural effusion. Lesion diagnosed as squamous cell carcinoma at histology.

At chest radiography, a solitary pulmonary nodule is seldom evident until it is at least 9 mm in diameter [7]. Average size at detection is approximately 2.5 cm by radiography. Tumour with hilar enlargement, chest wall invasion or bone destruction can be detected with radiography [8].

CT is widely available, fast, offers excellent spatial resolution and with current scanners is able to provide multiplanar reconstructions. CT of the chest should be performed in patients who have known or suspected lung carcinoma who are eligible for treatment [9].

Contrast enhanced computed tomography shows endobronchial lesions, lobar collapse and postobstructive pneumonitis due to bronchial obstruction. Computed tomography also provides information about pleural metastasis, mediastinal invasion and pleural effusion. Short axis of mediastinal lymph nodes greater than 1 cm considered abnormal and should be suspected for metastasis. Non-contrast enhanced computed tomography has an advantage of no contrast reactions and nephrotoxity with better adrenal lesion characterization however, it is difficult to detect hilar lymph nodes and vascular invasion [8].

MR imaging is reserved mostly for superior sulcus tumours, brachial plexus involvement, chest wall invasion and extrathoracic metastases. Advantages of MR imaging is superior soft tissue contrast and lack of ionising radiation. MR imaging is more vulnerable to motion artifacts than CT so cardiac pulsation and respiratory motion result in signal loss [9].

Although thoracic computed tomography has been considered the standard modality of choice for the assessment of intrathoracic spread of lung cancer [10], PET/CT and whole body MRI can be preferred as an alternative method. Whole body MRI is more useful for detecting brain and hepatic metastases, whereas PET/CT was more useful for detecting lymph node and soft-tissue metastases. All lymph nodes in the thorax and extrathoracic regions with abnormal FDG uptake (greater than mediastinal blood pool uptake) in the extrathoracic regions should be considered to be metastatic. Any nodule more than 10 mm in diameter with FDG uptake more than that of the mediastinal blood pool should be considered malignant [11]. Causes of false positive results are infections and sarcoidosis, false negative results are lesions smaller than 1 cm diameter, low grade adenocarcinomas, brochioloalveolar carcinoma and carcinoid tumour. In case of metastasis suspect brain MRI should be performed [8].

SMALL-CELL LUNG CANCER

The majority of patients with small cell carcinoma have metastatic disease at the time of presentation. In many cases, the primary tumour is not evident radiologically. There is typically a hilar or perihilar mass with extensive mediastinal lymphadenopaty. Small cell carcinoma usually invades adjacent structures (Fig. **4**) [5].

Primary pulmonary lesion often not detected radiographically. Tumour may collapse a lobe or entire lung. Lesion usually quite large at the time of diagnosis. Large mediastinal mass extending to at least one hilum is characteristic of small-cell lung cancer on radiography. Lobar consolidation and elevation of hemidiaphragm due to phrenic nevre involvement or pleural effusion can be seen on radiography [8].

Non enhanced computed tomography reveals bulky mediastinal mass, post-obstructive pneumonitis or collapse, bronchial encasement or obstruction, pleural effusion and pulmonary nodule. Contrast enhanced computed tomography demonstrates superior vena cava compression, invasion and pulmonary artery, aorta or great vessel enveloping. Role of PET remains controversial. Bone scan shows metastases as increased uptake areas [8].

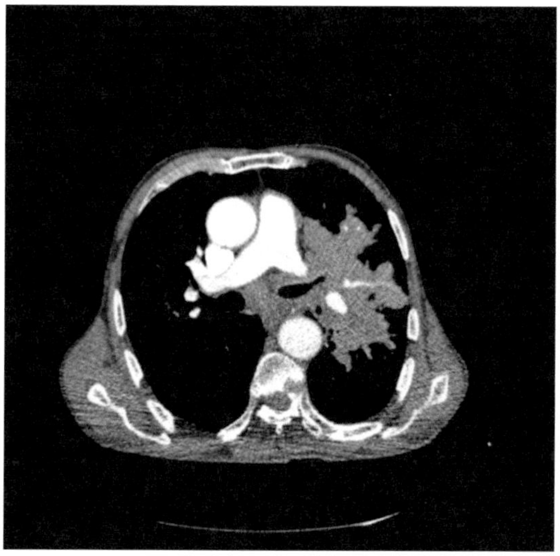

Figure 4: Axial CECT shows bulky mediastinal mass enveloping left main pulmonary artery. Lesion encasesleft main bronchus with mediastinal invasion.

BRONCHIAL CARCINOID

Bronchial carcinoid is a well defined lobular central mass which may have an endobronchial component and may be associated with recurrent pneumonia, atelectasis, bronchiectasis or mucoid impaction. Carcinoids may demonstrate intense contrast enhancement and variable patterns of calcification [6].

PULMONARY NODULE

A nodule is as a focal round or oval opacity that measured less than 30 mm in diameter. Most pulmonary nodules are found to be granulomas, lung cancers, or hamartomas [12,13]. Detection and work-up of solitary pulmonary nodules (SPNs) are critical because SPNs may be malignant [14].

Radiological goal is to separate benign from malignant nodules. Benign pattern calcification or presence of fat supports benign nodule. Positive fat is 94% sensitive for malignancy. 90% of nodules <2 cm are benign.

At chest radiography, it is difficult to detect a solitary pulmonary nodule smaller than 9 mm in diameter. Nodules shown to be stable at 2-year follow-up are considered benign and are no longer followed with CT [15].

With the improved technical quality of CT scans, more small lesions are now detectable in the lungs.

Some are normal intrapulmonary lymph nodes, which are typically small, round or oval, well-defined nodules in a subpleural location, most often in the lower lobes; others are granulomas which are not calcified [16]. The most common CT appearance of CT screening–detected lung cancers is an irregular semisolid or solid nodule [17].

Non-enhanced computed tomography determines pulmonary or extrapulmonary nodules. Although calcification and fat content supports benign process, 2% of lung cancers <3 cm have calcification. Osteogenic sarcoma and chondrosarcoma metastases have diffuse calcification [8]. If a lesion of this type has any of several defined patterns of calcification (concentric, uniform, popcorn, central), it can be classified confidently as benign. Certain other patterns of calcification (eg, eccentric, stippled) are indeterminate and should be considered potentially malignant [18]. Some malignancies, such as a metastasis from liposarcoma or renal cell carcinoma, may occasionally contain fat [19]. Contrast enhanced computed tomography have an advantage to detect lymph nodes, pleural, chest wall, liver and adrenal involvement [8].

PET for nodules 1-3 cm diameter have a sensitivity 94%, specifity 83% [20]. False negative results include small nodules, carcinoid, bronchioloalveolar cell carcinoma, cavitary nodules. False positive results include tuberculosis, histoplasmosis, sarcoidosis and rheumatoid nodules. Furthermore, sensitivity and specificity are not as high for nodules that are smaller than 1 cm in diameter [21].

PULMONARY METASTASES

Pulmonary metastases represent the most common neoplasms of the lung. Metastases are usually multifocal spherical nodules or masses with well defined borders and an angiocentric distribution. Metastases are more numerous in peripheral subpleural locations and the lower lobes [22].

ACKNOWLEDGEMENTS

Declared none.

CONFLICT OF INTEREST

The authors confirm that this article content has no conflict of interest.

REFERENCES

[1] Garland, LH (1961), 'Bronchial carcinomas: lobar distribution of lesions in 250 cases', *Calif Med*, no. 94, p. 7–8.
[2] Quinn D. Gianlupi A, Broste S (1996), 'The changing radiographic presentation of bronchogenic carcinoma with reference to cell types', *Chest*, no. 110, p. 1474–1479.
[3] Meniga IN *et al.* (2010), 'Prognostic value of computed tomography morphologic characteristics in stage I non-small-cell lung cancer', *Clin Lung Cancer*, no. 11(2), p. 98-104.
[4] Adler B, Padley S, Miller RR, Müller NN (1992), 'High-Resolution CT of bronchioloalveolar carcinoma', *AJR*, no. 159, p. 275-277.
[5] Rosado de Christenson ML, Templeton PA, Moran CA (1994), 'Bronchogenic Carcinoma: radiologic-pathologic correlation', *RadioGraphics*, no. 14, p. 429-446.
[6] Kirejczyk WM, Rosadp de Christenson ML, Travis WD, Olmedilla Arrequi G (1997), 'Bronchial Carcinoid: imaging features', *AJR*, no. 168 (3), Suppl: 109.
[7] Kundel HL (1981), 'Predictive value and threshold detectability of lung tumours', *Radiology*, no. 139, p. 25–29.
[8] Gurney JW, Winer-Muram HT, Stern EJ & Boiselle PM (2006), *Diagnostic Imaging Chest*, 1st ed., Amirsys Inc, Salt Lake City, Utah
[9] Godelman A, Haramati LB (2008), 'MR imaging in diagnosis and staging of pulmonary carcinoma', *Magn Reson Imaging Clin N Am*, no. 16, p. 309-317.
[10] 'Pretreatment evaluation of non-small-cell lung cancer: The American Thoracic Society and The European Respiratory Society', *Am J Respir Crit Care Med*, no. 156, p. 320–332.
[11] Yi CA, Shin KM, Lee KS *et al.* (2008), 'Non-small cell lung cancer staging: efficacy comparison of integrated PET/CT *versus* 3.0-T whole-body MR imaging', *Radiology*, no. 248, p. 632-642
[12] Bateson EM (1965),' An analysis of 155 solitary lung lesions illustrating the differential diagnosis of mixed tumours of the lung', *Clin Radiol*, no.16, p. 51–65.
[13] Murthy SC, Rice TW (2002), 'The solitary pulmonary nodule: a primer on differential diagnosis', *Semin Thorac Cardiovasc Surg*, no. 14, p. 239–249.
[14] Siegelman SS, Zerhouni EA, Leo FP, Khouri NF, Stitik FP (1980), 'CT of the solitary pulmonary nodule', *AJR*, no. 135, p. 1–13.
[15] Winer-Muram HT (2006), 'The solitary pulmonary nodule', *Radiology*, no. 239, p. 34-49.
[16] Keogan M, Tung K, Kaplan D, et al (1993), 'The significance of pulmonary nodules detected on CT staging for lung cancer', *Clin Radiol*, no. 48, p. 94-96.
[17] Lindell RM, Hartman TE, Swensen SJ et al (2007), 'Five-year lung cancer screening experience: CT appearance, growth rate, location, and histologic features of 61 lung cancers', *Radiology*, no. 242, p. 555-562

[18] Khan A, Herman P, Vorwecki P (1991), 'Solitary pulmonary nodules: comparison and classification with standard, thin section, and reference phantom CT', *Radiology*, no. 179, p. 477-481.

[19] Muram TM, Aisen A (2003), 'Fatty metastatic lesions in 2 patients with renal clear-cell carcinoma', *J Comput Assist Tomogr*, no. 27, p. 869–870.

[20] Gould MK, Maclean CC, Kuschner WG, Rydzak CE, Owens DK (2001), 'Accuracy of positron emission tomography for diagnosis of pulmonary nodules and mass lesions: a meta-analysis', *JAMA, no.* 285, p. 914–924.

[21] Goldsmith SJ, Kostakoglu L (2000), 'Nuclear medicine imaging of lung cancer', *Radiol Clin North Am*, no. 38, p. 511–524.

[22] Coppage L, Shaw C, Curtis AM (1987), 'Metastatic disease to the chest in patients with extrathoracic maignancy', *J Thorac Imag*, no. 2, p. 24-37.

Send Orders of Reprints at reprints@benthamscience.net
Lung Cancer: Clinical and Surgical Specifications, 2013, 129-164

CHAPTER 6

Current Scintigraphic Imaging of Lung Cancer

Tansel Ansal Balci*

Firat (Euphrates) University School of Medicine, Department of Nuclear Medicine, Elazig, Turkey

Abstract: In recent years, conventional scintigraphical techniques are rarely used in lung cancer patients except the whole body bone scanning and preoperative quantitative lung scintigraphy. With the introduction of positron emission tomography (PET) and more recently PET/CT, management of the lung cancer patients and of the patients with solitary pulmonary nodule has extremely changed from diagnosis to prognosis. The combination of PET with CT scanning allows the integration of metabolic and morphological image information. Nowadays, PET/CT is an accepted modality for lung cancer patients, for many cancer patients, in terms of diagnosis, staging, therapy/radiotherapy planning, prognostic prediction, response monitoring and assessment of recurrence, and becomes widespread throughout the world. In this chapter PET and PET/CT are mainly mentioned as the up-to-date nuclear medicine modalities for diagnostic and therapeutic management in lung cancer.

Keywords: Lung cancer, nuclear medicine, scintigraphy, preoperative evaluation, positron emission tomography, PET, PET/CT, fluorodeoxyglucose, FDG, standard uptake value, SUVmax, solitary pulmonary nodule, diagnosis, staging, therapy response, metastasis, recurrence, residual tissue assessment, survival assessment, radiation therapy planning, tumour hypoxia, neuroendocrine lung cancer.

INTRODUCTION

Lung cancer is the most common cancer and the main cause of death in many countries. Imaging plays a very important role for the whole management (*i.e.* screening, diagnosing, staging, and therapy following) of the patients with lung cancer. Although morphological imaging such as X-ray and CT are still used to get to these objectives, these modalities have some limitations especially at the

***Address correspondence to Tansel Ansal Balci:** Firat (Euphrates) University School of Medicine, Department of Nuclear Medicine, Elazig, Turkey; Tel: +90 424 2333555 / 2095; Fax: +90 2388096; E-mail: tansel_balci@yahoo.com point of the benign-malignant lesion differentiation, the possibility of metastases in normal-sized lymph nodes and the unsuspected distant metastases. The exact evaluation of the diagnosis and the staging is not achieved in these circumstances. Scintigraphic methods by using radiopharmaceuticals help anatomic imaging modalities in terms of determining the metabolic activity of the lesions. The whole body can be screened scintigraphically; planar or tomographic images (single photon emission computed tomography-SPECT) could be also obtained. There are many radiopharmaceuticals that are used for imaging of lung cancer. Some of these are Tc-99m labeled ones like sestamibi or tetrofosmin, Ga-67 citrate and Tl-201 (Fig. **1**). Additionally, the pulmonary metastases of other cancers can be visualized with these agents or some other radiopharmaceuticals such as radioactive iodine, MIBG (metaiodobenzylguanidine), octreotide, *etc.*

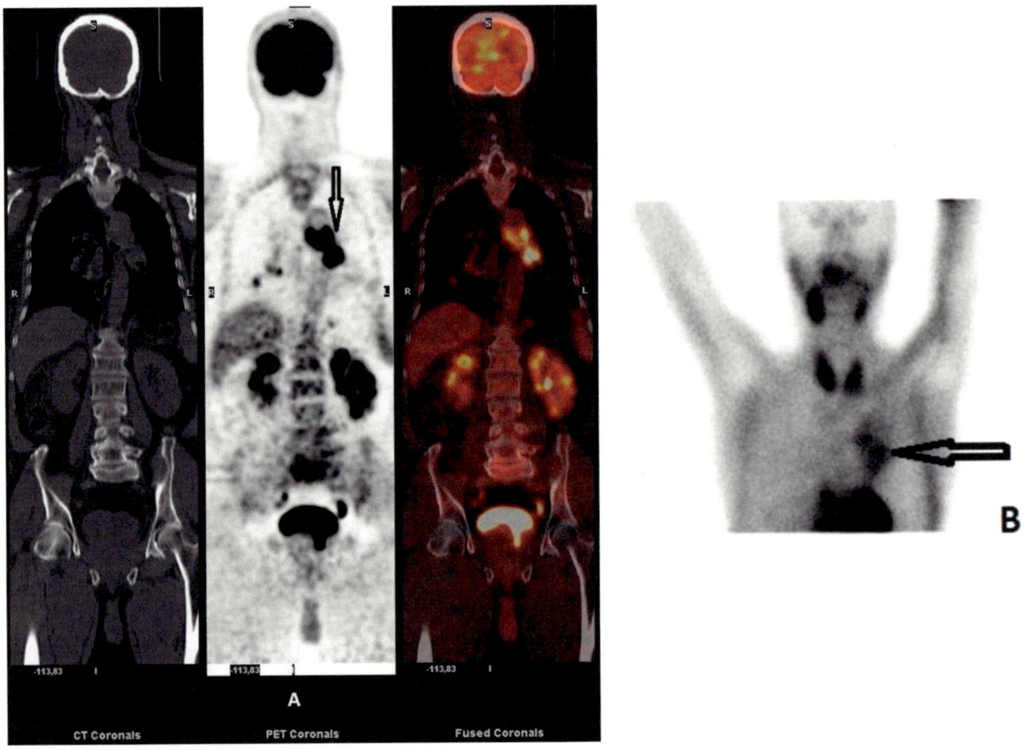

Figure 1: FDG (A) and Tc99m sestamibi (B) uptake in lung cancer (arrow). Sestamibi uptake is more insignificant compared to FDG.

Today, except for some cases in which these radiopharmaceuticals and these imaging techniques have to be definitely used, a new spectacular nuclear medicine modality which uses positron emitting radiopharmaceuticals replaced all of them. This is the positron emission tomography (PET). With the introduction of the PET systems, a new era in the field of oncology and also in lung cancer management has begun. There is a trend of shifting patients from conventional nuclear medicine to PET/CT not only for lung cancer but for the other oncological situations. PET provides metabolic information regarding tumour biology thus more accurate data about the nature and the behavior of tumour. CT or MRI plays a significant role in initial staging; but the morphological information is insufficient in many cases when compared to the metabolic or molecular information obtained by PET. The most common pharmaceutical that is used for imaging in PET is F-18 Flourodeoxyglucose (FDG). Tumours are usually seen as "hot spots" in FDG-PET/CT imaging. There are some other pharmaceuticals which are used less frequently and hence are less mentioned in this text. However main radiopharmaceutical that would be the subject in this chapter is F-18 FDG in terms of lung cancer. Integration of computerized tomography (CT) to PET device allows the integration of metabolic and morphological image information at high resolution. The combination of PET with CT increased accuracy of both of these techniques. PET/CT devices are gaining better spatial resolution and speed because of the developments in technology. Whole-body imaging from the head to the knees is accomplished in nearly 20 min. Spatial resolution reaches 4 mm. The standard whole-body imaging with PET/CT simplifies staging and speeds up decision processes for appropriate therapeutic strategies. Therefore, PET/CT is now considered as the most important imaging system for diagnosis, staging, radiation therapy planning, therapy response and also prognosis determination of the lung cancer, especially non-small cell lung cancer (NSCLC). The main goal of this chapter is to define the place of PET/CT beyond the other scintigraphical techniques in the management of lung cancer patients. First we mention in short about scintigraphical preoperative management of a patient with lung cancer. Then some technical issues on lung cancer imaging with PET/CT will be described. This is followed by the discussion of the different scintigraphic approaches, mainly FDG-PET including the benefits and limitations, about the imaging of the pulmonary malignancies after initial suspicion by chest CT. Future developments concerning lung cancer that can be expected in nuclear medicine will also be mentioned at the end of the chapter.

PREOPERATIVE SCINTIGRAPHIC EVALUATION OF LUNG CANCER PATIENTS

Quantitative lung perfusion or ventilation scintigraphy can be performed for the prediction of postoperative pulmonary function in preoperative period of lung cancer or the other lung pathologies [1, 2]. It is important especially for the patients with poor pulmonary function. Split lung functions can be assessed and the postoperative forced expiratory volume in 1 sec (FEV1) can be predicted by this imaging modality. According to ACCP guideline, in patients with a preoperative FEV1 or DLCO of lower than 80% predicted, predicted postoperative (ppo) lung function may be calculated by estimating the amount of functioning lung tissue that would be lost with the surgical resection [3]. Risk for perioperative complications of pulmonary surgery increases if predicted postoperative FEV_1 or DLCO is estimated as < 40%. One of the methods used for this aim is scintigraphic imaging and quantification, including ventilation scanning or perfusion scanning [1, 4, 5]. In patients with FEV1 or the diffusing capacity of the lung for carbon monoxide (DLCO) < 80% predicted, the probable postoperative pulmonary reserve should be estimated by either the perfusion scan method for pneumonectomy or the anatomic method for lobectomy [3]. The perfusion scintigraphy is preferred to estimate the PPO FEV1 and DLCO after pneumonectomy because the anatomic method tends to underestimate actual postoperative FEV1 values (Fig. **2**). However, after a lobectomy the anatomic method is recommended to estimate the pulmonary function [3]. Pulmonary perfusion scintigraphy is chosen rather than the ventilation scintigraphy because of the simplicity of it [6].

Whole-lung counts obtained from the posterior views on the perfusion scan were used to calculate predicted postpneumonectomy values for FEV1 and DLCO using the following formula [3]:

ppo FEV1% = preoperative FEV1% x (1 - functional contribution of affected lung)

Although, anatomic method is recommended for the predicted postlobectomy values, it can also be calculated based on perfusion scanning with a combination of the lateral and posteroanterior view counts [7]. At present, perfusion scintigraphy seems as a unique, simple, easy tolerable, accurate means for preoperative quantification.

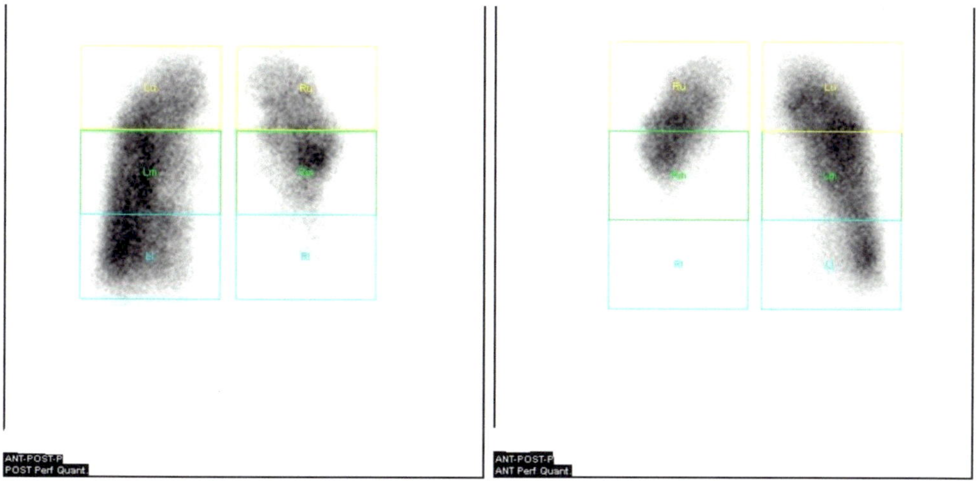

	Posterior Kct				Geometric Mean Kct				Anterior Kct			
	Left		Right		Left Lung		Right Lung		Right		Left	
	%	Kct	%	Kct	%	Kct	%	Kct	%	Kct	%	Kct
Upper Zone:	15,7	34,88	12,6	27,86	18,9	40,59	14,8	31,99	17,2	36,75	22,3	47,21
Middle Zone:	28,5	63,07	15,5	34,39	29,2	62,63	15,1	32,36	14,3	30,43	29,2	62,20
Lower Zone:	24,5	54,25	3,2	7,04	19,3	41,56	2,7	5,72	2,2	4,65	14,9	31,84
Total Lung:	68,7	152,20	31,3	69,28	67,4	144,78	32,6	70,07	33,7	71,83	66,3	141,26

Figure 2: Preoperative quantitative pulmonary perfusion scintigraphy of a patient with a large mass on middle and lower lobe of the right lung. The perfusion index of the right lung was quantified as 32.6% while the left lung was 67.4%.

PET/CT in LUNG CANCER

Imaging Technique

Patient Preparation

The most important part of patient's preparation step in all FDG-PET studies for optimal imaging is injecting the FDG while the plasma glucose level of the patient is in normal limits. Patients are warned to fast the night before or at least for 4-6 hours. Elevated plasma glucose levels prior to the study result with suboptimal image quality, so that glucose level is measured initially and if it is elevated (*e.g.* in case of diabetic status) insulin injection may even be required which was an undesired circumstance. Be aware that if the glucose level is high, rate of false negative results could be expected higher especially in oncological patients.

Imaging

After injection of the FDG, imaging should be started optimum 60 minutes later in order to improve image quality. It is also known that signal to noise ratio increases over time especially for malignant tumours. Even late images should be obtained if necessary because some of malignancies, especially solitary pulmonary nodules, manifest in the later phase.

From base of the cranium to the proximal femur is usually in field of view for oncological studies. However, for lung cancer imaging, there would be a benefit if the brain was included in the scanning because of the possibility of frequent brain metastasis of lung cancer.

Usually CT-based attenuation correction is applied to the images and we use corrected PET images for interpretation. But in some special instances which will be mentioned in this text, uncorrected data would be evaluated.

Interpretation

Interpretation of PET/CT images needs full information of patients' clinical situation; medical history and images of other techniques must be evaluated carefully prior to imaging. Some misinterpretations can be prevented with information obtained from patient (*e.g.* history of asbestos exposure or tuberculosis infection).

Corrected PET images in conjunction with CT images and fusion images should be examined carefully with uncorrected PET data if necessary. In case of attenuation correction artifacts, evaluating corrected images with uncorrected images would be appropriate. For thoracic imaging, segment charts of lung and mediastinal lymph node maps would be necessary.

Diaphragmatic artifacts may occur because of the vertical motion of diaphragm. Thus a pulmonary pathology localized on the lung basis can be evaluated as a liver pathology or on the contrary a hepatic pathology localized on the dome of the liver can be evaluated as lung pathology.

Physiological respiratory motion can also cause a motion artifact (Fig. **3**). In this manner, lesion may be visualized on the more anteriorly or posteriorly than it is visualized in CT images and the lesion would also be visualized as having less FDG uptake.

The nuclear medicine specialists have to be careful about these motion artifacts because they can cause false negative or false positive results.

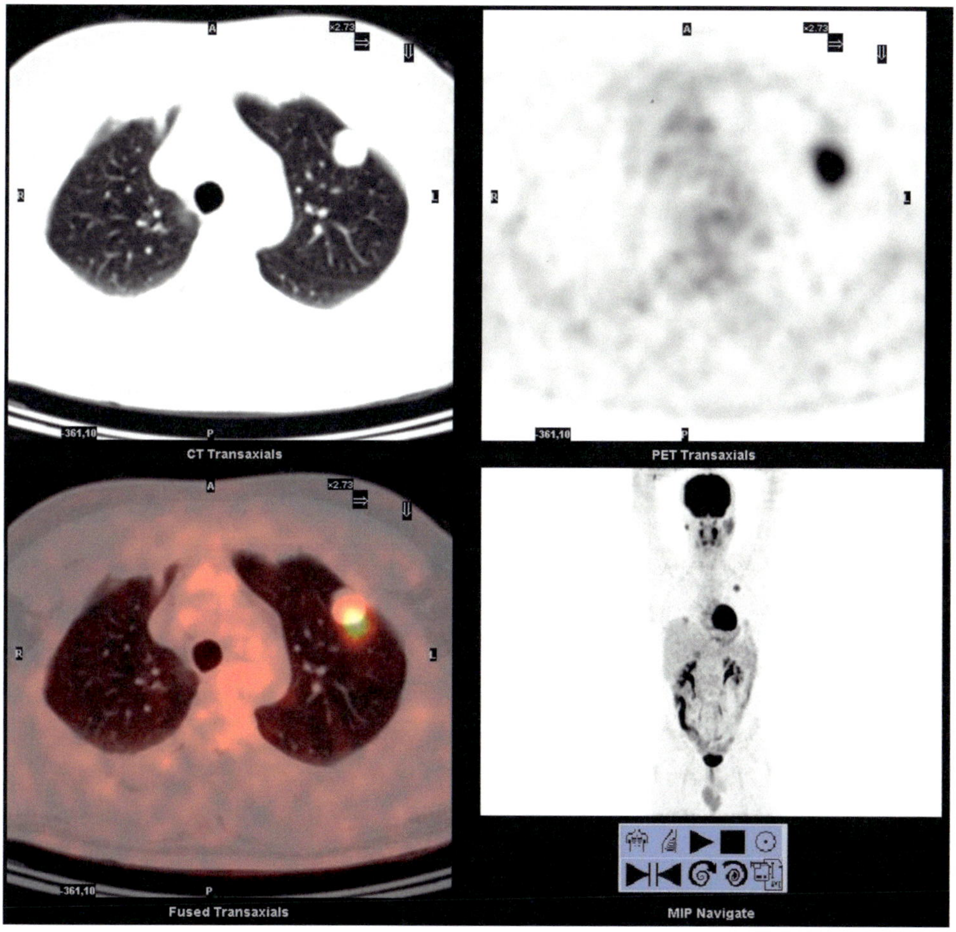

Figure 3: Respiratory motion can cause mismatch (as seen on the fused image at the left lower) between the real lesion place and the place of FDG uptake. Respiratory-gated study helps the localization.

Quantification

Standardized uptake value (SUV) reflects the uptake measurement of the region of interest according to injected dose and total body dose. Maximum SUV (SUVmax) is the most commonly used quantification unit for identifying what we see on images numerically. For most of the malignant tumours, SUVmax level above 2.5 was considered positive for malignancy. Increasing SUV between the early and late imaging suggests malignant pathology. In contrast, in benign pathologies SUV decreases over time. One of the most important applications of this quantification value is the evaluation of the treatment response and also obtaining prognostic information. Difference of the SUVmax values between pretreatment and post-treatment scans gives information about response to the treatment. But care should be taken in order to avoid mistakes. SUVmax has limitations such as dependency to several factors that may influence SUVmax results *i.e.* high glucose levels. Some authors also use cut-off levels for SUVmax according to some individual situations.

INDICATIONS OF PET/CT

1. SOLITARY PULMONARY NODULE

The solitary pulmonary nodule (SPN) is a frequent finding on the thoracic X-ray and CT. It is a lesion under 3 cm diameter surrounded by normal lung tissue [8]. Actually, SPN is the stage IA of lung cancer. Lesions bigger than 3 cm are not a SPN anymore, but mass lesion. A high percentage of the SPNs is malignant, *i.e.* primary lung cancer or metastasis of other tumours. There is no standardized protocol in the diagnosis and management of the SPN. CT has been used for the estimation of malignant or benign nature of a SPN for many years. However, it is impossible to decide exactly if a solitary pulmonary nodule is malignant by means of CT-based parameters. At the end of several investigations, excisional biopsy would generally be essential for patients because half of these nodules can be malignant [9]. While an initial high probability of benign diagnosis avoids the invasive treatment, the initial diagnosis of a malignant process will lead to further invasive investigations. Unfortunately there would be many unnecessary explorations in this kind of management. One of the first indications of PET/CT is solitary pulmonary nodule definition. SUVmax levels above 2.5 were considered malignant for solitary pulmonary nodules. Especially the spiculated nodules on CT with strongly positive FDG-PET are usually malignant. Average sensitivity and accuracy of PET/CT for nodule characterization is 96% and 94%, respectively according to the literature [10]. Specificity of FDG-PET for malignancy intensifies with increasing SUV (Fig. **4**). High negative predictive value of PET/CT can help like as an exclusion test (Fig. **5**). However, serial follow up scans are warranted. Histopathological data have to be obtained in case of positive PET/CT findings. For malignant SPNs, poor prognosis is expected between 5 to 10 SUV values.

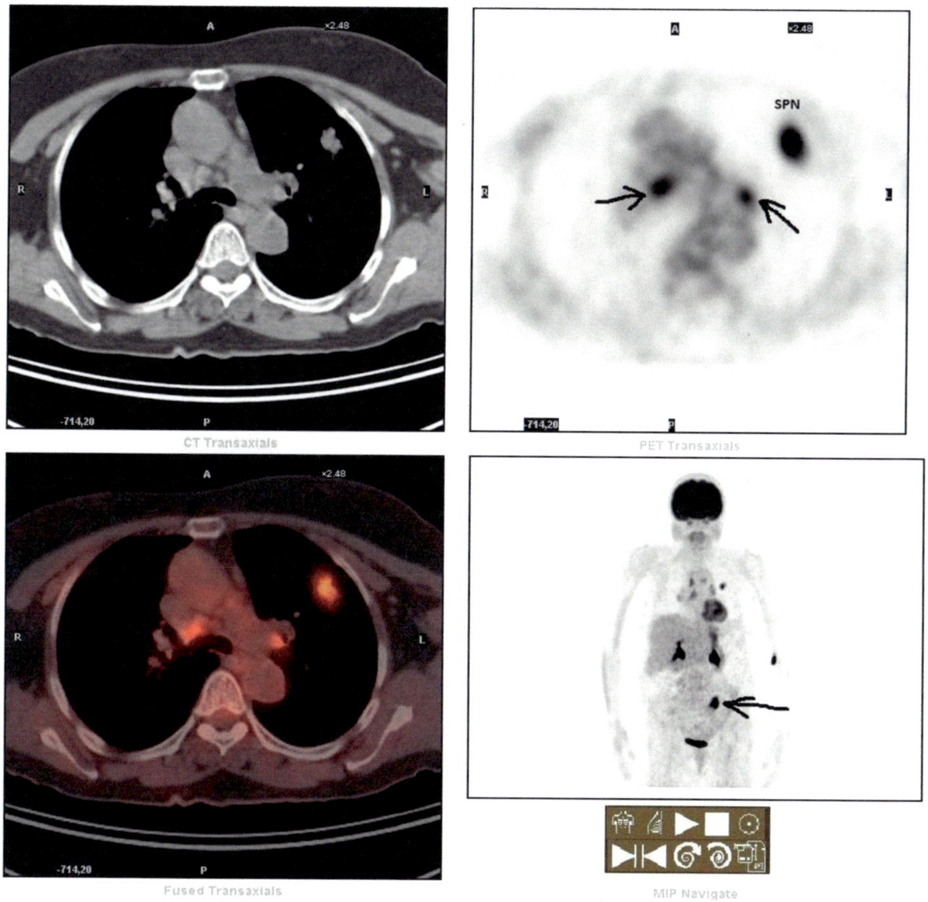

Figure 4: Malignant SPN on the upper lobe of the left lung with mediastinal lymph node involvements (arrows). SUVmax value of the SPN was 8. A very significant pathological FDG uptake (long arrow on the MIP image) on the sigmoid colon relating to a secondary malignancy (SUVmax was 10.5) was also visualized.

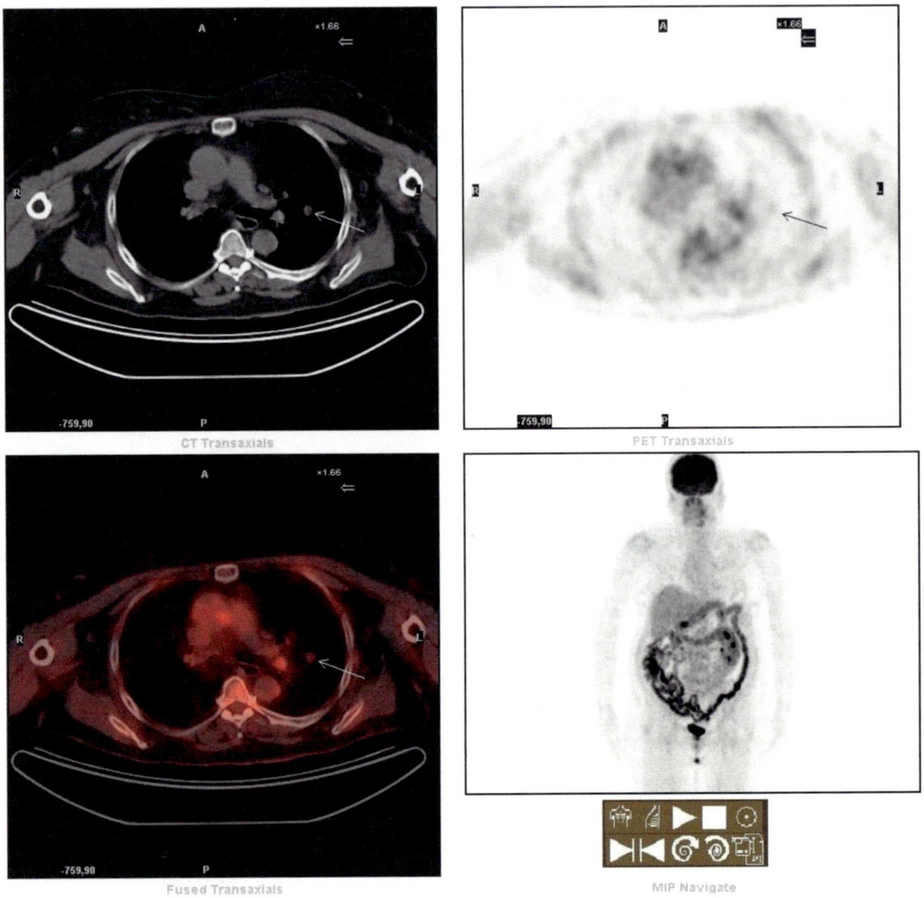

Figure 5: SUVmax (early) and SUVmax (late) of the well-defined nodular lesion on the upper lobe of the left lung (arrow) were 1 and 0.6, respectively. There was not another pathological FDG uptake suggesting malignancy throughout the body. With this appearance it is defined as a benign SPN.

PET/CT has resolution limitation and because of that it is not possible to evaluate nodules with less than 8-10 mm diameter [11]. Visualized activity is lower on the smaller lesions. This is called partial volume effect.

False positive interpretations may also be a consequence of some benign pathologies, such as inflammatory changes (*e.g.* abscess, granulomatous infections like tuberculosis, sarcoidosis, fungal disease), benign neoplasms (hamartomas), silicosis, infarction, *etc.* False negative results are due to small lesions and lack of avidity of tumour tissue to FDG. Certain lung carcinoma types (*i.e.* bronchoalveolar carcinoma, well-differentiated adenocarcinomas and some carcinoid tumours) are not FDG avid. False negative rate of a F-18 FDG PET study is given as 8-10% in a recent study and it was reported that visual assessment of non-attenuation corrected F-18 FDG PET images can be more accurate than classical studies in this instance [12]. These researchers suggested that a negative non-attenuation corrected PET study result may be discontinued following or followed infrequently.

18F-FLT (Fluoro-levo-thymidine) is a specific PET radiopharmaceutical indicating cell proliferation and the most important field of application of it is lung cancer. Thymidine is a deoxyribonucleic acid (DNA) base and actively joins into DNA during replication. 18F-FLT is thought to be more specific than FDG for oncological studies because it does not accumulate into inflammation. FDG-PET has an excellent sensitivity and good specificity for tumours but false positive results of it are mainly due to granulomatous and inflammatory disease [13, 14]. Differentiating malignant from benign solitary pulmonary nodes/lesions can be achieved more accurately by FLT-PET [15, 16, 17].

2. LUNG CANCER

Lung cancers are usually FDG avid and FDG-PET has a very low false negative rate for lung cancers. Most of the NSCLC and the small cell lung cancer (SCLC) can be visualized with great confidence by this imaging method. However, indolent lung cancers such as bronchoalveolar cancer, well-differentiated adenocarcinomas and some carcinoids could have low FDG avidity and also low SUVs. These types can be the reason for false negative interpretation. The other important false negativity reason is the size of the lesion. Lesions under the 8-10 mm in diameter usually cannot be identified by PET. Because of this reason, FDG-negative lesions under the resolution limits have to be followed using CT in terms of the enlargement of the dimensions. The reason of the false positive results is the same as in the SLN.

In this part it is especially mentioned about FDG PET/CT in the management of the NSCLC which is the most common type of lung cancer. The other types will take place at the end of the chapter on the other types heading.

2.1. Staging

Accurate pretreatment staging of lung cancer is an important issue because the existence of distant metastasis or contralateral lymph node makes the patient inoperable. The classical way of staging lung cancer was according to results of CT and mediastinoscopy before PET/CT has been introduced. Because histological assessment of the mediastinum is required for definitive therapy and mediastinoscopy serves up this opportunity, it is still considered as the gold standard although it is invasive. Comparative studies with mediastinoscopy results for mediastinal staging are still controversial and unfortunately the aim of replacing PET/CT with this invasive modality did not come true because of the limitations of it as mentioned above. However, PET/CT is accepted as the best non-invasive modality for the staging of lung cancer. It offers information of both tumour characteristics and local and distant metastasis in a single examination (Fig. **6**).

PET/CT appears superior for T, N and M staging of lung cancer patients compared with CT and PET individually. Major and also one the most important advantages of PET/CT is the opportunity to decrease the number of futile thoracotomies in all the series [18]. PET/CT changes stage of disease with an accurate staging of mediastinal lymph nodes and showing unexpected distant metastasis. This accurate staging results in changed patients' management and decreases the number of unnecessary explorations.

2.1.1. T Staging

CT imaging usually shows the large area of the entire mass, atelectasis and infection complex in especially central tumours but do not give an exact information regarding main tumour tissue. PET/CT correctly localizes metabolically active tumour tissue with adjacent atelectatic component. Thus identifying biopsy site and correct measurement of tumour tissue can be possible by means of PET/CT. Additionally PET/CT shows satellite nodules or pleural involvement [8] which in conclusion leads to accurate staging of tumour. The most important improvement with the addition of CT component to PET is in T staging of lung cancer; accuracy increases from 67% to 97% [19].

Specificity of FDG for tumour tissue is less than ideal because of its uptake in atelectatic and inflammatory tissue. Some new molecular imaging probes have been developed to get more specific tumour imaging and to improve and confirm the diagnostic confidence of FDG-PET imaging in tumours. 18F-deoxyfluorothymidine (FLT) which is a thymidine analog is one of the most accepted of them. Although it has been proposed especially for defining the therapy response, it has also been compared with FDG in terms of the diagnostic efficacy for the staging of lung cancer [14, 15, 20, 21]. FDG-PET was found to have higher sensitivity for characterization of primary tumour than FLT-PET in NSCLC [15]. However, FLT-PET has a high specificity for the detection of malignant lung tumours. It has been found less accurate compared with FDG for N-staging in patients with lung cancer and for detection of lung metastases [14, 20]. Because of its relatively low uptake in tumour tissue compared to FDG, detection of primary and metastatic NSCLC is limited by FLT-PET. FLT-PET is not recommended for staging and restaging of NSCLC [14, 20, 22].

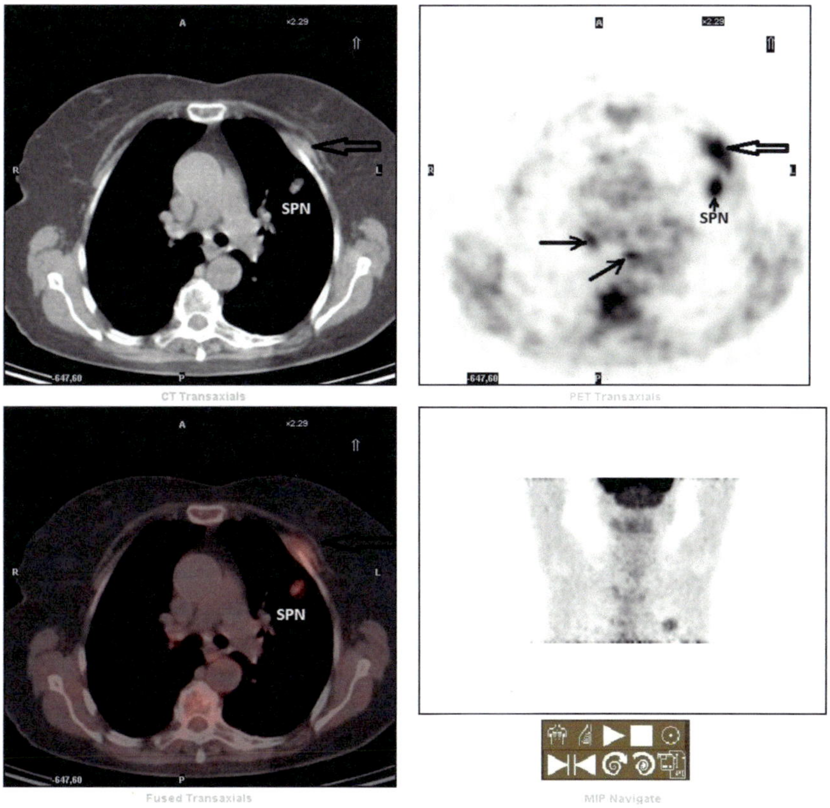

Figure 6: Malignant SPN with adjacent bone metastases (big arrow) and lymph nodes involvement (small arrows).

2.1.2. N Staging

Lymph node diameter was the main principle of CT-based staging as the evaluation of malignant involvement but large lymph nodes do not always contain malignant cells. Pieterman *et al.* compared PET and CT results for mediastinal staging of lung cancer and found sensitivity and specificity of 91% and 88%, respectively for PET and 75% and 66%, respectively for CT [23]. Some authors agree that patients should directly undergo operation without mediastinoscopy because of the high negative predictive value of PET/CT (*i.e.* accurate mediastinal lymph node staging) and the patients with positive PET/CT should be evaluated with mediastinoscopy before the surgery [24, 25]. Schimmer *et al.* reported the ranges of sensitivity, specificity, PPV, NPV and accuracy for FDG-PET 58-94%, 76-96%, 43-95%, 56-98% and 74-91%, respectively and for mediastinoscopy 80-96%, 100%, 100%, 92-97% and 94%, respectively in their meta-analysis [26]. PET decreases the need for mediastinoscopy in 65% of the patients according to guidelines [27]. PET/CT has the power of distinguishing N0-N1 disease from N2-3 disease which is the most important part of N staging [28]. Occult nodal metastasis (Fig. **7**) is another important issue that has been assessed in a recent literature; pathological staging of 144 patients was evaluated; percentage of nodal upstage with PET/CT was 14.3%, N1 occult nodal metastasis was 9.5% and N2 was 4.8% and SUVmax level of primary tumour was an independent predictor of occult metastasis according to this study [29]. However, mediastinoscopy is still accepted as the gold standard in ESTS guideline for the superior mediastinal lymph nodes for initial staging [27]. Invasive confirmation of mediastinal lymph nodes is not usually essential in patients with a peripheral clinical stage I NSCLC unless positive lymph nodes are visualized in PET scan according to ACCP guideline [30]. However, in case of central tumours, hilar N1 disease on PET, low FDG uptake on the primary tumour and lymph nodes larger or equal to 16 mm on CT, invasive staging is currently indicated. PET positive mediastinal lymph nodes have to be histologically confirmed [27].

Sensitivity and specificity of PET scanning for staging the mediastinum in lung cancer patients were reported as 74% and 85%, respectively although they were 51% and 86%, respectively with CT scanning [31].

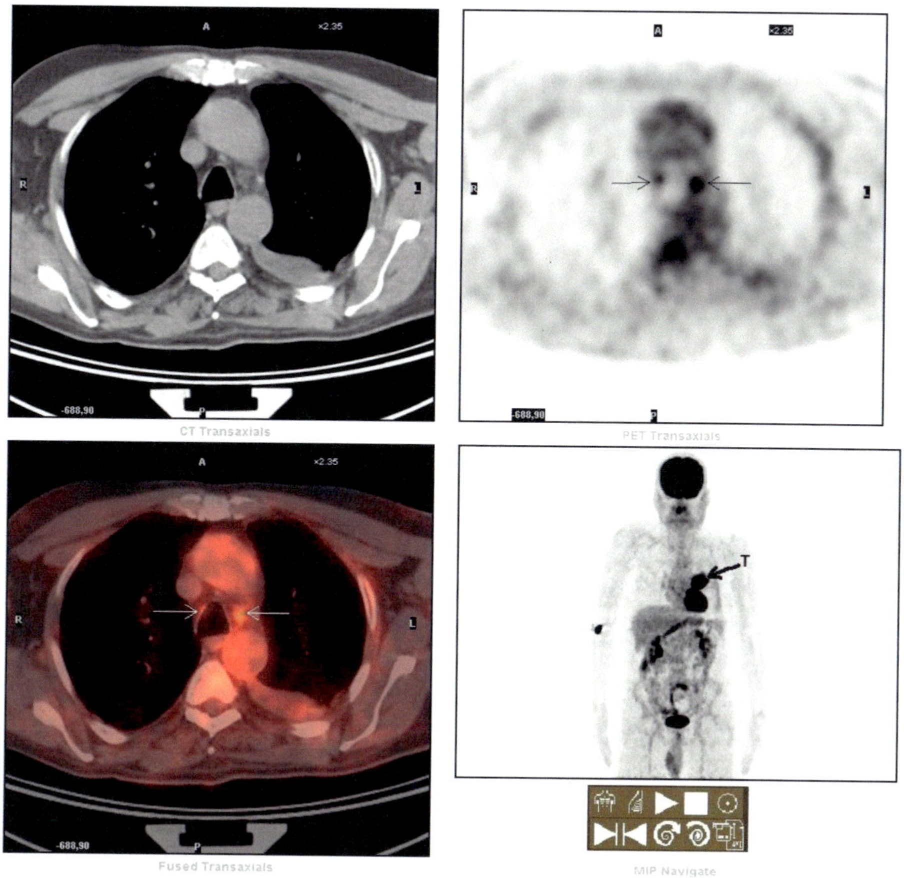

Figure 7: Bilateral small mediastinal lymph nodes with SUVmax 3.5 and 4.5 (arrows) appeared on PET/CT changed the N stage. Significantly increased FDG uptake within the tumour on the left lung-lower lobe (T with bold arrow on the MIP image) was visualized.

Dimension of lymph nodes is an important factor for false negative results. According to results of the study of Billé *et al.*, PET/CT identified 85.3% of lymph nodes >10 mm diameter *versus* 32.4% of <10 mm [32]. Perigaud *et al.* give a resolution limit of 5-6 mm for their PET/CT system and attribute most of false negatives to small size of lymph nodes and additionally long waiting times between PET/CT and surgery [33]. Same researchers identified a cut-off level of 5 for mediastinal lymph node involvement in PET/CT in order to decrease false positive interpretations. False positives are mostly a consequence of inflammatory changes especially due to granulomatous disease like tuberculosis or sarcoidosis. Overall in case of negative PET/CT according to distant metastasis and nodal involvement occult disease probability for N2 and N3 disease is given 6-9% in the literature, which is acceptable [34].

2.1.3. M Staging

Owing to the ability of imaging the whole body, valuable information about distant metastasis can be obtained in single examination by PET/CT (Fig. **8**). It is also stated that PET/CT usually upstages patients with showing unexpected distant metastasis and prevents unnecessary thoracotomies [18]. PET reveals 5-25% additional metastatic lesions particularly in stage III lung cancer patients [35, 36]. Distant metastasis regarding soft tissue can be diagnosed with PET/CT with accuracy of 96% [37].

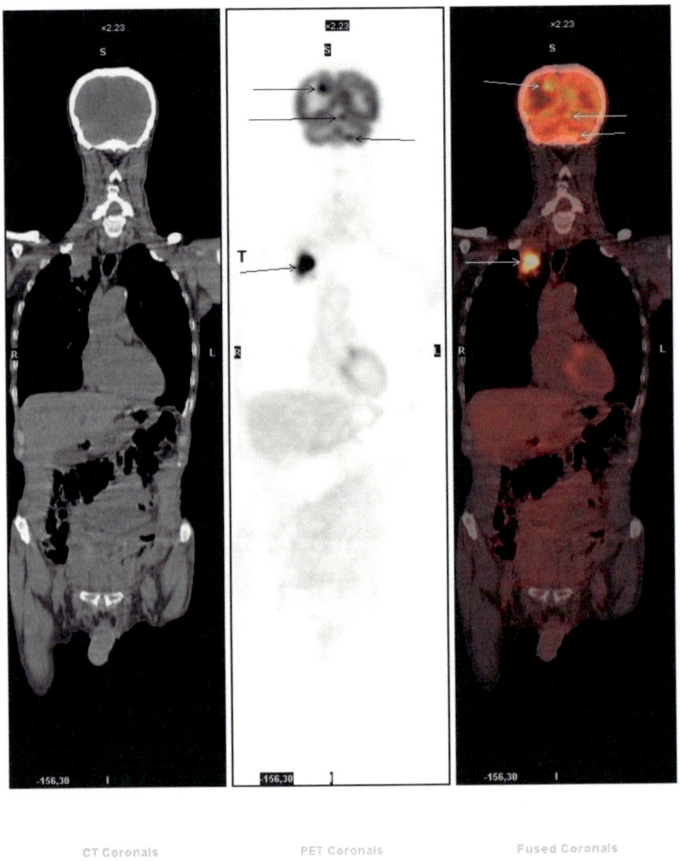

Figure 8: Cerebral and cerebellar metastases (arrows) of the lung cancer (T) with high FDG uptake. Central nervous system metastases can also be well defined although high physiologic uptake of FDG in brain.

Bone scanning with Tc-99m radiopharmaceuticals has been recommended to determine bone metastases because of its high negative predictive value. However, with the widespread usage of PET/CT devices and its excellent performance, PET scanning gains popularity also for evaluating bone metastases. Diagnostic power of PET/CT for bone metastasis showed similar sensitivity and increased specificity compared to bone scintigraphy [38, 39, 40]. Its sensitivity, specificity, NPV, PPV, and accuracy all exceed 90% [41].

Comparative studies between whole body MR with PET/CT and bone scintigraphy for diagnosis of bone metastasis showed that MR has higher specificity than both methods; however according to some recent meta-analyses, PET is still the best method to detect bone metastasis per-patient and per-lesion basis [42, 43]. Several studies indicated that less than 10% of the patients without neurologic symptoms have cerebral metastasis [44, 45]. Because of the high physiologic uptake of FDG in brain, diagnostic power of PET/CT for brain metastasis is low and MRI is the method of choice. Incidentalomas (*i.e.* incidentally found enlargement of adrenal gland) are frequent in CT scans of patients with lung cancer (10-15%); PET/CT also can eliminate benign ones with its low FDG uptake [8].

A recent research about the impact of F-18 FDG PET/CT to patient management including 537 NSCLC cancer patients reported that PET/CT changed patient management in 22% of the patients particularly those who received palliative treatment and changed the stage in 29.6% of them [46].

PET scan is recommended in the ACCP guidelines as grade IB standardized method for imaging of extrathoracic metastases [31]. According to that guideline, imaging for extrathoracic metastases should be performed if clinical evaluation is abnormal. Patients with lung cancer in clinical stage 1B-IIIB being treated with curative intent should undergo PET imaging for mediastinal and extrathoracic staging. If there is an abnormal result on FDG-PET scanning, abnormal mediastinal lymph node should be evaluated by biopsy before the surgical resection of the primary tumour. If there are specific symptoms of a certain organ/system, the most appropriate technique should be chosen to evaluate that site (*e.g.*, head CT/MRI, whole-body PET scanning or bone scintigraphy, abdominal CT, *etc.*). If the patient has clinical stage IIIA and IIIB disease, even there is no clinical evaluation finding, routine imaging for extrathoracic metastases (*e.g.*, head CT/MRI plus either whole-body PET scanning or bone scintigraphy plus abdominal CT) should be performed. In patients with clinical stage 1A lung cancer being treated with curative intent, PET scanning both for mediastinal and extrathoracic staging should be considered [31].

2.1.4. Other Lung Cancer Types

Adenocarcinoma shows significantly lower SUVmax level in comparison with NSLC types (squamous, large cell, pleomorphic carcinoma) and this level decreases with increasing bronchoalveolar component of adenocarcinoma tissue in terms of FDG affinity of various lung cancer types [47]. In the study of Higashi *et al.,* 57% of bronchoalveolar carcinoma (BAC) patients showed negative results on FDG PET [48]. They found significantly lower mean SUV in BAC (1.36 +/-0.821) than that of well-differentiated adenocarcinomas (2.92 +/-1.28) and mean SUV of well-differentiated adenocarcinomas was found significantly lower than that of moderately differentiated adenocarcinomas (4.63 +/-1.86). There is a correlation between FDG uptake and the degree of cell differentiation in adenocarcinoma of the lung. If there is an aspect suggesting BAC in CT, PET usually shows false-negative results. It is recommended in ACCP guideline that a PET scan with negative results should be followed by additional diagnostic tests to eliminate lung cancer [49]. C-11 acetate which is another tracer for PET in order to show FDG negative tumours, was shown sensitive for bronchoalveolar carcinoma and adenocarcinoma with bronchoalveolar component by Shibata *et al.* [50].

Neuroendocrine Lung Cancer

This group consists of typical and atypical carcinoids, large cell neuroendocrine tumour and SCLC. Aggressiveness increases, respectively. Typical carcinoid has favorable outcome. Because of these tumours contain somatostatin receptors, somatostatin receptor scintigraphy with 111In-DTPA-octreotide (Octreoscan) has been widely used in order to diagnose, stage and decide treatment option [51]. It has high sensitivity in the detection of neuroendocrine tumours and is classically used in the beginning of therapy to evaluate the biodistribution of the therapeutic octreotide that acts based on the connection to the sst2 receptor subtype. Tumours that have larger numbers of somatostatin receptors show more uptake in scintigraphy and greater benefit from octreotide therapy. The next step of the therapy is usually to use radiolabeled somatostatin analogs for metabolic radiotherapy in inoperable patients.

Their FDG affinity varies but it is lower than other groups except SCLC. Patients with SCLC can be clearly evaluated by means of PET/CT [52]. SCLC is considered in two stages: limited and extensive disease (*i.e.* whether disease is limited to thorax or not). PET has sensitivity of 89-100% and specificity of 78-95% for differentiation of these two stages [53]. PET/CT increased the specificity to 100% [11]. It was estimated a stage improvement to 17% by means of PET/CT in small cell carcinoma patients [54]. However, although whole-body bone scintigraphy is recommended in routine staging of SCLC (Grade of recommendation, 1B), PET does not [55]. Chong and colleagues investigated role of PET in neuroendocrine tumours and found that PET was useful for characterizing, staging and prediction of prognosis for this kind of tumours [56].

Because neuroendocrine tumours demonstrate an increased activity of L-DOPA decarboxylase they show a high uptake of 18F-DOPA [57]. Thus 18F-DOPA accumulates *via* a metabolic mechanism. 68Ga-DOTA-TOC/DOTA-NOC has been introduced as PET tracer for the imaging of neuroendocrine tumours [58]. This compound for PET imaging has a high affinity for sst2 and sst5 and their uptake is based on a receptor mechanism. PET with these agents is useful before metabolic radiotherapy in order to evaluate the biodistribution of the therapeutic compound as the 111In-DTPA-octreotide scanning. It has several advantages over 111In-Octreoscan: increased spatial resolution, the possibility of performing whole-body scanning with a short uptake time (60 min), relatively easy synthesis and increased diagnostic accuracy using hybrid PET/CT scanners [57, 59, 60].

Sensitivity, specificity and accuracy of Ga-68 DOTATOC were reported 97%, 92% and 96%, respectively [61]. Jindal *et al.* showed also that Ga-68 DOTATOC imaging provides proper staging and treatment planning [62]. Ga-68 DOTATOC PET/CT is useful in the evaluation of primary pulmonary carcinoids and should be included in the diagnostic work-up of these patients; its detection rate of carcinoids is 95% [62]. It was also shown that PET/CT with Ga-DOTA-NOC was useful in bronchial carcinoid patients because it led to a better evaluation of the extent of the disease [63].

2.2. Response Assessment

Although morphological imaging with CT is still the main visual technique for evaluating the response of lung cancer to therapy, PET/CT has gained an increased usage because of the high FDG uptake in tumour tissue and the decreased or absent uptake as a result of response to therapy. Among lung cancer patients who receive chemo-radiotherapy, local tumour failure is reported for 70% of the patients in literature [64]. The high percentage of recurrence brings the need for an optimal imaging modality. PET/CT has an advantage of showing metabolic changes thus showing early response or recurrence of tumour. A study from Velazquez *et al.* indicated that poor survival and patients who do not respond to radiotherapy can be identified by means of FDG-PET [65]. The Response Evaluation Criteria in Solid Tumours (RECIST) have been re-evaluated and according to RECIST 1.1 a new FDG-PET positive finding will be considered progression [66]. Obrzut *et al.* had concluded in their study that FDG-PET could show new metastatic lesions, particularly new nodal metastasis, and predicted a greater role for semiquantitative tumour response assessment [66]. Response assessment by means of SUVmax levels has some handicaps like some factors that influence quantification. All of the factors that impact on SUVmax levels have to be same for sequential scans of the patient in order to decide response by means of SUVmax. However, it was reported that if there was an 80% or more decrease of SUVmax of tumour, a complete pathologic response could be predicted with an accuracy of 96% [67]. Visual interpretation of PET images before and after therapy was considered more appropriate way of deciding the response (Fig. **9**). Complete response has been defined as returned FDG uptake of metabolic active tumour tissue to level of normal tissues by MacManus *et al.* [68]. Partial response generally was considered reduction of FDG uptake of tumour with existence of tumour tissue. SUV and metabolic tumour volume (MTV) changes between the before and after initial chemo-radiotherapy FDG PET/CT scans allow prediction of the treatment response in advanced NSCLC [69].

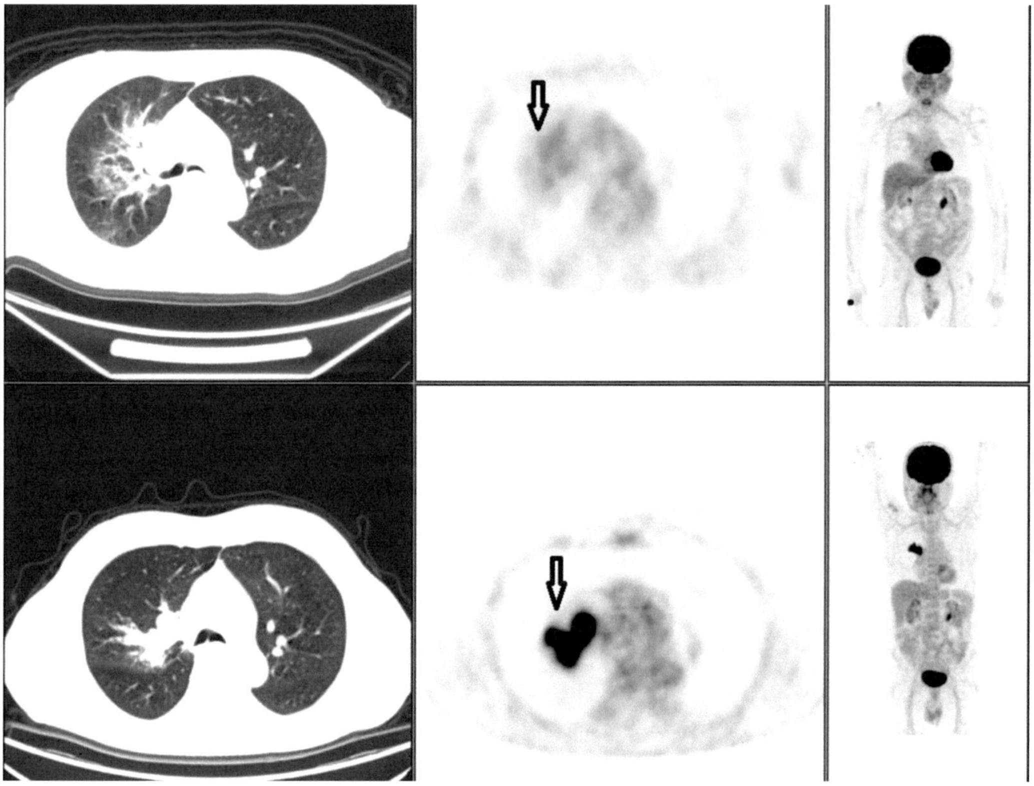

Figure 9: PET/CT images of a patient with NSCLCO in the right lung: before (lower line) and after chemo-radiotherapy (upper line). Significant FDG uptake (SUVmax:15) in tumour tissue (arrow) on the first imaging was disappeared on the imaging after therapy (SUVmax:2.3). It is evaluated as complete response.

PET has another indication of postoperative elevation of CEA levels to document metastasis according to a recent study [70]. Pottgen *et al.* showed in their study including 50 patients that PET/CT can predict response to neoadjuvant chemo-radiotherapy [71]. A new treatment option is radio-frequency ablation (RFA) for lung lesions [72]. A study concerning RFA of lung lesions showed that F-18 FDG can be used in order to predict treatment success and choose patients who may benefit from this treatment [73].

3'-deoxy-3'-(18F-fluorothymidine) (FLT) is a thymidine analog and a PET imaging marker of proliferation. FLT-PET has the capability of imaging and quantifying the proliferation fraction of tumours non-invasively. Proliferation dependent accumulation of FLT has been demonstrated for a variety of tumours including lung cancer. Although it did not show a performance as a tumour staging agent unlike FDG [14, 20], it has been suggested as an alternative to FDG for the assessment of response to treatment [21, 74-77].

The correlation between FLT uptake and cellular proliferation suggests its usage for the assessment of therapy response to anticancer drugs [77]. Tumour cell proliferation can also be assessed by immunohistochemistry such as Ki-67 or cyclin D1 staining. A significant correlation was observed between FLT uptake of pulmonary lesions and Ki-67 labeling index but not for FDG uptake [22]. Tumour FLT uptake was also found correlated by the cyclin D1 labeling index [21]. However, tumour imaging capability of FLT may be limited in human tumours without functional p53 [78].

FLT-PET imaging may represent an appropriate method for early prediction of response to treatment in patients with NSCLC and also adenocarcinoma of the lung according to studies designed with different drugs such as cetuximab, gefitinib, and erlotinib [74-77]. Although early FDG-PET predicts progression free survival (PFS), overall survival (OS), and nonprogression after 6 weeks of therapy with erlotinib in unselected, previously untreated patients with advanced NSCLC independent from EGFR mutational status, early FLT response predicted significantly longer PFS but not OS and was not predictive for nonprogression after 6 weeks of therapy [76].

18F-α-methyl tyrosine (18F-FMT) is a novel tracer for PET. In recent years it was studied by Kaira and colleagues in NSCLC [79-81]. FMT-PET has high specificity in the detection of primary tumour and lymph node metastasis and its uptake is well association with cellular proliferation [79, 80]. Although it has clear uptake in all types of NSCLC, uptake of FMT in primary lung tumours was found as an independent prognostic factor only in patients with lung adenocarcinoma [80]. Agreement of therapeutic response evaluated by RECIST was reported in more patients with FMT-PET than with FDG-PET (89% *versus* 56%, respectively) [81]. Thus FMT-PET was suggested as a promising PET tracer for monitoring response to chemoradiotherapy and for predicting the prognosis of patients with lung cancer.

2.3. Residual or Recurrent Tumour

PET/CT has several advantages at postoperative and post radiotherapy sites over conventional morphological imaging methods in terms of the differentiation of residual or recurrent tumour from the fibrous tissue. While residual or recurrent tumour tissue is FDG avid, fibrous tissue has no FDG uptake. However, it also has some limitations at postoperative period. There can be false positive results regarding inflammatory changes and 6-8 weeks of postoperative waiting period is necessary for PET/CT examination. Similarly, post-radiotherapy changes, like radiation pneumonia, make PET/CT images impossible to interpret before 3 months of waiting period.

According to a recent report, PET/CT has the sensitivity, specificity, accuracy, positive predictive value, and negative predictive value of 97%, 96%, 96%, 81%, and 99%, respectively in detecting recurrences in patients with NSCLC after potentially curative surgery [82].

Residual disease containing high FDG uptake means worse prognosis of patient. In order to decide prognosis and employ therapy options it is important to perform a PET scan because morphological changes of post-therapy or postoperative tissues make nearly impossible to decide residual disease by means of morphological imaging methods. There is not enough investigations regarding this issue, further studies are needed in this area.

2.4. Metastatic Lung Disease

Metastasectomy procedures are employed to patients with particularly single metastatic disease of lung. There is a limited data in the literature concerning preoperative approaches that can be applied to patients with lung metastasis. Since we know that PET/CT offers a whole body imaging of all structures, this technique will be important in this field. In addition, PET/CT shows unexpected metastasis in an important percentage of lung cancer patients and excludes unnecessary interventions. Unfortunately the only study about PET and pulmonary metastases concluded that sensitivity of PET in identifying pulmonary metastasis is low especially for small nodules [83]. They found true positivity and false negativity rates of FDG-PET as 67.5% and 32.5%, respectively for nodules.

Because of this high false negative percentage, negative FDG-PET result should not be used to rule out metastatic disease.

Detterbeck *et al.* recommend a PET scan prior to metastasectomy in their report in order to show unexpected metastasis [84]. Extrathoracic metastatic sites can be identified by PET in 10 to 15% of the patients. More prospective studies about management of metastatic lung cancer patients with PET/CT at preoperative and postoperative period are warranted.

2.5. Survival and Prognosis

Prognostification studies with PET/CT revealed excellent results. It is known that FDG uptake of lung cancer is strictly in relationship with prognosis of patients and predicts survival. In a recent literature it was observed that 12.5 and 9.7 as the cut-off SUVmax value for tumour and for lymph node metastasis, respectively, predicted worse prognosis for SCLC patients and these patients should receive a more aggressive treatment plan [85]. They also concluded that preoperative PET stage was a predictor of long-term outcome and SUV was a predictor of survival of SCLC patients. Al-Sarraf *et al.* did the same prognostification for NSCLC patients and concluded that SUV could serve as a predictor of prognosis and those patients who had SUVmax levels higher than 15 might benefit receiving neo-adjuvant chemotherapy [86]. Sasaki *et al.* showed that tumoural SUV value <5 was the most important indicator of longer disease-free interval and high survival rate [87].

It was reported by Saga and colleagues that pretreatment FLT uptake of patients, who developed recurrence and who died of lung cancer was significantly higher than that of patients who did not [88]. Pre-carbon-ion radiotherapy FLT-PET/CT was supposed to have a prognostic value and might contribute determining the treatment strategy.

2.6. Radiation Therapy Planning

To determine the area that will be irradiated with the most proper boundaries is especially important in terms of effective radiation therapy (RT). CT has been used traditionally in order to define tumour volumes and there are volumetric analysis options of CT systems. Since PET/CT has been introduced as a staging method for lung cancer patients it was inevitably applied to radiation therapy planning. This has been largely stimulated by widespread availability and integration of PET with treatment planning systems. Integrated PET/CT has excellent power of showing metabolically active part of tumour and discriminate tumour tissue from atelectasis or infectious part of complex (Fig. **10**). It leads to a change in gross tumour volume definition (GTV) and reduced inaccurate outlining of the GTV and/or to geographic misses in patients with NSCLC [89]. PET/CT fused images allow better contouring of primary tumours in 34% of thoracic cancers [90]. It provides advantages in virtual simulation compared with morphological contouring only with CT. Additionally, PET/CT accurately identifies malignant mediastinal lymph nodes and changes the radiation field. FDG PET-CT plays an increasing role in RT planning at the target selection and definition steps. Selective nodal irradiation of FDG positive nodes is the preferred treatment in NSCLC. This results in a more proper therapy margin, saves normal tissues from radiation exposure and provides the opportunity for dose escalation by leading to decreased normal tissue exposure [91]. Although there are limited data, first results in SCLC show similar results [92].

De Ruysscher *et al.* noted that FDG-PET also has the power to increase the radiation dose to real tumour tissue because of decreasing normal tissue volume included in the field. This improves local tumour control probability [93]. It preserves the organs at risk (*i.e.* esophagus). According to the results of the study by van Der Wel and colleagues, the PET/CT based planning decreases lung and esophagus doses considerably and allows significant radiation dose escalation in CT Stage N2-N3M0 NSCLC patients [94]. Local high-dose RT is the treatment of choice for the patients in early stage NSCLC who are unsuitable for resection. If there is no subclinical involvement of unsuspicious regional lymph nodes and exact staging can be done using PET/CT, local control rates up to 90% can be achieved by irradiating the primary T1/2 tumour alone especially for patients in good general condition [95].

The main problem with the lung tumours for RT is that they are non-stationary and can displace up to 2.5 cm during respiration. Because of that addition of extra margin around the tumour is usually used during RT treatment planning.

Nowadays a novel method is introduced to detect and track the tumour by respiratory-gated PET/CT images. Planning with respiratory-gated PET images can provide more accurate and effective RT treatment for lung cancer. The exact information about tumour movement during each respiratory cycle can be available in relatively short time by using this method and an excellent accuracy of 97% was obtained [96]. It was also stated that including PET in radiotherapy planning decreased interobserver variability of radiotherapy volumes [97].

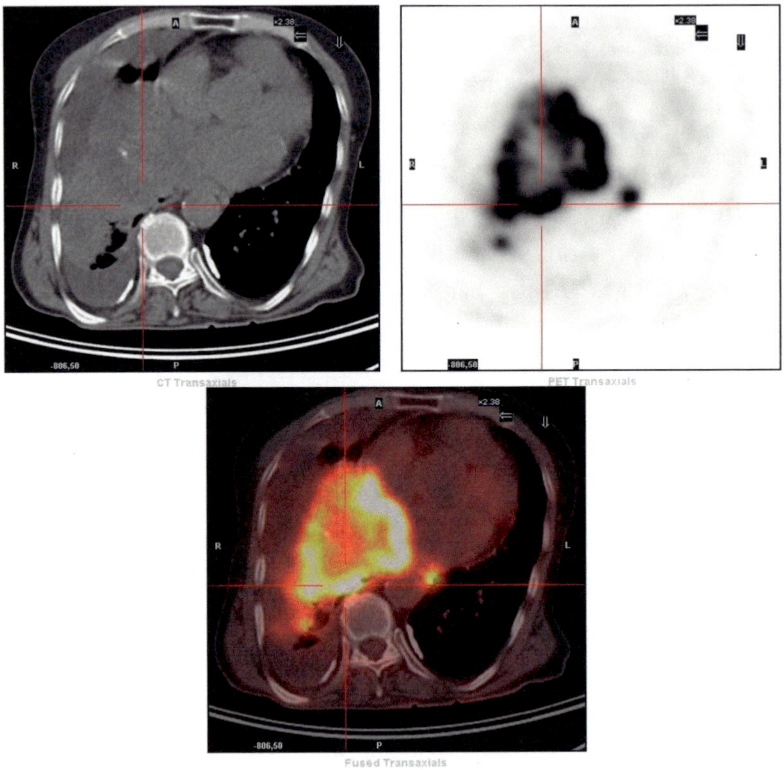

Figure 10: A gross lung tumour with lymph node metastases adjacent to the heart. FDG guides defining metabolically active tumour tissue for proper determination of GTV in RT planning.

In a recent study, it was shown that PET/CT performed for RT planning can detect disease progression better than staging PET/CT [98]. The mean scan interval between the PET/CT and RT was longer in patients with progression compared to patients without progression. Planning PET has detected progressive disease in 76%, 86% and 100% of the patients if the interval was 4, 5 and 6 weeks, respectively. Disease progression was defined as 33% when the interval was <4 weeks [98]. It was recommended that if the time-interval is 4 weeks or more, a new PET-CT should be done because of the possibility of upstaging of the disease [99, 100].

In all studies where "PET-assisted" and conventional target or treatment volumes were compared, there were major differences between PET and conventionally calculated volumes. Routine use of PET/CT for RT planning is recommended because PET-assisted staging is proven to be significantly more accurate than conventional staging and because all studies show major differences, in favor of PET, between PET-assisted and conventional treatment volumes in NSCLC.

2.6.1. Evaluation of Tumour Hypoxia by PET

Tumour hypoxia is one of most important characteristics of tumour tissue which determine treatment resistance. Hypoxic areas in tumour should be recognized before the RT and over-treated compared to non-hypoxic malignant tissues. Hypoxia inside big neoplastic tumours is especially important in terms of the efficiency of therapy. Imaging of tumour hypoxia has been addressed from several researches with different tracers. One of the most common tracers is imidazole compounds. F-18 Fluoromisonidazole (F-18 MISO) is formerly introduced as a hypoxia agent [101, 102]. FDG and F-MISO uptakes in lung cancer were found correlated during the RT but not pre-RT [103]. According to a recent study of Li *et al.*, uptake of a newly studied hypoxia marker named as 'F-18 Fluoroerytrhronitroimidazole' (FETNIM) is correlated well with FDG uptake in NSCLC tissue. FETNIM Tumour/Blood ratio was found as an independent prognostic factor. Although F-18 FETNIM predicts overall survival, F-18 FDG could not [104]. FETNIM is more hydrophilic than FMISO, and can be eliminated more rapidly from well-oxygenated tissues. This allows a higher tumour-to-background ratio. It was reported that F-18-labeled FETNIM could help detect tumour hypoxia and was easier to prepare, less costly, and more hydrophilic than F-18-labeled FMISO [105].

SUMMARY AND FUTURE DIRECTIONS

PET and PET/CT changed the algorithms in oncology. Solitary pulmonary nodule assessment and staging and management of NSCLC patients are the most common usages of PET/CT modality. In general, health care systems have approved the payment for PET or PET/CT for these indications. This technique is also cost-effective for those uses. The importance of PET/CT imaging comes from metabolic information which is derived from tumour tissue. This modality enables to characterize, quantify and follow up metabolic changes of lung cancer. A patient with solitary pulmonary nodule can be followed up in reliance on a negative PET/CT scan without any further operation. The whole body imaging obtained with PET/CT completely allows assessing possible metastatic involvements anywhere in the body. It can also identify unexpected metastases of the patients with lung cancer. One of the main impacts of PET/CT is reducing futile thoracotomies by accurate staging and thus changing patients' management. This impact results in both decreased costs and improvement in patients' survival. Mediastinoscopy, although it is invasive, is still considered as the gold standard for mediastinal staging of lung tumours. PET/CT can replace mediastinoscopy for nodal staging in the future but more prospective studies with both pathological and follow-up results are needed. Staging strategy in NSCLC with PET/CT can be extensively accepted as shown in Fig. **11** in the near future [106].

MR is introduced as an alternative for bone metastasis imaging of NSCLC patients but PET/CT has more advantages over MR both for bone metastasis and other staging requirements. More comparative studies have to be performed in this field. PET/CT may replace bone scintigraphy to define NSCLC patients' bone metastasis because it is more specific and gives additional information in a single examination. PET/CT can give excellent prognostic information. The initial SUVmax levels of tumours can predict patient's outcome and survival and change the patient's management. There are increasing numbers of metastasectomy procedures and PET/CT can guide these operations with showing all possible metastatic lesions in preoperative period. An important indication of PET/CT is to evaluate therapy response and a clear role has already been established. An early response assessment can be made by means of PET/CT. PET/CT guided radiotherapy procedures and volumetric analysis will probably continue to progress in the future and serve in patients' favor. Improving imaging protocols (*e.g.,* injection of contrast media, respiratory gating protocols) and advent of new and more specific PET tracers will further enhance the performance of PET-CT.

PET/CT and new PET-tracers with increasing availability will be more effective on overall management of lung cancer patients and take its proper place in guidelines.

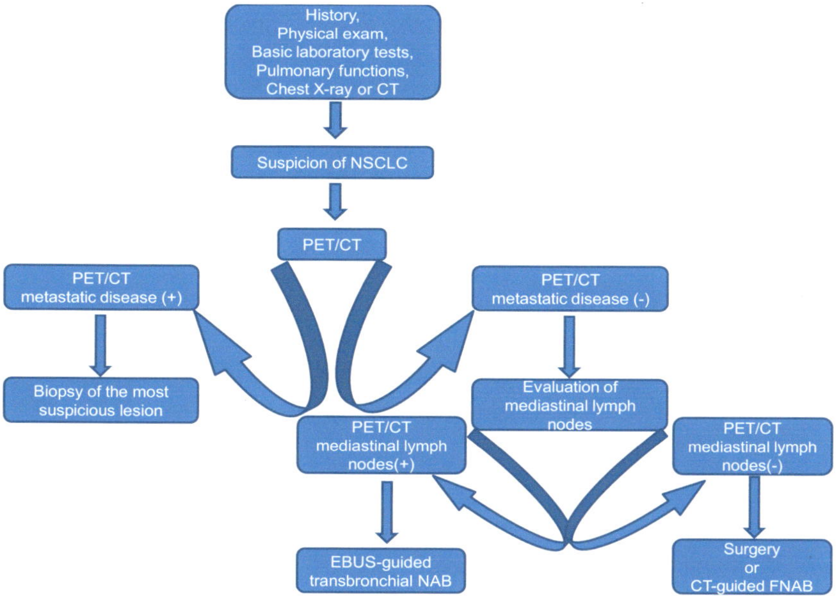

Figure 11: Suggested staging algorithm in NSCLC. (NAB: needle aspiration biopsy, FNAB: fine NAB).

ACKNOWLEDGEMENTS

I would like to thank Dr. Halil KOMEK from Diyarbakir Training Hospital for providing the PET/CT images and Dr. Z. Pinar KOC from Firat (Euphrates) University School of Medicine for her help towards this chapter.

CONFLICT OF INTEREST

The author confirms that this article content has no conflict of interest.

REFERENCES

[1] Corris PA, Ellis DA, Hawkins T, Gibson GJ. Use of radionuclide scanning in the preoperative estimation of pulmonary function after pneumonectomy. Thorax 1987;42(4):285-91.

[2] Mineo TC, Schillaci O, Pompeo E, Mineo D, Simonetti G. Usefulness of lung perfusion scintigraphy before lung cancer resection in patients with ventilatory obstruction. Ann Thorac Surg 2006;82(5):1828-34.
[3] Colice GL, Shafazand S, Griffin JP, Keenan R, Bolliger CT; American College of Chest Physicians. Physiologic evaluation of the patient with lung cancer being considered for resectional surgery: ACCP evidenced-based clinical practice guidelines (2nd edition). Chest 2007;132(3 Suppl):161S-77S.
[4] Bria WF, Kanarek DJ, Kazemi H. Prediction of postoperative pulmonary function following thoracic operations. J Thorac Cardiovasc Surg 1983;86(2):186-92.
[5] Pierce RJ, Copland JM, Sharpe K, Barter CE. Preoperative risk evaluation for lung cancer resection. Am J Respir Crit Care Med 1994;150(4):947-55.
[6] Cordiner A, De Carlo F, De Gennaro R, Pau F, Flore F. Prediction of postoperative pulmonary function following thoracic surgery for bronchial carcinoma. Angiology 1991;42(12):985-9.
[7] Markos J, Mullan BP, Hillman DR, *et al.* Preoperative assessment as a predictor of mortality and morbidity after lung resection. Am Rev Respir Dis 1989;139(4):902-10.
[8] Maldonado A, González-Alenda FJ, Alonso M, Sierra JM. Usefulness of positron emission tomography-computed tomography in respiratory medicine. Arch Bronconeumol 2007;43(10):562-72.
[9] Higgins GA, Shields TW, Keehn RJ. The solitary pulmonary nodule. Ten-year follow-up of Veterans Administration-Armed Forces Cooperative Study. Arch Surg 1975;110(5):570–5.
[10] Joshi SC, Pant I, Hamzah F, Kumar G, Shukla AN. Integrated positron emission tomography/computed tomography fusion imaging: an emerging gold standard in lung cancer. Indian J Cancer 2008;45(4):137-41.
[11] Hellwig D, Baum RP, Kirsch C. FDG-PET, PET/CT and conventional nuclear medicine procedures in the evaluation of lung cancer: a systematic review. Nuklearmedizin 2009;48(2):59-69.
[12] Huang YE, Pu YL, Huang YJ, *et al.* The utility of the nonattenuation corrected 18F-FDG PET images in the characterization of solitary pulmonary lesions. Nucl Med Commun. 2010;31(11):945-51.
[13] Buck AK, Halter G, Schirrmeister H, *et al.* Imaging proliferation in lung tumours with PET: 18F-FLT *versus* 18F-FDG. J Nucl Med 2003;44(9):1426-31.
[14] Buck AK, Hetzel M, Schirrmeister H, *et al.* Clinical relevance of imaging proliferative activity in lung nodules. Eur J Nucl Med Mol Imaging 2005;32(5):525-33.
[15] Yamamoto Y, Nishiyama Y, Ishikawa S, *et al.* 3'-Deoxy-3'-18F-fluorothymidine as a proliferation imaging tracer for diagnosis of lung tumours: comparison with 2-deoxy-2-18f-fluoro-D-glucose. J Comput Assist Tomogr 2008;32(3):432-7.
[16] Tian J, Yang X, Yu L, *et al.* A multicenter clinical trial on the diagnostic value of dual-tracer PET/CT in pulmonary lesions using 3'-deoxy-3'-18F-fluorothymidine and 18F-FDG. J Nucl Med 2008;49(2):186-94.
[17] Xu B, Guan Z, Liu C, *et al.* Can multimodality imaging using 18F-FDG/18F-FLT PET/CT benefit the diagnosis and management of patients with pulmonary lesions? Eur J Nucl Med Mol Imaging 2011;38(2):285-92.
[18] Van Tinteren H, Hoekstra OS, Smit EF *et al.* Effectiveness of positron emission tomography in the preoperative assessment of patients with suspected non-small-cell lung cancer: the PLUS multicentre randomised trial. Lancet 2002;359(9315):1388–93.

[19] Halpern BS, Schiepers C, Weber WA, *et al.* Presurgical staging of non-small cell lung cancer: positron emission tomography, integrated positron emission tomography/CT, and software image fusion. Chest 2005;128(4):2289-97.

[20] Cobben DC, Elsinga PH, Hoekstra HJ, *et al.* Is 18F-3'-fluoro-3'-deoxy-L-thymidine useful for the staging and restaging of non-small cell lung cancer? J Nucl Med 2004;45(10):1677-82.

[21] Yang W, Zhang Y, Fu Z, *et al.* Imaging of proliferation with 18F-FLT PET/CT *versus* 18F-FDG PET/CT in non-small-cell lung cancer. Eur J Nucl Med Mol Imaging 2010;37(7):1291-9.

[22] Yap CS, Czernin J, Fishbein MC, *et al.* Evaluation of thoracic tumours with 18F-fluorothymidine and 18F-fluorodeoxyglucose-positron emission tomography. Chest 2006;129(2):393-401.

[23] Pieterman RM, van Putten JW, Meuzelaar JJ, *et al.* Preoperative staging of non small-cell lung cancer with positron emission tomography. N Engl J Med 2000;343:254-61.

[24] Visioni A, Kim J. Positron emission tomography for benign and malignant disease. Surg Clin North Am 2011;91(1):249-66.

[25] Tasci E, Tezel C, Orki A, Akin O, Falay O, Kutlu CA. The role of integrated positron emission tomography and computed tomography in the assessment of nodal spread in cases with non-small cell lung cancer. Interact Cardiovasc Thorac Surg 2010;10(2):200-3.

[26] Schimmer C, Neukam K, Elert O. Staging of non-small lung cancer: clinical value of positron emission tomography and mediastinoscopy. Interact CardioVasc Thorac Surg 2006;5:418–23.

[27] De Leyn P, Lardinois D, Van Schil PE, *et al.* ESTS guidelines for preoperative lymph node staging for non-small cell lung cancer. Eur J Cardiothorac Surg 2007;32(1):1-8.

[28] Liu BJ, Dong JC, Xu CQ, *et al.* Accuracy of 18F-FDG PET/CT for lymph node staging in non-small-cell lung cancers. Chin Med J (Engl) 2009;122(15):1749-54.

[29] Park HK, Jeon K, Koh WJ, *et al.* Occult nodal metastasis in patients with non-small cell lung cancer at clinical stage IA by PET/CT. Respirology 2010;15(8):1179-84.

[30] Detterbeck FC, Jantz MA, Wallace M, Vansteenkiste J, Silvestri GA. Invasive Mediastinal Staging of Lung Cancer: ACCP Evidence-Based Clinical Practice Guidelines (2nd Edition) Chest 2007;132(3 suppl):202S-220S.

[31] Silvestri GA, Gould MK, Margolis ML, *et al*; American College of Chest Physicians. Noninvasive staging of non-small cell lung cancer: ACCP evidenced-based clinical practice guidelines (2nd edition). Chest 2007;132(3 Suppl):178S-201S.

[32] Billé A, Pelosi E, Skanjeti A, *et al.* Preoperative intrathoracic lymph node staging in patients with non-small-cell lung cancer: accuracy of integrated positron emission tomography and computed tomography. Eur J Cardiothorac Surg 2009;36(3):440-5.

[33] Perigaud C, Bridji B, Roussel JC, *et al.* Prospective preoperative mediastinal lymph node staging by integrated positron emission tomography-computerised tomography in patients with non-small-cell lung cancer. Eur J Cardiothorac Surg. 2009;36(4):731-6.

[34] Cerfolio RJ, Bryant AS, Ojha B, Eloubeidi M. Improving the inaccuracies of clinical staging of patients with NSCLC: a prospective trial. Ann Thorac Surg 2005;80(4):1207–13.

[35] Stroobants S, D'Hoore I, Dooms C, *et al.* Additional value of whole-body fluorodeoxyglucose positron emission tomography in the detection of distant metastases of non-small cell lung cancer. Clinical Lung Cancer 2003;4(4):242–7.

[36] Pieterman RM, Van Putten JW, Meuzelaar JJ, *et al.* Preoperative staging of non-small cell lung cancer with positron emission tomography. N Engl J Med 2000;343(4):254–61.

[37] Bury T, Barreto A, Daenen F, Barthelemy N, Ghaye B, Rigo P. FDG-PET for the detection of bone metastases in patients with NSCLC. Eur J Nucl Med 1998;25(9):1244-7.

[38] Cheran SK, Herndon JE II, Patz EF Jr. Comparison of wholebody FDG-PET to bone scan for detection of bone metastases in patients with a new diagnosis of lung cancer. Lung Cancer 2004;44(3):317–25.

[39] Gayed I, Vu T, Johnson M, Macapinlac H, Podoloff D. Comparison of bone and 2- deoxy-2-[18F]fluoro-D-glucose positron emission tomography in the evaluation of bony metastases in lung cancer. Mol Imaging Biol 2003;5(1):26–31.

[40] Hsia TC, Shen YY, Yen RF, Kao CH, Changlai SP. Comparing whole body 18F-2-deoxyglucose positron emission tomography and technetium- 99m methylene diophosphate bone scan to detect bone metastases in patients with non-small cell lung cancer. Neoplasma 2002;49(4):267–71.

[41] Marom E, McAdams H, Erasmus J, *et al.* Staging non-small cell lung cancer with whole-body PET. Radiology 1999;212(3):803-9.

[42] Takenaka D, Ohno Y, Matsumoto K, *et al.* Detection of bone metastases in non-small cell lung cancer patients: comparison of whole-body diffusion-weighted imaging (DWI), whole-body MR imaging without and with DWI, whole-body FDG-PET/CT, and bone scintigraphy. J Magn Reson Imaging 2009;30(2):298-308.

[43] Liu T, Xu JY, Xu W, Bai YR, Yan WL, Yang HL. Fluorine-18 deoxyglucose Positron Emission Tomography, Magnetic Resonance Imaging and Bone Scintigraphy for the Diagnosis of Bone Metastases in Patients with Lung Cancer: Which One is the Best? - a Meta-analysis. Clin Oncol (R Coll Radiol) 2011;23(5):350-8.

[44] Cole FH Jr, Thomas JE, Wilcox AB, *et al.* Cerebral imaging in the asymptomatic preoperative bronchogenic carcinoma patient: is it worthwhile? Ann Thorac Surg. 1994;57(4):838–40.

[45] Colice GL, Birkmeyer JD, Black WC, *et al.* Cost-effectiveness of head CT in patients with lung cancer without clinical evidence of metastases. Chest 1995;108(5):1264–71.

[46] Heo EY, Yang SC, Yoo CG, Han SK, Shim YS, Kim YW. Impact of whole-body ^{18}F-fluorodeoxyglucose positron emission tomography on therapeutic management of non-small cell lung cancer. Respirology 2010;15(8):1174-8.

[47] Casali C, Cucca M, Rossi G, *et al.* The variation of prognostic significance of Maximum Standardized Uptake Value of [18F]-fluoro-2-deoxy-glucose positron emission tomography in different histological subtypes and pathological stages of surgically resected Non-Small Cell Lung Carcinoma. Lung Cancer 2010;69(2):187-93.

[48] Higashi K, Ueda Y, Seki H, *et al.* Fluorine-18-FDG PET imaging is negative in bronchioloalveolar lung carcinoma. J Nucl Med 1998;39(6):1016-20.

[49] Arenberg D. Bronchioloalveolar Lung Cancer: ACCP Evidence-Based Clinical Practice Guidelines (2nd Edition) Chest 2007;132(3 suppl):306S-313S.

[50] Shibata H, Nomori H, Uno K, *et al.* 11C-acetate for positron emission tomography imaging of clinical stage IA lung vbadenocarcinoma: comparison with 18F-fluorodeoxyglucose for imaging and evaluation of tumour aggressiveness. Ann Nucl Med 2009;23(7):609-16.

[51] Cascini GL, Cuccurullo V, Mansi L. The non tumour uptake of (111)In-octreotide creates new clinical indications in benign diseases, but also in oncology. Q J Nucl Med Mol Imaging. 2010;54(1):24-36.

[52] Blum R, MacManus MP, Rischin D, Michael M, Ball D, Hicks RJ. Impact of positron emission tomography on the management of patients with small-cell lung cancer: preliminary experience. Am J Clin Oncol 2004;27(2):164-71.

[53] Ung YC, Maziak DE, Vanderveen JA, *et al.* 18F-fluorodeoxyglucose positron emission tomography in the diagnosis and staging of lung cancer: a systematic review. J Natl Cancer Inst 2007;99(23):1753–67.

[54] Fischer BM, Mortensen J, Langer SW, *et al.* A prospective study of PET/CT in initial staging of small-cell lung cancer: comparison with CT, bone scintigraphy and bone marrow analysis. Ann Oncol 2007;18(2):338–45.

[55] Simon GR, Turrisi A. Management of Small Cell Lung Cancer: ACCP Evidence-Based Clinical Practice Guidelines (2nd Edition). Chest 2007;132(3 suppl):324S-339S.

[56] Chong S, Lee KS. Spectrum of findings and usefulness of integrated PET/CT in patients with known or suspected neuroendocrine tumours of the lung. Cancer Imaging 2007;26(7):195-201.

[57] Hoegerle S, Nitzsche E, Altehoefer C, *et al.* Pheochromocytomas: Detection with 18F DOPA whole body PET--initial results. Radiology 2002;222(2):507-12.

[58] Wild D, Mäcke HR, Waser B, *et al.* 68Ga-DOTANOC: A first compound for PET imaging with high affinity for somatostatin receptor subtypes 2 and 5. Eur J Nucl Med Mol Imaging 2005;32(6):724.

[59] Brink I, Hoegerle S, Klisch J, Bley TA. Imaging of pheochromocytoma and paraganglioma. Fam Cancer 2005;4(1):61-8.

[60] Buchmann I, Henze M, Engelbrecht S, *et al.* Comparison of 68Ga-DOTATOC PET and 111In-DTPAOC (Octreoscan) SPECT in patients with neuroendocrine tumours. Eur J Nucl Med Mol Imaging 2007;34(10):1617-26.

[61] Gabriel M, Decristoforo C, Kendler D, *et al.* 68Ga-DOTA-Tyr3-octreotide PET in neuroendocrine tumours: comparison with somatostatin receptor scintigraphy and CT. J Nucl Med 2007;48(4):508–518.

[62] Jindal T, Kumar A, Venkitaraman B, Dutta R, Kumar R. Role of (68)Ga-DOTATOC PET/CT in the evaluation of primary pulmonary carcinoids. Korean J Intern Med 2010;25(4):386-91.

[63] Ambrosini V, Castellucci P, Rubello D, *et al.* 68Ga-DOTA-NOC: a new PET tracer for evaluating patients with bronchial carcinoid. Nucl Med Commun 2009;30(4):281-6.

[64] Zatloukal P, Petruzelka L, Zemanova M, *et al.* Concurrent *versus* sequential chemoradiotherapy with cisplatin and vinorelbine in locally advanced non-small cell lung cancer: A randomized study. Lung Cancer 2004;46(1):87–98.

[65] Velazquez ER, Aerts HJ, Oberije C, De Ruysscher D, Lambin P. Prediction of residual metabolic activity after treatment in NSCLC patients. Acta Oncol 2010;49(7):1033-9.

[66] Obrzut S, Bykowski J, Badran K, Hayeri MR, Hoh CK. Utility of fluorodeoxyglucose-positron emission tomography in the identification of new lesions in lung cancer patients for the assessment of therapy response. Nucl Med Commun 2010;31(12):1008-15.

[67] Cerfolio RJ, Bryant AS, Winokur TS, Ohja B, Bartolucci AA. Repeat FDG-PET after neoadjuvant therapy is a predictor of pathologic response in patients with non-small cell lung cancer. Ann Thorac Surg 2004;78(6):1903–9.

[68] MacManus MP, Hicks RJ, Matthews JP, *et al.* Positron emission tomography is superior to computed tomography scanning for response-assessment after radical radiotherapy or

chemoradiotherapy in patients with non-small-cell lung cancer. J Clin Oncol 2003;21(7):1285–92.

[69] Huang W, Zhou T, Ma L, *et al.* Standard uptake value and metabolic tumour volume of (18)F-FDG PET/CT predict short-term outcome early in the course of chemoradiotherapy in advanced non-small cell lung cancer. Eur J Nucl Med Mol Imaging 2011;38(9):1628-35.

[70] Isobe K, Hata Y, Takai Y, Shibuya K, Takagi K, Homma S. Usefulness of fluoro-2-deoxyglucose positron emission tomography for investigating unexplained rising carcinoembryonic antigen levels that occur during the postoperative surveillance of lung cancer patients. Int J Clin Oncol 2009;14(6):497-501.

[71] Pottgen C, Levegrun S, Theegarten D, *et al.* Value of 18F-fluoro-2-deoxy-D-glucose-positron emission tomography/computed tomography in non-small-cell lung cancer for prediction of pathologic response and times to relapse after neoadjuvant chemoradiotherapy. Clin Cancer Res 2006;12(1):97-106.

[72] Akeboshi M, Yamakado K, Nakatsuka A, *et al.* Percutaneous radiofrequency ablation of lung neoplasms: initial therapeutic response. J Vasc Interv Radiol 2004;15(5):463–70.

[73] Singnurkar A, Solomon SB, Gönen M, Larson SM, Schöder H. 18F-FDG PET/CT for the prediction and detection of local recurrence after radiofrequency ablation of malignant lung lesions. J Nucl Med 2010;51(12):1833-40.

[74] Sohn HJ, Yang YJ, Ryu JS, *et al.* [18F]Fluorothymidine positron emission tomography before and 7 days after gefitinib treatment predicts response in patients with advanced adenocarcinoma of the lung. Clin Cancer Res 2008;14(22):7423-9.

[75] Ullrich RT, Zander T, Neumaier B, *et al.* Early detection of erlotinib treatment response in NSCLC by 3'-deoxy-3'-[F]-fluoro-L-thymidine ([F]FLT) positron emission tomography (PET). PLoS One 2008;3(12):e3908.

[76] Zander T, Scheffler M, Nogova L, *et al.* Early prediction of nonprogression in advanced non-small-cell lung cancer treated with erlotinib by using [(18)F]fluorodeoxyglucose and [(18)F]fluorothymidine positron emission tomography. J Clin Oncol. 2011;29(13):1701-8.

[77] Takeuchi S, Zhao S, Kuge Y, *et al.* 18F-Fluorothymidine PET/CT as an early predictor of tumour response to treatment with cetuximab in human lung cancer xenografts. Oncol Rep 2011;26(3):725-30.

[78] Katz SI, Zhou L, Ferrara TA, *et al.* FLT-PET may not be a reliable indicator of therapeutic response in p53-null malignancy. Int J Oncol 2011;39(1):91-100.

[79] Kaira K, Oriuchi N, Otani Y, *et al.* Fluorine-18-alpha-methyltyrosine positron emission tomography for diagnosis and staging of lung cancer: a clinicopathologic study. Clin Cancer Res 2007;13(21):6369-78.

[80] Kaira K, Oriuchi N, Shimizu K, *et al.* 18F-FMT uptake seen within primary cancer on PET helps predict outcome of non-small cell lung cancer. J Nucl Med 2009;50(11):1770-6.

[81] Kaira K, Oriuchi N, Yanagitani N, *et al.* Assessment of therapy response in lung cancer with ^{18}F-α-methyl tyrosine PET. AJR Am J Roentgenol 2010;195(5):1204-11.

[82] Kanzaki R, Higashiyama M, Maeda J, *et al.* Clinical value of F18-fluorodeoxyglucose positron emission tomography-computed tomography in patients with non-small cell lung cancer after potentially curative surgery: experience with 241 patients. Interact Cardiovasc Thorac Surg 2010 Jun;10(6):1009-14.

[83] Fortes DL, Allen MS, Lowe VJ, *et al.* The sensitivity of 18F-fluorodeoxyglucose positron emission tomography in the evaluation of metastatic pulmonary nodules. Eur J Cardiothorac Surg 2008;34(6):1223-7.

[84] Detterbeck FC, Grodzki T, Gleeson F, Robert JH. Imaging requirements in the practice of pulmonary metastasectomy. J Thorac Oncol 2010;5(6 Suppl 2):S134-9.

[85] Okereke IC, Gangadharan SP, Kent MS, Nicotera SP, Shen C, DeCamp MM. Standard uptake value predicts survival in non-small cell lung cancer. Ann Thorac Surg 2009;88(3):911-5; discussion 915-6.

[86] Al-Sarraf N, Gately K, Lucey J, *et al.* Clinical implication and prognostic significance of standardised uptake value of primary non-small cell lung cancer on positron emission tomography: analysis of 176 cases. Eur J Cardiothorac Surg 2008;34(4):892-7.

[87] Sasaki R, Komaki R, Macapinlac H, *et al.* [18F]fluorodeoxyglucose uptake by positron emission tomography predicts outcome of non-small-cell lung cancer. J Clin Oncol 2005;23(6):1136-43.

[88] Saga T, Koizumi M, Inubushi M, *et al.* PET/CT with 3'-deoxy-3'-[18F]fluorothymidine for lung cancer patients receiving carbon-ion radiotherapy. Nucl Med Commun 2011;32(5):348-55.

[89] Spratt DE, Diaz R, McElmurray J, *et al.* Impact of FDG PET/CT on delineation of the gross tumour volume for radiation planning in non-small-cell lung cancer. Clin Nucl Med 2010;35(4):237-43.

[90] Vila A, Sánchez-Reyes A, Conill C, *et al.* Comparison of positron emission tomography (PET) and computed tomography (CT) for better target volume definition in radiation therapy planning. Clin Transl Oncol 2010;12(5):367-73.

[91] Greco C, Rosenzweig K, Cascini GL, Tamburrini O. Current status of PET/CT for tumour volume definition in radiotherapy treatment planning for non-small cell lung cancer (NSCLC). Lung Cancer 2007;57(2):125-34.

[92] van Loon J, van Baardwijk A, Boersma L, Ollers M, Lambin P, De Ruysscher D. Therapeutic implications of molecular imaging with PET in the combined modality treatment of lung cancer. Cancer Treat Rev 2011;37(5):331-43.

[93] De Ruysscher D, Wanders S, Minken A, *et al.* Effects of radiotherapy planning with a dedicated combined PET-CT-simulator of patients with non-small cell lung cancer on dose limiting normal tissues and radiation dose-escalation: a planning study. Radiother Oncol 2005;77(1):5–10.

[94] van Der Wel A, Nijsten S, Hochstenbag M, *et al.* Increased therapeutic ratio by 18FDG-PET CT planning in patients with clinical CT stage N2-N3M0 non-small-cell lung cancer: a modeling study. Int J Radiat Oncol Biol Phys 2005;61:649–55.

[95] Zimmermann F, Wulf J, Lax I, *et al.* Stereotactic body radiation therapy for early non-small cell lung cancer. Front Radiat Ther Oncol 2010;42:94-114.

[96] Gubbi J, Kanakatte A, Tomas K, *et al.* Automatic tumour volume delineation in respiratory-gated PET images. J Med Imaging Radiat Oncol 2011;55(1):65-76.

[97] Fox JL, Rengan R, O'Meara W, *et al.* Does registration of PET and planning CT images decrease interobserver and intraobserver variation in delineating tumour volumes for non--small cell lung cancer? Int J Radiat Oncol Biol Phys 2005;62:70-5.

[98] Lin P, Koh ES, Lin M, *et al.* Diagnostic and staging impact of radiotherapy planning FDG-PET-CT in non-small-cell lung cancer. Radiother Oncol 2011;101(2):284-90.

[99] Vanneste BG, Haas RL, Bard MP, Rijna H, Váldes Olmos RA, Belderbos JS. Involved field radiotherapy for locally advanced non-small cell lung cancer: isolated mediastinal nodal relapse. Lung Cancer 2010;70(2):218-20.

[100] Mohammed N, Kestin LL, Grills IS, *et al.* Rapid disease progression with delay in treatment of non-small-cell lung cancer. Int J Radiat Oncol Biol Phys 2011;79(2):466-72.

[101] Koh WJ, Bergman KS, Rasey JS, *et al.* Evaluation of oxygenation status during fractionated radiotherapy in human nonsmall cell lung cancers using [F-18]fluoromisonidazole positron emission tomography. Int J Radiat Oncol Biol Phys 1995;33(2):391-8.

[102] Vansteenkiste JF, Stroobants SG. Positron emission tomography in the management of non-small cell lung cancer. Hematol Oncol Clin North Am 2004;18(1):269-88.

[103] Vera P, Bohn P, Edet-Sanson A, *et al.* Simultaneous positron emission tomography (PET) assessment of metabolism with ^{18}F-fluoro-2-deoxy-d-glucose (FDG), proliferation with ^{18}F-fluoro-thymidine (FLT), and hypoxia with ^{18}fluoro-misonidazole (F-miso) before and during radiotherapy in patients with non-small-cell lung cancer (NSCLC): a pilot study. Radiother Oncol 2011;98(1):109-16.

[104] Li L, Hu M, Zhu H, Zhao W, Yang G, Yu J. Comparison of 18F-Fluoroerythronitroimidazole and 18F-fluorodeoxyglucose positron emission tomography and prognostic value in locally advanced non-small-cell lung cancer. Clin Lung Cancer 2010;11(5):335-40.

[105] Yang DJ, Wallace S, Cherif A, *et al.* Development of F-18-labeled fluoroerythronitroimidazole as a PET agent for imaging tumour hypoxia. Radiology 1995;194(3):795-800.

[106] Almeida FA, Uzbeck M, Ost D. Initial evaluation of the nonsmall cell lung cancer patient: diagnosis and staging. Curr Opin Pulm Med 2010;16(4):307-14.

Send Orders of Reprints at reprints@benthamscience.net
Lung Cancer: Clinical and Surgical Specifications, **2013, 165-174**

CHAPTER 7

Lung Cancer Staging

Serdar Erturan* and Günay Aydin

Istanbul University, Cerrahpasa Medical School, Department of Respiratory Diseases, Istanbul, Turkey

Abstract: Staging of lung cancer was first made in 1973 and was revised according to new information obtained by case series. The last staging was proposed by IASCL in 2007 [1] and accepted in 2009 [2]. New regulations are made in T and M descriptors in the new TNM staging but no change is made in N descriptor.

Keywords: Staging, TNM system, lung cancer, EUS, EUS, Bronchoscopy, regional lymph nodes, metastasis.

T (primary tumour)

T0: No primary tumour.

T1: Tumour ≤3 cm, surrounded by lung or visceral pleura, not more than lobar bronchus.

T1a: Tumour's largest diameter less than or equal to 2 cm.

T1b: Tumour's largest diameter is more than 2 cm but less than or equal to 3 cm.

T2: Tumour>3 cm but ≤7cm or tumour with any of the following.

Invades visceral pleura, involves main bronchus more than 2 cm distal to carina or:

Atelectasis/obstructive pneumonia extending to hilum but not the entire lung:

T2a: Tumour's largest diameter is more than 3 cm but less than or equal to 5 cm.

***Address correspondence to Serdar Erturan:** İstanbul University, Cerrahpasa Medical School, Department of Respiratory Diseases, Intanbul, Turkey; Tel: +90 212 4143000/21816; Fax: +90 212 6321216; E-mail: serdarerturan@mynet.com

T2b: Tumours largest diameter is more than 5 cm but less than or equal to 7 cm.

T3: Tumour's largest diameter>7 cm ($T3_{>7}$) or

Directly invading chest wall, diaphragm, phrenic nerve, mediastinal pleura or parietal pericardium ($T3_{inv}$) or

Tumour in the main bronchus less than 2 cm distal to carina ($T3_{cent}$) or

Atelectasis/obstructive pneumonia of entire lung ($T3_{cent}$) or

Separate tumour nodules in the same lobe ($T3_{satell}$).

T4: Tumour of any size with invasion of heart, great vessels, trachea, recurrent laryngeal nerve, esophagus, vertebral body or carina ($T4_{inv}$) or

Separate tumour nodule(s) in a different ipsilateral lobe ($T4_{ipsi\ nod}$).

N (regional lymph nodes).

N0: No regional node metastasis.

N1: Metastasis in ipsilateral peribronchial and/or perihilar lymph nodes and intrapulmonary nodes, including involvement by direct extension.

N2: Metastasis in ipsilateral mediastinal and/or subcarinal lymph nodes.

N3: Metastasis in contralateral mediastinal, contralateral hilar, ipsilateral or contralateral scalene, or supraclavicular lymph nodes.

M (distant metastasis).

M0: No distant metastasis.

M1a: Separate tumour nodules in a contralateral lobe($M1a_{contr\ nod}$) or

Tumour with pleural nodules or malignant pleural dissemination($M1a_{pl\ dissem}$).

M1b: Distant metastasis.

Stages according to TNM are shown in Table **1**.

Table 1: Stages according to TNM

T/M	**Subgroup**	**N0**	**N1**	**N2**	**N3**
T1	T1a	Ia	IIa	IIIa	IIIb
	T1b	Ia	IIa	IIIa	IIIb
T2	T2a	Ib	IIa	IIIa	IIIb
	T2b	IIa	IIb	IIIa	IIIb
T3	$T3_{>7}$	IIb	IIIa	IIIa	IIIb
	$T3_{inv}$	IIb	IIIa	IIIa	IIIb
	$T3_{satell}$	IIb	IIIa	IIIa	IIIb
T4	$T4_{inv}$	IIIa	IIIa	IIIb	IIIb
	$T4_{\text{ipsi nod}}$	IIIa	IIIa	IIIb	IIIb
M1	$M1a_{\text{contr nod}}$	IV	IV	IV	IV
	$M1a_{\text{pl yayım}}$	IV	IV	IV	IV
	M1b	IV	IV	IV	IV

Two staging assessments are commonly used. Clinical staging is done prior to any treatment using all the information available. Clinical staging can be done by history, physical examination, imaging techniques and surgical staging techniques such as mediastinoscopy. Pathological staging is assessment after surgical resection (Table **2**).

Table 2: Types of staging assessments

	Name	**Definition**
c	Clinical	Prior to initiation of any treatment
p	Pathologic	After resection, based on pathologic assessment
y	Restaging	After part or all of the treatment has been given
r	Recurrence	Stage at the time of recurrence
a	Autopsy	Stage as determined by autopsy

After surgical resection, negative surgical margins is represented by **R0,** microscopical positive margins are represented by **R1** and visible or palpable tumour remain is represented by **R2**.

Clinical Findings

Hoarseness, superior vena cava syndrome, chest pain give valuable information about intrathoracic dissemination of the tumour.

Loss of more than 5% of body mass in the last 6 months, bone pain, headache, syncope, epileptic seizures, hepatomegaly, peripheral lymphadenomegaly are signs and symptoms of metastacic disease.

Laboratory findings suggestive of metastasis are elevated AST, ALT, ALP and Ca levels.

Pleural effusion in lung cancer patients is mostly due to tumour. In these cases thoracentesis should be performed and the effusion should be cytologically assessed. VATS should be considered in highly suspected malignancy where plerural fluid cytology is negative [3].

Bronchoscopy

Bronchoscopy is the major diagnositcal method in the diagnosis of lung cancer. The rate of histopatological diagnosis of bronchoscopy is 79-98% in central tumours, whereas it drops to 48-80% in peripheric tumours [4]. Bronchoscopy can also be informative about the extent of the tumour. The accuracy of bronchoscopic staging can reach to 95% in intrabronchial tumours that can be reached by bronchoscope.

The following information can be obtained by bronchoscopy in TNM staging [5]:

T1: Tumour not visible endoscopically or has not reaced the proximal part of lobe bronchus.

T2: Tumour in main bronchus but the lesion is more than 2 cm distal to the carina.

T3: Tumour is closer than 2 cm but has not yet invaded the tracheal carina or atelectasis of entire lung.

T4: Tracheal carina invasion or tracheal invasion.

N1: Metastasis of ipsilateral peribronchial and hilar lymph nodes.

N2: Metastasis of ipsilateral mediastinal and/or subcarinal lymph nodes.

N3: Metastasis in contralateral mediastinal, contralateral hilar lymph nodes.

M1: Intrabronchial or intrapulmonary metastasis or lymphangitis carcinomatosis.

Needle aspirations from hilar and mediastinal lymph nodes adjacent to tracheobronchial tree can be done *via* bronchoscope. While practicing this procedure, the anatomy of tracheobronchial tree and the locations of lymph nodes and large vessels adjacent to the airways must be held in mind [6]. Although it is a minimally invasive procedure, it is not commonly used in daily practice. In USA, it has been reported that 10% of pulmonologists use this method commonly whereas 4% of pulmonologists use it rarely [7].

Needle aspirations from 11 different lymph nodes can be done by using four bronchoscopically defined areas (tracheal carina, right upper lobe bronchus, intermediary bronchus and left upper lobe branching). To minimize contamination, TBNA should be done before other samples are taken [8].

Sensitivity of TBNA is dependent on several factors:

1. TBNA can be done by either histologic or cytologic needles. The sensitivity of histologic needles is found to be higher than cytologic needles (57% *vs.* 41%) [9].

2. More positive results are obtained from aspirations of right paratracheal and subcarinal lymph nodes than other regions [9].

3. Sensitivity increases as the size of the lymph node increases. If the lymph node is larger than 10 mm in its shortest diameter, sensitivity is over 57%, negative predictive value is 80-91%. If ıt is larger than 15 mm, sensitivity is higher than 62% [9].

4. Sensitivity of TBNA is directly proportional to the number of aspirations. The rate of dedection of metastasis by the first aspiration is 42% whereas, after four aspirations sensitivity reaches up to 92%

[10]. For this reason, in order to gain efficient samples, at least four aspirations should be done for every lymph node.

5. Having a cytopathologist on-site, evaluation of the samples using rapid staining technique (rapid on site evaluation-ROSE) and conclusion of efficient material by a cytopathologist significantly increases diagnosic rates. It has been shown that the sensitivity of TBNA is elevated from 25% to 71% by the use of ROSE.

EBUS and EUS

Mediastinal structures can be visualized by ultrasonography. This can be achieved either by an esophagoscopy (endoscopic ultrasonography-EUS) or by bronchoscopy (endobronchial ultrasonography-EBUS). These methods are helpful in the visualization and aspiration of lymph nodes [11], evaluation of large vessel invasion [12] and the determination of the depth of bronchial wall invasion in early stage bronchial carcinomas [13,14].

By using EUS, paraesophageal region, aortopulmonary window, subcarinal region and areas adjacent to left atrium can be examined and EUS-controlled aspirations from 4L,5,7,8 and 9 lymph node stations can be made [11,15-17]. Due to the presence of air in trachea, right upper mediastinal region can not be assessed thoroughly. However, there are studies reporting aspiration results from 2R,4R,2L and 4L lymph nodes and even from surrenal gland [18].

By using EBUS, lymph nodes adjacent to tracheobronchial tree can be assessed and simultaneous TBNA can be performed. TBNA can be done using EBUS from right and left paratracheal, subcarinal and hilar lymph nodes [19] (Table **3**). In studies where sensitivity is reported higher than 90%, lymph node metastasis seems to be higher [20]. In cases with small lymph nodes sensitivity is lower [21]. More than 10% false negativity is reported so negative results should be reinforced with invasive methods such as mediastinoscopy [22].

Imaging Techniques

Chest CT should be obtained in every case. Chest CT should involve upper abdomen in order to evaluate liver and surrenal gland metastasis. Contrast material should be used and if possible multislice CT should be preferred. The size and location of the primary tumour and its relation to adjacent organs and fissures can be assessed by CT. Hilar and mediastinal lymph nodes can also be evaluated by CT. For a lymph node to have a shortest diameter longer than 10 mm is considered pathological. However, independent of the size, a small lymph node may be metastasized whereas an enlarged lymph node may be free of metastasis. This evaluation of CT based on side has sensitivity, specificity and positive predictive value varying between 58-79%, 78-82% and 56-83% respectively [23].

Table 3: Endoscopic mediastinal staging

	TBNA	EUS-NA	EBUS-TBNA
2R/L		±	+
3			+
4R	+	±	+
4L	+	+	+
5		+	+
6			
7	+	+	+
8		+	
9		+	
10	+		+
11-12	+		+

Although it has better results than CT in N staging, PET-CT has a high rate of false positivity (13-44%) [24, 25]. Positive mediastinal lymph node results obtained by PET-CT should be confirmed by invasive staging techniques. On the other hand, PET-CT can not distinguish central tumour and adjacent lymph node and overlooks microscopical metastasis which results in 5-23% false negativity in N staging [24-25]. However, in the case of a peripheral T1 tumour with high absorbtion of FDG and no hilar and mediastinal lymph node involvement in PET-CT and no findings of pathologically enlarged lymph nodes in chest CT has a negative predictive value more than 97%; invasive staging may not be necessary [26].

Re-evaluation of mediastinal lymph nodes by PET-CT after neoadjuvant treatment is less successful than primary staging of mediastinum. It has been suggested that waiting for 2 weeks after chemotherapy and 4 weeks after radiotherapy should be enough for restaging. PET-CT is suggested to be more effective than remediastinoscopy in restaging [27].

PET-CT is an effective method for demonstrating extra-cranial metastatic lesions. In a metaanalysis, sensitivity and specificity of PET-CT in demonstrating distant metastasis were 93% and 96%, respectively [28]. In the presence of solitary metastasis, other imaging techniques such as CT or MRI or biopsy should be used in order to avoid false positivity.

MRI is not a major imaging technique in evaluating intrathoracic staging of lung cancer. MRI may be useful in cases where there is suspicion of mediastinal, chest wall or vertebral invasion. MRI must be preferred in the evaluation of local invasion(brachial plexus invasion) in superior sulcus tumours [24].

Invasive Staging

In NSCLC patients with no distant metastasis and who are functionaly operable, the most important factor effecting survival is mediastinal lymph node metastasis.

In the presence of enlarged lymph nodes in chest CT, false negativity and positivity of PET-CT may rise up to 25% [25, 29]. For this reason, invasive mediastinal staging should be performed if there is enlarged mediastinal lymph nodes regardless of PET-CT results.

If chest CT reveals no enlarged mediastinal lymph nodes and if PET-CT is negative, rate of false positivity is considerably low. That's why in the case,of an epidermoid tumour clinically staged as T1N0, invasive staging may not be performed.

Bronchoscopic methods are the first choice in invasive staging. If the results are negative, because there is a risk of false negativity, surgical staging must be done [22]. Mediastinoscopy is the gold standard method in evaluating mediastinal lymph nodes. However there is 9% (4-16) chance of false negativity. The most common reason for false negativity is that pN2 lymph nodes are located outside mediastinoscopy field. Lymph nodes 1, 2R, 2L, 3, 4R, 4L and anterior 7 can be reached by mediastinoscopy. Depending on the location of the lymph node, extended mediastinoscopy (5 and 6 can be reached), mediastinotomy and VATS can be chosen [30].

ACKNOWLEDGEMENTS

Declared none.

CONFLICT OF INTEREST

The author confirms that this article content has no conflict of interest.

REFERENCES

[1] Groome PA, Bolejack V, Crowley JJ, *et al.* The IASLC lung cancer staging Project: Validation of the proposals for revision of the T, N, and M descriptors and consequent stage groupings in the forthcoming (seventh) edition of the TNM classification of malignant tumours. J Thorac Oncol 2007; 2: 694-705.
[2] Detterbeck FC, Boffa DJ, Tanoue LT. The new lung cancer staging system. Chest 2009; 136: 260-271.
[3] Neragi-Miandoab S. Malignant pleural effusion, current and evolving approaches for its diagnosis and management. Lung Cancer 2006; 54: 1-9.
[4] Mazzone P, Jain P, Arroliga AC, Matthay RA. Bronchoscopy and needle biopsy techniques for diagnosis and staging of lung cancer. Clin Chest Med 2002; 23: 137-58.
[5] Becker HD. Bronchoscopy for airway lesions. In: Wang KP, Mehta AC, Turner JF, eds. Flexible bronchoscopy. 2nd ed. Oxford: Blackwell; 2004: 71-88.
[6] Dasgupta A, Mehta AC. Transbronchial needle aspiration. An underused diagnostic technique. Clin Chest Med 1999; 20: 39-50.
[7] Haponik EF, Shure D. Underutilization of transbronchial needle aspiration. Experiences of current pulmonary fellows. Chest 1997; 112: 251-3.
[8] Wang KP, Mehta A, Turner JF. Transbronchial needle aspiration for cytology and histology specimens. In: Wang KP, Mehta AC, Turner JF, eds. Flexible bronchoscopy. 2nd ed. Oxford: Blackwell; 2004: 117-37.
[9] Harrow EM, Abi-Selah W, Blum J, *et al.* The utility of transbronchial needle aspiration in the staging of bronchogenic carcinoma. Am J Respir Crit Care Med 2000; 161: 601-7.
[10] Chin R, McCain TW, Lucia MA, *et al.* Transbronchial needle aspiration in diagnosing and staging lung cancer. How many aspirates are needed?.Am J Respir Crit Care Med 2002; 166: 377-81.
[11] Krasnik M. Endoscopic transesophageal and endoscopic transbronchial real-time ultrasound-guided biopsy. Respiration 2003; 70: 293-8.
[12] Okamoto H, Watanabe K, Nagatomo A, *et al.* Endobronchial ultrasonography for mediastinal and hilar lymph node metastases of lung cancer. Chest 2002; 121:1498-506.
[13] Falcone F, Fois F, Grosso D. Endobronchial ultrasound. Respiration 2003; 70: 179-94.

[14] Miyazu Y, Miyazawa T, Kurimoto N, *et al.* Endobronchial ultrasonography in the assessment of centrally located early-stage lung cancer before photodynamic therapy. Am J Respir Crit Care Med 2002; 165: 832-7.

[15] Wallace MB, Silvestri GA, Sahai AV, *et al.* Endoscopic ultrasound-guided fine needle aspiration for staging patients with carcinoma of the lung. Ann Thorac Surg 2001; 72: 1861-7.

[16] Wiersema MJ, Vazquez-Sequeiros E, Wiersema LM. Evaluation of mediastinal lymphadenopathy with endoscopic US-guided fine-needle aspiration biopsy. Radiology 2001; 219: 252-7.

[17] Larsen SS, Krasnik M, Vilmann P, *et al.* Endoscopic ultrasound guided biopsy of mediastinal lesions has a major impact on patient management. Thorax 2002; 57: 98-103.

[18] Larsen SS, Vilmann P, Krasnik M, *et al.* Endoscopic ultrasound guided biopsy *versus* mediastinoscopy for analysis of paratracheal and subcarinal lymph nodes in lung cancer staging. Lung Cancer 2005; 48: 85-92.

[19] Yasufuku K, Chiyo M, Sekine Y, *et al.* Real-time endobronchial ultrasound-guided transbronchial needle aspiration of mediastinal and hilar lymph nodes. Chest 2004; 126: 122-128.

[20] Herth FJ, Eberhardt R, Vilmann P, *et al.* Real-time endobronchial ultrasound guided transbronchial needle aspiration for sampling mediastinal lymph nodes. Thorax 2006; 61: 795-798.

[21] Herth FJ, Ernst A, Eberhardt R, *et al.* Endobronchial ultrasound-guided transbronchial needle aspiration of lymph nodes in the radiologically normal mediastinum. Eur Respir J 2006; 28: 910-914.

[22] Herth FJ, Becker HD, Ernst A. Ultrasound-guided transbronchial needle aspiration: An experience in 242 patients. Chest 2003; 123: 604-607.

[23] Toloza EM, Harpole L, McCrory D. Noninvasive staging of non-small cell lung cancer: a review of the current evidence. Chest 2003; 123: 137s-146s.

[24] Silvestri GA, Gould MK, Margolis MA, *et al.* Noninvasive staging of non-small cell lung cancer: ACCP evidence-based clinical practice guidelines. Chest 2007; 132(suppl 3): 178s-201s.

[25] Bellek E, Erturan SS, Halac M, ve ark. Küçük hücreli dışı akciğer kanserinde mediasten lenf nodu evrelemesinde PET-BT'nin yeri. Solunum 2010; 12: 13-20.

[26] Detterbeck F, Falen S, Rivera M, *et al.* Seeking a home for a PET, part 2: Defining the appropriate place for positron emission tomography imaging in the staging of patiets with suspected lung cancer. Chest 2004; 125: 2300-2308.

[27] De Leyn P; Stroobants S, De Wever W, *et al.* Prospective comparative study of integrated positron emission tomography-computed tomography scan compared with remediastinoscopy in the assessment of residual mediastinal lymph node disease after induction therapy for mediastinoscopy proven stage IIIA-N2 non-small cell lung cancer: A Leuven Lung Cancer Group Study. J Clin Oncol 2006; 24: 3333-3339.

[28] Mayor S. NICE issues guidance for diagnosis and treatment of lung cancer. Br Med J 2005; 330: 439.

[29] Nomori H, Watanabe K, Ohtsuka T, *et al.* The size of metastatic foci and lymph nodes yielding false-negative and false-positive lymph node staging with positron emission tomography in patients with lung cancer. J Thorac Cardiovasc Surg 2004; 127: 1087-1092.

[30] Toloza EM, Harpole L, Detterbeck F, *et al.* Invasive staging of non-small cell lung cancer: a review of the current evidence. Chest 2003; 123: 157s-166s.

CHAPTER 8

Pulmonary Nodules Less Than One Centimeter in Size

Dalokay Kiliç[*], Alper Findikçioğlu and Ahmet Hatipoğlu

Department of Thoracic Surgery, Baskent University Faculty of Medicine, Ankara Teaching and Medical Research Center, 5. Sokak No: 48, Kat: 0, 06490, Bahcelievler/Ankara, Turkey

Abstract: Solitary pulmonary nodule (SPN) is a challenging problem especially for the chest physicians and thoracic surgeons. Radiologic diagnosis and classification of an SPN in terms of margins, size and doubling time are very important but insufficient. Definitive diagnosis of an SPN depends on histopathologic examination. Differntial diagnosis of an SPN less than 10 mm is more difficult because sensitivity and accuracy of the diagnostic methods will also decrease with decreasing dimension. Conventional radiologic methods as chest X-ray and low dose CT have been widely used for screening high risk patients for lung cancer however this methods are insufficient for small SPN. Latest method, FDG PET CT, also depends on the size of the lesion. The sensitivity, specificity, and accuracy were 85%, 36% and 54% respectively for nodules smaller than 10 mm, compared to 91%, 47%, and 79% for nodules between 1.1-2.0 cm. Sensivity and accuracy of histopathologic diagnosis with fine needle biopsy for small SPN depend on the location of the lesion. The accuracy of the biopsy improves in peripheral nodules. Surgical excision of the SSPN *via* VATS can provide definitive diagnosis and treatment, however major lung resection and mediastinal lymph node dissection are the most effective treatment methods for malign nodules.

Keywords: Pulmonary nodule, Lung Cancer, Less than one centimeter, VATS.

INTRODUCTION

A solitary pulmonary nodule (SPN) is defined as a discrete, well-marginated, rounded opacity less than or equal to 3 cm in diameter that is completely

***Address correspondence to Dalokay Kiliç:** Department of Thoracic Surgery, Baskent University Faculty of Medicine, Ankara Teaching and Medical Research Center, 5. Sokak No: 48, Kat: 0, 06490, Bahcelievler/Ankara, Turkey; Tel: +90-312-2150552; Fax: +90-312-2132340;
E-mail: dalokay7@yahoo.com

surrounded by lung parenchyma, does not touch the hilum or mediastinum, and is not associated with atelectasis or pleural effusion. Patients with solitary pulmonary nodules are usually asymptomatic; however, solitary pulmonary nodules pose a challenge to both clinicians and patients. If the nodule is bigger than 1 cm in diameter, it can be seen with conventional radiologic methods as Thorax Computerized Tomography (Thorax CT) and X-ray. However, if the nodule is less than one cm "small solitary pulmonary nodule (SSPN)", it can be detected with widespread and high-resolution CT screening.

Most solitary pulmonary nodules are benign; however, they may represent an early stage of lung cancer. Lung cancer survival rates remain dismally low at 14% at 5 years. Early lung cancer, when the primary tumour is less than 3 cm in diameter (stage Ia), may lead to 5-year survival rates of 70-80%. Therefore, prompt diagnosis and management of early lung cancer manifesting, as solitary pulmonary nodule may be the only chance for cure. Unfortunately, these nodules can be found during the routine control for other chronic diseases.

SSPNs are frequently seen at screening CT performed in subjects at high risk of developing lung cancer, and although these nodules may show an increase in size at follow-up examinations Whether detected serendipitously or during a routine investigation, a nodule on a chest radiograph raises several questions: Is the nodule benign or malignant? Should it be investigated or observed? Should it be surgically resected?

Radiological Investigation

The many authors suggested that SPN (<1 cm) can be detected *via* a CT screening which has different techniques. Takashima S *et al.* mentioned qualitative (presence or absence of lobulation, spiculation, air bronchogram, cavity, satellite lesions, pleural tag, concave margins, polygonal shape, and peripheral subpleural lesion) and quantitative (lesion size, percentage of ground-glass opacity areas,) assessments in thin-section CT (two-and three-dimensional ratios of lesion) of 72 nodules (25 lung cancers, seven atypical adenomatous hyperplasias, and 40 benign lesions). In one study, small nodules were detected in 22% of high-risk patients, 90% of who proved to have benign lesions [1]. On the other hand, primary lung cancer was discovered in 38% of patients who underwent video-assisted thoracic surgery for nodules of 1 cm or smaller detected on Thorax CT [2]. Of the 27 lung cancers detected at screening lung CT, 15 (56%) were nodules of 1 cm or smaller [1]. Siegelman *et al.* found that 32 (28.7%) of 113 SPN (<1 cm) were malignant [3]. Wahidi *et al.* mentioned that 0 to 1% for nodules < 5 mm, 6 to 28% for nodules 5 to 10 mm, and 64 to 82% for nodules > 20 mm and screening-detected nodules showed that the risk for malignancy was approximately 20 to 30% in nodules with smooth edges; in nodules with irregular, lobulated, or spiculated borders, the rate of malignancy was higher but varied across studies from 33 to 100%. Nodules that were pure ground-glass opacities were more likely to be malignant (59 to 73%) than solid nodules (7 to 9%). Ahn *et al.* investigated that Baseline and follow-up thin-section multidetector Thorax CT scans obtained in 146 consecutive subjects at high risk for lung cancer (age range, 50–75 years; > 30 pack-year smoking history), in this study found none that had developed into lung cancer; this suggests that the malignancy potential of perifissural nodule is low [4]. Dong Ming Xu *et al.* evaluated noncalcified pulmonary nodules between 5 and 10 mm in diameter in 891 patients at 3 months and 1 year to assess growth and the authors founded In smooth or attached solid indeterminate nodules, no malignancies were found at 1-year follow-up [5]. In nonsmooth purely intraparenchymal nodules, size is the main baseline predictor for malignancy. When follow-up data are available, growth is a strong predictor for malignancy, especially at 1-year follow-up.

Veronrsi G *et al.* investigated a total of 5201 asymptomatic high-risk volunteers underwent screening with multidetector low-dose computed tomography. Nodules detected at baseline or new nodules at annual screening received repeat low-dose computed tomography at 1 year if less than 5 mm, repeat low-dose computed tomography 3 to 6 months later if between 5 and 8 mm, and fluorodeoxyglucose positron emission tomography if more than 8 mm. Growing nodules at the annual screening received low-dose computed tomography at 6 months and computed tomography-positron emission tomography or surgical biopsy according to doubling time, type, and size. During the first year of screening, 106 patients underwent lung biopsy and 91 lung cancers were identified (70% were stage I). Diagnosis was delayed (false-negative) in 6 patients (stage IIB in 1 patient, stage

IIIA in 3 patients, and stage IV in 2 patients), including 2 small cell cancers and 1 central lesion. Surgical biopsy revealed benign disease (false-positives) in 15 cases (14%). Positron emission tomography sensitivity was 88% for prevalent cancers and 70% for cancers diagnosed after first annual screening [6]. No needle biopsy procedures were performed in this cohort of patients. Low-dose computed tomography screening is effective for the early detection of lung cancers, but nodule management remains a challenge. Wormanns *et al.* reported that double reading increased the detection rate of pulmonary nodules from 63% to 74-79%, a considerable proportion of nodules remained undetected. No difference between sensitivities at standard-dose and low-dose multirow-detector CT for detection of small nodules [7]. Computed tomography-positron emission tomography is useful at baseline, but its sensitivity decreases significantly the subsequent year. Multidisciplinary management and experience are crucial for minimizing misdiagnoses.

A maximum intensity projection (MIP) is a computer visualization method for 3D data that projects in the visualization plane the voxels with maximum intensity that fall in the way of parallel rays traced from the viewpoint to the plane of projection. This implies that two MIP renderings from opposite viewpoints are symmetrical images [8]. Gruden *et al.* MIP processing reduces the number of overlooked small nodules, particularly in the central lung. Observer nodule detection remains imperfect even when lesions are clearly depicted on images [9, 10]. Some authors reported that, majority tumours of the lung, which were gone to surgery, were discovered incidentally [11-13].

The most of the authors supported that the hint poınts of detection and following SSPN, The persistence of nodular ground-glass opacity over time may be strongly suggestive of an early-stage malignancy, especially if the lesion increases in size or includes a solid component that increases in its extent. Persistent nodular ground-glass opacity may also remain stable in size but show increased attenuation. The more extensive the solid portions of the lesion, the higher the probability of malignancy and the poorer the prognosis. The awareness of the clinical setting, in addition to familiarity with the thin-section Thorax CT features of nodular ground-glass opacity at initial and follow-up imaging over several months, can help identify malignancy and achieve an accurate diagnosis. A meticulous evaluation of those Thorax CT features, and their correlation with specific histopathologic characteristics, may also enable a more accurate prognosis in cases of neoplastic disease.

Fluorine-18-FDG PET has been widely studied for its use in the accurate characterization of SPNs. An SUV cutoff of 2.5 or greater has been traditionally associated with malignant pulmonary nodules [14]. However, size does matter when evaluating SPN with PET CT. One of the major limitations is the resolution of the scanners used. Currently, the resolving limit of ^{18}F-FDG PET scanners is nodules that are 6-8 mm in size. Nodules smaller than this are not adequately evaluated with ^{18}F-FDG PET. Khalaf *et al.* reported that cutoff point 2.5 has minimal value for the nodules smaller than 1 cm. The sensitivity, specificity, and accuracy were 85%, 36% and 54% respectively for nodules smaller than 10 mm, compared to 91%, 47%, and 79% for nodules between 1.1-2.0 cm [15]. The value of PET CT tended to improve with increasing size of nodules.

Biopsy

Fine-needle biopsy by CT-guided and transbronchial CT guided floroscopic biopsy can be initial method for definitive diagnosis but the diagnostic acuracy was found 74% (li 76). Wallace *et al.* found that 0.8-1.0-cm lesions were considerably better (sensitivity, 88%; accuracy, 92%) than those for 10 lesions of 0.5-0.7-cm (sensitivity, 50%; accuracy, 70%). Sensitivity (75% *vs.* 87%) and accuracy (87% *vs.* 89%) were also improved when comparing subpleural (< or =1.0 cm from pleural surface,) with deeper (>1 cm from pleural surface, n = 27) pulmonary lesions [16]. Ng *et al.* mentioned that the sensitivity for malignancy and overall accuracy were 67.7 and 78.8% for CT-guided percutaneous fine-needle aspiration biopsy of pulmonary nodules measuring 10 mm or less. Therefore, the diagnostic accuracy cannot be 100 % for needle biopsy [17].

Surgical Approaches

Surgical removing "especially minimally invasive methods as video-assisted thoracic surgery (VATS)" is the most reliable methods for the definitive diagnosis of the SSPN. Metilen blue and hook-wire can be easily found during the VATS [18]. Pittet *et al.* advocated that VATS resection of SPN previously localized by a

CT-guided hook-wire system is related to a low conversion thoracotomy rate (4%), a short operation time, and few postoperative complications, and it is well suited for the clarification of SPN [19]. Kondo *et al.* developed a marking method for peripheral small pulmonary lesions about 10 mm. The solitary pulmonary nodules were marked with barium under CT guided bronchoscopy and then the lesions were resected *via* fluoroscopy-assisted thoracoscopy. All the SPNs were resected with sufficient margins [20, 21].

The SPNs less than 1 cm diagnosed with malign tumour must be considered as a lung cancer. Wedge resection and segmentectomy for the pulmonary malignant tumours have poor outcomes comparing with major pulmonary resections. The better survival rate and fewer recurrences can be obtained with lobectmy and mediastinal lymph node dissection [22, 23].

As a conclusion the most sensitive imaging modality for the detection of pulmonary nodules is computed tomography. Advances in radiologic techniques not only increase the number of nodules detected, but also the nodules that are identified smaller. With increasing use of spiral CT for lung cancer screening, there will be more SSPN that will require further diagnostic workup. Radiologic evaluation including repeat observational CT or CT contrast enhancement should be performed. Bronchoscopic or needle biopsy of the majority of SSPN is not practical. VATS is possible for SSPN but should be performed in a controlled manner to reduce the resection of benign lesions. An SSPN management algorithm is necessary to expedite resection of a malignant lesion and to minimize removal of benign disease.

ACKNOWLEDGEMENTS

Declared none.

CONFLICT OF INTEREST

The authors confirm that this article content has no conflict of interest.

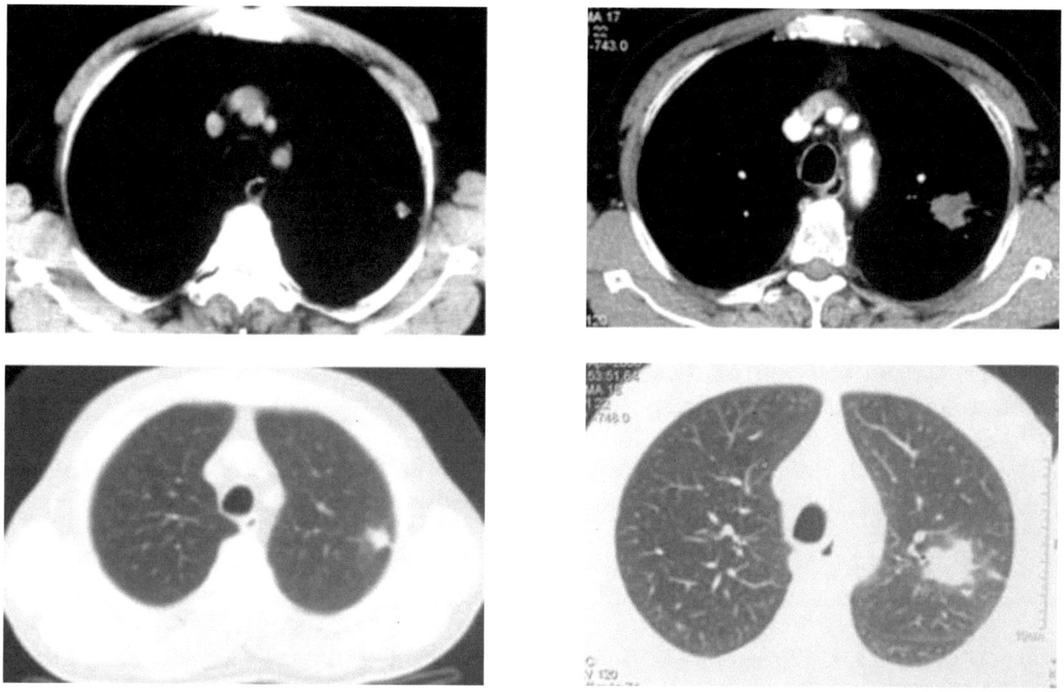

Figure 1: Thorax computed tomographic scan showing a small solitary pulmonary nodule on the left upper lobe (a) and the enlarged mass after 60 months (b).

REFERENCES

[1] Henschke CI, McCauley DI, Yankelevitz DF, *et al.* Early Lung Cancer Action Project: overall design and findings from baseline screening. Lancet. 1999; 354: 99-105.

[2] Munden RF, Pugatch R, Liptay MJ, Sugarbaker DJ, Le LU. Small pulmonary lesions detected at CT: clinical importance. Radiology. 1997; 202: 105-110.

[3] Siegelman SS, Zerhouni EA, Leo FP, Khouri NF, and Stitik FP CT of the solitary pulmonary nodule American Journal of Roentgenology. 1980; 135: 1-13.

[4] M. I. Ahn, T. G. Gleeson, I. H. Chan, A. M. McWilliams, S. L. MacDonald, S. Lam, S. Atkar-Khattra, and J. R. Mayo Perifissural Nodules Seen at CT Screening for Lung Cancer Radiology. 2010; 254: 949-56.

[5] Veronesi, G. Bellomi, M. Scanagatta, L. Preda, C. Rampinelli, J. Guarize, G. Pelosi, P. Maisonneuve, F. Leo, P. Solli. Difficulties encountered managing nodules detected during a computed tomography lung cancer-screening program. J. Thorac. Cardiovasc. Surg. 2008; 136: 611-17.

[6] Wormanns D, Ludwig K, Beyer F, Heindel W, Diederich S.Detection of pulmonary nodules at multirow-detector CT: effectiveness of double reading to improve sensitivity at standard-dose and low-dose chest CT. Eur Radiol. 2005; 15: 14-22.

[7] Wallis JW, Miller TR, Lerner CA, Kleerup EC (1989). "Three-dimensional display in nuclear medicine". IEEE Trans Med Imaging 8 (4): 297–303. 9. Gruden JF, Ouanounou S, Tigges S, Norris SD, Klausner TS.Incremental benefit of maximum-intensity-projection

images on observer detection of small pulmonary nodules revealed by multidetector CT. AJR Am J Roentgenol. 2002; 179: 149-57.

[8] 10. Truong MT, Sabloff BS, Ko JP. Multidetector CT of solitary pulmonary nodules. Thorac Surg Clin. 2010; 20: 9-23.

[9] 11. Lee PC, Korst RJ, Port JL, Kerem Y, Kansler AL, Altorki NK. Long-term survival and recurrence in patients with resected non-small cell lung cancer 1 cm or less in size. J Thorac Cardiovasc Surg. 2006; 132: 1382-9.

[10] 12. Takashima S, Sone S, Li F, Maruyama Y, Hasegawa M, Matsushita T, Takayama F, Kadoya M. Small solitary pulmonary nodules (< or =1 cm) detected at population-based CT screening for lung cancer: Reliable high-resolution CT features of benign lesions. AJR Am J Roentgenol. 2003; 180: 955-64.

[11] 13. Park, C. M. Goo J. M., Lee H. J., Lee C. H., Chun E. J. Nodular Ground-Glass Opacity at Thin-Section CT: Histologic Correlation and Evaluation of Change at Follow-up RadioGraphics. 2007; 27: 391-408.

[12] 14. Lowe VJ, Hoffman JM, DeLong DM, Patz EF, Jr, Coleman ER. Semiquantitative and visual analysis of FDG-PET images in pulmonary abnormalities. J Nucl Med. 1994; 35: 1771–6.

[13] 15. Khalaf M, Abdel-Nabi H, Baker J, Shao Y, Lamonica D, Gona J. Relation between nodule size and 18F-FDG-PET SUV for malignant and benign pulmonary nodules. J Hematol Oncol. 2008; 22: 13-9

[14] Wallace MJ, Krishnamurthy S, Broemeling LD, Gupta S, Ahrar K, Morello FA Jr, Hicks ME. CT-guided percutaneous fine-needle aspiration biopsy of small (< or =1-cm) pulmonary lesions. Radiology. 2002; 225: 823-8.

[15] Ng YL, Patsios D, Roberts H, Walsham A, Paul NS, Chung T, Herman S, Weisbrod G. CT-guided percutaneous fine-needle aspiration biopsy of pulmonary nodules measuring 10 mm or less. Clin Radiol. 2008; 63: 272-7.

[16] Paci M, Annessi V, Giovanardi F, Ferrari G, De Franco S, Casali C, Sgarbi G.Preoperative localization of indeterminate pulmonary nodules before videothoracoscopic resection. Surg Endosc. 2002; 16: 509-11.

[17] Pittet O, Christodoulou M, Pezzetta E, Schmidt S, Schnyder P, Ris HB.Video-assisted thoracoscopic resection of a small pulmonary nodule after computed tomography-guided localization with a hook-wire system. Experience in 45 consecutive patients. World J Surg. 2007; 31: 575-8.

[18] Kondo H, Kobayashi T. Fluoroscopy-assisted thoracoscopic surgery after computed tomography-guided bronchoscopic barium marking: a minimally invasive treatment for small peripheral early adenocarcinoma of the lungKyobu Geka. 2001; 54: 921-5.

[19] Okumura T, Kondo H, Suzuki K, Asamura H, Kobayashi T, Kaneko M, Tsuchiya R. Fluoroscopy-assisted thoracoscopic surgery after computed tomography-guided bronchoscopic barium marking. Ann Thorac Surg. 2001; 71: 439-42.

[20] Miller DL, Rowland CM, Deschamps C, Allen MS, Trastek VF, Pairolero PC. Surgical treatment of non-small cell lung cancer 1 cm or less in diameter. Ann Thorac Surg. 2002; 73: 1545-50.

[21] Xu DM., van der Zaag-Loonen HJ, Oudkerk M, Wang Y, Vliegenthart R., Scholten ET, Verschakelen J, Prokop M, Koning HJ. de, and Van Klaveren RJ. Smooth or Attached Solid Indeterminate Nodules Detected at Baseline CT Screening in the NELSON Study: Cancer Risk during 1 Year of Follow-up1 Radiology. 2009; 250: 264-272.

Send Orders of Reprints at reprints@benthamscience.net
Lung Cancer: Clinical and Surgical Specifications, **2013, 183-198**

CHAPTER 9

Invasive Surgical Techniques in the Mediastinal Staging in Non-Small Cell Lung Cancer

Mehmet Oğuzhan Özyurtkan*

Firat University, Faculty of Medicine, Department of Thoracic Surgery, 23119, Elazig, Turkey

Abstract: Non-small cell lung cancer is the most common malignancy in the world and accounts for an estimated 1 million deaths each year. Metastasis to the mediastinal lymph nodes is one of the most important factors in determining resectability and prognosis. It also influences staging algorithms. Non-invasive radiographic imaging investigations have their limitations, so tissue sampling is needed. Sampling can be achieved both by invasive surgical or non-surgical techniques. According to the ESTS guidelines, among invasive surgical techniques, mediastinoscopy is still considered to be the gold standard in the mediastinal staging in non-small cell lung cancer. This chapter deals with invasive surgical techniques.

Keywords: Invasive staging, lung cancer, mediastinoscopy.

INTRODUCTION

Correct staging of patients with non-small cell lung cancer (NSCLC) provides accurate information on the extent of disease and guides the choice of treatment. It is also fundamental for estimating prognosis and for comparison of studies. When there are no distant metastases, mediastinal lymph node involvement is the most important prognostic factor in patients with NSCLC and influences therapeutic strategies.

Primary mediastinal lymph node staging techniques include imaging [computed tomography (CT) of the chest, positron emission tomography (PET) or PET-CT scan], and invasive techniques. Invasive surgical staging modalities are the subject of this chapter and explained in details. There are also invasive non-

***Address correspondence to Mehmet Oğuzhan Özyurtkan:** Firat University, Faculty of Medicine, Department of Thoracic Surgery, 23119, Elazig, Turkey; Tel: +90 424 2333555/2136; Fax: +90 424 2388096; E-mail: moozyurtkan@hotmail.com

Akın Eraslan Balcı (Ed)

surgical techniques in the evaluation of the mediastinal lymph nodes. They include transbronchial needle aspiration (TBNA), endobronchial or esophageal ultrasound-guided fine needle aspiration (EBUS-TBNA and EUS-FNA, respectively).

It is evident that both in primary staging and restaging, not every staging technique is available in every centre. Therefore, the choice of the technique used is dependent on the availability and expertise of the centre.

Guidelines for Baseline Mediastinal Lymph Node Staging According to the ESTS Council (Figs. 1 and 2)

After a first successful workshop on intra-operative lymph node staging [1], the ESTS Council initiated a second workshop on preoperative mediastinal lymph node staging. The working group had three sessions in Zurich. Initial findings were presented and discussed at the postgraduate meeting of the EACTS—ESTS meeting in Barcelona (September 2005). The final paper was put on the website for discussion by all ESTS members [2].

- The accuracy of CT scans in the evaluation of mediastinal lymph nodes is insufficient to guide clinical decisions.

- Invasive staging can be omitted in patients with negative mediastinal PET images. However, in case of central tumours, PET hilar N1 disease, low FDG uptake of the primary tumour, invasive staging with mediastinoscopy remains indicated.

- PET positive mediastinal findings should be histologically or cytologically confirmed.

- TBNA, EBUS-TBNA and EUS-FNA are techniques that provide cytological/histological diagnosis and are minimally invasive. They can be complementary to surgical invasive staging technique. Their specificity is high, but their negative predictive value is low. Due to this, if they yield negative results, an invasive surgical technique is indicated.

- Cervical mediastinoscopy provides the advantage that a full mapping of mediastinal lymph nodes can be performed. At least one ipsilateral, one contralateral and the subcarinal lymph nodes should be biopsied.

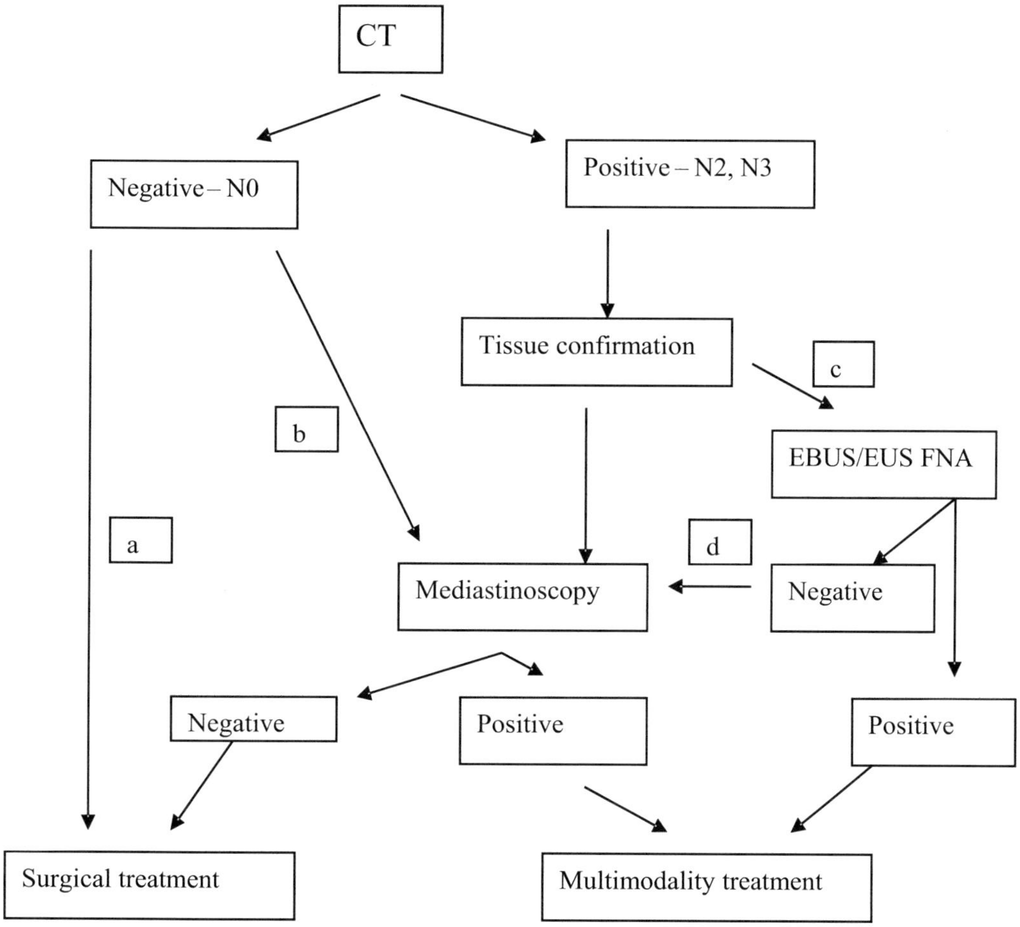

a: Only in T1N0 squamous cell tumours invasive staging is not necessary

b: In all other tumours, nodal metastasis need to be excluded by mediastinoscopy

c: Endoscopic techniques are minimally invasive and can be the first choice

d: Due to its higher negative predictive value mediastinoscopy remains indicated

Figure 1: The proposed algorithm to follow for primary mediastinal staging when PET scan is not available.

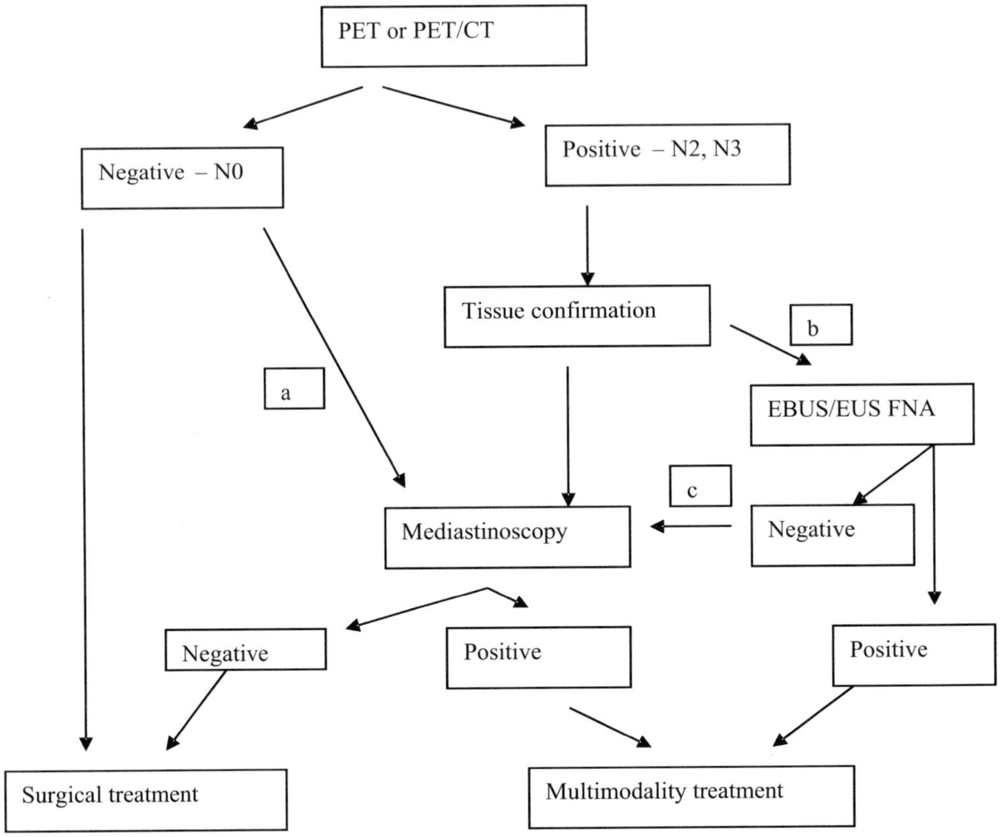

a: In central tumours, tumours with low FDG uptake, tumours with lymph nodes ≥ 1.6cm and/or PET N1 disease invasive staging is not necessary

b: Endoscopic techniques are minimally invasive and can be the first choice

c: Due to its higher negative predictive value mediastinoscopy remains indicated

Figure 2: The proposed algorithm to follow for primary mediastinal staging when PET or PET/CT is available.

MEDIASTINOSCOPY

Introduction

Mediastinoscopy is one of the most common operations performed in the general thoracic surgery. The procedure was very important in the diagnosis and the staging of lung cancer before the resection, but nowadays it is used more selectively as noninvasive imaging modalities such as CT and PET imaging have improved. However, it remains an integral part of the evaluation and staging of patients with suspected lung cancer. In the recent years, videomediastinoscopy gained popularity with the introduction of videoscopic technology. There is an increasing use of EBUS-TBNA and EUS-FNA. Although these increases may decrease the need for mediastinoscopy, mediastinoscopy is stil an important procedure in lung cancer and the other techniques should be considered complementary techniques.

History

Harken and associates [3] described an exploration way to the superior mediastinum from a lateral approach, after excision of the scalene fat pad, by using the Jackson laryngoscope in 1954. By using a supraclavicular incision they bluntly dissected through the cervical fascia into the superior mediastinum, sweeping the mediastinal pleura laterally, and reached the paratracheal lymph nodes. They either enucleated or biopsied enlarged lymph nodes using a laryngoscope and laryngeal biopsy forceps. A positive histologic diagnosis was obtained in 32% of the patients in their study. They advocated routine performance of this procedure in the evaluation of all patients with known or suspected bronchogenic carcinoma before thoracotomy.

Since pneumothorax and injury to subclavian and jugular veins were described following this procedure, it was not widely accepted. Later, Carlens [4] described the classic midline approach called cervical mediastinoscopy. By using an incision in the suprasternal notch he made blunt finger dissection to free the paratracheal nodes. Then with a specially designed mediastinoscope, a blunt-tipped aspirator, and forceps, he biopsied bilateral paratracheal and the subcarinal nodes. Beside the patients with known or suspected bronchogenic carsinoma, the procedure was applied for biopsy of other causes of mediastinal lymphadenopathy including sarcoidosis, lymphosarcoma, and Hodgkin's disease. There was no complications in Carlens' first 100 patients. Finally, this procedure has since become standard in the preoperative staging of patients with suspected mediastinal nodal involvement and non-small cell lung cancer.

Pearson and the Toronto surgical group [5] further developed the indications of the mediastinoscopy, and with their support, the use of the Carlens' procedure spread from Sweden to North America.

Indications

Mediastinoscopy is mostly used in the staging and the diagnosis of lung cancer. When enlarged mediastinal lymph nodes are detected by CT or PET, mediastinascopy is still the "gold standard" procedure to explore whether these lymph nodes are bening or malignant. Since the incidence of N2 disease has been increasing despite a normal CT scan, the application of mediastinoscopy is strongly suggested [6]. One of the advantages of mediastinoscopy is the ability to obtain a large fragment of tissue for histopathology or even entire small lymph nodes as compared to clusters of aspirated cells for cytologic examination.

In patients with clinical N0 disease, tumour size, location and histology are selective indications for mediastinoscopy. In 1994, Funatsu and colleagues [7] reported a study concerning 164 patients with T1 adenocarcinomas or T1 squamous cell carcinomas undergoing mediastinoscopy. Based on this study, true negative (TN) and true positive (TP) rates for tumours ≤2cm were 96% and 4% in comparison to large tumours (>2cm) with 84% TN and 14% TP rates. In another study reported by De Leyn and colleagues [8] concerning T1N0 patients (N0 defined by CT scan with diameter <1.5cm) having either adenocarcinomas or squamous cell carcinomas, the positivity was 9.5% in the adenocarcinoma group, and %0 in the squamous cell carcinoma group following mediastinoscopy.

A diameter larger than 1cm in the short axis is generally considered as the standard criterion for a suspicious lymph node [2]. According to the guidelines of the American College of Chest Physicians, based on a meta-analysis of 35 studies with a pooled population of 5,111 patients, the sensitivity of CT scan alone was 51%, and the specificity 86% [9]. The negative predictive value of PET scan is more than 90% in most lung cancer series [10-12]. If the patients underwent both PET and mediastinoscopy, the negative predictive value (NPV) for PET was 98.4% and the PPV 49% [13]. According to the study of de Langen and colleagues [14], based on a meta-analysis of 14 studies, PET scanning had a median sensitivity of 100% and a median specificity of 78% when utilized in the presence of enlarged nodes on CT scan.

Contraindications and Cautions

In the presence of huge cervical goiter, extensive calcification or aneurysm of the innominate artery, and permanent tracheostomy after laryngectomy and radiation, mediastinoscopy is contraindicated. Also several other factors may cause a difficult mediastinoscopy. In case of a carotid bruit, especially on the right side, the neck extension sould be minimized to avoid innomiate artery compression. In the presence of a prior sternotomy or a neck incision the midline may be hard to find, but since the pretracheal fascia is usualy intact, they do not generally affect the deeper dissection. However, there is a peritracheal fibrosis extending into the mediastinum in the patient with a prior mediastinoscopy. But repeat mediastinoscopy has been reported to be safe even in the setting of induction chemotherapy [15, 16]. As reported, mediastinoscopy can also be performed in the presence of superior vena caval obstruction [17].

Procedure

Cervical mediastinoscopy is generally performed as an outpatient procedure and can be combined with bronchoscopy, scalene biopsy, or anterior mediastinotomy as needed. Because of the possibility of significant bleeding, mediastinoscopy should probably be limited to hospital-based rather than free-standing facilities [18].

Since the technique of cervical mediastinoscopy is described in textbooks of general thoracic surgery, it is not detailed in this chapter but summarized. The procedure is performed under general anesthesia with an endotracheal tube. Correct positioning of the patient (neck extension, usage of an interscapular roll, slight elevation of the back of the operating table) is important to facilitate the insertion of the mediastinoscope into the pretracheal space. Following a 3-cm transverse skin incision 1cm above the sternoclovicular junctions, the avascular space between the strap muscles is opened vertically. When the deeper sternothyroid muscles are separated, the anterior wall of the trachea can be seen. If the length of trachea caudal to the thyroid isthmus is insufficient, the isthmus can be retracted cranially or rarely must be divided and ligated. The pretracheal fascia is incised and elevated. A tunnel is created in the pretracheal space using an index finger. Gentle advancement and lateral sweeping clear the pretracheal and paratracheal spaces. Finger dissection usually reaches a point 1 or 2cm proximal to the carina. During digital dissection, the surgeon creates a mental map of the surgical area (location of normal structures, lymphadenopathy, mass, or invasion).

According to the lymph-node map proposed by Montain and Dresler [19], the lymph- node stations that can be evaluated by cervical mediastinoscopy are the high mediastinal station (level 1), the right and left superior paratracheal station (level 2 right, level 2 left), the right and left lower paratracheal station (level 4 right, level 4 left), and the subcarinal station (level 7) (Fig. **3**). A metal suction catheter is used to dissect fascial planes. Aspirating the structure to be biopsied with a spinal needle (usually 20-gauge) may avoid a vascular damage if there is any doubt about the solid or vascular nature of the structure in question.

There is no internationally accepted recommendation on how many lymph node stations should be examined at cervical mediastinoscopy. The opinions vary among working groups and authors around the world:

- The American Thoracic Society stated that all reachable nodal stations should be explored, including the right and left superior paratracheal stations (levels 2R and 2L), right and left inferior paratracheal (levels 4R and 4L), right and left tracheobronchial (levels 10R and 10L) and subcarinal (level 7) stations.

- For Detterbeck and colleagues [20], the ideal exploration would include at least one node from the right and left, superior and inferior paratracheal and subcarinal stations, unless more nodes are present.

- Smulders and associates [21] suggest that the minimally acceptable exploration includes biopsy of nodes from the inferior paratracheal stations on both sides, and from the subcarinal station, with the addition of at least one contralateral lymph node.

- The ESTS working group recommends to systematically explore and biopsy always the right and left lower paratracheal nodes and the subcarinal nodes. Additionally, if present, the upper paratracheal lymph nodes should be sampled and biopsied [2].

Bleeding after biopsy is usually minor. Most bleeding can be controlled by packing with gauze, oxidized cellulose, or clipping if the bleeding vessel is visible. The power of cautery should be kept low to avoid arcing and thermal damage. The strap muscles are reapproximated in the midline using one or two absorbable sutures. The skin is closed subcutaneously. Drainage is not necessary.

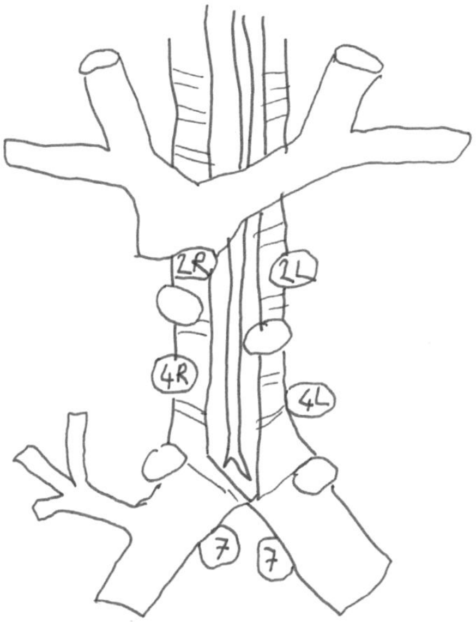

Figure 3: The procedure of standard cervical mediastinoscopy.

Extended cervical mediastinoscopy is a variation of mediastinoscopy, and used to reach aortopulmonary (level 5) and anterior mediastinal (level 6) nodes through the same cervical incision as described by Ginsberg [22]. After the clearing of the infraisthmic trachea, the space anterior to the aortic arch is digitally opened by piercing the fascia between the innominate and left common carotid arteries. Then the mediastinoscope is passed anterior to the aorta, and biopsy specimens are taken. Electrocautery is not used in the extended cervical mediastinoscopy to avoid injury to the vagus and phrenic nerves. The negative predictive value can increase by 10 to 20% when this procedure is added to the standard mediastinoscopy [23].

Complications

Mediastinoscopy is a safe procedure in experienced hands. The mortality rate ranges from 0 to 0.2%, and morbidity rates vary from 0.6 to 3.7% [23]. In a large series reported by Ginsberg (n= 2259) there was no mortality, and the morbidity rate was 2.0% [24]. A recent series of 2145 patients reported a morbidity rate of 1.07% and a mortality rate of 0.05% [25].

Massive hemorrhage, defined as any bleeding requiring additional surgery (thoracotomy or sternotomy) for control, is the most feared complication of mediastinoscopy. Hemorrhage can result from damage to the aortic arch or its branches, superior vena cava, azygos vein, or pulmonary artery. Lacerations in innominate and jugular vein are less common, and can be controlled more easily. Injury to a bronchial artery may produce significant but not massive bleeding unless the vessel has been avulsed from the aorta. Among the possible risk factors of hemorrhage are prior radiotherapy, induction therapy, prior surgical procedures in the mediastinum and re-mediastinoscopy [18, 26].

Park and colleagues [27] reported their study investigating the management of massive hemorrhage during a 12-year period at Memorial Sloan Kettering Cancer Center. They performed 3391 mediastinoscopy procedures, and encountered massive hemorrhage in 14 patients (0.4%). According to this series, the most common biopsy site resulting in major hemorrhage was the lower right paratracheal region (level 4R), and the most frequently injured vessels were the azygos vein and the pulmonary and innominate arteries.

In case of a major hemorrhage, the initial first step is gauze packing. The mediastinoscope should not be removed due to its rigidity that faciliates direct tamponade. If packing is unsuccessful and the hemorrhage is still ongoing, the surgical approach to repair the injury should be considered. When there is an aortic, innominate artery, main or left pulmonary artery, or medial caval injury, sternotomy is preferable. Right thoracotomy may be used for right pulmonary artery and azygos vein injuries [18, 26].

Tracheal or mainstem bronchial injuries are very rare complications of mediastinoscopy. The injury generally responds to packing with absorbable cellulose gauze and closes when the patient is extubated and the positive pressure ventilation finishes [28]. Esophageal perforation also is very rare, and occurs mainly during the biopsy in the subcarinal region. It may usually be detected earlier and corrected. The injury to the left recurrent laryngeal nerve is quite rare and, is due to the excessive dissection, sampling, or cautery at the left tracheobronchial angle. Pneumothorax, wound infections, and arrhythmias are other rare minor complications.

ANTERIOR MEDIASTINOTOMY

Anterior mediastinotomy, as described by McNeil and Chamberlain [29], is an alternative approach to biopsy the lymph nodes located in the aortopulmonary window. This approach can also be used on the right and offers access to the upper hilum, lung, and pleura on both sides. The sensitivity of anterior mediastinotomy is between 63 and 86% and the negative predictive values vary from 89 to 100%, when the procedure is directed by CT scan alone [23].

Indications and Contraindications

The most common indication for anterior mediastinotomy is the presence of an anterior mediastinal mass and a left upper lobe bronchogenic cancer. Left upper lobe drains mainly to the subaortic and anterior mediastinal stations (level 5 and 6), but also to the ipsilateral paratracheal nodes [30]. Anterior mediastinotomy may prevent a thoracotomy in 3.4% of the patients with suspected left-upper-lobe tumours, and yields one or more lymph nodes in 67% of patients as reported by Nechala and associates [31].

In a patient having a prior sternotomy, anterior mediastinotomy should be performed with great caution. However the procedure is contraindicated in the presence of a patent left internal mammary artery bypass graft [18].

Procedure

The technique of anterior mediastinotomy is summarized in this chapter since it is described in details in textbooks of general thoracic surgery. The procedure is performed under general anesthesia, and double-lumen endotracheal intubation may be helpful.

In the classic procedure a 6cm transvers parasternal incision was used with resection of the second and third costal cartilages. But in most cases, adequate exposure is achieved through the intercostal space and the cartilages are not removed. The pectoralis muscle is split to expose the cartilage. The injury to the internal mammary artery and vein should be avoided by retraction, the vessels are very rarely divided and ligated. Blunt dissection to the mediastinal pleura allows the access to the aortopulmonary window without entering the pleural space. The related regional lymph nodes are then biopsied using a mediastinoscope (Fig. **4**). Drainage is usually not needed.

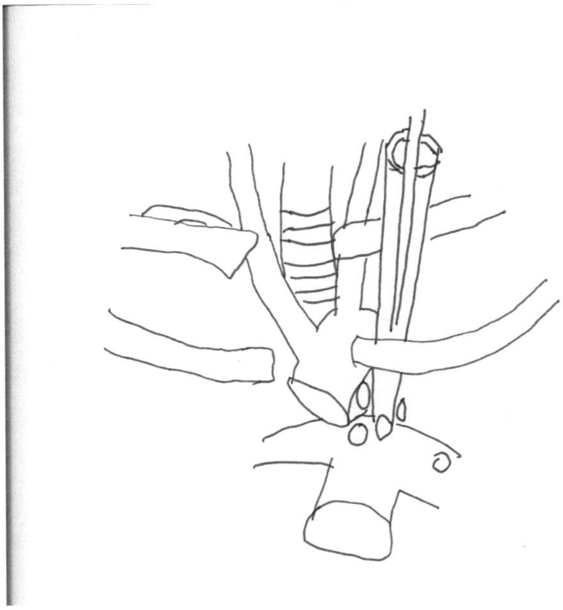

Figure 4: The technique of anterior mediastinotomy.

Complications

As reported by Nechala and associates [31], the complication rates of anterior mediastinotomy is 6.8% with no mortality in their retrospective series of 151 patients. Bleeding from the internal mammary vessels is a more common complication of the procedure, but can be controlled more easily. However, injury to the aorta, pulmonary artery, or superior pulmonary vein may cause significant bleeding. The procedure can also traumatize neural structures including the vagus, phrenic, and recurrent laryngeal nerves. Opening of the mediastinal pleura during the procedure may cause pneumothorax. Tumour seeding of the incision is rare [18, 26].

VIDEO-ASSISTED MEDIASTINOSCOPY AND MEDIASTINOSCOPIC LYMPHADENECTOMY

Sortini and associates [32] introduced and used video-assisted mediastinoscopy in 1994. In this technique, a mediastinoscope is connected to a video camera. This allows wide and magnified operative exposure. The surgeon then can dissect the normal and pathologic structures, and perform more precise biopsies. This technique is also an excellent teaching tool for the trainees. The series of Venissac and colleagues [33], which consisted of 240 patients, reported favorable results with a sensitivity of 97.3%, a specificity of 100%, and an accuracy of 98% for staging non-small-cell lung cancer. The complication rate was 0.83% in the same series with no mortalities. In a very recent study, Anraku and associates [34] compared video-assisted mediastinoscopy and standard cervical mediastinoscopy. The total number of dissected nodes was significantly higher in video-assisted mediastinoscopy. But this technique resulted in significantly higher morbidity rate compared to cervical mediastinoscopy.

Two new techniques for mediastinal lymphadenectomy using a cervicotomy approach are called video-assisted mediastinoscopic lymphadenectomy (VAMLA) [35], and transcervical extended mediastinal lymphadenectomy (TEMLA) [36]. Both techniques aim to perform a complete bilateral lymphadenectomy of the mediastinum including stations 2, 4, 7 and 8 (VAMLA) and stations 1, 2, 3A, 3P, 4, 5, 6, 7 and 8 (TEMLA) for staging purposes. Witte and colleagues [37] reported a sensitivity of 93.75% and a specificity of 100%, with a false-negative rate of 0.9% by using VAMLA. The sensitivity, specificity and accuracy of the TEMLA in detecting mediastinal node metastases were: 90, 100, and 96%, respectively, whereas the positive and negative predictive values were: 100 and 95%, respectively [36].

VIDEO-ASSISTED THORACOSCOPY

Video-assisted thoracoscopy is an other invasive method to assess all lymph node levels if performed on both right and left sides. It has been most frequently used to biopsy level 5 and 6 lymph nodes or when tumour invasion or pleural tumour seeding is suspected [26].

ACKNOWLEDGEMENTS

Declared none.

CONFLICT OF INTEREST

The author confirms that this article content has no conflict of interest.

REFERENCES

[1] Lardinois D, De Leyn P, Van Schil PE, Rami Porta R, Waller D, Passlick B, Zielinski M, Junker K, Rendina E, Ris HB, Hasse J, Detterbeck F, Lerut T, Weder W. ESTS guidelines for intraoperative lymph node staging in nonsmall cell lung cancer. Eur J Cardiothorac Surg 2006;30:787-92.

[2] De Leyn P, Lardinois D, Van Schil PE, Rami Porta R, Passlick B, Zielinski M, Waller DA, Lerut T, Weder W. ESTS guidelines for preoperative lymph node staging for non-small cell lung cancer. Eur J Cardiothorac Surg 2007;32:1-8.

[3] Harken DE, Black H, Clauss R, Farrand RE. A simple cervicomediastinal exploration for tissue diagnosis of intrathoracic disease. N Engl J Med 1954;251:1041-4.

[4] Carlens E. Mediastinoscopy: a method for inspection and tissue biopsy of the superior mediastinum. Dis Chest 1959;36:343-52.

[5] Pearson FG. An evaluation of mediastinoscopy in the management of presumably operable bronchial carcinoma. J Thorac Cardiovasc Surg 1968;55:617-25.

[6] Daly BD, Mueller JD, Faling LJ, Diehl JT, Bankoff MS, Karp DD, Rand WM. N2 lung cancer: outcome in patients with false-negative computed tomographic scans of the chest. J Thorac Cardiovasc Surg 1993;105:904-10.

[7] Funatsu T, Matsubara Y, Ikeda S, Hatakenaka R, Hanawa T, Ishida H. Preoperative mediastinoscopic assessment of N factors and the need for mediastinal lymph node dissection in T1 lung cancer. J Thorac Cardiovasc Surg 1994;108:321-8.

[8] De Leyn P, Vansteenkiste J, Cuypers P, Deneffe G, Van Raemdonck D, Coosemans W, Verschakelen J, Lerut T. Role of cervical mediastinoscopy in staging of non-small cell lung cancer without enlarged mediastinal lymph nodes on CT scan. Eur J Cardiothorac Surg 1997;12:706-12.

[9] Silvestri GA, Gould MK, Margolis ML, Tanoue LT, McCrory D, Toloza E, Detterbeck F; American College of Chest Physicians. Non-invasive staging of non–small cell lung cancer: ACCP evidenced-based clinical parctice guidelines. Chest 2007;132:178S-201S.

[10] Gupta NC, Graeber GM, Bishop HA. Comparative efficacy of positron emission tomography with fluorodeoxyglucose in evaluation of small (<1 cm), intermediate (1 to 3 cm) and large (>3 cm) lymph node lesions. Chest 2000;117:773-8.

[11] Kernstine KH, Mclaughlin KA, Menda Y, Rossi NP, Kahn DJ, Bushnell DL, Graham MM, Brown CK, Madsen MT. Can FDG-PET reduce the need for mediastinoscopy in potentially resectable non–small cell lung cancer? Ann Thorac Surg 2002;73:394-401.

[12] Poncelet AJ, Lonneux M, Coche E, Weynand B, Noirhomme P; Groupe d'Oncologie Thoracique des Cliniques Saint-Luc. PET-FDG scan enhances but does not replace

preoperative surgical staging in non-small cell lung cancer. Eur J Cardiothorac Surg 2001;20:468-74.
[13] Graeter TP, Hellwig D, Hoffmann K, Ukeda D, Kirsch CM, Schafers HJ. Mediastinal lymph node staging in suspected lung cancer: comparison of positron emission tomography with F-18 fluorodeoxyglucose and mediastinoscopy. Ann Thorac Surg 2003;75:231-5.
[14] de Langen AJ, Raijmakers P, Riphagen I, Paul MA, Hoekstra OS. The size of mediastinal lymph nodesand its relation with metastatic involvement: a metaanalysis. Eur J Cardiothorac Surg 2006;29:26-9.
[15] Mateu-Navarro M, Rami Porta R, Bastus Piulats R, Cirera Nogueras L, Gonzalez Pont G. Remediastinoscopy after induction chemotherapy in non–small cell lung cancer. Ann Thorac Surg 2000;70;391-5.
[16] Van Schil P, De Waele M, Hendriks J, Lauwers P. Remediastinoscopy. J Thorac Oncol 2007;2:365-6.
[17] Jahangiri M, Goldstraw P. The role of mediastinoscopy in superior vena caval obstruction. Ann Thorac Surg 1995;59:453-5.
[18] Ahmad US, Blum MG. Invasive diagnostic procedures. In Shields TW, LoCicero J, Reed CE, Feins RH (eds). General Thoracic Surgery. Philadelphia: Lippincott Williams&Wilkins; 2009, pp. 301-12.
[19] Mountain CF, Dresler CM. Regional lymph node classification for lung cancer staging. Chest 1997;111:1718-23.
[20] Detterbeck FC, Jones DR, Parker Jr LA. Intrathoracic staging. In: Detterbeck FC, Rivera MP, Socinski MA, Roseman JG (eds). Diagnosis and treatment of lung cancer. An evidence-based guide for the practicing clinician. Philadelphia: WB Saunders Company; 2001, pp. 73-93.
[21] Smulders SA, Smeenk FWJM, Janssen-Heijnen MLG, Wielders PL, de Munck DR, Postmus PE. Surgical mediastinal staging in daily practice. Lung Cancer 2005;47:243-51.
[22] Ginsberg RJ, Rice TW, Goldberg M, Waters PF, Schmocker BJ. Extended cervical mediastinoscopy: a single staging procedure for bronchogenic carcinoma of the left upper lobe. J Thorac Cardiovasc Surg 1987; 94:673-8.
[23] Toloza EM, Harpole L, Detterbeck F, McCrory DC. Invasive staging of non-small cell lung cancer: a review of the current evidence. Chest 2003;123:157-66.
[24] Ginsberg RJ. Evaluation of the mediastinum by invasive techniques. Surg Clin North Am 1987;67:1025-35.
[25] Lemaire A, Nikolic I, Petersen T, Haney JC, Toloza EM, Harpole DH Jr, D'Amico TA, Burfeind WR. Nine-year single center experience with cervical mediastinoscopy: complications and false negative rate. Ann Thorac Surg 2006;82:1185-9.
[26] Reed CE. The role for mediastinoscopy in the staging of nonsmall cell lung cancer. In Roth JA, Hong WK, Cox JD (eds). Lung Cancer. Massachusetts: Blackwell Publishing; 2008, pp. 169-79.
[27] Park BJ, Flores R, Downey RJ, Bains MS, Rusch VW. Management of major hemorrhage during mediastinoscopy. J Thorac Cardiovasc Surg 2003;126:726-31.
[28] Pubakka HJ. Complications of mediastinoscopy. J Laryngol Otol 1989;103:312-5.
[29] McNeill TM, Chamberlain JM. Diagnostic anterior mediastinotomy. Ann Thorac Surg 1966;2:532-9.
[30] Ginsberg RJ. The role of preoperative surgical staging in left upper lobe tumours. Ann Thorac Surg 1994;57:526.

[31] Nechala P, Graham AJ, McFadden SD, Grondin SC, Gelfand G. Retrospective analysis of the clinical performance of anterior mediastinotomy. Ann Thorac Surg 2006;82:2004-9.

[32] Sortini A, Navarra G, Santini M, Occhionorelli S, Sartori A, Bresadola V, Donini I. Video-assisted mediastinoscopy: a new application of television technology in surgery. Minerva Chir 1994;49:803-5.

[33] Venissac N, Alifano M, Mouroux J. Video-assisted mediastinoscopy: experience from 240 consecutive cases. Ann Thorac Surg 2003;76:208-12.

[34] Anraku M, Miyata R, Compeau C, Shargall Y. Video-assisted mediastinoscopy compared with conventional mediastinoscopy: are we doing better? Ann Thorac Surg 2010;89:1577-81.

[35] Hürtgen M, Friedel G, Tomes H, Fritz P. Radical video-assisted mediastinoscopic lymphadenectomy (VAMLA)-technique and first results. Eur J Cardiothorac Surg 2002;21:348-51.

[36] Kuzdzal J, Zielinski M, Papla B, Szlubowski A, Hauer L, Nabialek T, Sosnicki W, Pankowski J. Transcervical extended mediastinal lymphadenectomy- the new operative technique and early results in lung cancer staging. Eur J Cardiothorac Surg 2005;27:384-90.

[37] Witte B, Wolf M, Huertgen M, Toomes H. Video-assisted mediastinoscopic surgery: clinical feasibility and accuracy of mediastinal lymph node staging. Ann Thorac Surg 2006;82:1821-7.

CHAPTER 10

Lung Cancer Surgery

Part A: Pulmonary Artery Reconstruction

Akın Eraslan Balcı*

Euphrates University School of Medicine, Elazig, Turkey

Abstract: Reconstruction of the pulmonary artery in association with lung resection is technically feasible with some morbidity and mortality. To obtain complete resection is always main aim. Non-small cell carcinoma of the lung invading the PA has traditionally been treated by pneumonectomy. Sleeve resection and prosthetic reconstruction of the pulmonary artery (PA) has progressively gained acceptance as an alternative to pneumonectomy in lung cancer surgery. When the tumour involves the central PA, lobectomy associated with reconstruction of the PA with or without bronchoplasty is the only alternative to pneumonectomy. Pulmonary arterioplasty has come into more widespread use to achieve R0 resections while preserving lung parenchyma in patients with central primary cancers or metastatic N1 disease. This procedure preserves the lung parenchyma safely, resulting in a better postoperative quality of life.

Keywords: Lung cancer, pulmonary artery, sleeve, reconstruction.

INTRODUCTION

Surgical resection, which is offered for early-stage lung cancer, can be curative but is often associated with morbidity. Pneumonectomy confers significantly greater morbidity and mortality than pulmonary lobectomy and is also associated with a worse quality of life. Thoracic surgeons should perform lobectomy with sleeve resection of the bronchus or of the pulmonary artery (PA), or both, to avoid pneumonectomy if possible [1]. The technique and the principles of bronchial and pulmonary artery (PA) reconstruction were established in the late 1940s and early 1950's [2].

Pulmonary artery resection for lung cancer should include followings 1: (1)

***Address correspondence to Akın Eraslan Balcı:** Euphrates University School of Medicine, Elazig, Turkey; Tel: +90 424 2333555/2134; Fax: +90 424 2388096; E-mail: akineraslan.balci@hotmail.com proximal and distal control (by clamping the remaining pulmonary vein of the lobe[s] that is not resected) of the PA was obtained, (2) some part of the right or left PA was removed using a knife or scissors, and (3) the artery was reconstructed to reestablish blood flow to the remaining pulmonary parenchyma.

A NSCLC with hilar extension and have an infiltration to pulmonary artery may require reconstruction using a patch of various materials, such as sleeve resection and reconstruction by end-to-end anastomosis or reconstruction by a prosthetic conduit [3, 4]. A patient operated with a pulmonary vein graft can be free of disease for 1 year [2]. The primary indication is direct infiltration of the interlobar PA by the primary tumour. Even complete surgical reconstruction of the pulmonary arterial tree, it is possible to achieve a successful intervention with excellent early clinical and hemodynamic outcomes [5]. In a recent series, all repairs were performed with end-to-end anastomosis or direct suturing in patients who underwent a major lung cancer operation with pulmonary artery resection to avoid pneumonectomy for lung cancer surgery [6]. Parenchyma sparing resection through a variety of bronchoplastic modalities is a safe and advantageous procedure in selected patients with lung cancer and reduced pulmonary function as well as in non compromised patients with a suitable anatomy [7].

The pulmonary artery (PA) can be infiltrated by primary lung tumours or by metastatic hilar-mediastinal lymph nodes with extracapsular extension. When lung tumours involve not only the airway but also the central vascular structures, in particular the pulmonary artery, sleeve lobectomy associated with pulmonary artery reconstruction (double sleeve) remains as the only alternative to pneumonectomy [8]. Extracapsular nodal extension into the vessel can also be treated effectively by this technique. Approximately 70% of all PA reconstructions are performed for left upper lobe tumours and 20% for right upper lobe lesions. The remaining 10% require procedures performed on the main PA or on the lower lobes bilaterally. Frozen section must be sent for all resection margins, and if tumour infiltration is detected, pneumonectomy must be performed.

PREOPERATIVE PERIOD

Histopathological diagnostic specimens can be obtained by either fiberoptic bronchoscopy or computed tomography (CT)-guided needle biopsy. CT scans of each patient's chest and upper abdomen, bone scintigraphy, and a brain magnetic resonance imaging (MRI) study may be performed for noninvasive staging. Each patient may also be studied a pulmonary function test, electrocardiography, and arterial blood gas analysis to evaluate the operative risk. If there is any suspicion of N2 or N3 disease based on the CT scan, cervical mediastinoscopy or videoassisted thoracoscopy with histopathological examination of the mediastinal N2 lymph nodes is performed. Patients with biopsy-proven N2 disease undergo combined radiochemotherapy according to the current study's protocols. After reassessment of the tumour stage, patients with complete or partial remission are scheduled for surgery [1, 3, 4, 9].

In the preoperative period, to establish the indication for a PA reconstruction is not easy. PA angiography, computed tomography (CT) scan with injection of contrast material and magnetic resonance imaging (MRI) of the blood vessels (angio-MRI) can contribute to detection of the limits of the tumour infiltration. The decision for reconstructive surgery is generally established with intraoperative examination [5, 6, 7, 10].

TECHNIQUE CONSIDERATIONS

Techniques methods of the pulmonary artery patch reconstruction are autologous pericardium, bovine pericardium, azygos vein and synthetic material use for partial infiltration; pulmonary artery sleeve, end to end anastomosis, pericardial conduit and prostesis for complete circumferential infiltration; and reconstruction *via* cardiopulmonary bypass for infiltration of main pulmonary artery.

Most of the published cases have been performed by circumferential pulmonary artery sleeve resection and re-anastomosis or pericardial or prosthetic tissue reconstruction. Linear resection and closure of the main artery can be done. In this condition surgeon should be certain that the lumen of the artery is not considerably narrowed. Sometimes, to ensure lumen patency, the most appropriate approach may be to carry out a patch angioplasty with a piece of pericardium or bovine pericardium. A sleeve resection of the pulmonary artery can be done in conjunction with the sleeve lobectomy, and the arterial anastomosis is accomplished with fine monofilament suture in a continuous manner. The arterial anastomosis is done after the bronchial anastomosis has been completed to minimize retraction and handling of the vascular anastomosis. The divided artery permits excellent exposure for the bronchial anastomosis. Seldom, an extended arterial defect does not permit reanastomosis and a graft of autologous pericardium is constructed. Prosthetic material can also be utilized for the pulmonary artery conduit. Heparin (5.000 U) is given prior to a sleeve resection of the pulmonary artery. Heparin (3125 U) may also be administrated intravenously about 1 minute before vessel occlusion. Sucutanous heparin is maintained for 7 to 10 postoperative days. But administering an anticoagulation therapy is not a rule. Usually the PA was reconstructed using an end-to-end anastomosis. Postoperative computed tomography is useful in evaluating both PA patency as well as the oncologic status of the patient [1, 2, 4, 5, 7].

Proximal control of the main PA is obtained either extrapericardially or intrapericardially, and a Satinsky vascular clamp is placed on the proximal PA with/without administration of heparin or steroids. If the proximal control of the main PA is obtained extrapericardially. On the right side, proximal control is obtained posterior to the superior vena cava; and on the left side, it is obtained just distal to the ligamentous arteriosis. Care is taken to avoid the left recurrent laryngeal nerve. Subsequently, the distal part of the PA may be occluded using a bulldog or Satisnsky vascular clamp. Resection of the tumour-bearing lobe is carried out en bloc with the involved portion of the PA. A knife is used to cut out the part of the PA that has cancer invading its surface, and then the bronchus is cut as well. The large lobe with the cancer is removed from the operative field. This opens up the entire surgical field and affords more room for the surgeon to work. Frozen sections of the resected PA and/or bronchi are taken to ensure adequate resection margins. If both a PA and a bronchial sleeve resection are necessary, the PA anastomosis is performed in the right lung first, before bronchial anastomosis. In the left lung, a bronchial anastomosis first and subsequently reconstructed the PA because the operator is standing on the right side of the patient; thus, the operator reconstruct the most distant organ first, from the operator's viewpoint [1, 8, 11]. The PA is now examined from inside to determine if apartial or circumferential resection is needed. If removal of part of the PA narrows the lumen by more than 20% to 30% of its original size, a circumferential resection may be done. Another option is a patch angioplasty using a piece of bovine pericardium. If a circumferential resection is required the PA is sewn back together using 5–0 Prolene (Ethicon, Somerville, NJ). Just before reestablishing PA continuity, the distal clamp is taken off the pulmonary vein before tying the arterial sutures to help remove air from the pulmonary circuitry for a partial PA resection with primary repair. Then the proximal PA Satinsky clamp is removed to ensure hemostasis of the sewn PA. The bronchus is closed with interrupted sutures and is covered with an intercostal muscle flap that is harvested before chest retraction [1].

Direct occlusion of proximal and distal PA is still the primary technique used in PA reconstruction. Yin [11] and colleagues modified this technique and occluded the reserved PV instead of distal PA. In the event of proximal PA occlusion, on the left side and if only the interlobar PA was invaded, the PA trunk can be extrapericardially clamped just distal to the ligamentous arteriosis. In particular, careful attention to avoid the left recurrent laryngeal nerve is important. If the artery is infiltrated close to its origin, the pericardium must then be opened and proximal PA occlusion can be obtained intrapericardially. On the right side, if the tumour infiltrated very proximally, the anatomy of this region determined whether PN was usually unavoidable because of the invasion of the superior vena cava (SVC) or right atrium. Additionally, the distal of the PA is not occluded and backflow is avoided by occlusion of PV of the reserved lobe.

On the other hand, concerns of thoracic surgeons who continue to perform pneumonectomy in the circumstance of PA invasion or encroachment that is anatomically amenable to pulmonary artery resection and reconstruction have included the possibilites of intraoperative or postoperatife hemorrhage, pulmonary vascular thrombosis, and increased bronchial anastomotic complications [12]. For this reason lobectomy with tangential pulmonary artery resection can be an alternative. Partial infiltration of the arterial wall may be limited and require only simple, tangential resection and direct suture. This technique is regarded as a variation of standard lobectomy. This procedure demonstrated that it can be performed with minimal mortality and with morbidity less than that of pneumonectomy, even when most cases are performed by a simple tangential excision and primary repair technique without heparin.

Pulmonary artery primary repair is suitable only for small defects due to the resulting stenosis. Patch reconstruction is an effective method in the case of moderately extended defects. Left upper lobectomy and autologous patch reconstruction of the left pulmonary artery may be a good method for left upper lobe mass [13]. In series of Yin and collegues, PA reconstruction with end-to-end anastomosis was performed in 18 patients (52.9%); 7 patients (20.6%) required partial PA reconstruction with autologous pericardium patch and 5 patients (14.7%) with a lower lobe tumour required PA reconstruction with artery flap [14]. The calculated 5-year survival rates were 46% and 37% respectively. Politetrafluoroetilen for PA angioplasty is deemed to result in a high risk of thrombosis.

The right and left PAs can be involved to various extents and one of them can be involved to various degrees, from partial infiltration to a more extensive and even circumferential involvement. In the former case a simple tangential resection with direct suture is indicated, however, this procedure should not be considered as vascular reconstruction but rather as a simple variation of standard lobectomy [1]. Extensive defects in the arterial wall usually require patch reconstruction, end to end anastomosis, or interposition of a prosthetic conduit. Invasion of the main PA requires proximal reconstruction with the use of cardiopulmoary by pass. Reconstruction of the main PA *via* cardiopulmonary bypass is done only for patients with left T4 lung cancer. On the right side, the anatomic relationship of the PA to the SVC, right atrium, and ascending aorta makes these tumours invariably unresectable. PA resection may be performed more frequently for left-sided tumours because of the anatomical difference. Arterial resection can be successfully performed not only in the left side but also in the right side [5]. Right pneumonectomy should be avoided as thoroughly as possible because it is considered to cause more significant cardiopulmonary dysfunction and decrease in quality of life.

COMPLICATIONS

Atrial fibrillation is generally the most frequent morbidity [1, 11]. Local recurrence has to be considered as a major postoperative complication after bronchoplasty or angioplasty. Intra-operative microscopic assessment of the PA margin may not be routinely performed in all series; the area of resection is determined macroscopically in almost all cases. Intra-operative frozen-section examination was declared to be indispensable [5]. Bronchoarterial fistulae were reported as the most critical morbidity. Bronchopleural fistula may also be a cause for severe morbidity and mortality [11]. Several reports emphasized that a pedicled muscle flap was used to circumferentially cover the bronchial anastomotic site and that the procedure is indispensable. Total coverage, a muscle flap or a piece of fat tissue can be used for this. Intercostal muscle flap may be a good tool [11]. Separation is crucial to the protection of the PA suture line regardless of the bronchoplasty. Simple interposition of a biologic substitute can also prevent bronchoarterial fistula [5]. Acute respiratory distress syndrome (ARDS) is another severe postoperative complication. Warm ischemia for more than 60 minutes (PA oclusion time) may induce irreversible injury. In patients with this complication chest X-rays may reveal typical "ground-glass opacity" and pulmonary edema. The exceedingly long pericardial patch might induce kinking of the vessel and impairment of blood flow, especially in the upper lobe. Other complications include air leakage, atelectasis, and left recurrent laryngeal nerve neurapraxia.

Alifano [15] and coworkers performed lobectomy with pulmonary artery resection in 93 patients. Operative mortality was 5.4%. Postoperative complications occurred in 27 (29.0%) patients. Kojima [5] and colleagues reported 23% morbidity, no intra-operative death and two postoperative deaths (operative mortality was 3.3%). Causes of morbidity were arrhythmia requiring medication, pneumonia respiratory distress, bleeding from bronchial artery, air leakage requiring re-operation, empyema, and chylothorax. In one patient had empyema shortly after the operation and underwent completion pneumonectomy subsequently (postoperative day 19).

Although the postoperative course of bronchial sleeve resection depends to some extent on patient compliance and judicious clinical management, the short-term results of PA reconstruction depend mostly on operative judgment and technique. If the operation has been correctly performed, specific complications might be expected in no more than 5% of the patients. These essentially consist of leakage from the suture line and thrombosis. Bronchoarterial fistula is much more likely to be associated with bronchial sleeve resection and can be effectively prevented by interposing the intercostal muscle between the two structures.

Because the PA is a low-pressure vessel, leakage from the suture line may pass unnoticed intraoperatively. Also, the bleeding may start on the first or second postoperative day after a patch reconstruction. A blood loss of up to 800 to 1000 mL daily may occur after 1 or 2 days of no drainage. This may last for 1 or 2 days and then stop spontaneously, independently from anticoagulation. A possible explanation is that the autologous pericardium shrinks and curls markedly after harvesting, and it is difficult to place the suture bites at the appropriate distance. After declamping and distention, bites too wide apart may result. These would not cause bleeding immediately because the PA is stretched downward by the atelectatic lower lobe, and simple apposition of the tissue edges is enough to counteract the low PA pressure. However, in the postoperative period when the re-expansion of the lower lobe elevates the hilum, the rotation and kinking of the PA may distort the suture line and reopen the bleeding site. It is, therefore, very important, especially when using autologous pericardial patches, to carefully check the suture line and test the PA position after re-expansion of the residual lobe. The latter maneuver is also important to prevent thrombosis. After a patch reconstruction of the PA associated with a bronchial sleeve, the bronchial axis is shortened, and the length of the artery remains stationary. Some of the discrepancy is compensated by the elasticity of the vessel, but the PA may tend to kink and fold over on itself. The aforementioned repositioning of the PA caused by the re-expansion of the lower lobe further increases this risk. Impairment of blood flow may ensue, and thrombosis may be facilitated. Under these circumstances, it is better to cut the distorted segment away and proceed to an end-to-end anastomosis [8].

RESULTS

Lausberg and colleagues analyzed all their patients who underwent bronchial sleeve resection (group I, n = 104), bronchovascular sleeve resection (group II, n = 67), and pneumonectomy (group III, n = 63) for central lung cancer [16]. Early mortality was 1.9% in group I, 1.5% in group II, and 6.3% in group III. The rate of bronchial complications was 0.96% in group I, 0% in group II, and 7.9% in group III. Five-year survival was 46.1% in group I, 42.9% in group II, and 30.4% in group III. Freedom from local recurrence of disease (5 years) was 83.8% in group I, 84.2% in group II, and 88.7% in group III. Bronchovascular sleeve resections are as safe as bronchial sleeve resections for the treatment of central lung cancer.

Table 1: Reconstruction of the Pulmonary Artery in the Literature

Author (Year)	No. of Patients	Complete (%)	Technically Complete (%)	Mortality (%)	5-Year Survival (%)
Rendina (1999)	52	13.4	1.9	0	38.3
Icard (1999)	16	NS	NS	NS	39
Shrager (2000)	33	6.1	NS	NS	46.6
Lausberg (2000)	4	NS	0	NS	61.9
Okada (2000)	21	NS	0	0	48
Lausberg (2005)	67	NS	NS	1.5	42.9
Cerfolio (2007)	42	97.6	100		
Venuta (2009)	105	NS	NS	NS	44
Alifano (2009)	93	NS	NS	5.4	39.4
Yin (2010)	34	NS	NS	2.9	46 (end to end anstomosis)
37 (patch reconstruction)					
Yamashita (2010)	25	100	100	0	45
Kojima (2011)	61	98	NS	3.3	47

NS, not significant.

Venuta and colleagues performed pulmonary artery reconstruction in 105 patients with non-small cell lung cancer (tangential resections not included) [17]. Twenty-seven of their patients received induction therapy. They performed 47 pulmonary artery sleeve resections, 55 reconstructions by pericardial patch (with 3 left pneumonectomies under cardiopulmonary bypass), and 3 by pericardial conduit. In 65 patients, a bronchial sleeve resection was associated; in 6 cases superior vena caval reconstruction was also required. Fifteen patients had stage IB disease, 37 stage II, 31 IIIA, and 22 IIIB. Sixty-one patients had epidermoid carcinoma, and 38 adenocarinoma. Mean follow-up was 46±40 months. The procedure-related complications were 1 pulmonary artery thrombosis requiring completion pneumonectomy and 1 massive hemoptysis leading to death (operative mortality, 0.95%); 28 patients had other complications, with the most frequent prolonged air leakage. Overall 5-year survival was 44%. Five- and 10-year survivals for stages I and II *versus* stage III were, respectively, 60% *versus* 28% and 25% *versus* 12%. Five-year survivals were 52.6% for N0 and N1 nodal involvement *versus* 20% for N2; 10-year survivals were 28% *versus* 3%. Multivariate analysis yielded induction therapy, N2 status, adenocarcinoma, and isolated pulmonary artery reconstruction as negative prognostic factors. In Yin's11 study, as compared with the stage III patients, stage I patients had significantly greater 5-year survival (80% *vs.* 11%. Patients with pN0 disease also had greater 5-year survival than patients with pN2-3 disease (71% *vs.* 9%). Alifano [12] reported that tumour size of less than 3 cm; presence of vascular peritumoural emboli, intratumoural emboli, or both; and dyspnea influenced 5-year survival; the size of the primary tumour and the presence of vascular emboli were independent factors of worse outcome. Their indications for surgical intervention were non–small cell lung cancer in 87 patients and other malignancy in the remaining 6 patients. Bronchial sleeve resection was associated in 23 patients. Neoadjuvant chemotherapy had been administered in 34 cases because of cN2 disease. Median and 5-year survivals were 40 months and 39.4%, respectively. Disease-free survival was 41.4% at 5 years.

Puma and colleagues performed repair of PA using the tissue of the resected left superior PV in eight patients [18]. All patients were scheduled for pulmonary lobectomy and possibly pneumonectomy after a standard preoperative work-up. In the case of N2 disease, cisplatinum-based induction chemotherapy was administered; patients were then restaged at the end of medical treatment. Postoperative thromboembolic prophylaxis included subcutaneous Enoxaparin 4000 units once daily for a period of 21 days. Five left upper lobectomies (LUL), one bronchial sleeve LUL, and two LUL extended to the superior segment of the left lower lobe were performed. Mediastinal node dissection was always carried out prior to angioplasty. The PA wall was directly infiltrated by the tumour in 2/8 cases, and by metastatic lymph nodes in 5/8 cases; in one patient the PA wall resulted pathologically uninvolved. No perioperative mortality was recorded. Two postoperative complications occurred: left vocal cord paralysis and transient atrial fibrillation. The PA clamp time was 15 ± 4 min for the patch placement. The hospital stay lasted a mean of 8.8 days ranging from 8 to 10 (median 8.5 ± 1 day). Four patients are alive at 12, 24, 31, and 66 months without evidence of disease. They found only one local recurrence in the anterior chest wall, away from the reconstructed PA. They concluded: (1) the PV supplies superlative vascular tissue for angioplasty; (2) harvesting is very simple and quick; (3) no additional surgical trauma is required; (4) the procedure is safe and appears to be oncologically adequate.

Cerfolio [1] and colleagues were more liberal in the use of partial resection, used a lower dose of intraoperative heparin, avoided the use of postoperative heparin, and performed the procedures in patients who had undergone high-dose irradiation. PA resections were done in 42 patients, of whom 4 required a circumferential resection and 7 required bovine pericardium patch angioplasty. Six patients had a concomitant sleeve of the both the artery and the bronchus. An intercostal muscle was applied to the bronchial closure in 32 of the 42 patients, and in some, it acted as a buffer in between the vascular repair and the bronchial closure. In their study, patients who had biopsy-proven N2 disease underwent neoadjuvant radiochemotherapy. The indication for surgery was NSCLC in 41 (98%) of the 42 patients and for tuberculosis with a destroyed left upper lobe in 1 patient. In general, patients with N2 disease underwent neoadjuvant radiation and chemotherapy using doses of 60 Gy or higher of radiation, and patients with biopsy-proven N1 disease (with Wang needle biopsy during bronchoscopy) received neoadjuvant chemotherapy alone. All patients were restaged after neoadjuvant therapy, and resection was generally reserved for those who were down-staged. At the time of thoracotomy, all lymph nodesstations were completely removed. Median hospital stay was 4 days (range, 3 to 28 days). Median operative time was 2 hours and 25 minutes. One patient had to return to the operating room for a completion pneumonectomy on postoperative day 3 because final pathologic margins showed a positive proximal PA margin that had been called benign on frozen section pathology on the day of surgery. Five-year survival rate was 60%.

Yamashita [8] and colleagues performed 25 pulmonary angioplastic procedure for lung cancer surgery. Altogether, 13 patients had adenocarcinoma, and 11 had squamous cell carcinoma. The cancers were located in the left lung in 15 cases and in the right lung in 10 cases. The PA reconstructions comprised 4 circumferential resections and anastomoses, 18 wedge resections and end-to-end anastomoses, 2 tangential resections with direct suturing, and 1 wide wedge resection and autologous pericardial patch repair. Six patients underwent concomitant bronchoplasty with pulmonary artery reconstruction. The factors that led to PA plasty were tumour direct invasion in 14 cases and lymph node invasion in 11 cases. Prior to surgical treatment, seven patients had received neoadjuvant therapy. They routinely removed the all mediastinal lymph nodes according to Naruke's lymph node map. All patients who underwent partial or segmental PA resection had margin-negative R0 resections and lymphadenectomies. They had one case of induction chemotherapy and six cases of induction chemoradiotherapy. The radiation dose was 40–60 Gy. The pathological stages were I (n = 5), II (n = 7), and III (n = 13). The mean operating time was 277 ± 69 min, the PA clamping time was 32 ± 18 min, and the mean blood loss during operation was 391 ± 259 ml. No operative or in-hospital deaths occurred. Early postoperative complications occurred in eight patients (32%). Among seven induction cases, four patients had seven morbidities including one patient with major complications such as intrathoracic hemorrhage and cerebral infarction. The overall survival rate was 45% at 5 years. Disease recurrence developed in eight patients, and six patients died from their original cancer.

Kojima [5] and coworkers performed 61 pulmonary angioplasties. In their study the 5-year overall and disease-free survival rates were 76.0% and 62.9% for pN0 cases (n = 14), 45.7% and 43.5% for pN1 cases (n = 27), and 28.9% and 20.0% for pN2 + pN3 cases (n = 20). The influence of staging was significant on overall survivals, but was not significant on disease-free survivals. pN status was the only prognostic factor for both overall and disease-free survival. Although eight patients had local recurrence (five intrathoracic and three lymph nodes), no recurrence was observed along the PA suture line.

Pulmonary artery reconstruction was safe, with excellent long-term survival and their results supported this technique as an effective option for patients with lung cancer. On the other hand, complications may be in high rate, severe and fatal. Most operative complications after PA reconstruction were controllable despite the high morbidity rate.

ACKNOWLEDGEMENTS

Declared none.

CONFLICT OF INTEREST

The author confirms that this article content has no conflict of interest.

REFERENCES

[1] Cerfolio RJ, Bryant AS. Surgical techniques and results for partial or circumferential sleeve resection of the pulmonary artery for patients with non-small cell lung cancer. Ann Thorac Surg 2007; 83: 1971–7

[2] Venuta F. Rendina EA. Combined pulmonary artery and bronchial sleeve resection. Operative Techniques in Thoracic and Cardiovascular Surgery, 2008: 13: 260-273

[3] Cerezo F, Cano JR, Espinoza D, Salvatierra A. New technique for pulmonary artery reconstruction. European Journal of Cardiot-thoracic Surgery. 2009; 36: 422-423.

[4] Venuta F, Ciccone AM. Reconstruction of the Pulmonary Artery. Seminars in Thoracic and Cardiovascular Surgery, Volume 18, Issue 2, Summer 2006, Pages 104-108

[5] Al-Khaldi A, Mohammed Y, Tamimi O, Alharbi A. Early Outcomes of Total Pulmonary Arterial Reconstruction in Patients With Arterial Tortuosity Syndrome. Ann Thorac Surg 2011 [Epub ahead of print].

[6] Kojima F, Yamamoto K, Matsuoka K, Ueda M, Hamada H, Imanishi N, Miyamoto Y. Factors affecting survival after lobectomy with pulmonary artery resection for primary lung cancer. Eur J Cardiothorac Surg 2011; 40: e13-e20.

[7] Veronesi G, Solli PG, Leo F, Aiuto MD, Pelosi G, Leon ME, De Braud F, Spaggiari L, Pastorino U. Low morbidity of bronchoplastic procedures after chemotherapy for lung cancer. Lung Cancer 2002; 36: 91-97

[8] Ma Z, Dong A, Fan J, Cheng H. Does sleeve lobectomy concomitant with or without pulmonary artery reconstruction (doulbe sleeve) have favorable results for non-small cell lung cancer compared with pneumonectomy? A meta analysis. European Journal of Cardiot-thoracic Surgery 2007: 32: 20-28

[9] Yamashita M, Komori E, Sawada S, Suehisa H, Nozaki I, Kurita A, Takashima S. Pulmonary angioplastic procedure for lung cancer surgery. Gen Thorac Cardiovasc Surg. 2010; 58: 19-24.

[10] Rendina EA, Venuta F. Reconstruction of the pulmonary artery. In: Patterson GA, Cooper JD, Deslauriers J, Lerut EMR, Luketich JD, Rice TW, eds. Pearson's Thoracic & Esophageal surgery. 3rd edition. Philadelphia, PA: Churchill Livingstone; 2008: 909-922.

[11] Deslauriers J, Gregorie J, Jacques LF, Paraux M, Guojin L, Lacasse. Sleeve lobectomy *versus* pneumonectomy for lung cancer: a comparative analysis of survival and sites or recurrences. Ann Thorac Surg 2004;77:1152–6.

[12] Shrager J, Lambright ES, McGrath CM, Wahl PM, Deeb ME, Friedberg JS, Kaiser LR. Lobectomy with tangential pulmonary artery resection without regard to pulmonary function. Ann Thorac Surg 2000; 70: 734-9.

[13] Haciibrahimoglu G, Cansever L, Bedirhan MA. Autologous patch reconstruction to pulmonary artery for left upper lobe tumour. Acta Chir Belg 2006;106:734-5.

[14] Yin R, Xu L, Ren B, Jiang F, Fan X, Zhang Z, Li M, Hu Z. Clinical Experience of Lobectomy With Pulmonary Artery Reconstruction for Central Non–Small-Cell Lung Cancer. Clin Lung Cancer. 2010;11:120-5.

[15] Alifano M, Cusumano G, Strano S, Magdeleinat P, Bobbio A, Giraud F, Lebeau B, Régnard JF. Lobectomy with pulmonary artery resection: morbidity, mortality, and long-term survival. J Thorac Cardiovasc Surg 2009; 137:1400-5.

[16] Lausberg HF, Graeter TP, Tscholl D, Wendler O, Schafers HJ. Bronchovascular *versus* bronchial sleeve resection for central lung tumours. Ann Thorac Surg 2005; 79: 1147-52.

[17] Venuta F, Ciccone AM, Anile M, İbrahim M, Giacomo TD, Coloni GF, Rendina EA. Reconstruction of the Pulmonary Artery for Lung Cancer: Long-term Results. J Thorac Cardiovasc Surg 2009; 138: 1185-91

[18] Puma F, Capozzi R, Daddi N, Ragusa M, Cagini L, Quintili A, Vannucci J. Experience with the autologous pulmonary vein for pulmonary arterioplasty. Eur J Cardiothorac Surg 2011 Jun 14. [Epub ahead of print]. doi:10.1016/j.ejcts.2011.05.012

Send Orders of Reprints at reprints@benthamscience.net
Lung Cancer: Clinical and Surgical Specifications, **2013, 213-258**

CHAPTER 10

Part B: Methods and Results of Extended Pulmonary Resections'

Akın Eraslan Balcı*

Euphrates University Thoracic Surgery, Elazig, Turkey

Abstract: The results of resection of non-small cell lung cancer depend on its stage. The 5-year survival of patients with stage I and II non-small cell lung cancer is 70 and 50%, respectively; therefore, surgical treatment is thought to be indicated in these patients. However, in patients with stage IIIa and IIIb non-small cell lung cancer 5-year survival is as low as 20 and 6%, respectively. There are especially few long-term survivors with stage IIIb non-small cell lung cancer. On the other hand, stage IIIb non-small cell lung cancer can be classified into T4 and N3, with the former considered to be operable in selected patients. The symptoms and prognosis of T4 cancer vary depending on the region invaded: trachea, esophagus, vertebral column, superior vena cava (SVC), aorta, left atrium (LA). Good survival rates are obtained by upfront resection (excluding pancoast tumours) of T4 tumours in cases of NO or N1 nodal status and if complete resection is achieved, and resection should be recommended in patients fit for surgery. Therefore, the indications for surgical operation should be determined by taking into consideration the region of invasion, the degree of invasion, lymph node involvement and curability by surgery [1-4]. Most of these cancers are staged T3 or T4. Therefore, it is mandatory that all patients undergo extensive staging, including mediastinoscopy, before an attempt at resection. Operative planning is critical because only a complete resection provides the patient with any opportunity for cure.

Keywords: Lung cancer, extended resection.

EXTENDED PULMONARY RESECTIONS OF THORACIC MALIGNANCIES WITH CARDIO-PULMONARY BYPASS

Conventional techniques frequently do not allow for complete resection of advanced pulmonary tumours invading the heart or great vessels. Thus for non-small cell lung cancer invading the mediastinum with infiltration of the great vessels complete resection has been reported in only 30-40% of such cases [5,

***Address correspondence to Akın Eraslan Balcı:** Euphrates University Thoracic Surgery, Elazig, Turkey; Tel: +90 424 2333555/2134; Fax: +90 424 2388096; E-mail: akineraslan.balci@hotmail.com

6]. For these cases extended pulmonary resections with support of cardio-pulmonary bypass (CPB) are occasionally applied in many specialized thoracic surgical centers in order to achieve complete resection or to manage intraoperative complications [7-10]. CPB is an established alternative to ventilation during extended resections; it provides both oxygenation and hemodynamic stability.

These operations may include the potential mortality and morbidity, the poor prognosis or technical considerations [11]. The key issue for a favorable outcome justifying extended resection of advanced thoracic malignancies on CPBP is patient selection. Unfortunately, there are no clear guidelines for this, it must be based on an individual basis. It may be anticipated that if pulmonary resection is limited to lobectomy and the time of CPB is kept short, no major increase in pulmonary complications will have to be expected. However, extended pneumonectomies with CPB support remain to be associated with a substantial risk of pulmonary complications.

CPB cannot be avoided if the surgical resection of a malignancy extends into the heart and requires opening of 1 of the cardiac cavities or if it infiltrates the aortic arch or the pulmonary trunk. Carefully selected patients may be resected on CPB with acceptable mortality and morbidity, which allows the achievement of good palliation and long-term survival in a few [7].

Median sternotomy is the most often used approach to combine thoracic and cardiac procedures. For some of the complex cases, a clamp-shell incision, as used in pulmonary transplantation is used to offer the best exposure. Posterolateral thoracotomy incision can also be done. Bicaval venous canulation should be practiced routinely. In case of tumour preventing caval access, femoral vein or pulmonary artery canulation can be alternative ways of connecting the extracorporal bypass [11]. The common pulmonary artery, the right atrium, the right ventricle, the aorta, and the coronary arteries can be resected enbloc with the pulmonary tumour. For reconstruction of cardiac structures, autologous pericardium can be used. In addition, aortic and pulmonary homografts and polytetrafluoroethylene (PTFE) prosthetic material can also be used. Mediastinal lymph nodes infiltrating the trachea may prevent complete resection [11].

Morbidity rate after standard pneumonectomies is 11 to 49% and mortality rate is 5.4%. Extended pneumonectomies and prolonged anesthetic time is associated with the highest rates of complications. For extended resections with CPB, postoperative pulmonary complications were 38%, the 30-day mortality was 15% [11]. Five-year survival for these patients ranged between 20% to 40% and it was the best (62.5%) in sarcomas that are known for the resistance for chemotherapy and radiotherapy [1, 12, 13].

Despite its advanteges, CPB has several disadvantages, such as increased need for blood products for full heparinization of the patient, the danger of potential tumour cell spilling through the suction system, and the proven immunosuppressive effect of the device itself. In this situation, venoarterial extracorporeal membrane oxygenation (ECMO) offers an attractive alternative. It does not require full heparinization; it acts through closed-loop extracorporeal circulation without suction of blood and is considered to be more biocompatible [14, 15]. ECMO can be initiated through the left side of the groin, and the aorta was cross clamped under the base of the left subclavian artery and above the diaphragm. The upper half of the body was perfused by the patient's heart, whereas the lower part of the body was perfused by ECMO. ECMO bypass can also be established with cannulation of the abdominal part of the IVC and the ascending aorta. The IVC can be crossclamped close to the right atrium and above the entrance to the renal veins [14]. In this method, 1 of 9 patients died, median time for intensive care unit was 1 day. The only complication directly related to the use of ECMO was a lymphatic fistula in the left side of the groin which required surgical revision. Median hospital time was 10 days and patients returned to normal life [14].

CHEST WALL INVASION

Invasion of the parietal pleura, the subpleural soft tissue, or the bony structure of the chest wall occurs in 5 to 8% of patients with non-small cell lung cancer who are undergoing surgical treatment [16-18] and alters the TNM classification, staging, and planned treatment approaches [19]. In the absence of metastatic spread, en-bloc anatomic surgical resection of the involved lung and chest wall is the primary treatment for most patients. These lesions are T3 tumours and, because of the favorable survival following surgical resection of T3N0 tumours, they have been reclassified as stage IIB disease. If lymph node involvement is present, the overall survival following resection of T3 tumours is reduced such that T3 N1 to 2 tumours remain in the stage IIIA category. Factors that influence survival in this group of patients include completeness of resection, the extent of chest wall invasion, and the presence of regional lymph node metastasis [20].

Among locally advanced lung cancers involving the neighboring structures, tumours invading chest wall are the most common and an extended surgical resection is considered to be the only curative method for patients with this disease, especially in cases with no lymph node metastases [21]. Parietal pleura and Luschka's fascia make up a natural barrier to cancer involvement and usually are interested by an `adhering' more than `infiltrating' process and therefore quite a few of these tumours may be detached from chest wall by extrapleural dissection. The overcoming of such a barrier by the neoplasm requires a more extended procedure that will encompass all involved ribs and chest wall soft tissue with a safety resection edge of at least 3±4 cm [22].

Some series advocated that en bloc resection of the chest wall and lung is the procedure of choice to obtain complete resection in lung cancer invading the chest wall [23-25]. On the other hand, some surgeons have advocated the extrapleural dissection of the tumour from the chest wall (the extrapleural dissection of the tumour from the chest wall with removal of the lung parenchyma and a portion of the overlying parietal pleura with the removal of the lung parenchyma and a portion of the overlying parietal pleura), if possible [26-28]. But no statistical difference was detected between two surgical methods [22, 29].

The most reliable predictor of chest wall invasion is chest pain. Pain is a highly specific (>90%) clinical sign for chest wall infiltration [18]. It is the clinical sign leading patients to consult their doctors. The pain was burning and continuous (Paulson called it 'excruciating') and did not respond effectively to high doses of analgesics [18]. Peripheral lung cancers invading the parietal pleura which do not cause chest pain are detected by other clinical signs (*e.g.,* pneumonia or haemoptysis) or incidentally, by extensive use of chest radiographs [18]. Radiographic demonstration of the chest wall invasion is not reliable unless clear evidence of chest wall soft tissue or bony invasion is demonstrated by computed tomography (CT) or magnetic resonance imaging (MRI) [30]. Because MRI can detect differences in intensity between tumour and normal tissues, including bone, soft tissues, fat, and vascular structures, it may be more accurate than CT scanning in delineating direct tumour invasion of the mediastinum, chest wall, diaphragm, or vertebral bodies [31]. Exploratory video-assisted thoracoscopy may be clearly better than computed tomography and/or magnetic resonance imaging for detecting chest wall invasion [32]. In a study ultrasound has been found to have good sensitivity (89%) and specificity (95%) in assessing chest wall involvement [19]. Positron emission tomography (PET) using C-i 1-labeledL-methionine(11C-L-Met) can detect chest well invasion [33].

If resection is contemplated, accurate staging is essential. N2 disease must be excluded. Since the prognosis of patients with mediastinal lymph node metastases and chest wall infiltration is worse (T3N2M0, < 10%), the histological proof of N2 disease should lead to the recommendation of definitive non-surgical treatment such as radio-chemotherapy; in the case of Pancoast tumours, ipsilateral supraclavicular lymph node metastases do not preclude trimodality treatment [18, 30]. PET has proven to be an effective tool to stage lung cancer concerning lymph nodes and distant sites. It can be recommended as a basic investigation technique in combination with MRI of the brain. The suspicion of mediastinal lenf node metastases has to be confirmed by mediastinoscopy [18, 30].

The goal of surgery when lung cancer invades the chest wall is complete resection and reconstruction of the chest wall when necessary. Four clinical situations are possible when the tumour reaches the chest wall [18]: (1). The tumour infiltrates the soft tissue or bones of the chest wall. Complete chest wall resection is clearly necessary to achieve a radical operation. (2). The tumour has only penetrated the visceral and parietal pleura. Extrapleural lobectomy might be possible for histologically documented complete resection. (3). The tumour and the visceral pleural are fixed to the parietal pleura by inflammatory adhesion induced by the tumour or by previous pleurisy. Extrapleural lobectomy is sufficient for radical resection. (4). The lung and the tumour are not fixed to the chest wall. Standard lobectomy would be an adequate operation. Frequently, reconstruction is not required because the chest wall defect is often beneath the scapula or chest wall musculature and does not require reconstruction for cosmesis or chest wall stability. However, for anterolateral or anterior defects, standard techniques of reconstruction are employed [30].

In cases in which chest wall invasion is suspected, the chest initially is explored through an aspect of the incision that is away from the area of suspected invasion. Careful digital palpation of the pleural surface will confirm the location and extent of the tumour [30]. the decision of performing extrapleural lobectomy or chest wall resection was made intraoperatively by the surgeon trusting in his personal experience. The rate of extrapleural resection ranges from 30 to 60%. Stoelben [18] recommend being aware of a T3 tumour in every case of a tumour making contact with the parietal pleura and if in doubt to use further investigation such as high-resolution CT, MRI or ultrasound. If the surgeon finds the tumour fixed to parietal pleura and this fixation is not obviously produced by an inflammatory reaction, parietal infiltration is likely. In these cases, full-thickness resection of the chest wall is recommended to reach a higher 5-year survival rate. Chest wall invasion is usually evident by the degree of fixation of the primary tumour to the chest wall. If fixation is not firm, the adhesion is likely due to inflammatory fibrosis. In this situation, an extrapleural plane can easily be developed over the area of adherence. If the parietal pleura dissects away easily, tumour invasion farther into the chest wall is usually not present. Frozen section examination of the pleural surface under suspicion is essential to confirm tumour-free margins on the outer pleural surface [18].

The need for chest wall reconstruction depends on the size and location of the defect. The main reasons to reconstruct the chest wall are to protect vital underlying structures and to prevent paradoxical chest wall motion and respiratory compromise [20]. For defects greater than three ribs or 5 cm, some type of chest wall reconstruction is usually warranted. Very small defects of one to two ribs, or defects located posteriorly beneath the scapula, usually do not require reconstruction. However, if a posterior chest wall resection extends to the fifth rib or lower, chest wall reconstruction should be performed to prevent the scapula from caving into the chest. For posterior and lateral defects beneath the scapula, chest wall reconstruction is not required. However, if the fifth rib is removed, some sort of prosthetic replacement using Marlex, Gore-Tex, or Dacron is employed to prevent the scapular tip from falling into the chest over the top of the posterior sixth rib [30]. If reconstruction is undertaken for posterior superior defects, curved chest contour is not required. However, for more anterior or lateral defects, a contoured rigid reconstruction is preferable and can be accomplished by a combination of Marlex and methylmethacrylate [30]. PTFE net was also found successful for reconstruction of the chest wall [18]. Titanium rib osteosynthesis in combination with Dualmesh can easily and safely be used in a one-stage procedure for major chest wall defects after resection [34].

RESULTS

Several reports have demonstrated acceptable long-term survival in patients undergoing resection of bronchogenic carcinoma with chest wall invasion. But opposite results have presented also: the 5-year, 10-year, and median survivals were 61%, 50%, and 90 months, respectively, in the Chemo-RT group *versus* 22%, 14%, and 22 months, respectively, in the surgery group, so aggressive treatment of node-negative invasive T3 and T4 NSCLC with induction chemoradiotherapy may significantly prolong survival [35]. Operative morbidity and mortality 34% and 2.1%, respectively, in patients who underwent radical en-bloc lung and chest wall resection for NSCLC; overall and disease-free survivals were significantly influenced by N-status; five-year overall survival in radically resected patients (resection margins are clear) was 73% [36]. In addition, analysis proved presence of micrometastasis and microinfiltration of the resection margins as the only factors influencing overall and disease-free survival rates. The 5-year overall survival rate of T3 and T4 tumours was 45.7%; age of 70 years or more, tumour length more than 5 cm, lymph node metastases, incomplete resection, and histology of non-adenocarcinoma were significantly associated with an unfavorable prognosis; older age, incomplete resection, and lymph node metastases were independent predictors of shorter survival [37]. Heterogeneity existed among the chest wall invasion, *i.e.* pleural invasion showed most favorable survival rate, whereas rib destruction exerted unfavorable prognosis. Especially, Pancoast type lung cancer showed poorest survival rate [38].

Radical surgery including chest wall resection may result in a 5-year survival rate of up to 50% in T3N1 disease [39]. Adjuvant chemotherapy is recommended and radiotherapy is reserved for cases with unclear resection margins. Clinical trials of preoperatively proven N2 patients could show a better outcome when downstaging is achieved after neoadjuvant chemo- or chemoradiotherapy prior to surgery. Patients who may need a pneumonectomy should be selected with caution since some centers experience a high perioperative mortality rate. If unforeseen N2 disease is found during surgery, an adjuvant therapy is recommended [39].

VERTEBRAL INVASION

Locally advanced resectable non-small cell lung cancer (NSCLC) should be resected; however, the treatment of patients for NSCLC with vertebral body invasion remains challenging. NSCLC with substantial invasion of vertebral bodies was usually considered a contraindication to operation due to poor long-term survival. Additionally, vertebral involvement by bronchogenic carcinoma has represented a specific contraindication to resection because of the low likelihood of complete margins and the associated morbidity of vertebral resection [30]. Under most circumstances vertebral body invasion is considered T4 disease and thus unresectable [40]. However, technical developments and the introduction of spinal surgery into lung cancer operations made the extensive operations for NSCLC feasible with an acceptable long-term survival and morbidity. But limited survival suggests that the problem of incomplete resection has not been resolved. An aggressive multidisciplinary approach to NSCLC with vertebral invasion can lead to longterm survival with acceptable morbidity. The recent advances in chemotherapy and/or radiotherapy have made it possible to control distant metastasis or local recurrence. Furthermore, the recent evolution of sophisticated spinal stabilization techniques has allowed larger portions of the vertebral body to be resected successfully and safely [41]. If complete surgical resection is possible with or without induction therapy, then surgery itself will be the therapy of choice for NSCLC with vertebral invasion [42].

There have been many variations of the methods of resection and reconstruction, which are always done in conjunction with orthopedic surgeons and neurosurgeons. DeMeester and colleagues [43] described a technique of partial vertebral resection for tumours fixed to the paravertebral fascia. They use a tangential osteotomy through the transverse process, costotransverse foramen and superficial vertebral body. This approach is not suitable for patients with radiographic evidence of bone destruction. Spinal canal invasion was an absolute contraindication to resection [44, 45].

An en-bloc hemivertebrectomy or total vertebrectomy is ideal. En bloc total vertebrectomy can be done succesfully. In this method, a long posterior thoracotomy incision is made, allowing the section of the chest wall in tumour-free margins [42]. At thoracotomy, a right fourth rib is resected and preserved for bone grafting for vertebral body reconstrution. Intervertebal discs of T1/2 and T3/4 are curetted and the thoracotomy is temporarily closed. Then, in a prone position a median posterior incision from the level of C5 to that of T7 is performed. Pedicle screws are inserted bilaterally at C7, T1, T5, and T6 using a computer assisted navigation system, and laminectomy from T1 to T4 is performed. Transverse processes and pedicles from T2 to T4 are resected, and the costovertebral joints are disarticulated (T2-T4), which allowes to reach the anterior aspect of the vertebrae. Vertebral body reconstruction is achieved with a placement of titanium mesh cage packed with bone chips made of an autogenous fourth rib which was resected at thoracotomy [42].

The vertebral resection can be performed piecemeal (*versus* en bloc). Gandhi and colleagues [46] performed total and partial vertebrectomies with a multidisciplinary approach in patients with superior sulcus tumours invading the vertebra. Approach is through an extended posterolateral thoracotomy with occasional addition of a posterior midline incision for tumours with significant vertebral involvement. They also advocate an endolesional approach to resection in which the tumour is resected off the vertebral body, allowing a more careful evaluation of the extent of vertebral involvement. They performed total vertebrectomy in 7 patients (42%), partial vertebrectomy in 7 patients (42%). Three (18%) patients underwent neural foramina or transverse process resection. The median hospital stay was 11 days. Postoperative complications occurred in 7 patients (42%) and included pneumonia (6, 36%), arrhythmia (2, 12%), cerebrospinal fluid leak (2, 12%), wound breakdown (1, 6%), and reoperation for bleeding (1, 6%). Sixteen out of total 17 patients received preoperative or postoperative radiation therapy. No perioperative mortality occurred. All patients remained ambulatory after spinal reconstruction. Overall actuarial survival at 2 years was 54%, with 11 patients still alive 2 to 50 months after resection. Locoregional tumour recurrence was noted in all 6 patients who had positive surgical margins, as opposed to 1 out of 11 patients (9%) with negative margins. The 2-year actuarial survival of patients with negative microscopic margins was 80% *versus* 0% for positive margins.

Schirren and colleagues [47] retrospectively reviewed their prospective database of all patients, who underwent lung resection with *en bloc* hemivertebrectomy or total vertebrectomy for NSCLC. Those they determined the preconditions for the resection of NSCLC invading the spine areas are as follows: (1) histologically proven diagnosis of NSCLC; (2) no N2-disease; (3) no distant metastases; (4) radiological criteria of spine infiltration; (5) no infiltration of the plexus above C8; and (6) neo-adjuvant treatment, as appropriate, depending on tumour board decision. In this the newest study, the steps of their surgical approach are as follows 1. Posterior midline incision with dorsal release for hemivertebrectomy or total vertebrectomy. 2. Posterolateral thoracotomy with en bloc resection of the chest wall, spine and lung including systematic lymph node dissection. 3. Stabilization of the spine. 4. Reconstruction of the chest wall. Eight of their 28 patients were inoperable at the time of diagnosis.The contraindication for surgery included tumour invasion into the spinal canal at multiple levels (n = 3), unfitness for anesthesia and surgery at the time of diagnosis (n = 2), multilevel N2-disease (n = 2), and pre-existing paraplegia (n = 1). Complete resection (R0) could be achieved in 16 patients (80%). The mean and 5-year survival for patients, who underwent surgery, were 46.0 ± 7.6 months and 47%, respectively. Inoperable patients had poorer survival (14.2 ± 5.0 months). Incomplete resections and sublobar resections were associated with inferior survival. They concluded that multimodality treatment including *en bloc* lung resection with hemivertebrectomy or total vertebrectomy offers promising long-term survival in highly selected patients. Addititonaly they favored chemoradiotherapy in the adjuvant setting to address the possible local and systemic residual disease in patients without mediastinal nodal disease. There is a lack of prospective randomized trials providing answers to this debatable issue about the timing of the non-surgical treatment options within a multimodality treatment.

AORTIC INVASION

Lung tumours invading mediastinal structures (T4) generally considered unresectable. Curative resection is usually limited by locoregional tumour extension. Moreover, more than two-thirds of the patients undergoing complete tumour resection die due to systemic recurrence [48]. Aorta involvement by lung cancer has long been considered a technical and oncological contraindication to surgical treatment. However, in recent years, several reports regarding SVC and aorta resection and replacement as well as advances in anesthesiology and surgical techniques have increased interest in these extended operations [49-51]. In case of direct invasion by the tumour of SVC or aorta as the only mediastinal structure involved, an en block resection may be attempted. The main issue that must be debated is the long-term benefit that can be attained with such an extensive operation. Under certain circumstances T4 tumours may be completely resected improving the long-term survival rate for some patients. Specifically, patients with localized tumour in growth and low node stage are expected to benefit from a combined resection of the lung and the involved aortic or SVC segment [51]. Full-thickness involvement of the aortic wall is generally considered a contraindication to resection. Unfortunately, determination of such involvement is very difficult before resection. For such central lesions, direct aortic invasion and frequent nodal metastasis make complete resection and cure unlikely. In most patients, resectability cannot be determined until the time of exploration. It may be possible to develop a plane of dissection within the aortic adventitia and to accomplish a complete resection. Fukuse and colleagues1 had 13 patients with invasion of the aorta. They performed total replacement of the aorta with a Dacron graft in 3 patients and a closure with a Dacron patch graft for repair of the defect. The tumour was, enucleated leaving behind part of the invaded focus in 9 patients. Two patients with invasion of the subclavian artery had total replacement of the artery with a Dacron graft.

Involvement of the aorta is not uncommon for left-sided lung cancers. Accurate preoperative diagnosis of the extend and degree of infiltration of the aorta and of the SVC is essential. Aortic invasion can be suspected when the tumour is in apposition to the aorta, when it is more than 25% of aortic circumference, or when the fat plane is lost between the aorta and the tumour [52]. The extent of the disease was clinically determined in each patient on the basis of the results of bronchoscopy, computed tomography, gallium-67 scanning, magnetic resonance imaging, and selective pulmonary angiography. Modern imaging technologies have proved extremely useful in defining the extend of aortic or SVC involvement and the resectability of the affected tissues. Moreover, ruling out N2 disease and distant metastases is also needed. Positron emission tomography may be mandatory in this group of patients with IIIB NSCLC. Aortic invasion in patients with NSCLC identified preoperatively at CT or MRI is not a contraindication if aortic inner layer is intact. Involvement of the aortic arch, with or without left recurrent nerve palsy, is usually due to extensive mediastinal adenopathy. Primary involvement of the aorta by a left-sided T4 N0-1 lung cancer is uncommon. In most instances, it is limited to the adventitia of the vessel and may be suitable for subadventitial dissection. Deep invasion of the aorta is extremely rare and difficult to identify by spiral CT or MRI of the chest. Cine computed tomography has been proposed as a way to differentiate between invasive and fibrous or inflammatory adhesion [53]. Radical resection can be done without increase of operative risk. Additionally, no influence on long-term survival was recorded. Patients with NSCLC invading aorta are classified in stage IIIB, which have dismal prognosis. This is maybe inaccurate, since radical resection of the primary tumour along with aortic involvement disclosed favorable long-term survival comparable to stage IIB-IIIA. The methods for resecting tumours that invade the aortic area include a subadventitial dissection, a partial resection with patch, or a total tubular resection with reconstruction. The latter approach requires at least partial bypass or other techniques to maintain distal circulation.

Saitoh and colleagues [48] were classified the lung tumours according to their clinical extent of invasion as Type A (invading the anterior mediastinum including the central part of the pulmonary artery), Type B (invading upwardly to the mediastinum through the aortic window) or Type C (invading the posterior mediastinum including the thoracic aorta or esophagus). Complete resection was performed in eight patients, and incomplete resection in three. Adjacent mediastinal structures included in the resection were the intrapericardial pulmonary artery in five patients, thoracic aorta in three, and esophagus in one. The recurrent nerve was resected in nine patients. Hoarseness was observed in all these patients, but aspiration pneumonia did not develop. Postoperative arrhythmia (paroxysmal atrial tachycardia) was observed in one patient, and an empyema due to a minor leak of the main bronchial stump developed in one patient. They concluded that the patients with type A invasion are considered good candidates for surgical treatment.

Suziki and colleagues [54] performed neoadjuvant chemotherapy followed by en bloc resection of the tumour, lung, chest wall and aortic arch in 54 year-old patient with squamous cell carcinoma, T4N0M0. Perfusion was maintained through femoral-femoral cardiopulmonary bypass, with permanent bypass to the arch vessels to avoid separate extracorporeal cerebral circulation. Total reconstructions of the chest wall and aortic arch were completed without the need for cardiac arrest. The patient was discharged without major complications and has been free of disease for 20 months postoperatively. Pneumonectomy with en bloc resection of aortic adventitia and media was accomplished after thoracic aorta endovascular stent graft placement. The aortic defect was reinforced with an extrathoracic muscle flap. Berna and colleagues [55] described a wise technique: they placed a thoracic endovascular stent graft under general anesthesia through a retrograde femoral approach. Then pneumonectomy with en bloc resection of aortic adventitia and media (8-cm length) was done during the same anesthesia and in the same operating room. The patient was disease-free at 23-month follow-up. Klepetko and colleagues [56] reported their experience in 7 patients undergoing resection of lung tumours involving the aorta. Six of these seven resections were conducted with the assistance of cardiopulmonary bypass, and in 1 patient a temporary interposition graft was employed. Aortic reconstruction was performed by tube graft or pericardial patch for small noncircumferential defects. Long-term survival was limited, with only 2 of the 7 patients alive without disease. The combined resection should be performed without cardiopulmonary bypass. The combined pneumonectomy and aortic wall resection for lung cancer can be successfully performed using a heparinized bypass tube [57]. In this technique, the tumour was first resected with pneumonectomy to facilitate the operation, its invading portion being cut as close as possible to the aortic wall. Then a heparinized tube was inserted from the proximal to the distal descending aorta for a temporary bypass. The aorta was cross-clamped proximal and distal to the invaded wall without systemic heparinization. The invaded anterior aortic wall was partially resected, and the defect was closed with a polyethylene terephthalate fiber prosthetic patch. Complete mediastinal lymphadenectomy was performed.

Misthos and collegues [51] performed lung resection in 13 patients with their cancers had aortic invasion. In three cases (23%) the tumour was adhered to the parietal pleura overlying descending aorta, which was resected en block with tumour-associated lung parenchyma. Aortic adventitia invasion by tumour led to local resection of adventitia (<1 cm^2) in nine patients (69%). Invasion deeper than adventitia was encountered in one case (8%), which was managed with aortic partial occlusion, resection of aortic wall and repair of the defect with Gore graft patch. In three patients (33%) the SVC wall was involved by the tumour 1-3 cm in length and 2-4mm of the circumference. The defect was repaired with direct suturing. In five patients (56%) the area of SVC wall that was invaded was 3 cm×2 cm. The defect was repaired with Dacron patch. In 1 patient (11%) an arterial 14 graft was end-to-end interposed. All resections were radical (R0). Neither associated postoperative complications nor operative mortality was recorded. Five-year survival was 30.7% for the cases with aortic invasion and 11% for the ones with SVC involvement. In their study, surgery was indicated in case of absence of intraluminal extension. Their all patiens were cN2 negative. They have used adjuvant chemotherapy and radiotherapy in all patients. They have no patients who have entered into a neoadjuvant chemotherapy protocol and the study had the small number of patients. However, there is a powerful trend towards improved survival rates for the patients with aortic invasion who were surgically managed [51]. Tsuchiya and colleagues [58] performed a subadventitial resection in 20 patients and full-thickness resection and aortic replacement in 7 patients. Only 1 patient with full-thickness resection was a long-term survivor. Among the 21 patients with aortic adventitial resection, 11 had incomplete resections and all of these patients did poorly. Ten patients had a complete subadventitial resection, but 4 of these patients developed recurrent disease. Nakahara and colleagues [59] reported results in 3 patients who underwent en-bloc resection of left-sided lung cancers and the aorta. Two of these patients died of metastatic disease within 1 year. In their experience, there was only one intermediate-term survivor. Ohta and colleagues [60] performed combined resection of the thoracic aorta and primary lung cancer in 16 patients: there were six left pneumonectomies, nine left upper lobectomies, and one partial lung resection. Cardiopulmonary bypass was utilized in 10 cases, and a shunt between the ascending and descending aorta was used in 4 cases. Operative morbidity was 31%, and the mortality rate was 12.5%. Five-year survival was 70% for patients with N0 disease and 16.7% for those with N2 or N3 disease. Shiraishi and colleagues [61].

Extended aortic resection with primary lung cancer is complex and possibly high risk, but can achieve long-term survival in selected patients. Surgical resection should be considered as a treatment option for T4 lung cancer for this T4 subcategory.

ATRIUM INVOLVEMENT BY LUNG CANCER

In the surgical removal of primary lung cancers, associated partial resection of thc left atrium occasionally is indicated in patients in whom a tumour invades the intrapericardial portion of the pulmonary vein or the left atrium. There are limited reports of curative resection for bronchogenic carcinoma involving the left atrium. Because left atrial invasion by lung cancer is rare and occurs by direct penetration or *via* the pulmonary veins. Several cases of intracardiac extension of systemic malignancies through the inferior vena cava have been described, but fairly less frequently pulmonary neoplasms may invade the left atrium through the pulmonary veins [62].

Tumours that directly invade the left atrium belong to T4 of the TNM classification, suggesting that the tumour is inoperable. However, indication of surgical resection of lung cancers has been expanded to some T4 patients, and long-term survival has been reported in T4 patients with N0 (no regional lymph node metastasis) or N1 (lymph node metastasis in the peribronchial or the ipsilateral hilar region or both) who underwent expanded resection of the cardiovascular system associated with a primary lung tumour. Thus assessment of invasion of the intrapericardial pulmonary vein and the left atrium by lung cancer is necessary to determine whether or not partial resection of the left atrium is needed. In general, evaluation of pulmonary veins on various images is difficult due to their compromised anatomical features: superposition by the pulmonary artery and the thoracic aorta, difficulty in taking a direct approach using a catheter, and decrease in the flow of the pulmonary veins in cases in which lung cancers invade the arteries of the same segment. Takahashi [63] and colleagues hypothesized that gadolinium-enhanced three-dimensional (3D) MR angiography consisting of coronal source images is useful in the assessment of the pulmonary vein. Transesophageal echocardiography can reveal tumour present in the pulmonary veins that extended into the left atrium. This condition can be confirmed by magnetic resonance imaging. patients with pulmonary malignancy who have a systemic embolic event, tumour emboli from the pulmonary vein should be included in the differential diagnosis of possible causes of the event [64]. More favorable results could be expected by the routine preoperative use of positron emission tomographic scan staging in these patients [65].

On the right side, the anterior left atrial wall can be lengthened significantly by opening the interatrial groove, thus increasing the margin of resection and the likelihood of an adequate cuff for primary atrial closure. Tanimura [66] and colleagues used neoadjuvant chemotherapy and surgery successfully. After the massive tumour extending into the left atrium was diagnosed by computed tomography (CT), brushing cytology by broncoscopy showed squamous cell carcinoma and its stage was IIIB. Chemothrapy using cisplatin, paclitaxel and gemcitabine hydrochloride was given 8 courses during 6 months. The effect of the chemotherapy was complete response, enabling the surgical treatment. They performed the right pneumonectomy with partial resection of the left atrium by using vascular clamp. The defect of the left atrium could be sutured directly. The patient has been well for 3 years and 6 months after surgery.

Selection criteria for extended pneumonectomy with partial resection of the left atrium are [67]: (1) patients younger than 75 years of age, (2) patients who were motivated and fully informed about the proposed surgery, (3) a thorough, cardiorespiratory evaluation. Patients would be excluded if they presented with cardiac diseases, chronic renal and hepatic insufficiencies, or a predicted postoperative forced expiratory volume in 1 second of less than 40%. Oncologic criteria are: (1) Bulky N2 disease (ie, invasion of the mediastinal structures) was a definitive contraindication to surgical resection, even when there was a good response to preoperative chemotherapy, (2) Metastases (diagnosed by mediastinoscopy) in R2 and L2 were absolute contraindications to surgical resection, even when there was a good response to preoperative chemotherapy, because of evidence of extensive metastatic disease, (3) Intranodal metastases in R4 and 7 stations (diagnosed by mediastinoscopy) indicated induction chemotherapy, followed by surgery if there was a response.

Bobbio [68] and colleagues reviewed their 23 patients who underwent atrial resection. A complete resection was achieved in nineteen patients (83%). With respect to nodal staging, there were 13 N0, 5 N1 and 4 N2 cases, respectively. Two deaths occurred during the one month postoperative period (9%). Three patients had postoperative atrial fibrillation. Two other patients had postpneumonectomy empyema without bronchopleural fistula and recovered, one after thoracoscopic debridement and the second after open window thoracostomy. Median survival, excluding the perioperative mortality, was 20 months (range 4 - 62 months). The calculated survival ratc was 63% at 1 year, 2 % at 3 years and 10% at 5 years. Lymph node stage and completeness of resection were not independent prognostic factors. Tsuchiya and colleagues stated that a favorable 5 year survival rate of 22% was achieved in T4 cases in which associated resection were limited to the left atrium [69]. They also reported on their experience with 44 patients who underwent resection of the left atrium alone or in combination with other major vascular structures [70]. They found the most important factors affecting survival defined by multivariate analysis were postoperative pneumonia, complete resection, postoperative bleeding, and opposite of Bobbio's study, lymph node metastasis. All of these resections were conducted without cardiopulmonary bypass using vascular clamps.

Spaggiari [67] and colleagues performed extended pneumonectomy with partial resection of the left atrium for lung cancer in 15 patients, without cardiopulmonary bypass. Six of 15 patients (40%) underwent preoperative invasive mediastinal staging. Nine patients (60%) underwent induction chemotherapy. Nine patients (60%) underwent right pneumonectomy. There are 8 patients (53%) with N2 disease, 5 patients (33%) with N1 disease, and 2 patients with N0 disease. The T status was T4 in 10 patients, pT3 in 3 patients, and T0 in the remaining 2 patients. The median intensive care unit and hospital stay were 1 day and 6.4 days, respectively. There were two (15.3%) minor postoperative complications (atrial arrhythmias), which were successfully treated medically. There was no postoperative mortality. Nine of 15 patients (60%) were still alive, with 8 showing no evidence of disease. The remaining 6 died because of systemic recurrences. The 3-year probability of survival was 39%. Ratto and colleagues reported a 5-year overall survival rate of 14% with a median survival of 25 months on 19 patients over a 12-year period [65]. The 3 patients with N2 disease who underwent induction chemotherapy were alive and disease-free at 30, 15, and 11 months from surgery. Among these 3 patients, the one who survived longest was staged down by induction chemotherapy to N1 disease. Survival was not affected by histology, type of surgery, or completeness of resection. Three patients with residual cancer in the atrial resection margin underwent postoperative chemoradiotherapy and are alive at 25, 17, and 15 months after surgery.

Fukuse and colleagues1 had 14 patients with cancer invasion to the left atrium. surgery could be performed with the use of vascular clamps only. In the remaining patient, the resection was carried out by opening the atrium using a cardiopulmonary bypass Ferguson and Reardon [71] needed cardiopulmonary bypass to resect the tumour. They performed a right thoracotomy that revealed a mass that was anterior and adherent to the right inferior pulmonary vein. The pericardium was opened, and intrapericardial involvement was discovered. The left atrium was mobilized intrapericardially, but a vascular clamp could not be placed around the edge of the tumour because the mass extended into the interatrial septum. When the left atrium was opened, the tumour was found to involve the interatrial septum, the left atrium, and the right atrium. They resected the tumour en bloc and then performed primary closure of the atria. A pericardial defect was replaced with a Gore-Tex® sheet (W.L. Gore and Associates, Inc.; Flagstaff, Ariz). Pathologic analysis of the specimen confirmed a Stage IIIB (T4 N0 M0), moderately differentiated squamous cell carcinoma of the lung. The resection margins were found to be free of tumour. When they reported, the patient was at 24-month follow-up and chest CT showed no evidence of recurrence.

Primary or metastatic neoplasms of the lung are reported to be the more common source of cardiogenic embolus of the neoplastic origin; a cerebral embolic episode can be the only clinical presentation of patients with metastatic cardiac tumour [72].

In cases of NSCLC with left atrial invasion complete resection is technically feasible in most instances without cardiopulmonary bypass. The acceptable operative risk and the encouraging long-term survival observed in this series suggest that NSCLC invading the left atrium should not be systematically considered as a definitive contraindication to surgery. Whenever technically feasible, nonsmall cell lung carcinoma that has invaded the left atrium without distal metastases should be resected. For better results, a more-extensive assessment of atrial invasion, the application of induction chemotherapy in patients with N2 disease, and postoperative chemoradiotherapy in patients with tumours abutting the atrial resection margin should be performed. The results of surgery may be improved by induction treatments.

SUPERIOR AND INFERIOR VENA CAVA INVASION

Bronchogenic carcinoma can involve the superior vena cava by direct extension of the primary tumour or by nodal metastasis [52, 73]. The patterns of involvement of the SVC system may be important in survival of the patients. ıf a lung cancer is centrally located and involves the SVC directly, the prognosis of the patients would be relatively promising. In contrast, if a tumour is located peripherally and metastatic lymph nodes involve the SVC, the prognosis would be dismal [74].

SVC resection and patch or prosthetic reconstruction is a feasible and safe technique allowing radical surgical treatment in selected patients. It has been suggested, that among patients with T4 tumours, those with SVC invasion may have a better prognosis, when the tumour is surgically resected, as compared to those with tumours invading the esophagus, myocardium or aorta [75, 76]. Several factors have been found to influence survival in the majority of studies: (1) existence of N2 disease was correlated with significantly worse prognosis; (2) incomplete (R1/R2) resection resulted in extremely poor prognosis; (3) higher degree of SVC invasion by the cancer, usually as evidenced by a need for total

SVC resection, correlated with worse prognosis. In the absence of evident extra-thoracic metastases, the existence of positive ipsilateral mediastinal lymph nodes should not be considered an absolute contra-indication to surgical resection. In our experience, patients with N2 disease who were treated with induction therapy experienced nearly comparable survival to those with N1-0 disease [76]. Among patients with lung cancer, rate of combined resection of the SVC is 1.1% [74].

There are two possible techniques for resecting the superior vena cava. It may be performed en bloc with the pulmonary resection. Whichever method is used, the overall goals are to relieve symptoms, minimize the risk of complications, and ensure long-term patency of the SVC. The pattern of SVC invasion in NSCLC will allow for safe proximal and distal cross-clamping of the SVC in most patients, with adequate resection margins [52, 77]. Innominate vein to right atrium shunt is always an option, and should be considered whenever SVC clamping is not considered safe, due for either technical or oncological reasons. For minimal involvement, a side-biting clamp can be applied and the vena cava simply oversewn or patched if the lumen is compromised. Patches can include Gore-Tex or pericardium. For full reconstruction, a ringed Gore-Tex sleeve patch may be preferred [78]. Some authors have advocated the use of larger (18-20mm) grafts; but relatively small grafts to replace the resected SVC (mostly 8-12 mm) can be used [76]. The risk of occlusion of grafts depends on the number of reconstructions or the caliber of the lumen of the grafts. Two vascular reconstructions would be vulnerable to vascular occlusion, and a small-caliber prosthesis would also lead to vascular troubles. Thus isolated reconstruction of the SVC system with a large-lumen prosthesis can be a preference [74]. Fukusel and colleagues had the 11 patients with invasion of the SVC. Three of them had replacement with a spiral polytetrafluoroethylene (PTFE) graft and 5 patients had a partial resection. The tumour was enucleated leaving behind part of the invaded SVC in 3 patients. Of the 2 patients with invasion of the innominate vein, 1 had total and the other partial resection. The replacement of the SVC by a stapled bovine pericardial conduit may be a good solution in selected cases, as it is a simple, expeditious, and economic solution [75].

The optimal strategy for SVC reconstruction remains controversial. Among the synthetic materials employed for graftreconstruction of the SVC (Dacron, polytetrafluoroethylene (PTFE), and Gore-Tex), the PTFE is the option of choice [52, 73, 76, 78]. Although the deal approach for superior vena cava reconstruction is a sternotomy or hemiclamshell, often this is encountered at the time of thoracotomy; and the incision is appropriately extended to allow appropriate control of vessels. In Suzuki's study, lung carcinoma was resected through a median sternotomy in 7 patients (18%) and through a right thoracotomy in 33 patients (82%; Table **1**). A median sternotomy approach was used mainly for making an intraoperative shunt between the left brachiocephalic vein and the right atrium. If the shunt is patent, combined resection of the SVC can be performed more simply because a crossclamp of the SVC is safely performed [74].

The degree of SVC infiltration dictates the type of resection. Direct repair is the simplest reconstruction, but it is acceptable only when the caliber of the repaired SVC is 50% or more of the original one. When that is not the case, but SVC is not circumferentially resected, SVC can be cross-clamped and repaired by an autologous pericardial patch, which does not require long-term anticoagulation. When a circumferential SVC resection is performed, a prosthetic replacement should be performed immediately afterward. Historically, the gold standard of SVC prosthetic replacement was PTFE. Thc main problems of PTFE replacement are the need for long-term anticoagulation therapy and thrombosis [77, 79].

A right pneumonectomy or right upper lobectomy is typically performed en bloc with the superior vena cava. A truncular replacement of the vena cava requires that the confluence of both innominate veins be tumour-free [52]. In the case of bovine pericardial conduit for replacement of the superior vena cava, the distal anastomosisis performed first, with a 5/0 polypropylene suture, starting from the posterior aspect of the prosthesis.The proximal anastomosisis subsequently performed with the same technique and the mechanical suture line helps to keep the graft properly positioned and aligned. Furthermore, the intrinsic rigidity of the pericardium and staple line grant patency of the graft without the need for any reinforcement. For an interposition graft of Gore-Tex is placed between this confluence and the proximal superior vena cava stump. Alternatively, if the confluence of the innominate veins is involved with tumour, then either the right, left, or both innominate veins may be revascularized with individual ringed Gore-Tex grafts from the right atrium. Clamping the superior vena cava can be associated with several adverse consequences, including decreased cardiac output resulting from decreased venous return and increased venous pressures in the cerebral territories. SVC resection is feasible without cardiopulmonary support in all patients, if selection is appropriate. Venous clamp times must be kept as short as possible. There is poor tolerance when SVC clamping time exceeded 45 minutes. Strict full anti-coagulation for up to 6 months postoperatively and higher flow rate through small grafts appear to provide adequate protection against graft thrombosis [52, 67, 75, 76].

Ringed PTFE grafts have been reported to remain patent for several years, and some authors believe that the PTFE prosthesis has the advantage of rings', which avoid graft collapse when the central venous pressure becomes negative; according to others, the rigidity of the reconstruction does not allow compression due to surrounding structures at closure (sternum) and is not modified when mediastinal fibrosis due to surgical scars or radiotherapy occurs. Furthermore, shortly after its implantation, it becomes re-epitheliarized with autogenous epithelial cells in humans,has low risk of infection, less platelet deposition, and less thrombogenicity of the flow surface in comparison with Dacron grafts.Other conduit options include tubularized bovine pericardium, spiral saphenous vein graft and, more recently, cryopreserved arterial allograft [75].

More than one reconstruction may also need [74]: Number of reconstructions was 44 in 40 patients; the SVC pathway was reconstructed with two vascular grafts in 4 patients (10%). The SVC system was totally and partially resected in 11 patients (28%) and 29 patients (72%), respectively. For all of the former patients, a replacement with vascular grafts was performed. For the latter patients, autologous pericardial patch was used in 8 patients, and running direct suture was performed in 21 patients. Replacement of the SVC or brachiocephalic vein was performed with Gore-Tex bypass grafts (W.L. Gore & Associates, Inc, Naperville, IL). The size of the grafts ranged from 10 to 14 mm for the reconstruction for the SVC, and 10 to 12 mm for the left brachiocephalic vein. Resection and reconstruction of the SVC system is a major technical challenge because of possible detrimental effects of clamping a patent vessel. A venous catheter in the lower limbs is usually necessary for maintaining volume during clamping. They performed a partial clamp of the SVC system in 19 patients (48%), and a crossclamp in 7 patients (18%). Among the 7 patients who underwent cross-clamping, just 1 patient underwent total replacement of the SVC. In the remaining 6 patients, they performed a direct running suture of the SVC in 3 patients, and pericardial patch in 3 patients. Therefore total replacement of the SVC was performed using extraluminal shunt in most cases. The time for cross-clamping ranged from 10 to 44 minutes, with a median of 33 minutes. Postoperative neurologic complications were not observed. For the other patients vascular shunts were used to reduce the harmful effect of clamping the SVC. Intraluminal shunts were used in 3 patients, and extraluminal shunts in 12 patients. When total replacement of the SVC is necessary, they preferred making shunts to reduce the potential risk of cross-clamping of the SVC [74].

RESULTS

Ciccone and colleagues performed operations using superior vena cava prosthetic conduits. Artificial prosthesis of the superior vena cava (SVC) may occlude with time. For this reason, they proposed in 2003 the use of a biological material (bovine pericardium) and devised an original technique to construct the prosthetic conduit. They reported the long-term results in 15 patients [80]. They observed one (6%) major postoperative complication for heart failure. Minor (non-life-threatening) postoperative complications developed in two (13%) patients (one chest wall hematoma and one atrial fibrillation). There were no intraoperative or postoperative complications related to the reconstructive procedures. They did not observe late complications. Postoperative in hospital stay ranged from 5 to 13 days. Postoperative mortality was 6% (n = 1) due to heart failure in a 76-year-old patient preoperatively treated with six cycles of induction chemotherapy for T4 lung cancer. Three patients died between 2 and 5 years after surgery as a result of metastatic disease. Postoperative morbidity was negatively affected by older age (>60-year old *vs.* <60-year-old) and by epidermoidal histology (*vs.* non-epidermoidal) showing a statistically significant difference, whereas, postoperative morbidity was not negatively affected by preoperative chemotherapy, gender, type of surgical approach (thoracothomy *vs.* sternotomy), clamping time, and intra-operative by pass. Eleven patients are still alive: 10 disease free and one is alive with local recurrence at 35 months from the operation. All caval grafts were open at follow up. Mean follow-up was 46 months (range: 6-70 months). One-and 5-year overall survival was 93% and 73%, respectively.

Spaggiari and colleagues described their experience in 25 patients who underwent resection of the superior vena caval system for non-small cell lung cancer [49]. This report included patients from four centers, collected over a period of 37 years. Among those patients, 28 underwent total SVC resection, with subsequent reconstruction by a prosthetic graft. The overall 5-year probability of survival for patients undergoing partial or total SVC resection was 32 and 15%, respectively. Interestingly, all 28 patients undergoing total resection were operated on during the last 15 years of the study. The earlier surgical interventions in this series included therefore only partial SVC resections. Seven patients had complete resection of the superior vena cava with graft interposition. Twelve patients underwent tangential resection of the superior vena cava, and 1 patient had a pericardial patch. Five patients underwent resection of the right innominate and subclavian veins without vessel reconstruction. Most patients had N2 disease, and 20% of patients had an incomplete resection. Operative mortality was 12%, median survival was 11.5 months, and 5-year actuarial survival was 29%. There were only 4 patients alive at 5 years. The central location of non-small cell lung cancers involving the vena cava often mandates extended resections of other structures, including the airway.

Suzuki [74] and colleagues performed resection and reconstruction of the SVC in 40 patients with lung cancer infiltrating SVC. All lung cancers were located at right side. Preoperative treatment was performed in 6 patients: preoperative chemotherapy for 2, radiotherapy for 1, and chemoradiotherapy for 3, and none of them underwent the multimodal strategy in clinical trial setting. Postoperative treatment was performed in 7 patients. Chemotherapy was performed for 1 patient and radiotherapy for 6 patients. Histologic typing of resected lung carcinoma resulted in 17 adenocarcinomas, 15 squamous cell carcinomas, 4 large cell carcinomas, and 4 other histologic types. The maximum tumour dimension ranged from 1.8 to 11 cm, with a mean of 5.6 cm. No patients were pathologically classified as stage I, 5 were classed as stage IIB, 6 as stage IIIA, 26 as stage IIIB, and 3 as stage IV. As to T factor, T4 disease was found in 26 patients, and mediastinal lymph node metastases were found in 27 patients. Pneumonectomy was performed in 21 patients (53%) and lobectomy in 19 patients (47%). Bronchoplasty procedures were necessary in 20 patients (50%), and sleeve pneumonectomy was performed in 15 of these patients (75%). Surgical margin was negative macroscopically and microscopically in 33 patients (83%) and 28 patients (70%), respectively. There were two vascular occlusions (5%) with a median follow-up period for patency of the graft of 67 months. One occlusion occurred as a result of a locoregional recurrence of lung cancer 9 months after surgery, and the other was caused by a thrombosis 13 months after surgery. Postoperative major morbidity and 30-day mortality were 40% and 10%, respectively. There were three bronchopleural fistulas with one postoperative death, three major pneumonias with one fatal sequence, 4 patients with thoracic empyema, 3 patients with postoperative bleeding, one fatal bronchoarterial fistula, and one fatal Mallory-Weiss syndrome. Among 16 patients with major complications, 11 patients underwent bronchoplastic procedures. Furthermore, 8 patients underwent sleeve pneumonectomy. The overall 5-year survival rate for 40 resected lung cancer patients was 24% with the median follow-up period for living patients of 67 months. Univariate analyses revealed no significant prognostic factors except the patterns of involvement of the SVC system. The 5-year survival rate of patients with SVC invasion by direct tumour extension was 36% and those with SVC invasion by metastatic lymph nodes was 6.6%, and this difference was statistically significant. Interestingly, nodal status (N0 to N1 *vs.* N2 to N3) was not a significant prognostic factor.

On the contrary to this, Spaggiari [77] (2007) and colleagues has found that 5-year survival was affected by mediastinal nodal status (5-year survival in N0-N1 patients 52%, 21% in N2 patients, 0 in N3 patients). They had 70 consecutive patients (52 with lung cancer and 18 with mediastinal tumours) underwent SVC system resection. There were 25 replacements (36%) of the SVC system by prosthesis, whereas the remaining underwent partial resection. Major postoperative morbidity and mortality rates in lung cancer patients were 23% and 7.7%, respectively (50% and 5.6% in mediastinal tumours).

Replacement of the SVC can also be performed with low mortality and morbidity for effective treatment of superior vena cava compression (SVCC) secondary to benign disease that fails to respond to medical therapy. Picquet [73] and colleagues performed SVC reconstruction using ringed e-PTFE vascular grafts in 11 patients with SVCC. All 11 patients presenting clinical signs of SVCC improved rapidly after SVC reconstruction. Ten of these symptomatic patients had benign or malignant mediastinal disease, and 1 had a bronchopulmonary neoplasm.

Lung cancer infiltrating the SVC frequently involves the bronchial tree, especially the carina, and lobectomy with bronchoplasty or pneumonectomy is often necessary to resect such lung tumours. Therefore surgical morbidity and mortality is not negligible. Complete resection is also reported to be a significant prognostic factor. Thus, to operate on patients with lung cancer infiltrating the SVC, the selection of surgical candidates is quite important. Infiltration of SVC can achieve satisfactory long-term results after neoadjuvant chemotherapy, only when pathologic N2 disease is excluded by preoperative mediastinoscopy [74, 77].

Invasion of the inferior vena cava by resectable bronchogenic carcinoma is exceedingly rare. Roberts [81] and coworkers reported their experience with an interesting patient who presented with a lesion involving the right lower lobe and intrapericardial inferior vena cava. Kuehl [82] and colleagues performed extended resection of malignant tumours invading the vena cava inferior and superior in 35 patients. There were invasion of the hepatic and suprahepatic segment of the inferior vena cava (IVC) in 14 patients, When the tumour invasion is more than 180° of the circumference of the vessel wall they performed segmental caval resection. They performed partial excision of the vessel wall in 21 cases, followed by direct suturing of the vessel in 17 patients or patch repair with Dacron patches in 4 cases. Thirteen patients underwent reconstruction of the vena cava by using ringed, rifampicin-tinctured polytetrafluoroethylene grafts. The operative mortality rate was 6%. There were three intraoperative complications: one patient who had a myocardial infarction and two patients with major hemorrhage. Minor complications occurred in 12 patients (34%). The graft patency rate was 85%, and there was no graft-related perioperative morbidity. The 1-, 3-, and 5-year survival rates were 76%, 32%, and 21%, respectively, with a median survival of 29 months. Incomplete resection and cardiopulmonary risk have a significant negative effect on survival.

Patients with advanced tumour growth and invasion of the superior or inferior vena cava should be considered for surgical treatment, even when tumour infiltration necessitates segmental resection of the vena cava followed by graft reconstruction [82]. Survival is significantly better in patients with complete resection, and morbidity and mortality rates are acceptable. Especially in patients with assumed microscopic radical tumour resection, surgical treatment should be considered.

TRACHEAL CARINA (BIFURCATIO) INVASION

Sleeve lobectomy and carinal resection are widely accepted as beneficial alternatives to pneumonectomy. Carinal resection has been regarded as a potential curative treatment for selected bronchial nonsmall-cell lung cancer (NSCLC) invading the tracheobronchial bifurcation, but with the associated high morbidity and mortality and poor long-term outcome [83]. This operation offer maximal preservation of lung function, allowing radical operations in patients who would not tolerate pneumonectomy.

Liu [84] and colleagues reported an experience with 15 carinal resections without mortality. Mitchell [85] and coworkers determined that postoperative mechanical ventilation, length of resected airway, and development of anastomotic complication were all significant predictors of postoperative mortality after carinal resection. They have performed 60 carinal resections for bronchogenic carcinoma: 18 isolated carinal resections for tumour confined to the carinal or proximal main stem bronchus; 35 carinal pneumonectomies; 5 carinal plus lobar resections, and 2 carinal resections for stump recurrence after prior pneumonectomy. Thirteen patients (22%) had a history of lung or airway surgery. The overall operative mortality was 15%, improved from the first half of the series (20%) to the second half (10%), and varied according to the type of resection performed. Adult respiratory distress syndrome was responsible for 5 early deaths, and all late deaths were related to anastomotic complications. In 34 patients, all lymph nodes were negative for metastatic disease; 15 patients had positive N1 nodes, and 11 patients had positive N2/N3 nodes. The overall 5-year survival including operative mortality was 42%, with 19 absolute 5-year survivors. Survival was highest after isolated carinal resection (51%). Lymph node involvement had a strong influence on survival: patients without nodal involvement had a 5-year survival of 51%, compared with 32% for patients with N1 disease and 12% for those with N2/N3 disease. In de Perrot's [87] report there were 119 patients underwent carinal resection for carcinoma. The main clinical symptoms at presentation were hemoptysis (n = 44) and dyspnea (n = 29). Indications for surgical intervention were non-small cell lung carcinoma (NSCLC) in 100 patients, adenoid cystic carcinoma in 8 patients, neuroendocrine carcinoma (carcinoid tumour) in 5 patients, mucoepidermoid carcinoma in 4 patients, and metastatic renal cell carcinoma in 2 patients. The 5- and 10-year survivals were 44% and 25%, respectively, for patients with bronchogenic carcinoma. Not surprisingly, long-term survival was significantly influenced by nodal status. Survival was significantly better in patients with N0 or N1 disease (n = 73) than in those with N2 or N3 disease (n = 27; 53% *vs.* 15% at 5 years, respectively). Their overall operative mortality was 7.6%.

The largest series of carinal resections come from Porhanov [86] and associates, who reported on 231 carinal resections, 151 of which were performed for bronchogenic carcinoma. Carinal resection following pneumonectomy was performed in 28 cases, isolated resection of bronchial bifurcation was performed in 25 cases, and in 15 cases they combined lobectomy and resection of bifurcation. Complications were observed in 82 patients (35.4%), dominated by anastomotic problems which occurred in 58 cases (25.1%). Intraoperatively, there were injuries to great vessels in four patients (1.7%): pulmonary artery in two patients, and superior vena cava in two patients. Impaired anastomotic healing was observed in 58 cases (25.1%). There was a complete dehiscence in 21 patients (9.1%): 17 had undergone a carinal pneumonectomy (7.3%), three a neo-carina operation (1.3%), and one a complex reconstruction (0.43%). Another 29 patients (50%) were found to have a microfistula, measuring from 1 to 3 mm, disclosed by endoscopy between 3 and 14 days postoperatively. Local necrosis of anastomosis without visible disturbance of its integrity was observed in eight patients (13.7%). Pleural empyema and local mediastinitis developed in 34 patients (41.6%), and five patients (6.1%) had sepsis. All patients were drained. Intrapleural bleeding and clotted hemothorax were found in nine patients (10.9%); re-thoracotomy was required in five cases (55%) and re-sternotomy was required in one case (11%). Sputum retention and lung atelectasis developed in 49 patients (59.7%). In addition to fibrobronchoscopy we performed microtracheostomy in 19 patients. Cardiac arrhythmia occurred in 24 patients: the disorder appeared intraoperatively in 19 cases (79%), and 11 events (58%) developed during left pneumonectomy. Among three patients with resection extended to the esophageal muscular wall, one (33%) was found to have esophageal-pleural fistula on postoperative day 12. He died of associated sepsis. Operative mortality was 16% and was mostly related to respiratory distress syndrome, and anastomotic complications and complications were observed in 35%. Mortality and complications were correlated to the length of resection, laryngeal nerve injuries, and the mode of intraoperative ventilation (jet ventilation). Several strategies have been developed to maintain viability of the remaining proximal and distal airway and reduce tension on the airway anastomosis. Most authors advocate coverage of the airway anastomosis with vascularized pericardial fat pad, pericardium, or omentum.

Carinal resection without sacrifice of pulmonary parenchyma and left-sided carinal pneumonectomies are usually approached through a median sternotomy [87]. Right-sided lesions necessitating a carinal resection with sacrifice of the pulmonary parenchyma are best approached through an ipsilateral, muscle-sparing dorsal thoracotomy in the fifth intercostal space. Ventilation strategy is the important point of the operation. The patient is initially intubated with an extra-long oral endotracheal tube that can be advanced into the opposite bronchus if single-lung ventilation is desired. Once the carina has been resected, the opposite main bronchus is intubated with a cross-field sterile endotracheal tube connected to a sterile tubing system. After the trachea and bronchi are anastomosed, the cross-field tube is withdrawn, and the patient is ventilated through the endotracheal tube left in place above the anstomosis. Patients can be ventilated through low tidal volume controlled techniques except during airway resection and reconstruction, during which the apneic (hyper) oxygenation techniques are used. Just before airway section, and during resection and reconstruction, patients were managed with the apneic (hyper) oxygenation technique. High inspiratory oxygen concentrations, multiple collapse and reexpansions, hypoperfusion of the ipsilateral lung, and fluid overload are avoided. Patients are being tried to extubate in the operating room [83]. For carinal pneumonectomy, the end-to-end reconstruction started on the deepest anastomotic part of the left half of both cartilaginous walls or left margin of the membraneous portion. For carinal lobectomies, the choice to reimplant the residual bilobe end to side either into the trachea or left main bronchus depended on the length of the residual intermedius bronchus, the status of the trachea (fibrotic, malacic, and so forth), the extent of node dissection, and the degree of traction on hilus residual vessels [83].

Despite advances, long-term survival may show variety. In Macchiarini's report [83] actuarial 5-year and disease-free survivals were 51% and 47%, respectively. Disease-free survival was significantly affected by endobronchial extension (tracheobronchial angle invasion *versus* less than 0.5 cm from carina) and nodal status (N0 *versus* N1-2) in the multivariate analysis. Operative mortality (less than 30 days) was 4% and included a massive myocardial infarction and a lung embolism. Complications were observed in 18 patients (36%) and were supraventricular arrhythmias (n = 7), cerebral transient ischemic attack (n = 1), cardiac luxation requiring surgical intervention (n = 1), anticoagulation-related bleeding (n = 1), and anastomotic leaks in 8 patients successfully managed either conservatively (temporary drainage of the ipsilateral cavity, n = 4) or through immediate reoperation and anastomosing (n =3) or tissue engineered airway interposition (n = 1). Beyond the 2 operative deaths, the 2 patients having a transient ischemic attack and cardiac luxation required mechanical ventilation postoperatively for 3 days. All their 50 patients but 1 (98%) with residual microscopic disease (R1) on the ipsilateral residual pulmonary artery stump were completely resected.

Carinal resection for carcinoma is relatively safe in experienced centers and can be associated with good long-term survival. The feasibility of carinal resection is limited by the patient's functional status and extension of tumour growth. Patients presenting with bronchogenic carcinoma and negative mediastinal nodes should be considered for carinal resection without any induction therapy. However, mediastinoscopy at the time of the planned operation is important because the presence of positive N2 disease should be considered a potential contraindication to carinal resection because of the poor long-term survival [83, 87].

Contraindications include patients whose tumours are so extensive that reconstruction would be under tension and those with involved precarinal and paratracheal nodes. Patients with diseased subcarinal nodes might benefit from surgery. Right carinal pneumonectomy is the most common carinal procedure, and the safe limit of resection is approximately 4 cm between the lower trachea and contralateral main bronchus. Small lesions involving the carina only may be resected without pulmonary resection with somewhat greater resectional limits. Right upper lobe tumours involving the carina may also be completely resected by saving the right middle and lower lobes and fashioning a new carina. Fatal early (noncardiogenic pulmonary edema) and late (anastomotic dehiscence or separation) complications after carinal pneumonectomy may be preventable by limiting mediastinal lymphatic dissection and perioperative intravascular fluid overload. A limited tailored thoracoplasty and transposition of the latissimus and serratus muscles into the postpneumonectomy pleural space can mitigate anastomotic complications [88].

DIAPHRAGM INVASION

Diaphragmatic invasion by otherwise resectable non-small cell lung cancer is exceedingly rare. Diagnosis of isolated diaphragmatic invasion is difficult. Symptoms are usually absent, and imaging is of limited value in determining diaphragmatic invasion. Thoracoscopic examination has been suggested as a means to detect diaphragmatic invasion in suspected cases.

Yokoi [89] and associates identified 63 patients who underwent resection lung cancer invading the diaphragm. Tumour invasion to the diaphragm was diagnosed before operation only in 17 patients (27.0%). Complete resections of the primary lung tumours with the invaded diaphragm were performed in 55 patients (87.3%). The operative mortality was 1.6% in all patients. The 5-year survival of patients with complete resection was 22.6%, but there was no 4-year survivor in patients with incomplete resection. The survivals of patients with completely resected T3 N1-2 M0 tumours were 28.3% and 18.1%, respectively. In those patients, the depth of diaphragmatic involvement significantly affected the prognosis. The 5-

year survival of the patients with shallow invasion (parietal pleura or subpleural tissue involvement) was 33.0%, whereas that of the patients with deep invasion (muscle or peritoneal infiltration) was 14.3%.

Rocco [90] and colleagues reported 15 patients, treated by en bloc resection (14 patients) and only explored (1 patient). A partial infiltration of the diaphragm was observed in 3 patients, whereas full-depth invasion was found in 12. Diaphragmatic reconstruction was done primarily in 9 patients, and, by prosthetic material in 5. Overall, 5-year actuarial survival was 20% and only 27% for patients without nodal metastasis. Interestingly, these authors found a correlation between need for prosthetic diaphragmatic replacement and survival, suggesting that wider margins of resection conferred some survival benefit.

COMPLETION PNEUMONECTOMY

Completion pneumonectomy refers to the resection of the remaining lung tissue after a previous pulmonary resection. The characteristic feature of pulmonary metastasectomy is parenchyma-sparing resection, thus making multiple resectional procedures of metachronously occurring metastases possible. Recurrent lung cancer and second primary lung cancer were discriminated using the following criteria: a second primary tumour was of different histology or if histology was the same, the disease-free interval between cancers was at least 2 years or the second cancer was in the different lobe but with no cancer in common lymphatic or extrapulmonary metastasis at the time of diagnosis. The risk of developing a second primary is approximately 2% per patient per year in early stage lung cancer while the frequency of recurrence in the same area as the first site of failure after resection ranges from 3 to 9% for stage IA to 32% for stage IIIA with positive surgical margins [91]. Regarding diffusely or centrally located metastases-recurrences-second primaries of the lung, in individual cases primary pneumonectomy is necessary, although this procedure is considered an aggressive and risky measure as well as technically demanding, and is associated with a considerably greater mortality (12%) compared to standard pneumonectomy, where mortality rates are 6.2% [92]. The indication for CP is rare, only 10% of all pneumonectomies are CPs. When recurrent metastases of the lung reoccur ipsilaterally, only completion pneumonectomy (CP) may leave a tumour-free state [52, 93].

The indications for a completion pneumonectomy have expanded with the increased incidence of lung cancer, increased survival of patients undergoing previous lung resections, increased survival in patients with long-term pulmonary infections, and an increased demand for repeat resection of metastatic disease to the lungs. The best indication may be left-sided elective surgery for a metachronous cancer occurring. 2 years after the treatment of an initial bronchogenic carcinoma, managed by surgery alone at that time [94].

Previous resections, radiation therapy, or past infections or inflammatory processes may obliterate the pleural and pericardial spaces and lead to a difficult operation. The time from operation of the primary tumour to the first metastasectomy is approximately 37 months [93]. The first metastasectomy may include lobe resection, segment resection and wedge resections, and contralateral resections may be performed. The time from the first metastasectomy to the second metastasectomy is approximately 12 months [93].

Intrapericardial control is optimal if adhesions and scarring involve the hilar vessels. Haraguchi [95] and coleagues performed intrapericardial dissection of vessels in 14 of their 17 patients (87.5%). In cases of obliteration of the pericardial space, the pulmonary artery may be exposed posteriorly by first dividing the bronchus [53]. On the right the pulmonary artery may also be isolated by dividing the posterior pericardium between the superior vena cava and the ascending aorta. After a completion pneumonectomy, a larga bronchopleural fistula may develop; in this setting carinal sleeve resection may treat the fistula completely [96]. Right side CPs may hava a higher mortality rate (29.8 *vs.* 7.7% [92]) similar to standart pneumonectomies.

Guggino [94] and coworkers reported 55 patients undergoing completion pneumonectomy (42 for malignancy and 13 for benign disease). Before completion pneumonectomy, 50 patients had had a lobectomy, three a bilobectomy, and two lesser resections. The mean interval between the two procedures was 51 months for the whole group, 60 months for lung cancer, 43 months for pulmonary metastases and 29 months for non-malignant disorders. The surgical approaches were a posterolateral thoracotomy in 50 cases (91%) and a lateral thoracotomy in five cases (9%). Intrapericardial route was used in 49 patients (89%). Five patients had an extended resection (2 chest wall, 1 diaphragm, 1 subclavian artery and 1 superior vena cava). Operative mortality was 16.4%: 11.9% for malignant disease and 30.8% for benign disease: Operative mortality was 20% for right completion pneumonectomies and 10% for left-sided procedures. Twenty three patients (42%) experienced non-fatal major complications. Actuarial 3- and 5-year survival rates from the time of completion pneumonectomy were 48.4 and 35.2% for the entire group. Three- and five-year survival for patients with bronchogenic carcinoma were 56.9 and 43.4%, respectively. In the study of Junkraithmayr [93] and colleagues, the mean survival was 21 months. Patients were recurrence free for 13 months (4-26 months). Five-year survival was 31% following the first metastasectomy, while 3-year survival after CP was 34%. The actual survival was 33% (3/9). The recurrence-free survival was 11% (1/9). Three patients died of metastatic disease of the contralateral lung, two patients died of brain metastases and another patient died of a different extrapulmonary metastatic disease. performed completion pneumonectomy in 17 patients, 15 of them (94%) underwent lung resection for primary lung cancer. Terzi [91] and colleagues had 59 patients underwent completion pneumonectomy for lung cancer, classified second primary or recurrence/metastasis according to a modified form of Martini's criteria, after a mean interval from first resection of 60 months for second primary lung cancers and 19 months for recurrences/metastases. Operative mortality was 3.4% and complications occurred in 30% of patients. Five-year survival rate for completely resected patients was 25% (median 20 months). No significant difference in long-term survival was detected between second primary and recurrent tumours; survival was not adversely affected by a resection interval of less than 2 years or less than 12 months. Fujimoto [97] and coworkers reported on 66 completion pneumonectomies. The indication was malignancy in 49 patients and benign disease in 17. In patients with malignant indications there were 14 local recurrences, 4 second primary tumours, 5 metastatic diseases, and 26 indications because of incomplete initial resection. Intrapericardial vessel ligation was done in 62% of cases. Complications were encountered in 32 (53%) patients, without any significant difference between benign indication (71%) and malignant indication (47%). Bronchopleural fistula was encountered in 5 (7.6%) patients, and empyema was encountered in 7 (11%) patients. There were no intraoperative deaths, and the postoperative mortality rate was 7.6%. Five-year actuarial survival was 65% for benign indications and 54% for malignant disease. Chataigner [98] and cowerkers identified 69 patients, who accounted for 17.8% of all pneumonectomies during the study period; 22 had benign disease and 47malignant disease (second primary lung cancer, n = 19; local recurrence, n = 17; ormetastasis, n = 11). Therewere 50 males and 19 females with a mean age of 60 years (range, 29-80 years). Postoperative mortality was 12% and postoperative morbidity 41%. Factors associated with postoperative mortality included obesity, coronary artery disease, removal of the right lung, advanced age, and renal failure. Preoperative renal failure was the only significant risk factor for mortality by multivariate analysis. Bronchopleural fistula developed in seven patients, with risk factors being removal of the right lung and mechanical stump closure. Overall survival was 65% after 3 years and 46% after 5 years. Long-term survival was not affected by the reason for completion pneumonectomy. They conluded that Although long-term survival was acceptable, postoperative mortality and morbidity rates remained high, confirming the reputation of completion pneumonectomy as a challenging procedure. Significant comorbidities and removal of the right lung were the main risk factors for postoperative mortality. Improved patient selection and better management of preoperative renal failure may improve the postoperative outcomes of this procedure, which offers a chance for prolonged survival.

CONTRALATERAL RESECTION AFTER PNEUMONECTOMY

Resections for lung cancer on a single remaining lung after previously performed pneumonectomy are rare in common thoracic practice. Metachronous primary lung cancers occur at a rate of 0.3% to 3% per year in patients who have undergone prior curative resection for lung cancer [52, 99]. There is a great deal of uncertainty regarding surgical mortality and morbidity in this group of patients; their functional results as well as long-term survival rate. Many physicians consider resection of a lesion in the remaining lung contraindicated. If the prior resection was pneumonectomy, resection of a subsequent contralateral lesion is often contraindicated because of the extent of the lesion. General indications for lung cancer resection after a pneumonectomy include clinical stage I disease, resectability by wedge or segmentectomy, and adequate pulmonary reserve present. Grodzki [99] and colleagues treated 18 patients by subsequent resection of the lung cancer invading the contralateral lung remaining after previously performed pneumonectomy due to NSCLC. Their acceptance rate of patients with lung cancer in the contralateral lung after previously performed pneumonectomy was 18%. Incision was contralateral postero-lateral approach (incision was usually shorter than for pneumonectomy and was 7-12 cm long). Anesthesia was based on single lumen tube intubation with FiO2 30-100% ventilation. All patients were treated by wedge resection not larger than single segmentectomy. In two patients, single rib resected due to suspicion of chest wall invasion confirmed postoperatively. The survival rates were as follows: 11 patients survived 2 years (61%) while 8 patients survived 5 years (44%). The majority of patients died due to lung cancer (70%) but all the rest (30%) due to circulatory or respiratory insufficiency. There was a significant difference in 5-year survival for N0-N1 *vs.* N2 status (63% *vs.* 14% - 1 patient) and also regarding the time interval between surgeries: less than 12 months *vs.* more than 12 months (0% *vs.* 63%).

Donington [100] and colleagues had 24 patients. Median preoperative forced expiratory volume in 1 second of these patients was 1.47 L (range, 0.66 to 2.55 L). Subsequent pulmonary resection was performed 2 to 213 months after pneumonectomy (median, 23 months). Wedge excision was performed in 20 patients, segmentectomy in 3, and lobectomy in 1. Diagnosis was a metachronous lung cancer in 14 patients and metastatic lung cancer in 10. Mortality and morbidity were 8.3% and 44% respectively. Overall 1-, 3-, and 5-year survivals were 87%, 61%, and 40%, respectively. Five-year survival of patients undergoing resection for a metachronous lung cancer (50%) was better than the survival of patients who underwent resection for metastatic cancer (14%). Five-year survival after a solitary wedge excision was 46% compared with 25% after a more extensive resection.

Patients who have a lung cancer in the residual lung after pneumonectomy should not be automatically excluded for surgical consideration [52, 67, 101, 102]. These patients should be carefully staged. Meticulous staging with chest CT, PET, brain

MRI, and mediastinoscopy should be able to successfully exclude metastatic disease, multifocal disease, or locally advanced tumours [100]. Only patients who have stage I disease may be candidates for this type of extended resection. Ideally, these patients should have small peripheral tumours that can be encompassed with a low-volume wedge resection. More extended resections, such as segmentectomy or right middle lobectomy, may be considered in some patients but seem to bear a higher operative morbidity and mortality. The need for an upper or lower lobectomy after contralateral pneumonectomy is probably an absolute contraindication to surgical resection. To tolerate pulmonary resection after pneumonectomy, and to obtain the desired survival benefit, patients should have a good to excellent performance status, no serious comorbidities, and a ppoFEV1 greater than 1.0 L/second. In these highly selected patients, pulmonary resection after pneumonectomy can be accomplished with an acceptable operative morbidity and mortality and, in true cases of metachronous second primary lung cancers, may achieve a 5-year survival rate of up to 50% [101]. Long-term survival is possible, especially in patients with a metachronous cancer [100].

SYNCHRONOUS PRIMARY LUNG CANCERS

With the recent advancement in diagnostic imaging techniques, such as multi-slice spiral computed tomography (CT) and positron emission tomography-computed tomography (PET-CT) scan, thoracic surgeons are increasingly facing the problem of synchronous multiple lung nodules [102]. The distinction of synchronous primary lung cancers from primary lung cancer with pulmonary metastasis is important because the prognosis and treatments are different. Few selected patients with synchronous multiple lung cancer can benefit from surgery, but the difficult diagnostic definition in the clinical setting makes the selection for surgery controversial. Immunostaining is an even more widely adopted tool to achieve a diagnosis, but its preoperative usefulness is impaired by the difficulty to obtain adequate specimens from all foci of tumours. Synchronous primary lung cancers can be identified with the following clinical and pathologic criteria modified from Martini and Melamed [103, 104]: (1). Presence of tumours with different histologies (*e.g.*, adenocarcinoma *versus* squamous cell carcinoma). (2). Tumours of different histologic subtypes:(*e.g.*, different estimated percentages of acinar *versus* bronchoalveolar *versus* papillary adenocarcinoma), regardless of nodal status. (3). Tumours of similar histology but arising from separate foci (*e.g.*, in the case of squamous cell carcinoma, the presence of *in situ* carcinoma in both tumours). (4). Tumours of similar histology in the absence of metastatic disease in intervening regional or mediastinal lymph node stations and the absence of extrathoracic disease. Voltalini [102] and colleagues selected the patients with more than one physically distinct tumour, located in a different lobe or lung for the operation. All the patients with synchronous lesions within the same lobe as the primary tumour had been excluded. PET scan was performed in all patients. For bilateral lesions, their surgical policy favoured sequential lobectomies over sublobar resections. In case of unilateral resection, they tried to perform lobectomy and wedge resection, avoiding pneumonectomy. Sublobar resections (*e.g.*, segmentectomy and wedge resection) and lymph node sampling were preferred for small peripheral tumours (<2 cm) in patients with limited pulmonary function tests, especially after the first operation. The second surgery was performed only when the patient had fully recovered, as demonstrated by a fresh spirometry and in the absence of progressive disease at re-staging with CT of the chest, brain and upper abdomen. In their study, 50 patients were found to have unilateral (other lobe) (n=15) or bilateral (n=35) synchronous multiple lung cancers, representing 3.2% of all their pulmonary resections. In patients with unilateral disease (n=15), lobectomy and sublobar resection (n=8), sublobar resection (n=2), bilobectomy (n=2) and pneumonectomy (n=3) were done. In patients with bilateral disease (n=28), Bilateral sublobar resection (n=2), lobectomy and sublobar resection (n=13), bilateral lobectomy (n=10), pneumonectomy and sublobar resection (n=3). Morbidity was 37%. The most frequent complication was prolonged air leak, which was observed in six cases, followed by supraventicular arrhythmia in two cases; pulmonary oedema in two cases; and pneumonia, haemothorax requiring re-thoracotomy, empyema and atelectasis requiring bronchoscopy in one case. The operative mortality was 7% (n = 3). Acute respiratory distress syndrome (ARDS) was the cause of death in two patients and pulmonary embolism in one. Histology was identical in 27 patients (60%): adenocarcinoma and squamous cell carcinoma were the predominant histologic types, 65% and 25%, respectively. Two patients in the bilateral group had a bronchioloalveolar carcinoma in only one side. The highest pN factor was pN0 in 18 patients, pN1 in seven and pN2 in three patients in the bilateral group, and pN0 in seven patients, pN1 in two and pN2 in six patients in the unilateral group. Survival analysis of all 50 patients with synchronous multiple lung cancers showed a 3-year and 5-year survival of 40% and 31%, respectively, with a median survival of 30 months. The 5-year survival was 57% and 0% for patients without (n = 25) and with (n = 18) lymph node metastasis, respectively. They speculated that improved results reflect a better selection process related to PET-CT scan.

Finley [103] and colleagues performed single or more operations for 175 patients with sychronous primary lung cancers. Roughly half of the patients (n = 91, 52%) were diagnosed preoperatively as having SPLC, whereas 42% (73 of 175) had additional lesions discovered at the time of operation for a single lesion. In all cases, complete resection was performed while maintaining optimal lung parenchymal preservation. The majority of patients (148 of 175, 84%), regardless of whether they underwent single or multiple operations, had either a single lobectomy (100 of 175, 57%) and/or sublobar resections (48 of 175, 27%). Ten patients underwent sequential bilateral lobectomies, and 13 patients required bilobectomy. Pneumonectomy was rarely performed (5 of 175, 3%). Operative morbidity was 33%, the majority of which was grade 1 or 2 (91 of 99 complications), and in-hospital mortality was 1.2%. Most patients received no additional therapy after complete resection. Twenty-five patients (14%) received adjuvant therapy with 17 undergoing chemotherapy and eight having external beam radiotherapy. Median survival was 67.4 months. Survival revealed that decreasing size of the largest tumour, fewer pack-years of cigarettes smoked, female gender, and T-, N-, and overall pathologic stage were associated with improved survival. Tumour location, tumour histology, and time of diagnosis (preoperative *versus* intraoperative) did not seem to influence survival. Patients with stage IA disease had a significantly better survival than patients with higher stage disease. Patients with stages IB, II, and III disease did not have statistically significantly different survival, although there was a trend toward worse survival.

De Leyn [105] and colleagues analysed their all patients with bilateral synchronous lung lesions: Thirty-six patients underwent bilateral resection for synchronous multiple primary lung cancer. All resections were performed as sequential procedures. In 23 patients, one side was anatomically resected (2 pneumonectomies) and the contralateral side was resected by limited resection. In

10 patients a bilateral lobectomy was performed, and 3 patients had bilateral limited resections. Postoperative mortality was 2.8%. Eighteen patients had a tumour with a different histological pattern, confirmed by comparing both specimens by an experienced senior pathologist. The median survival after resection of synchronous bilateral lung cancer in our series was 25.4 months with a 5-year survival rate of 38%. There was no significant difference in survival between patients with different *versus* same histology. This survival is much higher compared to the survival of assumed stage IV disease.

Surgical resection of synchronous multiple lung cancers could be recommendable after an extensive work-up (including PET scan and mediastinoscopy routinely) to select node-negative patients. In about one quarter of the patients that were planned for bilateral resection, this might not be performed due to oncological or medical reasons [105]. In patients with bilateral lesions, sequential delayed resections are safer and can be performed with acceptable morbidity and mortality. Lobectomy may be performed in presence of optimal respiratory reserve, although sublobar resections are an acceptable alternative for patients with resectable disease but marginal cardiopulmonary function tests.

ACKNOWLEDGEMENTS

Declared none.

CONFLICT OF INTEREST

The author confirms that this article content has no conflict of interest.

REFERENCES

[1] Fukuse T, Wada H, Hitomi S. Extended operation for non-small cell lung cancer invading great vessels and left atrium. Eur J Cardiothorac Surg 1997;11:664-669

[2] Naruke T, Goya T, Tsuchiya R, Suemasu K. Prognosis and survival in resected lung carcinoma based on the new international staging system. J Thorac Cardiovasc Surg 1988; 96: 440-447.

[3] Raemdonck DE, Schneider A, Ginsberg RJ. Surgical treatment for higher stage non-small cell lung cancer. Ann Thorac Surg 1992;54:99-1013.

[4] Chambers A, Routledge T, Bille A, Scarci M. Does surgery have a role in T4N0 and T4N1 lung cancer? Interactive CardioVascular and Thoracic Surgery 2010; 11: 473-479.

[5] Pitz CCM, de la Riviere AB, v Swieten HA,Westermann CJJ, Lammers JWJ, van den Bosch JMM. Results of surgical treatment of T4 non-small cell lung cancer. Eur J Cardiothorac Surg 2003; 24: 1013-8.

[6] Martini N, Yellin A, Ginsberg RJ, Bains MS, Burt ME, McCormack PM, Rusch VW. Management of non-small cell cancer with direct mediastinal involvement. Ann Thorac Surg 1994; 58: 1447-51.

[7] Weder W. Extended pulmonary resections of advanced thoracic malignancies with support of cardio-pulmonary bypass - is surgery justified? Eur J Cardiothorac Surg 2006; 29: 577-578

[8] Vaporciayan AA, Rice D, Correra AM, Walsh G, Putnam JB, Swisher S, Smythe R, Roth J. Resection of advanced thoracic malignancies requiring cardiopulmonary bypass. Eur J Cardiothorac Surg 2002;22:47-52.

[9] Byrne JG, Leacche M, Agnihotri AK, Subroto P, Bueno R, Mathisen DJ, Sugarbaker DJ. The use of cardiopulmonary bypass during resection of locally advanced thoracic malignancies. Chest 2004;125: 1581-6.

[10] Park JB, Bacchetta M, Bains MS, Downey RJ, Flores R, Ruch VW, Girardi LN. Surgical management of thoracic malignancies invading the heart or great vessels. Ann Thorac Surg 2004;78:1024-30.

[11] Wiebe K, Baraki H, Macchiarini P, Haverich A. Extended pulmonary resections of advanced thoracic malignancies with support of cardiopulmonary bypass. Eur J Cardiothorac Surg 2006;29:571-578

[12] De Perrot M, Fadel E, Mussot S, De Palma A, Chapelier A, Dartevelle P. Resection of locally advanced (T4) non-small cell lung cancer with cardiopulmonary bypass. Ann Thorac Surg 2005;79:1691-7.

[13] Tsuchiya R, Asamura H, Kondo H, Goya T, Naruke T. Extended resection of the left atrium, great vessels, or both for lung cancer. Ann Thorac Surg 1994;57:960-5.

[14] Lang G, Taghavi S, Aigner C, Charchian R, Matilla JR, Sano A, Klepetko W. Extracorporeal membrane oxygenation support for resection of locally advanced thoracic tumours. Ann Thorac Surg 2011;92:264 -71.

[15] Fromes Y, Gaillard D, Ponzio O, *et al.* Reduction of the inflammatory response following coronary bypass grafting with total minimal extracorporeal circulation. Eur J Cardiothorac Surg 2002;22:527-33.

[16] Grillo HC. Technical consideration in stage III disease: pleural and chest wall involvement. In: Delarue NC, Eschapasse H, eds. International trends in general thoracic surgery. New York, NY: Saunders, 1985; 134-138

[17] McCaughan BC, Martini N, Bains MS, *et al.* Chest wall invasion in carcinoma of the lung: therapeutic and prognostic implications. J Thorac Cardiovasc Surg 1985; 89:836-841.

[18] Stoelben E, Ludwig C. Chest wall resection for lung cancer: indications and techniques. Eur J Cardiothorac Surg 2009; 35: 450-456.

[19] Bandi V, Lunn V, Ernst A, Eberhardt R, Hoffmann H, Herth FJF. Ultrasound *vs.* CT in Detecting Chest Wall Invasion by Tumour. A Prospective Study. Chest 2008; 133:881-886.

[20] Kozower BD. Chest Wall Resection and Reconstruction for Non-Small-Cell Lung Cancer. Operative Techniques in Thoracic and Cardiovascular Surgery. 2007; 12: 279-285

[21] McCaughan BC, Martini N, Bains MS, *et al.* Chest wall invasion in carcinoma of the lung. Therapeutic and prognostic implications. J Thorac Cardiovasc Surg 1985;89:836-41.

[22] Elia S, Griffo S, Gentile M, Costabile R, Ferrante G. Surgical treatment of lung cancer invading chest wall: a retrospective analysis of 110 patients. Eur J Cardiothorac Surg 2001;20:556-360

[23] Ramsey HE, Cliffion EE. Chest wall resection for primary carcinoma of the lung. Ann Surg 1968;167:34:2-51.

[24] Albertucci M, DeMeester TR, Rothberg M, Hagen JA, Santoscoy R, Smyrk TC. Surgery and the management of peripheral lung tumours adherent to the parietal pleura. J Thorac Cardiovasc Surg 1992;103:8-13.

[25] Facciolo F, Cardillo G, Lopergolo M, Pallone G, Sera F, Martelli M. Chest wall invasion in non-small cell lung caricinoma: a rationale for en bloc resection. J Thorac Cardiovasc Surg 2001;121:649-56.

[26] Downey RJ, Martini N, RuschVW, *et al.* Extent of chestwall invasion and survival in patients with lung cancer. Ann Thorac Surg 1999;68:188-93.

[27] Magdeleinat P, Alifano M, Benbrahem C, *et al.* Surgical treatment of lung cancer invading the chest wall: results and prognostic factors. Ann Thorac Surg 2001;71:1094-9.

[28] Matsuoka H, Nishio W, Okada M, *et al.* Resection of chest wall invasion in patients with non-small cell lung cancer. Eur J Cardiothorac Surg 2004;26:1200-4.

[29] Kawaguchi K, Mori S, Usami N, Fukui T, Mitsudomi T, Yokoi K. Preoperative evaluation of the depth of chest wall invasion and the extent of combined resections in lung cancer patients. Lung Cancer 2009: 64: 41-44

[30] Fernandez FG. Extended pulmonary resections. In: Patterson GA, Cooper JD, Deslauriers J, Lerut EMR, Luketich JD, Rice TW, eds. Pearson's Thoracic & Esophageal surgery. 3rd edition. Philadelphia, PA: Churchill Livingstone; 2008: 941-956.

[31] Silvestri GA, Gould MK, Margolis ML, Tanoue LT, McCrory D, Toloza E, Detterbeck F. Noninvasive Staging of Non-small Cell Lung Cancer ACCP Evidenced-Based Clinical Practice Guidelines (2nd Edition). Chest 2007; 132:178S-201S.

[32] Valera GG, Ramirez AT, Congregado M, Merchan RJ, Jarne FJA, Loscertales J. Usefulness of Video-assisted Thoracoscopy for Correctly Staging Tumours as T3 Because of Chest Wall Invasion. Archivos de Bronconeumología (English Edition) 2009; 45: 325-328.

[33] Kubota K, Matsuzawa T, Ito M, Fujiwara T, Abe Y, Yoshioaka S, Fukuda H, Hatazawa J, Iwata R, Watanuki S, Ido T. Lung Tumour Imaging by Positron EmissionTomography Using C-i 1 L-Methionine. J NuclMed 1985; 26:37-42.

[34] Berthet JP, CanaudL, D'Annoville T, Alric P, Ane CHM. Titanium Plates and Dualmesh: A Modern Combination for Reconstructing Very Large Chest Wall Defects Ann Thorac Surg 2011;91:1709 -1716.

[35] Daly BDT, Ebright MI, Walkey AJ, Fernando HC, Zaner KS, Morelli DM, Kachnic LA. Impact of neoadjuvant chemoradiotherapy followed by surgical resection on node-negative T3 and T4 non-small cell lung cancer. J Thorac Cardiovasc Surg 2011; 141: 1392-1397.

[36] Mineo TC, Ambrogi V, Pompeo E, Baldi A. Immunohistochemistry-detected microscopic tumour spread affects outcome in en-bloc resection for T3-chest wall lung cancer. Eur J Cardiothorac Surg 2007; 31: 1120-1124.

[37] Iyoda A, Hiroshima K, Moriya Y, Yoshida S, Suzuki M, Shibuya K, Yoshino I. Predictors of Postoperative Survival in Patients with Locally Advanced Non-Small Cell Lung Carcinoma. Surg Today 2010; 40: 725-728.

[38] Watanabe Y. Surgical outcomes of N2 and T3-4 non-small cell lung cancer. Lung Cancer. 2003; 42: S23-S28

[39] Hillinger S, Weder W. Extended surgical resection in stage III non-small cell lung cancer. Front Radiat Ther Oncol. 2010;42:115-21. Epub 2009 Nov 24

[40] LoCicero J. Surgical treatment of non-small-cell lung cancer. In: Shields TW, LoCicero III J, Reed CE, Feins RH, eds. General Thoracic Surgery. Seventh edition. Philadelphia, PA: Lippincott Williams&Wilkins; 2009: 1387-1425.

[41] Mazel Ch, Grunenwald D, Laudrin P, Marmorat JL. Radical excision in the management of thoracic and cervicothoracic tumours involving the spine: results in a series of 36 cases. Spine 2003;28:782-92.

[42] Chen F, Takahashi A, Omasa M, Neo M, Fujibayashi S, Wada H, Bando T. En bloc total vertebrectomy for lung cancer invading the spine. Lung Cancer 2008; 61: 137-139.

[43] DeMeester TR, Albertucci M, Dawson PJ, Montner SM. Management of tumour adherent to the vertebral column. J Thorac Cardiovasc Surg. 1989; 97: 373-8.

[44] Grunenwald D, Mazel C, Baldeyrou P, Girard P: En bloc resection of lung cancer invading the spine. *Ann Thorac Surg* 1996; 61:1878-1879.

[45] Dartevelle P, Missenard G, Macchiarini P, et al: Invited commentary. *J Thorac Cardiovasc Surg* 1996; 102:259.

[46] Gandhi S, Walsch GL, Komaki R, Gokaslan ZL, Nesbitt JC, Putnam JB, Roth JA, Merriman KW, McCutcheon IE, Munden RF, Swisher SG. A Multidisciplinary Surgical Approach to Superior Sulcus Tumours With Vertebral Invasion. Ann Thorac Surg 1999;68:1778-85

[47] Schirren J, Donges T, Melzer M, Schonmayr R, Eberlein M, Bolukbas S. En bloc resectionofnon-small-cell lungcancer invading the spine. Eur J Cardio-thorac Surg 2011; doi:10.1016/j.ejcts.2010.12.046.

[48] Saitoh Y, Minami K, Tokunou M, Omiya H, Umemoto M, Imamura H, Yonezu S, Okamura A. Results of surgery for bronchogenic carcinoma located in the aortic window. Lung Cancer; 1997; 18: 47-56

[49] Spaggiari L, Regnard JF, Magdeleinat P, Jauffret B, Puyo P, Levasseur P. Extended resections for bronchogenic carcinoma invading the superior vena cava system. Ann Thorac Surg 2000;69:233-6.

[50] McCormack PM. Extended pulmonary resections. In: Pearson FG, Deslauriers J, Ginsberg RJ, Hiebert CA, McKneally MF, Urschel HC, editors. Thoracic surgery. New York: Churchill Livingstone; 1995. p. 897-908.

[51] Misthos P, Papagiannakis G, Kokotsakis J, Lazopoulos G, Skouteli E, Lioulias A. Surgical management of lung cancer invading the aorta or the superior vena cava. Lung Cancer 2007; 56: 223-227.

[52] Fernandez FG. Extended pulmonary resections. In: Patterson GA, Cooper JD, Deslauriers J, Lerut EMR, Luketich JD, Rice TW, eds. Pearson's Thoracic & Esophageal surgery. 3rd edition. Philadelphia, PA: Churchill Livingstone; 2008: 941-956.

[53] Pastorino U. Extended resections for lung cancer: indications and results. Surgical Oncology 2002; 11: 207-216.

[54] Suzuki H, Sekine Y, Ko E, Sunazawa T, Lida H, Kishi H, Saitoh Y. Permanent Cerebral Bypass Approach for Lung Cancer Resection with Aortic Arch Invasion. Thorac Cardiovasc Surg. 2011 Jul 15. [Epub ahead of print]

[55] Berna P, Began P, Dominicis FD, Dayen C, Douadi Y, Riquet M. Aortic Endostent Followed by Extended Pneumonectomy for T4 Lung Cancer. Ann Thorac Surg 2011;91:591-3

[56] Klepetko W, Wisser W, Birsan T, et al: T4 lung tumours with infiltration of the thoracic aorta: Is an operation reasonable?. *Ann Thorac Surg* 1999; 67:340-344.

[57] Shimokawa S, Uehara K, Watanabe S, Taira A. Combined pneumonectomy and aortic wall resection for lung cancer with the use of a heparinized bypass tube: a case report (English abstract). Nippon Kokyuki Geka Gakkai Zasshi 1988; 2:66-70.

[58] Tsuchiya R, Asamura H, Kondo H, et al: Extended resection of the left atrium, great vessels, or both for lung cancer. *Ann Thorac Surg* 1994; 57:960-965.

[59] Nakahara K, Ohno K, Mastumura A, et al: Extended operation for lung cancer invading the aortic arch and superior vena cava. *J Thorac Cardiovasc Surg* 1989; 97:428-433.

[60] Ohta M, Hirabayasi H, Shiono H, et al: Surgical resection for lung cancer with infiltration of the thoracic aorta. *J Thorac Cardiovasc Surg* 2005; 129:804-808.

[61] Shiraishi T, Shirakusa T, Miyoshi T, Yamamoto S, Hiratsuka M, Iwasaki A, Kawahara K. Extended resection of T4 lung cancer with invasion of the aorta: is it justified? Thorac Cardiovasc Surg. 2005; 53: 375-9.

[62] Lestuzzi C, Viel E, Mimo R, Meneguzzo N. Left atrial invasion by lung carcinoma through a pulmonary vein. The International Journal of Cardiovascular Imaging 2001; 17: 107-110.

[63] Takahashi K, Furuse M, Hanaoka H, Yamada T, Mineta M, Ono H, Nagasawa K, Aburano T. Pulmonary Vein and Left Atrial Invasion by Lung Cancer: Assessment by Breath-Hold Gadolinium-Enhanced Three-Dimensional MR Angiography. J Comput Assist Tomogr. 2000; 24: 557-61.

[64] Gandhi AK, Pearson AC, Orsinelli DA. Tumour invasion of the pulmonary veins: a unique source of systemic embolism detected by transesophageal echocardiography. J Am Soc Echocardiogr. 1995; 8: 97-9.

[65] Ratto GB, Costa R, Vassallo G, Alloisio A, Maineri P, Bruzzi P. Twelve-year experience with left atrial resection in the treatment of non-small cell lung cancer. Ann Thorac Surg. 2004;78:234-7.

[66] Tanimura S, Tsutsumi K, Okura M, Tanaka N, Yamamoto H, Honma K, Aida Y. Successful removal of T4 lung cancer with left atrial invasion after induction chemotherapy. Kyobu Geka. 2005;58:988-91.

[67] Spaggiari L, D'Aiuto M, Veronesi G, et al: Extended pneumonectomy with partial resection of the left atrium, without cardiopulmonary bypass, for lung cancer. *Ann Thorac Surg* 2005; 79:234-240.

[68] Bobbio A, Carbognani P, Grapeggia M, Rusca M, Sartori F, Bobbio P, Rea F. Surgical outcome of combined pulmonary and atrial resection for lung cancer. Thorac Cardiovasc Surg. 2004; 52: 180-2.

[69] Tsuchiya R. Extended resection for lung cancer. Nihon Geka Gakkai Zasshi. 1997; 98: 26-30

[70] Tsuchiya R, Asamura H, Kondo H, Goya T, Naruke T. Extended resection of the left atrium, great vessels, or both for lung cancer. Ann Thorac Surg. 1994; 57: 960-5.

[71] Ferguson ER, Reardon MJ. Atrial Resection in Advanced Lung Carcinoma Under Total Cardiopulmonary Bypass. Tex Heart Inst J. 2000; 27: 110-112.

[72] Park JH, Seo HS, Park SK, Suh J, Kim DH, Cho YH, Lee NH. Spontaneous systemic tumour embolism caused by tumour invasion of pulmonary vein in a patient with advanced lung cancer. J Cardiovasc Ultrasound. 2010; 18: 148-50.

[73] Picquet J, Blin V, Dussaussoy C, Jousset Y, Papon X, Enon B. Surgical reconstruction of the superior vena cava system: Indications and results. Surgery 2009;145:93-9.

[74] Suzuki K, Asamura H, Watanabe S, Tsuchiya R. Combined Resection of Superior Vena Cava for Lung Carcinoma: Prognostic Significance of Patterns of Superior Vena Cava Invasion. Ann Thorac Surg 2004;78:1184 -9.

[75] Cicconne AM, Venuta F, D'Andrilli A, Andreetti C, Ibrahim M, Giacomo TD, Masullo D, Rendina EA. Long-term patency of the stapled bovine pericardial conduit for replacement of the superior vena cava. Eur J Cardiothorac Surg (2011),doi:10.1016/j.ejcts.2011.03.008
[76] Shargall Y, Perrot MD, Keshavjee S, Darling G, Ginsberg R, Johnston M, Pierre A, Wadell TK. 15 years single center experience with surgical resection of the superior vena cava for non-small cell lung cancer. Lung Cancer 2004; 45: 357-363.
[77] Spaggiari L, Leo F, Veronesi G, Solli P, Galetta D, Tatani B, Petrella F, Radice D. Superior Vena Cava Resection for Lung and Mediastinal Malignancies: A Single-Center Experience With 70 Cases. Ann Thorac Surg 2007;83:223-30.
[78] Dartevelle P, Macchiarini P, Chapelier A, et al: *Superior Vena Cava Resection and Reconstruction*, Philadelphia, WB Saunders, 1995.
[79] Lanuti M, Delva PED, Gaissert HA, Wright CD, Wain JC, Allan JS, Donahue DM, Mathisen DJ. Review of Superior Vena Cava Resection in the Management of Benign Disease and Pulmonary or Mediastinal Malignancies. Ann Thorac Surg 2009;88:392- 8
[80] Ciccone AM, Venuta F, D'Andrilli A, Andretti C, Ibrahim M, Giacomo TD, Masullo D, Rendina EA. Long-term patency of the stapled bovine pericardial conduit for replacement of the superior vena cava. Eur J Cardiothorac Surg 2011: 40: 1487-1491.
[81] Liu D, Guo Y, Shi B, Tian Y, Song Z, Ma Q, Zhang Z, Ge B. Tracheal carinal reconstruction and bronchovasculoplasty in central type bronchogenic carcinoma. Zhongguo Fei Ai Za Zhi. 2010; 13: 352-6.
[82] Kuehnl A, Schmidt M, Hornung HM, Graser A, Jauch KW, Kopp R. Resection of malignant tumours invading the vena cava: perioperative complications and long-term follow-up. J Vasc Surg. 2007; 46: 533-40.
[83] Macchiarini P, Altmayer M, Go T, Walles T, Schulze K, Wildfang I, Haverich A, Hardin M; Hannover Interdisciplinary Intrathoracic Tumour Task Force Group. Technical innovations of carinal resection for nonsmall-cell lung cancer. Ann Thorac Surg. 2006 Dec;82(6):1989-97.
[84] Liu D, Guo Y, Shi B, Tian Y, Song Z, Ma Q, Zhang Z, Ge B. Tracheal carinal reconstruction and bronchovasculoplasty in central type bronchogenic carcinoma. Zhongguo Fei Ai Za Zhi. 2010; 13: 352-6.
[85] Mitchell JD, Mathisen DJ, Wright CD, Wain JC, Donahue DM, Allan JS, Moncure AC, Grillo HC. Resection for bronchogenic carcinoma involving the carina: long-term results and effect of nodal status on outcome. J Thorac Cardiovasc Surg. 2001; 121: 465-71
[86] Porhanov VA, Poliakov IS, Selvaschuk AP, Grechishkin AI, Sitnik SD, Nikolaev IF, Efimtsev JP, Marchenko LG. Indications and results of sleeve carinal resection. Eur J Cardiothorac Surg. 2002; 22: 685-94.
[87] de Perrot M, Fadel E, Mercier O, Mussot S, Chapelier A, Dartevelle P. Long-term results after carinal resection for carcinoma: does the benefit warrant the risk? J Thorac Cardiovasc Surg. 2006; 131: 81-9.
[88] Dartevelle P, Macchiarini P. Carinal resection for bronchogenic cancer. Semin Thorac Cardiovasc Surg. 1996; 8: 414-25.
[89] Yokoi K, Tsuchiya R, Mori T, Nagai K, Furukawa T, Fujimura S, Nakagawa K, Ichinose Y. Results of surgical treatment of lung cancer involving the diaphragm. J Thorac Cardiovasc Surg. 2000; 120: 799-805
[90] Rocco G, Rendina EA, Meroni A, Venuta F, Della Pona C, De Giacomo T, Robustellini M, Rossi G, Massera F, Vertemati G, Rizzi A, Coloni GF. Prognostic factors after surgical treatment of lung cancer invading the diaphragm. Ann Thorac Surg. 1999; 68: 2065-8.

[91] Terzi A, Lonardoni A, Falezza G, Scanagatta P, Santo A, Furlan G, Calabrò F. Completion pneumonectomy for non-small cell lung cancer: experience with 59 cases. Eur J Cardiothorac Surg. 2002; 22: 30-4.

[92] Jungraithmayr W, Hasse J, Olschewski M, Stoelben E. Indications and results of completion pneumonectomy. Eur J Cardiothorac Surg. 2004; 26: 189-96.

[93] Jungraithmayr W, Hasse J, Stoelben E. Completion pneumonectomy for lung metastases. Eur J Surg Oncol. 2004; 30: 1113-7.

[94] Guggino G, Doddoli C, Barlesi F, Acri P, Chetaille B, Thomas P, Giudicelli R, Fuentes P. Completion pneumonectomy in cancer patients: experience with 55 cases. Eur J Cardiothorac Surg. 2004; 25: 449-55.

[95] Haraguchi S, Koizumi K, Hirata T, Hirai K, Mikami I, Kubokura H, Shimizu K. Surgical results of completion pneumonectomy. Ann Thorac Cardiovasc Surg. 2011; 17: 24-8.

[96] Chan V, Shamji F, Sundaresan SR. Carinal sleeve resection for persistent bronchopleural fistula after completion right pneumonectomy. Ann Thorac Surg. 2010; 89: 1266-8.

[97] Fujimoto T, Zaboura G, Fechner S, Hillejan L, Schröder T, Marra A, Krbek T, Hinterthaner M, Greschuchna D, Stamatis G. Completion pneumonectomy: current indications, complications, and results. J Thorac Cardiovasc Surg. 2001; 121: 484-90

[98] Chataigner O, Fadel E, Yildizeli B, Achir A, Mussot S, Fabre D, Mercier O, Dartevelle PG. Factors affecting early and long-term outcomes after completion pneumonectomy. Eur J Cardiothorac Surg. 2008;33:837-43

[99] Grodzki T, Alchimowicz J, Kozak A, Kubisa B, Pierog J, Wojcik J, Bielewicz M, Witkowska D. Additional pulmonary resections after pneumonectomy: actual long-term survival and functional results. Eur J Cardiothorac Surg 2008; 34: 493-498.

[100] Donington JS, Miller DL, Rowland CC, Deschamps C, Allen MS, Trastek VF, Pairolero PC. Subsequent pulmonary resection for bronchogenic carcinoma after pneumonectomy. Ann Thorac Surg. 2002; 74: 154-8

[101] Wood DE. Pulmonary resection after pneumonectomy. Thorac Surg Clin. 2004; 14: 173-82.

[102] Voltolini L, Rapicetta C, Luzzi L, Ghiribelli C, Paladini P, Granato F, Gallazzi M, Gotti G. Surgical treatment of synchronous multiple lung cancer located in a different lobe or lung: high survival in node-negative subgroup. Eur J Cardiothorac Surg. 2010; 37: 1198-204.

[103] Finley DJ, Yoshizawa A, Travis W, Zhou Q, Seshan VE, Bains MS, Flores RM, Rizk N, Rusch VW, Park BJ. Predictors of outcomes after surgical treatment of synchronous primary lung cancers. J Thorac Oncol. 2010; 5: 197-205.

[104] Martini N, Melamed MR. Multiple primary lung cancers. J Thorac Cardiovasc Surg 1975;70:606-612.

[105] De Leyn P, Moons J, Vansteenkiste J, Verbeken E, Van Raemdonck D, Nafteux P, Decaluwe H, Lerut T. Survival after resection of synchronous bilateral lung cancer. Eur J Cardiothorac Surg. 2008; 34: 1215-22.

CHAPTER 10

Part C: Segmentectomy and Wedge Resection in the Surgical Treatment of NSCLC

Ahmet Demirkaya* **and Kamil Kaynak**

Istanbul University Cerrahpasa Medical Faculty, Department of Thoracic Surgery, Kocamustafapasa/Fatih Istanbul, 34303 Turkey

Abstract: The standard treatment for stage I NSCLC is lobectomy with mediastinal lymph node sampling or dissection. The role of limited resection for stage IA lesions, especially those ≤ 2 cm in diameter is controversial despite many proponents. Patients with physiologic limitation prohibiting lobectomy should be evaluated for sublobar resection, as it seems to offer increasingly similar overall and cancer-free survival rates. Limited resection should be done with systematic or complete lymph node sampling.

As limited resection leads to better postoperative lung function of pulmonary function and decreased morbidity, it may become the preferred strategy for these patients in the future. Non-randomized series comparing patients undergoing sublobar resection because of compromised lung function and those undergoing formal lobectomy show similar long-term survival and cancer-free survival especially for stage IA tumours less than 2 cm.

Keywords: Lung cancer, limited resection, wedge resection, segmentectomy.

INTRODUCTION

The standard surgical treatment modality for stage I NSCLC is lobectomy with mediastinal lymph node sampling or dissection [1-3]. The role of limited resection for stage IA lesions, especially those ≤ 2 cm in diameter is controversial despite many proponents. Current recommendations for anatomic lobectomy for these patients are based on the results of a single trial in which 267 patients with stage IA tumours ≤ 3 cm were randomly assigned to lobectomy or limited

***Address correspondence to Ahmet Demirkaya:** Istanbul University Cerrahpasa Medical Faculty, Department of Thoracic Surgery, Kocamustafapasa/Fatih Istanbul, 34303 Turkey; Tel: +90 212 4143590; Fax: +90 212 6328474; E-mail: drdemirkaya@yahoo.com

Resection [4]. This study showed that the lobectomy group had a significantly lower rate of loco-regional recurrence and a trend towards better survival. However, several more recent retrospective studies have suggested that limited resection and lobectomy could provide similar outcomes among patients with smaller [≤2 cm] stage I NSCLC [5-9]. Since, the limited resection associate with lesser reducing of pulmonary function, reduced morbidity and disability and increased likelihood of surgical intervention in the event of a secondary primary lung cancer, it could be recommended in select patients [8].

Accordingly, some evidence suggests that limited resection may be equally effective for patients with smaller tumours or in the elderly [6-9]. Several studies have shown that the cutoff of 3 cm for T1 tumours may be arbitrary since survival appears to be significantly better in patients whose tumours are less than 1.5 or 2 cm [10-12]. These findings is not unexpected, since T stage for tumours<2 cm is T1a according to new staging system [13].

Therefore, smaller tumours have a better prognosis and may be amenable to a less extensive resection with similar outcomes. Additionally, a number of retrospective studies from the United States and Japan have suggested the survival equivalency of limited resection and lobectomy for tumours ≤2 cm in size [5-8]. It was reported that the overall 5-year survival following lobectomy was not significantly different from the survival after more limited segmentectomy for patients with T1a tumours [7].

Similarly, Kodama *et al.* reported that the 5-year survival, after intentional limited resection, was 93% and essentially identical to that achieved by lobectomy in a stage matched group [14].

However, the majority of these studies evaluated a small number of patients recruited from single institutions and did not use advanced techniques to overcome of selection bias. A larger study, investigating stage I and II patients of all sizes from the SEER registries, suggested that lobectomy may not confer an additional survival benefit over limited resection among patients ≤71 years of age. Conversely, limited resection may be an adequate alternative to full resection, in patients with multiple comorbidities or limited life expectancy. Future studies should analyze whether outcomes following limited resection are similar regardless of patient's age. In the United States, a recently initiated randomized ACOSOG controlled trial including approximately 1200 patients is comparing lobectomy *versus* limited resection for the treatment of patients with NSCLC ≤2 cm [15].

A similar study is comparing lobectomy to limited resection for the treatment of adenocarcinomas ≤2 cm size with a predominant solid component on chest computed tomography [16]. Patients with a predicted postoperative forced expiratory volume in 1 second or diffusion capacity ≤40% predicted are thought to have an increased risk for perioperative complications and full resection may result in high morbidity and mortality rate, low postoperative pulmonary function and these subjects are more likely to have limited resection [17].

In summary, these data suggests that limited resection and lobectomy may lead to similar survival among patients with T1a tumours. As limited resection leads to better postoperative lung function of pulmonary function and decreased morbidity, it may become the preferred strategy for these patients in the future. However, confirmation of these suggestions with larger randomized trials is warranted.

TYPES OF LIMITED RESECTION

Wedge resection is the removal of a part of the lung without considering its anatomical margins. A part of a segment or a section of lung parenchyma is resected in this procedure. This procedure can also be named as 'atypical' resection. Segmentectomy refers to the removal of an anatomical pulmonary unit with its own arteriole, bronchus and venule. Identification and dissection of the segmental bronchus and artery should be done. They are sutured and ligated, respectively, and the identification of the common vein of the two adjacent segments, which must be preserved when possible. The tributary veins from the resected segment must be ligated only as they appear in the intersegmental plane. A segmentectomy is a kind of anatomical lung resection such as lobectomy, bilobectomy and pneumonectomy. In extended segmentectomy, the affected segment and adjacent subsegments are resected and mediastinal and hilar lymph node exploration with dissection, is added to the procedure to confirm pN0 status with 'frozen section' examination.

In sleeve segmentectomies, segmental bronchus is removed with part of the lobar bronchus, and then the airway is reconstructed with an end-to-end anastomosis. This procedure is useful in cases when the tumour is so close to the origin of the segmental bronchus that a standard segmentectomy may produce a positive bronchial margin, such a procedure can provide an opportunity to avoid a lobectomy [18,19].

Limited resections can be performed both as an open or videothoracoscopic procedure but videothoracoscopic interventions have been found to reduce hospital stay compared with open procedures [20-22].

IMPACT OF TUMOUR SIZE

There is an agreement on 2-cm landmark in studies investigating the impact of limited resections. Okada *et al.* [23] suggested that extended segmentectomy was an alternative to lobectomy in patients with clinical T1N0M0 tumours of ≤ 2 cm in diameter. In this study 5-yr survival rates after extended segmentectomy and after lobectomy were 87.3% and 77.7%, respectively [p=0.1644]. The 5-yr survival rates of their pathological T1N0M0 group were 87.1% for extended segmentectomy whereas it was 87.8% for lobectomy [p=0.8008].Warren *et al.* [24], Koike *et al.* [25], Watanabe *et al.* [26] and Sienel *et al.* [27] reported similar results in this group of patients with T1a tumours.

IMPACT OF AGE

Age of the patient is also an important factor for the outcome of limited resections. In the study of Mery *et al.* [28] patients who underwent lobectomy, pneumonectomy and wedge resection were divided into 3 groups depending on their ages [65yo, 65-74yo, ≥75yo]. Survival was found to be significant better for lobectomy in patients of the first two age groups. Whereas lobectomy and wedge resection resulted similar survival rates in patients older than 75 years.

SEGMENTECTOMY *VERSUS* WEDGE RESECTION

Two retrospective studies that compares segmentectomy and wedge resection have been published [29,30]. In the study of El-Sherif *et al.* [29] reported that local recurrence was significantly higher when resection margin was <1 cm.

Wedge resections have a risk of closer resection margins so this procedure is associated with higher local recurrence. But there were no relationship between resection margin and regional or distant recurrence.

In the second study [30], segmentectomy was found to be associated with a significantly better cancer-related 5-yr survival compared with wedge resection [71% and 48%, respectively]. Local recurrence was significantly lower in segmentectomy [16%] than in wedge resection [55%]. The results were same with tumours ≤2 cm in diameter. Five-year survival rates were found as 80% for segmentectomy and 48% for wedge resection. Local recurrence rates were 11% for segmentectomy and 40% for wedge resection.

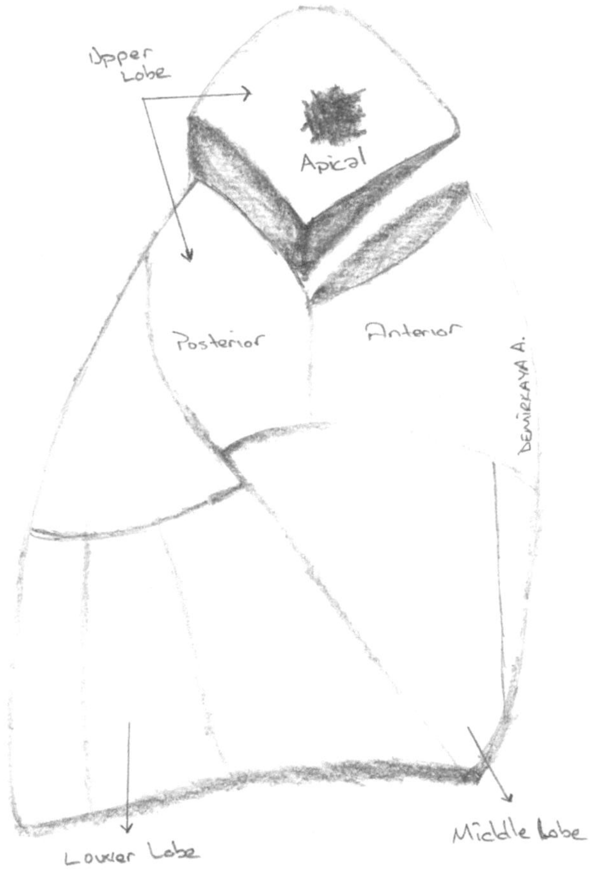

Figure 1: Segmentectomy.

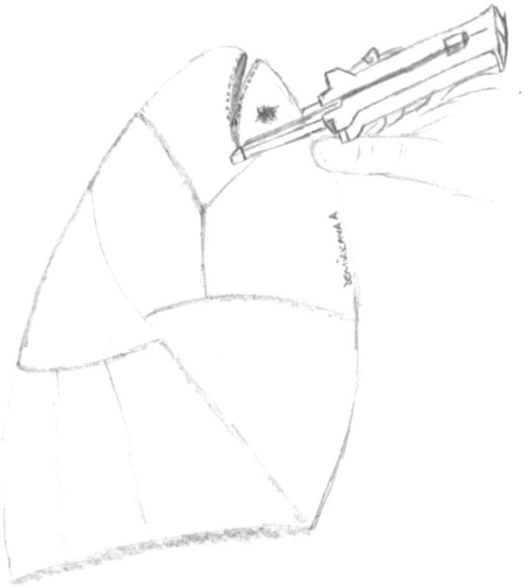

Figure 2: Wedge Resection.

POST-OPERATIVE PULMONARY FUNCTION

Impaired pulmonary function is the most common indication for limited resection. In the report of Takizawa *et al.* [31] pre-operative forced vital capacity [FVC] and preoperative FEV_1 were similar in lobectomy and segmentectomy groups. 2 weeks postoperatively, FVC was significantly higher in the segmentectomy group [72.7% *versus* 67.2%], but 1 year after the operation there were similar values in both groups.[94.9% *versus* 91.0%]. But there were significant benefit at 2 weeks post-operatively in FEV1 in the group of patients who had undergone segmentectomy [73.0% *versus* 66.6%] and it was maintained at 1 year [93.3% *versus* 87.3%].

The study of Harada *et al.* [32] showed that, the post-operative reduction of FVC and FEV_1 was significantly smaller in the segmentectomy group than that of in the lobectomy group. These two studies were performed in patients with good pre-operative pulmonary function. In patients with lung disease, careful evaluation of the type, degree and location of the lung abnormalities is necessary in order to select the best lung resection. This is particularly relevant in patients with emphysema of the upper lobes in whom a lobectomy will have a lung volume reduction effect, with improvement of postoperative lung function, whereas a segmentectomy would not provide amelioration [33]. Conversely, the preservation of lung function in patients with small lung cancers and anticipated long survival is important, considering the possibility of further lung resections to treat second primary lung tumours.

CONCLUSION

The standard of surgical resection type for patients with stage I non-small cell lung cancer remains anatomic lobectomy, since it causes lower local recurrence rate when compared with lesser resection in a randomized trial and has been confirmed in many prospective and retrospective studies. Patients with physiologic limitation prohibiting lobectomy should be evaluated for sublobar resection, as it seems to offer increasingly similar overall and cancer-free survival rates.

Limited resection should be done with systematic or complete lymph node sampling. Best outcomes were found to achieve when tumour size is ≤2cm and margins should be ≥2cm. Retrospective series comparing patients undergoing sublobar resection because of compromised lung function and those undergoing formal lobectomy show similar long-term survival and cancer-free survival especially for stage IA tumours less than 2 cm [34].

ACKNOWLEDGEMENTS

Declared none.

CONFLICT OF INTEREST

The authors confirm that this article content has no conflict of interest.

REFERENCES

[1] Wisnivesky JP *et al.* Limited resection for the treatment of patients with stage IA lung cancer. Ann Surg. 2010 Mar;251[3]:550-4.

[2] Spiro SG, Porter JC. Lung cancer–where are we today? Current advances in staging and nonsurgical treatment. Am J Respir Crit Care Med. 2002;166[9]: 1166–1196.

[3] Spira A, Ettinger DS. Multidisciplinary management of lung cancer. N Engl J Med. 2004;350[4]:379 –392.

[4] Ginsberg RJ, Rubinstein LV. Randomized trial of lobectomy *versus* limited resection for T1 N0 non-small cell lung cancer. Lung Cancer Study Group. Ann Thorac Surg. 1995;60[3]:615–22; discussion 622–623.

[5] Koike T, Yamato Y, Yoshiya K, *et al.* Intentional limited pulmonary resection for peripheral T1 N0 M0 small-sized lung cancer. J Thorac Cardiovasc Surg. 2003;125[4]:924 –928.

[6] Mery CM, Pappas AN, Bueno R, *et al.* Similar long-term survival of elderly patients with non-small cell lung cancer treated with lobectomy or wedge resection within the surveillance, epidemiology, and end results database. Chest. 2005;128[1]:237–245.

[7] Warren WH, Faber LP. Segmentectomy *versus* lobectomy in patients with stage I pulmonary carcinoma. Five-year survival and patterns of intrathoracic recurrence. J Thorac Cardiovasc Surg. 1994;107[4]:1087–93; discussion 1093–1094.

[8] Keenan RJ, Landreneau RJ, Maley RH, Jr., *et al.* Segmental resection spares pulmonary function in patients with stage I lung cancer. Ann Thorac Surg. 2004;78[1]:228 –33; discussion 228–233.

[9] Nakamura H, Kawasaki N, Taguchi M, *et al.* Survival following lobectomy vs limited resection for stage I lung cancer: a meta-analysis. Br J Cancer. 2005;92[6]:1033–1037.

[10] Wisnivesky JP, Yankelevitz D, Henschke CI. The effect of tumour size on curability of stage I non-small cell lung cancers. Chest. 2004;126[3]:761–765.

[11] Gajra A, Newman N, Gamble GP, *et al.* Impact of tumour size on survival in stage IA non-small cell lung cancer: a case for subdividing stage IA disease.Lung Cancer. 2003;42[1]:51–7.

[12] Koike T, Terashima M, Takizawa T, *et al.* Clinical analysis of small-sized peripheral lung cancer. J Thorac Cardiovasc Surg. 1998;115[5]:1015–1020.

[13] Rami-Porta R, Ball D, Crowley J, *et al.* The IASLC Lung Cancer Staging Project: proposals for the revision of the T descriptors in the forthcoming [seventh] edition of the TNM classification for lung cancer. J Thorac Oncol. 2007;2[7]:593– 602.

[14] Kodama K, Doi O, Higashiyama M, *et al.* Intentional limited resection for selected patients with T1 N0 M0 non-small-cell lung cancer: a single institution study. J Thorac Cardiovasc Surg. 1997;114[3]:347–353.

[15] Comparison of Different Types of Surgery in Treating Patients With Stage IA Non-Small CellLungCancer.http://clinicaltrials.gov/ct2/show/NCT00499330?term_calgb_140503&rank_1. Accessed July 7, 2008.

[16] Rusch VW, Tsuchiya R, Tsuboi M, *et al.* Surgery for bronchioloalveolar carcinoma and "very early" adenocarcinoma: an evolving standard of care? J Thorac Oncol. 2006; 1[9]: S27–S31.

[17] Beckles MA, Spiro SG, Colice GL, *et al.* The physiologic evaluation of patients with lung cancer being considered for resectional surgery. Chest. 2003;123[1 Suppl]:105S–114S.

[18] Rami-Porta R, Tsuboi M. Sublobar resection for lung cancer. Eur Respir J. 2009 Feb;33[2]:426-35.

[19] Okada M, Nishio W, Sakamoto T, *et al.* Sleeve segmentectomy for non-small cell lung carcinoma. J Thorac Cardiovasc Surg 2004; 128: 420–424.

[20] Shiraishi T, Shirakusa T, Iwasaki A *et al.* Video-assisted thoracoscopic surgery [VATS] segmentectomy for small peripheral lung cancer tumours. Surg Endos 2004; 18: 1657–1662.

[21] Okada M, Mimura T, Ikegaki J *et al.* A novel video-assisted anatomic segmentectomy technique: selective segmental inflation *via* bronchofiberoptic jet followed by cautery cutting. J Thorac Cardiovasc Surg 2007; 133: 753–758.

[22] Atkins BZ, Harpole Jr DH, Mangum JH *et al.* Pulmonary segmentectomy by thoracotomy or thoracoscopy: reduced hospital length of stay with a minimally-invasive approach. Ann Thorac Surg 2007; 84: 1107–1113.

[23] Okada M, Yoshikawa K, Hatta T, Tsubota N. Is segmentectomy with lymph node assessment an alternative to lobectomy for non-small cell lung cancer of 2 cm or smaller? Ann Thorac Surg 2001; 71: 956–961.

[24] Warren WH, Faber LP. Segmentectomy *versus* lobectomy in patients with stage I pulmonary carcinoma. Five-year survival and patterns of intrathoracic recurrence. J Thorac Cardiovasc Surg 1994; 107: 1087–1094.

[25] Koike T, Yamato Y, Yoshiya K, *et al.* Intentional limited pulmonary resection for peripheral T1N0M0 small-sized lung cancer. J Thorac Cardiovasc Surg 2003; 125: 924–928.

[26] Watanabe T, Okada A, Imakiire T *et al.* Intentional limited resection for small peripheral lung cancer based on intraoperative pathologic exploration. Jpn J Thorac Cardiovasc Surg 2005; 53: 29–35.

[27] Sienel W, Stremmel C, Kirschbaum A, *et al.* Frequency of local recurrence following segmentectomy of stage IA nonsmall cell lung cancer is influenced by segment localisation and width of resection margins – implications for patient selection for segmentectomy. Eur J Cardiothorac Surg 2007; 31: 522–528.

[28] Mery CM, Pappas AN, Bueno R, *et al.* Similar long-term survival of elderly patients with non-small cell lung cancer treated with lobectomy or wedge resection within the Surveillance, Epidemiology, and End Results database. Chest 2005; 128: 237–245.

[29] El-Sherif A, Fernando HC, Santos R, *et al.* Margin and local recurrence after sublobar resection of non-small cell lung cancer. Ann Surg Oncol 2007; 14: 2400–2405.

[30] Sienel W, Dango S, Kirschbaum A, *et al.* Sublobar resections in stage IA non-small cell lung cancer: segmentectomies result in significantly better cancer-related survival than wedge resections. Eur J Cardiothorac Surg 2008; 33: 728–734.

[31] Takizawa T, Haga M, Yagi N, *et al.* Pulmonary function after segmentectomy for small peripheral carcinoma of the lung. J Thorac Cardiovasc Surg 1999; 118: 538–541.

[32] Harada H, Okada M, Sakamoto T, *et al.* Functional advantage after radical segmentectomy *versus* lobectomy for lung cancer. Ann Thorac Surg 2005; 80: 2041– 2045.

[33] Santambrogio L, Nosotti M, Baisi A, *et al.* Pulmonary lobectomy for lung cancer: a prospective study to compare patients with forced expiratory volume in 1 s more or less than 80% of predicted. Eur J Cardiothorac Surg 2001; 20: 684–687.

[34] Bilfinger TV, Baram D. Review. Sublobar resection in nonsmall cell lung carcinoma. Curr Opin Pulm Med. 2008 Jul;14[4]:292-6.

CHAPTER 10

Part D: Lobectomies

Kamil Kaynak* **and Ahmet Demirkaya**

Istanbul University Cerrahpasa Medical Faculty, Department of Thoracic Surgery, Kocamustafapasa/Fatih Istanbul, 34303 Turkey

Abstract: The aim of surgical treatment of NSLC is complete resection. Lobectomy remains the definitive resections because it is an anatomic resection that assures the regional lymph nodes that course along the lobar bronchus and thus provides the best staging information and local control. The risk of pulmonary resection depends on both patient characteristics (*i.e.* FEV1, DLCO *etc.*), and type of resection (*i.e.* pneumonectomy, lobectomy, segmentectomy; open thoracotomy *vs.* VATS). The posterolateral position is used for lobectomy because it gives the surgeon the greatest maneuverability. Key points in the performance of lobectomy are mobilization of the lobe, fissure dissection and management of the vessels and bronchus.

Keywords: Lung carcinoma, resection, lobe.

INTRODUCTION

The aim of surgical treatment of NSLC is a complete resection. Lobectomy is the gold standard for localized lung cancer [1]. Lobectomy remains the definitive resection because it is an anatomic resection that assures the regional lymph nodes that course along the lobar bronchus and thus provides the best staging information and local control. Lobectomy is the ideal operation of a lung cancer performed to the parenchyma of a single lobe. Lobectomy is generally well tolerated, usually leaves sufficient lung volume to fill the pleural space left by resection. Lobectomy is associated with about half the operative mortality of pneumonectomy (about 2% *vs.* 4%), as reported by Ginsberg [2] and Wada [3] and their associates. Pagni and associates [4] reported operative mortality rate of

***Address correspondence to Kamil Kaynak:** Istanbul University Cerrahpasa Medical Faculty, Department of Thoracic Surgery, Kocamustafapasa/Fatih Istanbul, 34303 Turkey; Tel: +90 212 4143590; Fax: +90 212 6328474; E-mail: kamil@istanbul.edu.tr

1.9% in patients >75 years of age and a long-term survival no different from those patients between 65 and 75 years of age.

The risk of pulmonary resection depends on both patient characteristics (*i.e.* FEV1, DLCO *etc.*), and type of resection (*i.e.* pneumonectomy, lobectomy, segmentectomy; open thoracotomy *vs.* VATS). The problem in patients with limited pulmonary reserve is perioperative mortality and no long-term functional capacity. Most studies [5, 6] have shown good long-term functional status after conventional resection in pts with poor PFT's. Several studies indicated that long-term functional impairment was usually due to random events (*e.g.* ARDS). There are some percentages that should be considered for selection of lung resection criteria;

- ppo-FEV_1 < 40% -Most extensively documented Mortality ~30%.
- pre-DLCO <60% or ppo-DLCO <50% -Reasonable amount of data mortality ~25%.
- VO_{2max} < 15 ml/kg/min Limited data, usually pts with good FEV1, DLCO Mortality~15%.

Risk for Lobectomy increases from 2% to 8% for age < 60 to > 80

Risk for pneumonectomy increases from 7% tp 28% for age < 70 to > 80

ppo FEV1 should not to be used alone to select patients with lung cancer for lung resection, particularly patients with moderate to severe COPD. A ppo FEV1 value of predicted 30% is suggested to be a high risk threshold for this parameter when included in an algorithm for assessment of pulmonary reserve before surgery. DLCO should be routinely measured during pre-operative evaluation of lung resection candidates regardless of whether the spirometric evaluation is abnormal. Shuttle walk test should not be used alone to select patients for operation. It could be used as a screening test: patients walking less than 400m may have peakVO^2 lower than 15 ml/kg/min. Standardized symptom-limited stair climbing test should be used as a first line functional screening test to select those patients that may undergo safely to operation (height of ascent > 22m) or those who need more sophisticated exercise tests (cf paragraph 2-3-3) in order to optimize their perioperative management. The 6-min walk test should not be used to select patients for operation.

Lobectomy is a more difficult operation to perform than other procedures and also in the most serious group in terms of morbidity and mortality. The posterolateral position is used for lobectomy because it gives the surgeon the greatest maneuverability. Anterolateral thoracotomy, median sternotomy except for the left lower lobe and muscle sparing lateral or axillary thoracotomy are also used. With the lateral position, a fourth intercostal space incision is used for upper lobectomies and a fifth or sixth interspace incision is used for the right middle lobe, lingula and lower lobe resections. Key points in the performance of lobectomy are mobilization of the lobe, fissure dissection and management of the vessels and bronchus [7]. Meticulous technique to prevent air leak reduces pleural space problems and patients length of stay [8].

Operative mortality with lung resection varies with surgeon specialty. Some, but not all, of this variation in operative mortality are attributable to hospital and surgeon volume [9]. In USA, female gender is associated with decreased mortality and morbidity after lung cancer resections. Complication rates are lower for black, Hispanic, and Asian patients. Low socioeconomic status increases the risk of in-hospital death. These factors should be considered during patient risk stratification for lung cancer resection [10].

RIGHT UPPER LOBECTOMY

Viewed from the patient's side, the anatomy of the right hilum is a triangle with the pulmonary artery at the apex, the vein anterior, and the bronchus posterior. The mediastinal pleura is incised around the hilum of the right lung, lateral to the superior vena cava inferior to the azygos vein, continuing posteriorly over the bronchus, anterior to bronchus intermedius. The procedure is to divide the segmental arteries first, then the veins, and finally the upper lobe bronchus. The azygos vein caps the triangle. It is often adhesed to the bronchus, the artery, or both and can be divided as a first step to gain proximal control of the pulmonary artery and to perform the paratracheal lymphadenectomy. İnferior to the

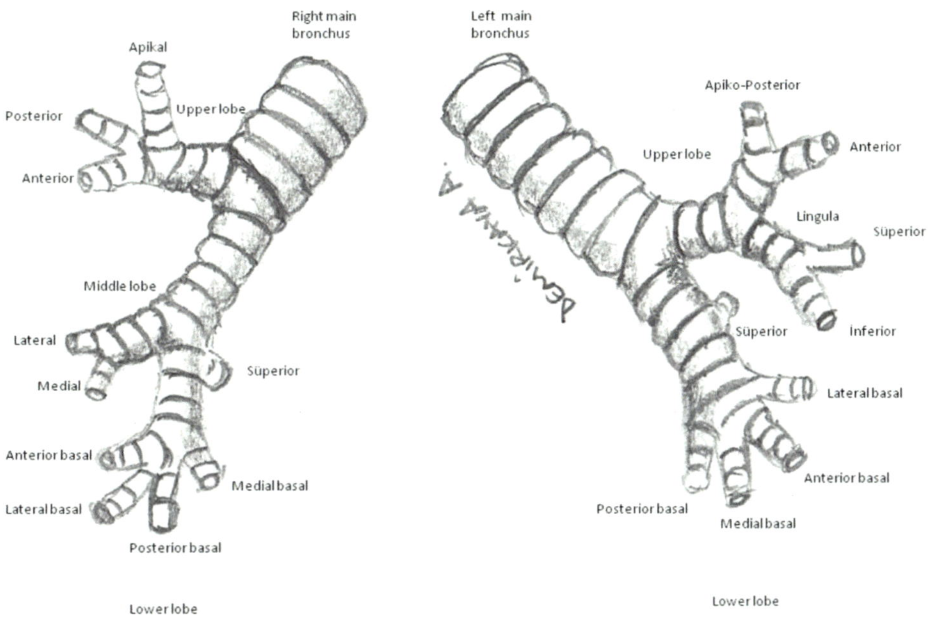

Figure A: The Anatomy of Bronchus.

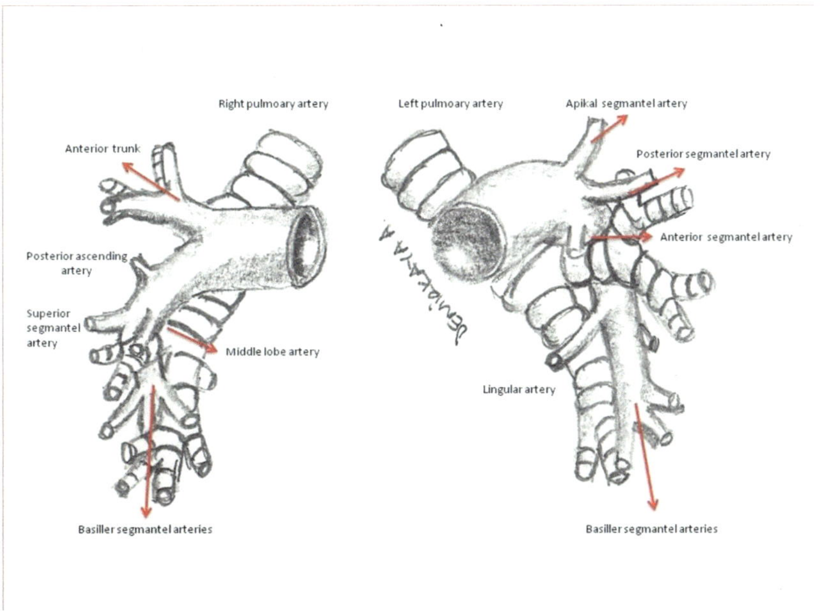

Figure B: The Anatomy of Pulmonary Arteries.

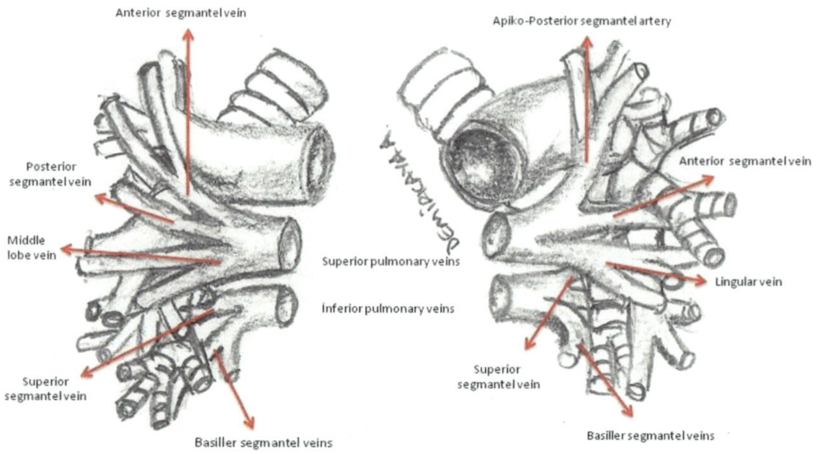

Figure C: The Anatomy of Pulmonary Veins.

azygos-caval junction a lymph node found just below this lymph node is the upper border of the pulmonary artery. The apical vein which lies on the apicoposterior artery and complicated to dissection is ligated and divided. Superior arterial trunk and its apical and anterior segmental branches are dissected. The superior arterial trunk is doubly tied, the apical and segmental branches are tied and then divided.Vascular stapler (2.0 mm) that concurrently ligates and divides the vessels can be used. After division of the superior trunk of the pulmonary artery the common stem of the apical and anterior segmental veins dissected and divided. After dividing the veins to the right upper lobe posterior segment of upper lobe is usually much smaller than the main branch of the ascending branch and recognizable in many patients. The posterior segmental artery arises within the fissure. Three approaches have been described: an anterior approach, an approach through the oblique fissure, and a retrograde approach. In such cases, posterior segmental artery arises anteriorly and arteries do not originate from the upper lobe within the major fissure. After the division of upper lobe arteries the lung is retracted posteriorly and the hilar region is visible. Pleura is opened from the outside of phrenic nerve, upper lobe veins and branches are dissected. The middle lobe veins which enter the inferior portion of the right superior pulmonary vein must be carefully handled to protect the middle lobe vein interlobar artery which lies directly beneath the upper and middle stems of the superior pulmonary vein and therefore, this dissection must be performed cautiously.

After dividing vessels bronchus is dissected carefully. In the bifurcation of the upper lobe and the intermediate bronchus a lymph node is located. It is dissected towards the upper lobe so inferior border of the right upper lobe bronchus is cleared. Due to the possibility of posterior ascending artery injury clamp usage is not recommended. A scissor dissection of the medial surface of the bronchus was performed. A right angle clamp may then be passed safely around the right upper lobe bronchus. If a bronchial stapler is used, it must be placed carefully to avoid narrowing the right mainstem or intermediate bronchus and the stapler's long axis should lie along the axis of the membranous trachea. By doing so, the flexible membranous trachea will seal the cartilaginous trachea. A semb clamp is used to widen the peribronchial space, allowing the passage of a 4.8-mm stapling device. The bronchus is either stapled and divided or manually sutured. The parenchyma then is divided and sealed. The other upper lobe bronchial artery may arise between the upper division of pulmonary artery and the posterior segment artery must be known and lifted up and investigated. The anterior (minor) fissure between the upper and lower lobes is sometimes absent or is incomplete. In this case, a stapler can be used to divide the parenchyma between the upper and lower lobes or with selective inflation the upper lobe can be excised, and air leaks and bleeding points can be controlled with sutures. After the specimen removed and bronchial closure tested the pulmonary ligament is divided. To prevent torsion of the middle lobe the edges of the partially expanded middle and lower lobes are sutured as shown in Figs. **A**, **B** and **C**.

MIDDLE LOBECTOMY

The first step is to open the major fissure and expose the interlobar portion of the pulmonary artery. The superior segmental artery and posterior segmental artery of upper lobe is exposed and two or three middle lobe arteries are first determined then dissected and divided. Usually there is a single common trunk and the middle lobe bronchus is quite obvious just behind it. The possibility of an anomalous branch of a middle lobe artery to the upper lobe must be kept in mind. After division of the middle lobe arteries the table is rotated posteriorly and the anterior aspect of the hilum is dissected isolating and ligating the middle lobe vein, which enters the lower portion of the süperior pulmonary vein. The tissue deep into the vein then should be cleaned posteriorly to reveal the middle lobe bronchus Figs. **A**, **B** and **C**. It should be stapled or divided and then closed with interrupted absorbable sutures. Its closure should be accomplished to avoid encroachment on the lumen of the main bronchial trunk or the superior segmental bronchus. The parenchyma between the upper and middle lobes is then divided with multiple firings of the stapler, the major fissure between middle lobe and lower lobe is easily divided with the use of sponge sticks and dissection with a long curved hemostat. After completion of the fissure and removel of the specimen, the raw surfaces of the upper lobe may be approximated to the lower lobe by several ties or sutures to help seal air leak.

RIGHT LOWER LOBECTOMY

The oblique fissure is opened while retracting the right upper and middle lobes anteriorly and the lower lobe posteriorly. The interlobar portion of the pulmonary artery is exposed to the depths of the fissure, and the dissection is carried to approximately the extent shown to detect possible anomalous branches between the lobes. The artery to the lower lobe branches into two trunks—the superior segmental and the basilar segment arteries. The middle lobe artery, originating from the anteromedial surface of the interlobar artery, must be demonstrated. An exactly opposite and posterolaterally lies the superior segmental artery. The one or two branches of the superior segmental artery arise from the same level from where the middle lobe arterial supply is ligated and divided. The basal arteries may have a short common trunk from where two branches originate: one supplying the anterior and medial segments and the other supplying the posterior and lateral segments. After identifying the middle lobe artery, which is preserved, the basilar segmental artery is encircled and divided. The lobe is retracted anteriorly and superiorly. The inferior pulmonary ligament is divided up to the lymph node at the lower border of the inferior pulmonary vein. The phrenic nerve lies close to the anterior aspect of the ligament and must be protected and preserved. The inferior vein is then encircled and either divided with a vascular load stapler or clamped and oversewn with a running prolene suture. The parenchyma is divided anteriorly and posteriorly with a stapler. The lower lobe bronchus is then dissected. As the middle lobe bronchus and the superior segmental bronchus originate from the intermediate bronchus almost at the same level, it may be necessary to close the basal segmental bronchus and the superior segmental bronchus separately to avoid obstructing the middle lobe bronchus Figs. **A**, **B** and **C**.

LEFT UPPER LOBECTOMY

The upper left lobectomy is performed in a hard area. With the upper lobe retracted downward and backward, the anterosuperior portion of the pleura is incised and seperated. The procedure is to divide the segmental arteries first, then the veins, and finally the upper lobe bronchus. The most common anatomic variation encountered during upper left lobectomy is the number of segmental arterial branches, which vary from three to eight. The arteries to the apical and posterior segments are on the anterosuperior surface of the primary hilum. The arteries to the anterior and lingular segments are found within the fissure between the upper and lower lobes, except for those instances in which the anterior segmental artery branches off proximal to the apical posterior artery. Proximal control of left pulmonary artery is recommended for safety. The main pulmonary artery lies in the left pleural space from the arch of the aorta. Both are close to the recurrent nerve and to the phrenic nevre. These proximal branches are often the last to be dissected and divided. As the fissure dissection proceeds the posterior segmental arteries are noted opposite to the superior segmental artery. With the lower lobe retracted inferiorly and upper lobe retracted superiorly the lingular branches are isolated and divided. The posterior segmental branches are ligated and divided by clockwise rotation of the upper lobe. The apical and anterior branches arise from the convex surface of the pulmonary artery often as a short trunk, slightly anterior to the middle point of the artery. These branches are the last to be divided. The lung is retracted posteriorly for dissection of the superior pulmonary vein. This step is usually deferred until all the upper lobe arteries have been divided and may be important if the patient has had recent bleeding from the lobe. Three or four branches entering the superior pulmonary vein are encircled with ligatures. Safe ligation of pulmonary vein is often unsuitable because of extrapericardial length of the pulmonary vein and for that reason vascular stapler may be useful in this area. If branches are not tied a vascular clamp is applied proximally and the vein is divided and then closed with a vascular suture. After dividing the arteries and veins the upper lobe bronchus is the only important structure remaining. The bronchus is freed by blunt dissection unless the peribronchial lymph nodes are unusually adherent. The upper left lobe bronchus is short and encroachment on the remaining airway to the lower lobe must be avoided. The bronchus stapler should be placed at least 1.5 to 2 cm from the main bronchial trunk usually at the bifurcation of the upper and lower divisional bronchi. After devising stapler differential inflation it should be ensured that the lower lobe bronchus does not compromise when the stapler is fired and the bronchus is transected by protecting the vein. The most common technical accident associated with upper left lobectomy is the injury to the main trunk of the pulmonary artery as it curves around the upper lobe bronchus. Injury is most likely to occur during dissection of an incomplete fissure or freeing of an adherent bronchus. The inferior pulmonary ligament is divided to allow the lower left lobe to advance upward to better fill the thoracic cavity Figs. **A**, **B** and **C**.

LEFT LOWER LOBECTOMY

Generally, oblique fissure is complete and vascular anomalies are not commonly noted. The first step is to open the fissure. The upper lobe is retracted anteriorly and superiorly, exposing the lower two thirds of the interlobar portion of the pulmonary artery. After the upper lobe and lingula artery, the superior segment artery is found at 1-2 cm proximally below lingula artery, which is dissected and divided. If the fissure is obliterated by adhesions, dissection of the posterior segment of upper lobe takes place by dissecting interlobar pulmonary artery from the overlying parenchyma, as well as by the creation of a tunnel so that a stapling device or clamps may be inserted to complete enough of the fissure to allow further exposure of the interlobar artery. The main basal trunk is then followed downward and the basal segmental branches are exposed. Arteries are ligated and divided separately to ensure adequate length of the proximal stump. The inferior pulmonary vein is exposed by retracting the lung anteriorly, opening the posterior hilar pleura and dividing the pulmonary ligament. The extrapericardial portion of the left inferior pulmonary vein is longer than the right; double proximal ligation is acceptable. Stapling the cardiac end of the vein or using a vascular stapler and suture is recommended. The upper and lower lobes below the bronchus are often strongly adherent and must be separated. A stapling instrument or the clamp and suture technique may be used without appreciably altering the contour of the upper lobe. The bronchus is cleared of alveolar tissue and the crotch below the upper lobe bronchus is dissected. The stapling device is applied just distal to the upper lobe bronchus to avoid occluding Figs. **A**, **B** and **C**. It is normally simple to advance the pleura overlying the aorta to covert the bronchus.

ACKNOWLEDGEMENTS

Declared none.

CONFLICT OF INTEREST

The authors confirm that this article content has no conflict of interest.

REFERENCES

[1] Albain KS, Rusch VW, Crowley JJ et al:Concurrent cisplatin/etoposide plus chest radiotherapy followed by surgery for stage IIIA(N2) and IIIB.JClin Oncol13:1880-1392,1995.
[2] Ginsberg RJ,*et al.*Modern 30 day operative mortality for surgical resections in lung cancer.J Thorac Cardiovasc Surg.1983;86-654
[3] Wada *et al.* Thirty day operative mortality for thoracotomy in lung cancer.J Thorac. Cardiovasc. Surg 1998;115:70.
[4] Pagni S, Frederico JA, Ponn RB. Pulmonary resection for lung cancer in octogenerians.Ann. Thorac. Surg 1997;63-785.
[5] Brunelli A, Refai M, Salati M *et al.* Predicted *vs.* observed FEV1 and DLCO after major lung resection: a prospective evaluation at different postoperative periods. Ann Thorac Surg. 2007 Mar;83(3):1134-9
[6] Brunelli A, Charloux A, Bolliger CT *et al.* The European Respiratory Society and European Society of Thoracic Surgeons clinical guidelines for evaluating fitness for radical treatment (surgery and chemoradiotherapy) in patients with lung cancer. European Respiratory Society; European Society of Thoracic Surgeons Joint Task Force on Fitness For Radical Therapy.Eur J CT Surg 2009;36:181-184
[7] Stanley C. Fell, Malcolm M. De Camp Jr Technical Aspects of Lobectomy.421-444 Shields 2009.
[8] Ginsberg RJ, Rubinstein LV:Randomized trial of lobectomy *vs.* limitied resection for T1N0M0 nonsmall cell lung cancer.Lung Cancer Study Group.Ann Thorac Surg 60:615-623,1995.

[9] Goodney PP, Lucas FL, Stukel TA, Birkmeyer JD. Surgeon specialty and operative mortality with lung resection. Ann Surg 241:179-84,2005.

[10] Lapar DJ, Bhamidipati CM, Harris DA *et al.* Gender, Race, and Socioeconomic Status Affects Outcomes After Lung Cancer Resections in the United States. Department of Surgery, Division of Thoracic and Cardiovascular Surgery, University of Virginia Health System, Charlottesville, Virginia. Ann Thorac Surg. 2011 Jun 24.

Lung Cancer: Clinical and Surgical Specifications, 2013, 279-288

CHAPTER 10

Part E: Pneumonectomy

Ahmet Demirkaya[1,*], Kamil Kaynak[1] and Ezel Ersen[2]

[1]Istanbul University Cerrahpasa Medical Faculty, Department of Thoracic Surgery, Kocamustafapasa/Fatih Istanbul, 34303 Turkey; and [2]Thoracic Surgery Department, State Hospital, Kocaeli, Turkey

Abstract: The aim of surgical treatment of non-small cell lung cancer is complete resection. Lately, the number of patients in whom pneumonectomy is necessary is decreasing attributable to advances in diagnostic imaging and improved techniques for surgery such as bronchoplasty. The risk of pulmonary resection depends on both patient characteristics, and type of resection. The type of surgical procedure affects mortality. The fact that patients undergoing a right-sided pneumonectomy have a higher mortality than those undergoing a left one. Patients who will undergo pneumonectomy first must undergo preoperative staging. Considering the prominent decreases in quality of life after pneumonectomy, most surgeons tend to avoid the indication of pneumonectomy whenever possible.

Keywords: Lung cancer, resection, mortality, pneumonectomy.

INTRODUCTION

Lately, the number of patients in whom pneumonectomy is necessary is decreasing attributable to advances in diagnostic imaging and improved techniques for surgery such as bronchoplasty. Considering the prominent decreases in quality of life after pneumonectomy, most surgeons tend to avoid the indication of pneumonectomy whenever possible. However, since there are always some patients in whom pneumonectomy is required and is the most appropriate treatment, surgeons should excel the procedure of pneumonectomy as a basic surgical technique.

***Address correspondence to Ahmet Demirkaya:** Istanbul University Cerrahpasa Medical Faculty, Department of Thoracic Surgery, Kocamustafapasa/Fatih Istanbul, 34303 Turkey; Tel: +90 212 4143590; Fax: +90 212 6328474; E-mail: drdemirkaya@yahoo.com

Akın Eraslan Balcı (Ed)

Rudolph Nissen performed the first successful pneumonectomy in 1931 [1]. The patient was a 12-year-old girl who had been struck by a horsedrawn cart in 1930, sustaining a crushing injury of the left chest with multiple rib fractures and mediastinal and subcutaneous emphysema Graham performed the first successful one-stage pneumonectomy on April 5, 1933 and presented his case at Sixteenth Annual Meeting of the AATS held on May 9–11, 1933 [1].

Three months after Edward Archibald at the Royal Victoria Hospital in Montreal performed the first pneumonectomy by individual ligation of the hilar vessels and bronchus [1].

On July 24, 1933, William F. Rienhoff, Jr., performed the first of two successful left pneumonectomies by hilar Dissection. Rienhoff stated that in order to prevent infection, mass suture and cauterization of the bronchus must be abandoned. In 1953, Brewer presented his method for buttressing bronchial stump with the pericardial tissue and reducing the incidence of bronchopleural fistula [1].

PREOPERATIVE EVALUATION AND MANAGEMENT

Staging

Patients who will undergo pneumonectomy first must undergo preoperative staging. At this time, a complete history and a physical examination that focuses on the identification of lymph nodes and liver masses, followed by a chest CT scan and a PET scan, are appropriate. This evaluation will rule out distant metastases other than brain metastases. Patients without symptoms of headache are unlikely to have brain metastases, and brain CT scans or MRIs are not obligatory. However, the risk of the procedure supports appropriate evaluation to rule out brain metastases.

Cardiopulmonary Evaluation

Various modalities exist which can be used to evaluate preoperative lung function as a means to predict postoperative complications. A preoperative forced expiratory volume in 1 second [FEV_1] of more than 2.0 L has been relatively arbitrarily chosen as minimal requirement for resection without further pulmonary evaluation and has been confirmed by experience.

Because of the obstructive nature of cancers that may lead to pneumonectomy, many patients have less than 50% perfusion to the affected lung. Quantitative perfusion scanning has been used successfully for almost 30 years to determine the relative contribution of each lung to the patient's lung function [2] Patients with a predicted postoperative FEV_1 of more than 800 mL are considered to have adequate pulmonary reserve to undergo resection. This technique has been found to be accurate in long-term follow-up [up to 5 years] [3], especially with respect to predicting the postoperative FEV_1 [4,5].

Right Pneumonectomy

Patients who undergo right pneumonectomy are more likely to die from this procedure than left pneumonectomy patients. Mortality typically is the result of complications of surgery rather than the surgery itself. Consequently, for right pneumonectomy, postoperative management is crucial.

Right pneumonectomy is performed with an incision which is similar to that selected for right upper lobectomy. Incision site is decided regarding characteristics of the patient and the choice of the surgeon.

In patients with a known or suspected lung cancer, lymph node biopsies must be performed intraoperatively and evaluated by frozen section to determine whether resection is appropriate. To ensure the technical feasibility of a complete resection pulmonary artery and vein must be fully assessed.

Upon deciding to proceed with right pneumonectomy, the pulmonary ligament is mobilized to the level of the inferior pulmonary vein. Also pleura surrounding the hilum must be dissected. Both pulmonary veins are dissected circumferentially to perform an extrapericardial pneumonectomy, right pulmonary artery is then dissected circumferentially to the level of the pericardial reflection. Unlike pulmonary arteries, the veins are not only relatively resistant to injury during dissection, but can easily be repaired in the case of such an injury. The pulmonary artery can easily be ruptured so every effort must be made to avoid any type of injury such as tearing. The safest instrument to use to encircle the pulmonary artery is their own index finger.

Injuries to the proximal right pulmonary artery are challenging to control. There is very little room available to permit placement of an occluding vascular clamp, and positioning such a clamp too close to the point of injury may serve to extend the injury more proximally on the vessel. One technique for gaining control of the vessel is to dissect between the superior vena cava and the ascending aorta, entering the pericardium and cross clamping the right pulmonary artery at its takeoff from the pulmonary trunk. In some situations it is appropriate to dissect intra-pericardially to obtain control of the vessels. Typical indications include a tumour that encroaches on any of the three main vessels close to the pericardial reflection, pericardial involvement by a bulky proximal tumour, and extensive fibrosis and inflammation after radiation therapy. Minimal dissection of the veins and artery are usually enough to encircle after proper exposure is obtained. After the dissection of the vessels, occluding the pulmonary artery using a tape or a clamp for a couple of minutes prior its permanent occlusion can be useful to ensure whether the patient can tolerate loss of the lung or not. The vessels are then occluded and divided. Under appropriate circumstances the vessel is sectioned by a vascular stapler, or is divided using a linear cutting stapler. If cost is an important issue, or if there is not sufficient normal vessel dissected to permit placement of a vascular stapler, the medial portion of the vessel is clamped and is oversewn with a running stitch using a permanent monofilament suture such as polypropylene. The pulmonary end of the vessel is ligated by a suture.Than bronchus is dissected circumferentially, and care must be taken not to devascularize the trachea or left mainstem bronchus. Also subcarinal nodes must be completely removed to prepare the bronchus for division and closure. If the tumour is very proximal and encroaches on the azygos, the azygos arch is resected with the lung to provide better exposure of the origin of the right mainstem bronchus. If a right-sided double lumen tube has been used for lung isolation, which performed very rarely in this setting, the tube must be withdrawn into the trachea at this time. The right mainstem bronchus is then closed with a stapler, occluded distally with a bronchial clamp, and divided Fig. **1**.

An alternative to use of this stapled closure is application of a linear cutting stapler (*i.e.*, endoscopic stapler), which completely seals both ends of the cut bronchus and helps limit pleural space contamination as the bronchus is divided.

In patients in whom there is tumour close to the carina, the bronchus is divided at the carina without clamping across the tumour. The bronchus then is closed with interrupted absorbable sutures such as polyglactin.

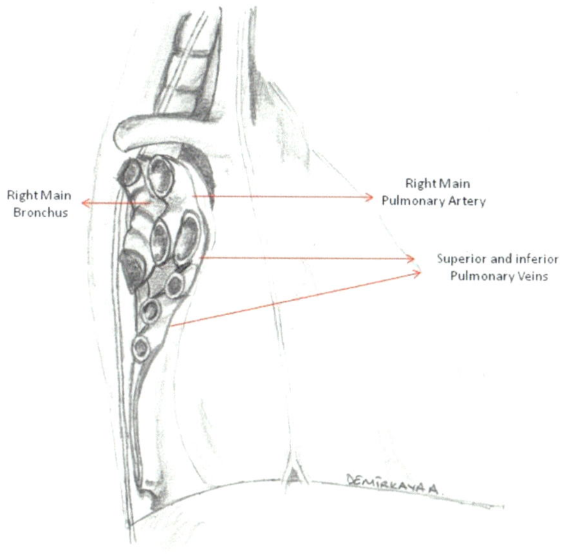

Figure 1: The anatomy of right main bronchus, artery and veins for pneumonectomy.

The stump can be covered with a flap of vascularized tissue to reduce the risk of stump leak. Pericardial fat, pleura, pericardium, azygos vein, and intercostal muscle can be utilized.

Pericardium must be closed after performing an intrapericardial pneumonectomy to avoid cardiac herniation in two sides. Primary closure is essential if possible, and also a patch can be used. Use of a small patch, such as expanded polytetrafluoroethylene [PTFE], prevents cardiac herniation and decreases the risk of pericardial restrictive effects in the immediate postoperative period.

Putting a drain in the pneumonectomy space is controversial. One advantage of a drain is that it may be used after the thoracotomy incision is closed to balance the mediastinum in the center of the chest. This is done by first positioning the still-intubated and sedated patient supine on the operating table. The pleural drainage system is placed at the level of the right heart and on water seal only. The contralateral lung is inflated and maintained at a constant airway pressure of about 30 cm H_20 for up to 10 seconds. After excess air is evacuated from the pneumonectomy space during this breath, the drainage tube is clamped before the inspiratory cycle is terminated. The drainage tube is then left clamped if there is not a tension hemothorax develops on the side of the pneumonectomy, which can be relieved by temporarily unclamping the chest tube but nevertheless requires urgent return to the operating room. Disadvantage of placing a chest tube is that there is increased risk of contaminating the pleural space, leading to postpneumonectomy empyema. Another technique to balance the mediastinum is to insert a catheter through the incision as it is being closed, the tube is placed under water seal and the patient is given a sustained breath as previously described. If the excess air has been evacuated, the tube is quickly removed and normal ventilation is resumed. If these techniques fail, an appropriate volume of air is insuflated or removed with the use of an angiocath as necessary to achieve the desired result.

Left Pneumonectomy

Left pneumonectomy generally is safer than right pneumonectomy in terms of overall perioperative postoperative mortality. However, the procedure may be technically more demanding, especially in patients with large hilar masses. Hilar tumours are truly in challenging territory adjacent to the main pulmonary artery, aorta, and esophagus.

These lesions can be near to the aortic arch, recurrent laryngeal nerve, phrenic nerve, pericardium, and the main pulmonary artery before it bifurcates into the right and left main pulmonary arteries (the intrapericardial portion of left main pulmonary artery is very short). The primary procedures are described separately to account for the varying anatomy and dissections used on the left and right sides. We then discuss factors that can complicate the procedure.

The left pulmonary artery is dissected circumferentially lateral to the ligamentum arteriosum. When tumour involves the left main pulmonary artery intrapericardially it is necessary to divide the ligamentum arteriosum and complete the circumferential dissection of the left pulmonary artery close to its takeoff from the main pulmonary artery. The vessels are occluded and divided using stapler or oversewing techniques.

The bronchus is dissected circumferentially at its origin, one should not devascularize the trachea. Traction on the lung and left mainstem bronchus is sometimes required to enable the dissection to be developed medially enough to reach the carina. Also subcarinal nodes must be completely cleared to prepare the bronchus for division and closure. Prior to applying a clamp or stapler to the bronchus, the surgeon must be sure that the endotracheal tube has been withdrawn into the trachea. The left mainstem bronchus is then closed with a stapler, occluded distally with a bronchial clamp, and divided Fig. **2**.

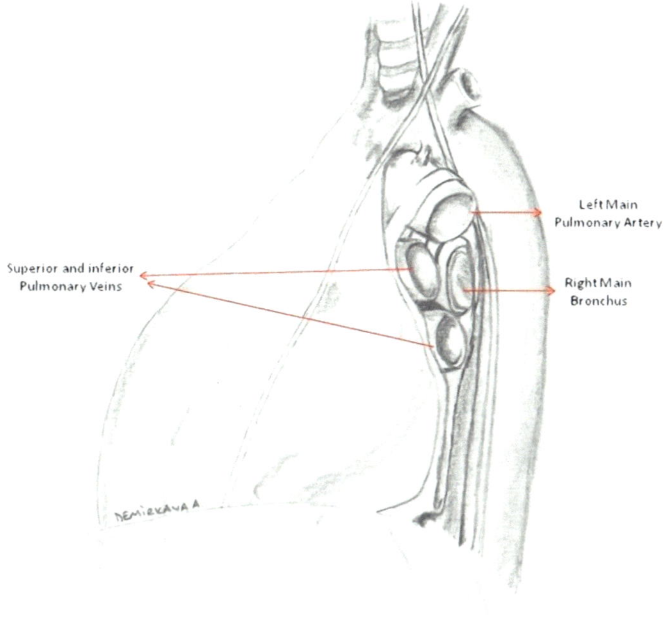

Figure 2: The anatomy of left main bronchus, artery and veins for pneumonectomy.

When a right pneumonectomy is performed, during which a left-sided double lumen tube is used for lung isolation, division of the bronchus and oversewing the proximal stump is straightforward because of continued isolation of the right mainstem bronchus. If a left-sided double lumen tube is used for a left pneumonectomy, withdrawing the tube into the trachea prior to division of the left mainstem bronchus results in loss of isolation of the left lung, and the majority of the ventilatory volume will flow through the opened mainstem bronchus. This situation is obviously untenable because of inadequate ventilation of the patient and because of the contamination of the left pneumonectomy space by airway secretions. As a result, closed management of the left mainstem bronchus is most appropriate. When the margins are close for a lung cancer resection, initial consideration should be given to use of a right-sided double lumen tube for managing the airway.

It is not usually required to cover the bronchial stump for the development of certain tissue flaps especially when it is compared with right pneumonectomy. As the mainstem bronchus is cut in the vicinity of the carina, the stump may sink back into the mediastinum once the bronchus is cut. Soft tissues that are attached to the stump are closed over the latter with interrupted sutures. In certain conditions (*e.g.* following induction chemotherapy or radiation therapy and in cases where the mediastinum is frozen and the stump does not retract) a pleural or pericardial fat pad flap can be introduced in order to support the closure of the stump.

On the other hand, the pericardium should be closed after a left intrapericardial pneumonectomy to avoid cardiac herniation since the left ventricle is more inclined to herniate even through minor pericardial defects. In order to reduce the risk of causing an iatrogenic restrictive process that is poorly tolerated in the postpneumonectomy patients, a patch can be used to close the pericardial defect. Once sufficient hemostasis is reached, the incision should be closed through the usage of one of the mediastium centering techniques that are summarized in the right pneumonectomy section.

Operative Mortality

The Lung Cancer Study Group published their detailed analysis on 30-day operative mortality for lung resections in a large population of lung cancer patients in North America, and stated that mortality of pneumonectomy should be less than 8% to comply with modern standards [5,6]. During the past decade, mortality rates below 5% have been reported [7,8,9]. Underlying lung disease, particularly chronic obstructive pulmonary disease, has been consistently shown to be a very important risk factor.

The type of surgical procedure appears to affect mortality. Patients undergoing pleuropneumonectomy are at increased risk for death. Completion pneumonectomy, as well, is also associated with a higher mortality rate. These statements are widely accepted because are based upon good sense. Conversely, the fact that patients undergoing a right-sided pneumonectomy have a higher mortality than those undergoing a left one has not always received great attention both in the past, and currently. Present day mortality rates for right-sided procedures range from 10 to 12%, while rates for left-sided procedures range from 1 to 3.5% [10].

ACKNOWLEDGEMENTS

Declared none.

CONFLICT OF INTEREST

The authors confirm that this article content has no conflict of interest.

REFERENCES

[1] Stanley C. Fell Special article: A brief history of pneumonectomy Chest Surg Clin N Am 2002; 12: 541– 563

[2] Boysen PG, Block AJ, Olsen GN, et al: Prospective evaluation for pneumonectomy using the 99m technetium quantitative perfusion lung scan. Chest 1977; 72:422–5,

[3] Boysen PG, Harris JO, Block AJ, Olsen GN: Prospective evaluation for pneumonectomy using perfusion scanning: Follow-up beyond one year. Chest 1981; 80:163–6

[4] Taube K, Konietzko N: Prediction of postoperative cardiopulmonary function in patients undergoing pneumonectomy. Thorac Cardiovasc Surg 1980; 28:348–51

[5] Pulmonary Procedures. Mark K Ferguson. Chapter 3 Thoracic Surgery Atlas Ed: Mark K Ferguson, Philadelphia 2007; 48-108

[6] Pierre Antoine Fuentes. Pneumonectomy: historical perspective and prospective insight. European Journal of Cardio-thoracic Surgery 2003; 23:439–445

[7] Ginsberg RJ, Hill LD, Eagan RT, *et al.*30-day operative mortality for surgical resections in lung cancer. J Thorac Cardiovasc Surg 1983;86:654–8.

[8] Mitsudomi T, Mizoue T, Yoshimatsu T, *et al.* Postoperative complications after Pneumonectomy for treatment of lung cancer: multivariate analysis. J Surg Oncol 1996;61:218–22.

[9] Harpole DH, Liptay MJ, DeCamp Jr MM, *et al.* Prospective analysis of pneumonectomy: risk factors for major morbidity and cardiac dysrhythmias. Ann Thorac Surg 1996;61:977–82.

[10] Wada H, Nakamura T, Nakamoto K, Maeda M, *et al.* operative mortality for thoracotomy in lung cancer. J Thorac Cardiovasc Surg 1998;115:70–3.

[11] Kopec SE, Irwin RS, Umali *et al.*The postpneumonectomy state Chest 1998;114:1158– 84

Send Orders of Reprints at reprints@benthamscience.net
Lung Cancer: Clinical and Surgical Specifications, 2013, 289-299

CHAPTER 10

Part F: Surgical Treatment Modalities for Pulmonary Metastases

Mustafa Yüksel* **and Hasan Volkan Kara**

Marmara University, School of Medicine, Department of Thoracic Surgery, Istanbul, Turkey

Abstract: Pulmonary metastasectomy has been widely used treatment modality in selected patients with pulmonary metastases due to primary tumour, initiated at some other site. Presence of any metastases in a view may yield an uncontrolled tumoural disease, isolated pulmonary metastases do not consistently represent a systemic or untreatable spread of a primary neoplasm. Making an appropriate surgical resection for isolated pulmonary metastases may help in patients' survival positively. Approach to pulmonary metastases including patient selection, surgical treatment modalities and outcomes of surgery will be discussed in this chapter.

Keywords: Pulmonary metastases, surgery.

INTRODUCTION

Though the combined treatment modalities in primary malignant tumours are improving the success for treatment, metastatic disease in the follow up period is possible risk for many of these patients [1]. Presence of any metastases in a view may yield an uncontrolled tumoural disease and may represent a rapid systemic progression of the malignancy. This may decrease trust about the curative potential of surgical resection of pulmonary metastases, this thought is still announced to be possible by some oncologists [2] Lungs are common places for some neoplastic situations. Pulmonary metastasectomy had become a popular treatment method in the end of 20th century for selected patients with pulmonary metastases due to another primary cancer [1]. Isolated pulmonary metastases do not consistently represent a systemic or untreatable spread of a primary neoplasm as thought so [3]. These patients are thought to have a more favourable tumour biology and much more susceptible to local and systemic treatment than patients with other multiorgan metastases [1, 3]. Improvement of surgical techniques and

***Address correspondence to Mustafa Yüksel:** Marmara University, School of Medicine, Department of Thoracic Surgery, Istanbul, Turkey; Tel: +90 216 6254545; E-mail: drmustafayuksel@gmail.com proven safety and efficacy of limited lung resections including pulmonary metastasectomy gained greater popularity [4, 5]. Depending on the current data of retrospective series, patients who have complete resection of all metastases have a longer survival than patients who have pulmonary metastases left behind. The evaluation and surgical treatment ways will be discussed in this chapter.

Background

The first resection of a single lung metastatis was performed in late 1882 by Weinlechner for a metastatic rib sarcoma, in which successful resection of the lung and the associated chest wall was performed [6]. Resection of multiple pulmonary metastases from a patient with osteochondromas was reported in 1952. Martini and co-workers, noted the value of multiple resections (multiple sequential operations) in the treatment of osteogenic sarcoma in 1971. In an autopsy series of the patients who died of any malignancies, the lung was found to be the second most common metastatic locus [6,7]. In the mid-1960s, resection of lung metastases was performed infrequently and only in highly selected patients in a few centres [3,8]. In the 1970s, experience from major thoracic surgical centres suggesting a proof for curative potential of metastasectomy was achieved in childhood osteosarcoma in which fatal lung metastases occurred in 80% of patients after amputation of the primary tumour [6]. The International Registry of Lung Metastases was established in 1991 and accrued 5,206 patients of pulmonary metastasectomy. The results of these analyzes showed that complete resection, short disease-free interval and single lesion in the lungs were favourable measurements for long term survival. This was a supporting data for the physicians to refer their patients with metastases in the lungs to surgical pulmonary metastasectomy [2].

Symptoms

In patients with pulmonary metastases, clinical symptoms rarely appears. Only very few (<5%) patients with metastases present with clinical symptoms like dyspnea, pain, cough, or hemoptysis secondary to bronchial or vessel erosion and mediastinal syndrome resulting from nodal metastases. This silent process makes early diagnosis much more important to plan any surgical intervention.

Diagnosis

Most pulmonary metastatic lesions are detected on the routinely performed chest X – rays in the follow up period, after the intervention towards the primary neoplasm. Thus these patients are generally asymptomatic as mentioned before [3].

Metastases in the lung parenchyma may appear as single or multiple nodules. They may be well-circumscribed or diffuse opacities, and they may be tiny or massive in appearance. Routine chest X-rays(CXRs) are very valuable for screening in the followup of these patients. But it should be kept in mind that any suspicious lesion in the lungs may also have the possibility for being a related diagnosis such as histoplasmosis, tuberculosis, or other malignant diseases such as lung cancer [1,5]. There are still no pathognomonic radiographic criteria for pulmonary metastatic disease. Computed Tomography (CT) of the chest is the current appropriate diagnostic procedure for clarifying the nature of any suspicious nodular density on the CXR [9]. Patients without any detected lesion on CXR may have a demonstrated lesion on CT. This provides a more sensitive but less specific examination than CXR for demonstrating the probable metastatic lesion.

Patients with known metastases on chest radiographs should undergo CT to identify the precise location of the known metastases and to identify other smaller, potentially occult metastases. Also CT provides a consistent anatomical reference for resection. CT may demonstrate nodules as small as 3 mm. When the patient is clinically correlated with the age, prior history of malignancy, and prior treatment, a clinical diagnosis of pulmonary metastases can easily be clarified [10].

Magnetic Resonance Imaging(MRI) may be as sensitive as CT scans for identifying pulmonary metastases but adds very little additional information, as observed by Feuerstein (1992) and Wyttenbach (1998) and their associates. Thus MRI is not performed in the presence of CT in the daily practice [9].

^{18}F-fluorodeoxyglucose (FDG) Positron Emission Tomography (PET) is a newer diagnostic method and can be used to identify patients with metastases. FDG – PET, could identify local and distant recurrence or metastases of any primary tumour (except brain).

All these diagnostic methods should be used in a complementary fashion to identify the extent of disease initially and during follow-up [8,11].

A solitary lesion which is seen on the CXR should be considered as a metastasis unless it histologically shows another diagnosis. The probability of a new primary tumour is related to the type and also to the stage of the previous cancer [8,9].

The surgeon must select the appropriate radiographic imaging or scanning techniques that will provide the necessary and complete clinical information required for treatment-planning decisions[1,8,10]

The technique chosen should be helpful in:

1. Identifying the size, location and characteristics of pulmonary metastases (nodules).

2. Characterising the solitary squamous cell carcinoma (or adenocarcinoma) metastasis from a primary NSCLC.

3. Evaluating for extrathoracic metastatic disease (other sites of hematogenous spread, metastasis to regional lymph nodes, or other tumours).

4. Evaluating the potential for local invasion.

Preoperative definitive diagnosis of the lesion may be done by fiber optic bronchoscopy, percutaneous needle aspiration biopsy or also thoracoscopy in some cases.

The role of mediastinal staging in pulmonary metastases is unclear and is not performed routinely preoperatively in the daily practice. Ercan *et al.* in their series defend the adverse effect of metastatic disease in regional lymph nodes on the survival and underlying the importance of complete lymph node dissection to better define their prognosis and potentially guide adjuvant therapy [4].

Treatment

In the treatment of pulmonary metastases, radiation therapy or chemotherapy is frequently used, inconsistent response rarely leads to consistent control or cure. Patients in whom the undercontrol primary tumour and metastases have been confined to the lungs, resection of all visualised or palpable metastases may be considered [6]. Complete resection of isolated pulmonary metastases is generally associated with improved patient survival regardless of primary histology [11].

Selection of Patients for Resection

Patients with isolated pulmonary metastases may be candidates for surgical resection. Clinical criteria have been proposed to identify and select patients who can benefit optimally from resection of their pulmonary metastases by McCormack (1978), Mountain (1984), and Pastorino (1997) and their co-workers as well as by the author (JBP) and Roth (1990) as follows:

1. Pulmonary nodules consistent with metastases
2. Control of primary tumour at the time of planned resection
3. All nodules potentially possibly resectable with planned surgery
4. Adequate postoperative pulmonary reserve anticipated
5. No extrathoracic other organ metastases

In patients being considered or planned for resection, a detailed physical examination including evaluation of cardiac and renal function is performed. Also sufficient lung reserve evaluation, radiographic examination, and physiologic assessment(primarily the lung capacity) are performed to estimate the extent of resection and to determine whether the planned procedure can be safely performed.

Surgical Approach

Posterolateral thoracotomy has been a standard and familiar surgical approach to pulmonary metastasectomies [1,8]. Posterolateral Thoracotomy may provide better exposure for metastases located more medially, or more posteriorly near the hilum on the left side. Also for patients with bulky metastases, a posterolateral thoracotomy provides good exposure thus accessing for faster resection and optimal sparing of lung parenchyma. Since 1990 limited skin incisions and muscle-sparing thoracotomies have become more popular. These procedures result in less functional damage of thoracic muscles and nerves, lessen post operative pain, enable earlier mobilisation of the patient and reduce pleural adhesions which would be facilitating any possible future reoperations. The surgeon is limited to operating in one hemithorax. For bilateral lesions, two sequential operations are performed, this may be done in one or two hospitalisation times. Bilateral thoracotomies are rarely performed at the same time, only there are some examples of left thoracotomy followed by median sternotomy in selected patients at the same operation time [1,12,13].

Median sternotomy incision is an alternative approach for resection of bilateral metastases. Here, both lungs can be examined at the same time, midsternal split prevents surgical damage of thoracic muscles, nerves and disruption of the chest wall parietal pleura and causes fewer pleural adhesions [13].

The advantage of this technique is that the lungs are sequentially deflated and can easily be palpated for the known and possible unknown masses. Metastases are identified and resected surgically. Exposure of the left lower lobe by median sternotomy may be difficult than the other lobes because of the overlying heart [14]. There are maneuveurs for better visualising the lung, as surgical packs behind the hilum of the deflated lung to elevate the parenchyma or an internal mammary artery retractor to expose basilar tumours or posterior hilar left lower lobe masses. In osteogenic or soft tissue sarcomas, median sternotomy is helpful exploration for lungs even in case of documented unilateral mass lesion. It has been demonstrated that 30 to 50 % cases with unilateral metastases sternotomy revealed bilateral metastases. Most cases of sarcomas can be operated by this medial approach but if a left lobe segmentectomy or lobectomy is required it may be difficult technically because mobilisation of the lung may trigger transient arrhythmias [8]. Relative contraindications for median sternotomy include; obesity, chronic obstructive pulmonary disease, elevated hemidiaphragm (particularly on the left), and cardiomegaly.

Patients with metastases involving the left hilum or the posterior or medial portions of the left lower lobe may benefit from bilateral staged thoracotomies, rather than median sternotomy [1,3].

Bilateral anterior thoracotomy with or without transverse sternotomy also called the *clamshell incision*, was described by Bains and co-workers (1994) [1,15]. This is a combination for advantages of sternotomy allowing access to both lungs and providing adequate exposure to all lobes of both lungs. For patients with numerous or centrally located lesions involving both lungs or with mediastinal adenopathies a sequential lateral approach may facilitate resection and prevent acute lung injury [14,15].

Video-assisted thorocoscopic surgery (VATS) uses high-resolution video imaging, and may be used for resection of pulmonary metastases. VATS gained popularity during the last decade of 20th century [3]. But majority of the thoracic surgeons believe to make a complete metastasectomy, for which palpation of the entire lung is essential. So its affectivity is limited on the surface of the lung. Lesions within the lung parenchyma may be missed. Creating adequate tumour free margins also requires palpation of the lesion so that the stapling device may be placed properly, open manual suture or precision dissection may better fit in size and location of the nodule. This challenging situation is discussed in an elegant study done by Mc Cormack and colleagues. In this prospective study using VATS in pulmonary metastasectomy, all patients underwent an open surgical technique following VATS intervention. In the result, more nodules were diagnosed in the open method and was noted that VATS failed to identify all the nodules [16]. At present, VATS can be advocated only for diagnosis and staging of the extent of the metastases for many surgeons [1,16]. Complications of a performed VATS may be failure to resect all metastases, positive surgical margins or pleural seeding with extraction of the metastases [8]. The advantages and disadvantages are summarised in Table **1**.

Laser-assisted pulmonary resection, using the neodymium:yttrium-aluminum-garnet (Nd:YAG) laser, may provide a better means of resecting pulmonary metastases than the surgical stapler. The advantage in use of the laser may enhance preservation of lung parenchyma with less distortion. Disadvantages of laser resection include longer operating time and potential for prolonged postoperative air leaks. Even some authors identified that the use of the laser reduced hospital stay, air leak and tissue loss; however, a survival advantage was not proved [1,8].

Table 1: Advantages and Disadvantages of Different Surgical Procedures

Surgical Procedure	*Advantages*	*Disadvantages*
Median sternotomy	Bilateral thoracic explorations done with one incision and one operating session Less patient discomfort.	Difficulty in resection of lesions posterior and medial (near the hilum) Difficult exposure to the left lower lobe in patients with obesity, congestive heart failure, or chronic obstructive pulmonary disease (increased thoracic anteroposterior diameter)
Transverse sternotomy or clamshell sternotomy	Bilateral thoracic explorations with one incision Good exposure to all aspects of both right and left thoraces Access to both right and left hila and to left lower lobe.	Larger incision Patient discomfort (postoperatively)
Posterolateral thoracotomy	Standard approach Excellent exposure of the hemithorax A second operation is needed for bilateral metastases.	Patient discomfort Only one hemithorax may be explored per operation
Video-assisted thoracic surgery(VATS)	Potentially less immunosuppressive Excellent visualisation (diagnostic) Excellent exposure for visceral pleural metastases May identify unresectable metastases, Extra-pleural disease, pleural studding, *etc.* Early postoperative mobilisation Less patient discomfort.	Unable to fully evaluate metastases fully in the lung parenchyma Late chest wall port recurrences Does not identify occult nodules

Techniques for Resection

The aim of lung metastasectomy is excision of all detectable lesions, allowing clear surgical margins and preserving as much healthy lung tissue as possible. The thoracic surgeon should palpate the lungs both in inflated and deflated phases to achieve macroscopically complete resection. A sublobar resection as wedge or atypical tangential resection is usually adequate [4]. A Frozen section may help to decide the proper volume of resection. For multiple metastases that are centrally located and larger solitary lesions suggestive of primary lung tumours, segmentectomy or lobectomy may be necessary to obtain a complete resection [3,8]. Pneumonectomy or other extended resections may be performed in patients with associated long term disease-free survival. Preoperative lung function test values should be adequate enough for a good quality of life after surgery. The rate of patients need to have extended resection is less than 3%. En bloc resections of chest wall, pericardiumor diaphragm during metastasectomy are still associated with satisfactory long-term survival.

Results of Surgery

Pastorino and colleagues had analysed 5206 patients with pulmonary metastases with the known largest group according to the results of survival for completely resected patients 36% for 5 years and 26% for 10 years (median survival 3 years) [2]. Incompletely resected patients 5 years' survival was 13% and 10 year survival only 7%. Different series mention about different adverse prognostic factors. These prognostic indicators are clinical, biological and molecular based depending on the patient and association with prolonged survival [1, 2, 18]. It has been mentioned that age, gender, histology, grade and location of the primary tumour, disease free survival, number of nodules on preoperative radiologic studies, unilateral or bilateral metastases, tumour doubling time, synchronous or metachronous metastases are the preoperatively evaluated indicators. Post operatively extent of resectability, technique of resection, nodal spread, number of metastases and location, re-resection post-thoracotomy disease-free survival, and overall survival may be additional criteria [4,12,14].

In resectable patients longer diasease – free interval, longer tumour doubling time and less number and solitary metastases are associated with prolonged postresection survival.

CONCLUSION

Pulmonary metastasectomy is a commonly used procedure in the treatment of a variety of primary solid tumours as they are diagnosed with pulmonary metastases

[3]. The most of the current data is from retrospective analysis of the series of patients. Technical aspects of pulmonary metastasectomy, such as the best surgical approach, the role of advantages and disadvantages of minimal invasive techiniques and mediastinal lympadenectomy are not clear for every clinician. Complete resection is the crucial characteristic associated with long-term survival regardless of primary tumour histology [17]. The fundamental biology of the neoplastic and metastatic process is unchanged by resection so surgery may not be helpful for prolonged survival to every patient. Improved adjuvant therapies or new novel strategies directed at biological and molecular events in life cycle of the metastatic cell may have a positive effect on the benefit of surgery [1,19,20].

There is still a need for more randomised prospective data about effects on the survival to convince some authors about the positive effect of metastasectomy. Combinations of chemotherapy and surgery may be considered and may offer more to the patients the potential for optimal local and systemic control of their disease process. Important selection of ideal therapy for patients with pulmonary metastases isolated to the lung requires multidisciplinary evaluation in all but the simplest of situations.

ACKNOWLEDGEMENTS

Declared none.

CONFLICT OF INTEREST

The authors confirm that this article content has no conflict of interest.

REFERENCES

[1] Putnam JB. Pulmonary Metastases.In: L. Franco, Putnam JB Advanced Therapy In Thoracic Surgery London B.C. Decker Inc. Hamilton 1998:117-125

[2] Pastorino U, Buyse M, Friedel G, *et al.* Long-term results of lung metastasectomy: prognostic analyses based on 5206 cases. J Thorac Cardiovasc Surg 1997;113:37–49.

[3] Putnam JB. Secondary tumours of the lung. In: Shields TW, LoCicero J, Ponn RB, eds. General Thoracic Surgery, 5th ed. Philadelphia: Lippincott Williams & Wilkins, 2000:1555–76.

[4] Ercan S, Nichols FC 3rd, Trastek VF, *et al.* Prognostic significance of lymph node metastasis found during pulmonary metastasectomy for extrapulmonary carcinoma. Ann Thorac Surg 2004;77:1786–91.

[5] Martini N, McCormack PM. Evolution of the surgical management of pulmonary metastases. Chest Surg Clin North Am 1998;8:13–27.

[6] Martini N, Huvos AG, Mike V, Marcove RC, Beattie EJ Jr. Multiple pulmonar y resections in the treatment of osteogenic sarcoma. Ann Thorac Surg 1971;12:271–80.

[7] Meade RH. A history of thoracic surgery. Springfield, IL: Charles C Thomas, 1961:194–7.

[8] Pastorino L. Pullmonary Metastases In:. Pearson, FG, Deslauriers J, Ginsberg RJ, Hiebert CA, McKneally MF, Urschel HC (eds). Thoracic Surgery 2nd edition Churchill Livingstone, New York, 1999:962-973.

[9] Feuerstein IM, Jicha DL, Pass HI, *et al.* Pulmonary metastases: MR imaging with surgical correlation—a prospective study. Radiology 1992;182:123–9.

[10] Pass HI, Dwyer A, Makuch R, Roth JA. Detection of pulmonary metastases in patients with osteogenic and soft-tissue sarcomas: the superiority of CT scans compared with conventional linear tomograms using dynamic analysis. J Clin Oncol 1985;3:1261–5.

[11] Pulmonary metastasectomy: a survey of current practice amongst members of the European Society of Thoracic Surgeons. Internullo E, Cassivi SD, Van Raemdonck D, Friedel G, Treasure T; ESTS Pulmonary Metastasectomy Working Group.J Thorac Oncol. 2008 Nov;3(11):1257-66.

[12] Putnam JB Jr, Suell DM, Natarajan G, Roth JA. Extended resection of pulmonary metastases. Is the risk justified? Ann Thorac Surg 1993;55:1440–6.

[13] Johnston MR. Median sternotomy for resection of pulmonary metastases. J Thorac Cardiovasc Surg 1983; 85:516–22.

[14] Roth JA, Pass HI, Wesley MN, *et al.* Comparison of mediansternotomy and thoracotomy for resection of pulmonary metastases in patients with adult soft-tissue sarcomas. Ann Thorac Surg 1986;42:134–8.

[15] Bains MS, Ginsberg RJ, Jones WG, *et al.* The clamshell incision: an improved approach to bilateral pulmonary and mediastinal tumour. Ann Thorac Surg 1994;58:30–32.(discussion 33).

[16] Girard P, Baldeyrou P, Le Chevalier T, *et al.* Surgical resection of pulmonary metastases. Up to what number? Am J Respir Crit Care Med 1994;149:469–76.

[17] McCormack PM, Bains MS, Begg CB, *et al.* Role of video-assisted thoracic surgery in the treatment of pulmonary metastases: results of a prospective trial. Ann Thorac Surg 1996; 62:213–6.

[18] Pastorino U, Buyse M, Friedel G, *et al.* Long-term results of lung metastasectomy: prognostic analyses based on 5206 cases. J Thorac Cardiovasc Surg 1997;113:37–49.

[19] Treasure T.Pulmonary metastasectomy: a common practice based on weak evidence.Ann R Coll Surg Engl. 2007 Nov;89(8):744-8

[20] Pfannschmidt J, Dienemann H, Hoffmann H Surgical resection of pulmonary metastases from colorectal cancer: a systematic review of published series. Ann Thorac Surg. 2007 Jul;84(1):324-38

Lung Cancer: Clinical and Surgical Specifications, 2013, 300-310

CHAPTER 10

Part G: Superior Sulcus Tumours

Mustafa Yüksel* **and Hasan Volkan Kara**

Marmara University, School of Medicine, Department of Thoracic Surgery, Istanbul, Turkey

Abstract: Superior sulcus tumours were first described by "a radiologist" Henry Pancoast. These rare tumours have typical presentation as causing "Pancoast-Tobias" syndrome. The management and outcome of superior sulcus tumours remained nearly unchanged in the last 40 years. Patients with, extrathoracic metastases, proven N2 disease, invasion of the superior and middle trunk of the brachial plexus, spinal canal, esophagus and trachea are not suitable for resection. All the diagnosed patients who do not have absolute contraindications for surgery should be evaluated for combined therapy including surgical excision.

In this chapter, we discussed the superior sulcus tumours with diagnosis, treatment and results with the current literature.

Keywords: Superior sulcus tumours, pancoast, surgery.

HISTORICAL

Dr. Henry Pancoast, "a radiologist", described an unusual but apparently a rare mass growth in the apical region of the lung in 1924 [1]. This was the first documentation of superior sulcus tumours in the literature. In 1932, including Pancoast [2] also Tobias [3] reported other groups of patients having notable features of the syndrome such as a characteristic and constant phenomenon of pain in the distribution of first and second thoracic spinal nerve, Horners Syndrome (composed of ptosis, meiosis and anhydrosis), minor and major destruction of ribs and vertebral infiltration with a lesion located at the apex of the lung [2,4].

This clinical situation is defined as "Pancoast –Tobias Syndrome". The most common cause of Pancoast –Tobias Syndrome is primary bronchogenic carcinomas. These tumours are known as *superior sulcus* or *Pancoast tumours* when they

***Address correspondence to Mustafa Yüksel:** Marmara University, School of Medicine, Department of Thoracic Surgery, Istanbul, Turkey; Tel:+90 216 6254545; E-mail: drmustafayuksel@gmail.com

Akın Eraslan Balcı (Ed)

involve the apex of the thoracic cavity and cause pain in the perscapular region or arm [5].

CLINICAL PRESENTATION

Superior Sulcus Tumours represent less than 5% of all bronchogenic carcinomas [6]. Until the 1950 s superior sulcus tumours were characteristically rapidly mortal [4]. Chardack and Mac Callum performed a lobectomy and chest wall excision followed by radiation therapy. This patient achieved a 5 year survival after the combined therapy following surgery [7]. In 1966, Paulson and *et al.* reported a group of 18 patients who had preoperative radiation followed by surgical resection of the superior sulcus tumour [8]. This radiosurgical approach became a standard approach in the management of superior sulcus tumours in the following years offering better disease control and survival to the patients.

The pain related to superior sulcus tumours may lead to a prolonged time period from its onset to definitive diagnosis. Thus, any patient having signs and symptoms evoking the involvement of the thoracic inlet should be evaluated quickly for diagnosis for any mass lesion and further availability of resectability if a tumour is found in evaluation.

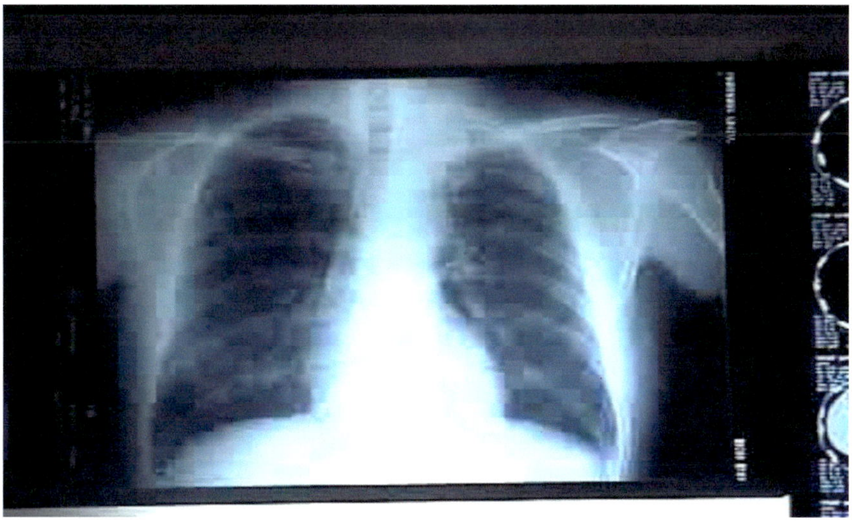

Figure 1: Chest X-ray of 63 year old male-patient (Patient 1) with superior sulcus tumour on the left hemithorax. The patient had the diagnosis of non small cell lung cancer by transthoracic fine needle aspiration biopsy.

The diagnosis is established by patient's history, physical examination, blood tests, chest X- rays, fiber optic bronchoscopy(FOB) and sputum cytology, fine needle transthoracic or transcutaneous biopsy and aspiration from any suspicuous lesion by using computed tomography (CT). Bone scan, and Magnetic Resonance Imaging(MRI) of the chest and Fluorodeoxyglucose Positron Emission Tomography (FDG-PET) and additional invasive diagnostic tools may be applied for staging thus determining the availability of surgical resection [9]. Also, patients should be evaluated by physical status including cardiopulmonary function tests.

In routinely performed chest X- rays superior sulcus tumours are peripherally located apical densities with speculations (Fig. **1**).

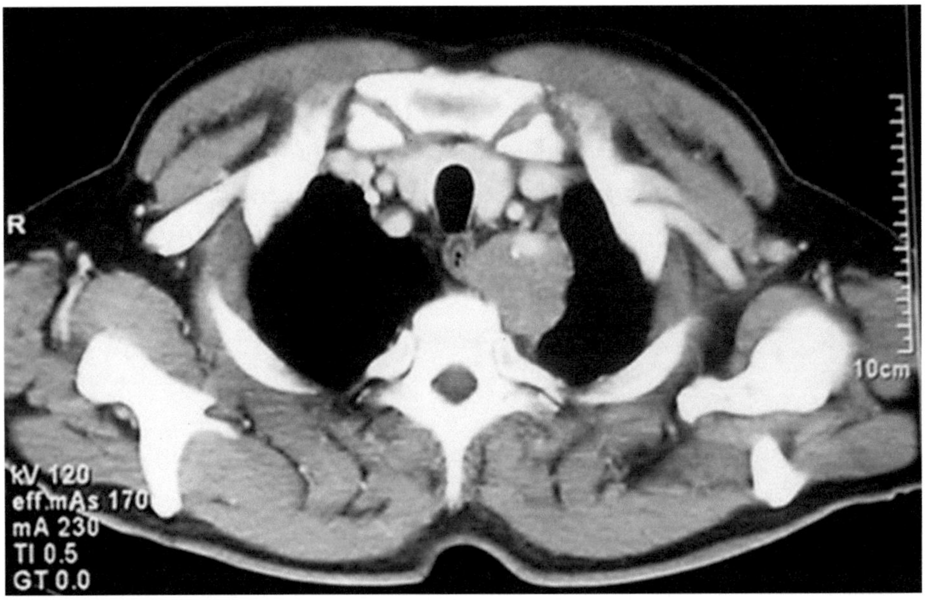

Figure 2: Pre operative MRI of Patient 1. The patient had 2 cycles of chemotherapy (CT) and, 5000 cGY Radiotherapy(RT).

They may even represent as a hidden lesion behind the clavicle and first rib. CT of the thorax is mandatory for visualising the lesion and also making fine needle aspiration biopsy [4] also abdominal CT is done to checkout any possible mass lesion correlated to metastases. Due to the positioning of the tumours, bronchoscopy and cytology are helpful in the diagnosis of only 10-20% of patients [10]. A video assisted thoracoscopy might be indicated to obtain tissue for definitive diagnosis if other method fails to do so, also visualising the presence of any pleural metastases. Mediastinal staging for any N2 disease is important and done by mediastinoscopy. Any proven N2 disease in this patient group is also known to have poor prognosis [2,11]. MRI of the chest and magnetic resonance angiography [12] are helpful to define the extent of the tumour and surgical resectability concerning involvement of branchial plexus, neural foramina, vertebral bodies and arteriovenous involvement [4] (Fig. **2**).

The use of PET in either mediastinal staging or defining distant metastases has the parallel conflicting and helpful results as the other non-small cell lung cancer cases (Fig. **3**).

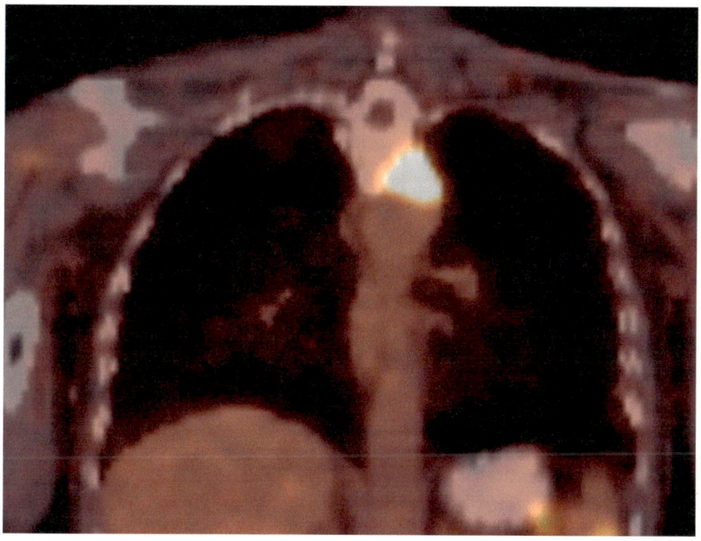

Figure 3: The PET-CT of Patient 1. 18x32 mm Lesion in left upper lobe in the posterior segment with a SUVmax value 5,1.

DIAGNOSIS

Surgical resection for superior sulcus tumours is generally limited to lobectomy. Resection also includes chest wall, involved adjacent structures. The only aim of the surgery is to establish a complete and en bloc resection with upper lung lobe invaded ribs, transverse processes, subclavian vessels, T1 nerve root, upper dorsal sympathetic chain and prevertebral muscles [13].

SURGICAL TREATMENT

Patients with, extrathoracic metastases, proven N2 disease, invasion of the superior and middle trunk (above T1) of the brachial plexus, spinal canal, esophagus and trachea are not suitable for resection [2]. Extensive involvement of the subclavian vessels is not a contraindication thus a complete surgical resection can be still anticipated and accepted [10].

As a general rule superior sulcus tumours that are not invading the thoracic inlet are completely resectable through the classical approach of Shaw – Paulson alone [5]. The lesion having a suspicion of any invasion of the thoracic inlet should be first explored by an anterior transcervical approach possibility, followed by the previous mentioned Shaw-Paulson approach to continue the resection [5]. The main goal of any chosen surgical approach in superior sulcus tumours is to make a complete resection with tumour free surgical margins.

General anesthesia using one-lung anesthesia greatly facilitates exposure within the chest. During the operation full monitoring is established by continuous recording of arterial blood pressure (arterial line opposite the lesion), oxygen saturation, cardiac rhythm, central blood pressure, urine output and at least 2 venous lines for volume expansion in case of need [15]. In posterolateral approach, known as "Shaw-Paulson" [14] the patient is placed in the lateral decubitus position with the affected side uppermost.

A long posterolateral thoracotomy incision is done from midway between the spinous process of the seventh cervical vertebra and posterior aspect of the scapula superiorly, like an arc between the thoracic spinous processes and the medial margin of the scapula that extends downwards 2 cm below the inferior angle of the scapula, ends just lateral to breast in women also 2 cm beyond scapula. This approach is quite satisfactory as mentioned before when dealing with posteriorly located tumours but it should be kept in mind that it is not fully adequate in the presence of invasion of anteriorly located structures (especially subclavian vessels and their branches) [16] (Fig. **4**).

According to the need of additional techniques different types of modified anterior approaches have been used by surgeons. These can be listed as:

Hemi-Clamshell incision or Trapdoor incision; as a partial sternotomy prolonged into an anterior thoracotomy [17]

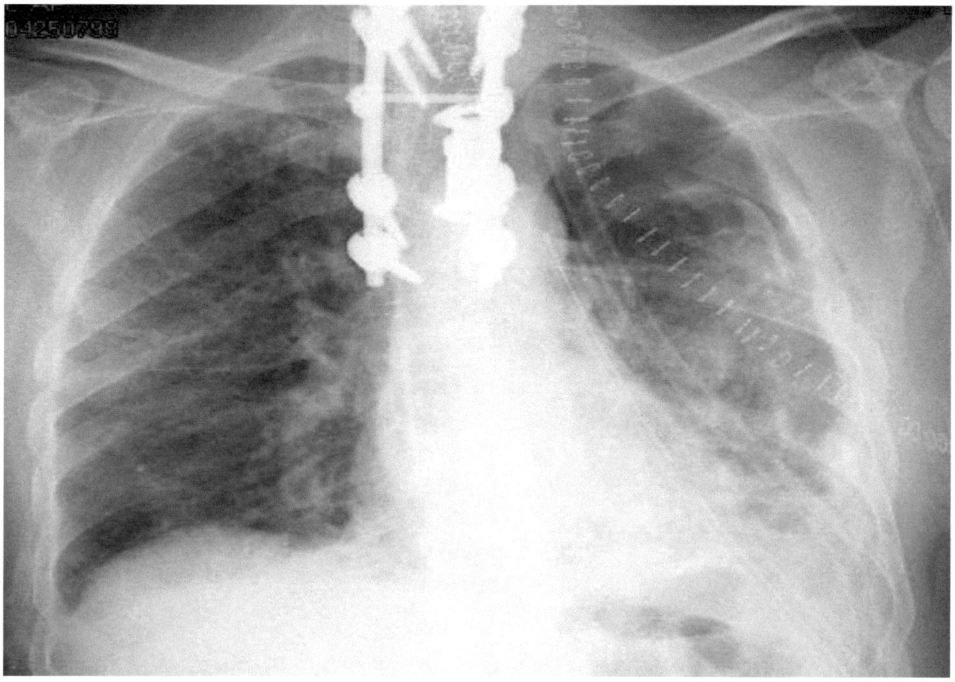

Figure 4: Post operative chest X –Ray of Patient 1. The patient had Rigid Bronchoscopy + Left Upper Lobectomy + Mediastinal Lymph node dissection + Hemivertebrectomy + Distractable Cage implantation and stabilization.

Masaoka incision; approximal median sternotomy continuing downwards with an incision in the anterior fourth intercostal space and upwards with a transverse cervical incision at the base of the neck [18]

Tatsamura incision; can be the approach for long tumours invading the thoracic inlet including an incision at the level of spinal process of the 2nd or 3rd thoracic vertebrae, it continues downwards along the paravertebral line and the tip of scapula and continues upward to the nipple level following the axillary line up to the level of sternoclavicular joint [19].

Also, *Dartevelle* described an *anterior transcervical–thoracic approach;* which involves an incision along the anterior border of the sternocleidomastoid muscle that continues laterally over the clavicle [5,6] (Figs. **5-6 and 7**).

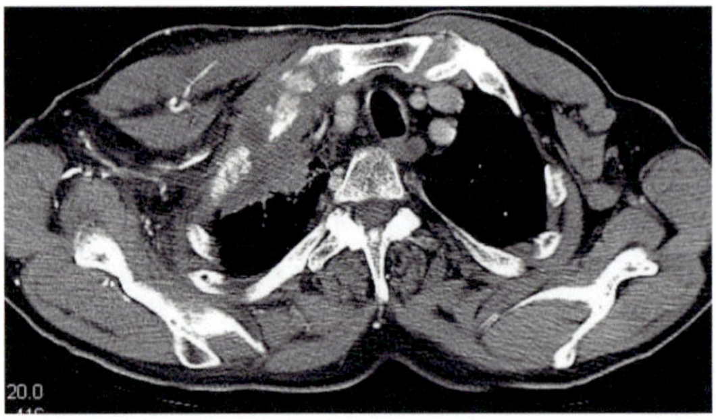

Figure 5: 56 Year old patient with right superior sulcus tumour of histologically documented NSCLC (Patient 2).

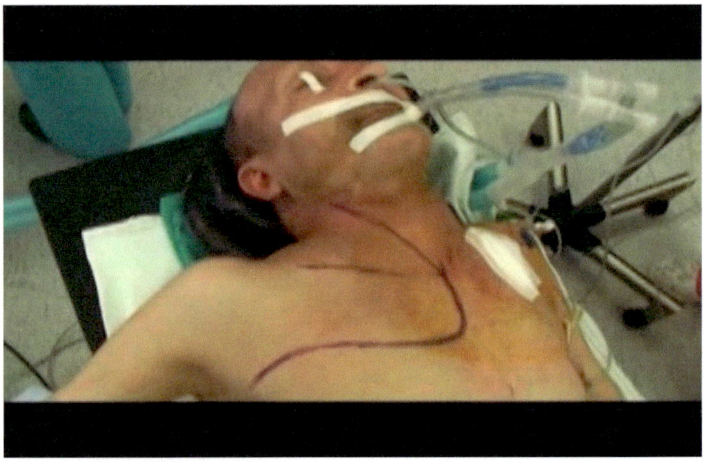

Figure 6: Patient 2 had Dartavelle incision an example of anterior approach.

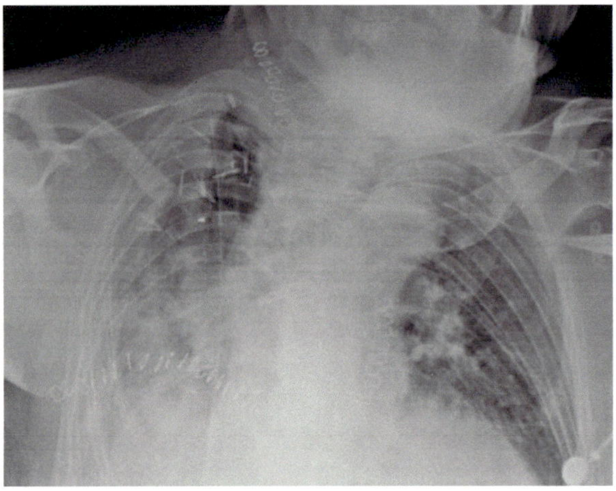

Figure 7: Post operative Chest X-Ray of Patient 2. The patient had en-bloc right upper lobectomy + 1-2. Rib resection + mediastinal lymph node dissection +chest wall reconstruction.

Despite the type of the approach for resections chosen the, main goal of the surgery is considering en bloc resection and excision of the following anatomical structures [15]:

1. Chest wall: Entire first rib and posterior parts of other involved ribs(most often the second and third ribs). Portions of upper thoracic vertebrae (up to one quarter of the body can be removed without undue stability) including the transverse process if needed. Removal of more than 3 ribs requires chest wall reconstruction generally.

2. Corresponding nerve roots up to the intervertebral foramen.

3. Portion of the lower trunk of the brachial plexus with sacrifice of the first thoracic nerve and usually with preservation of the 8th cervical nerver root.

4. A portion of the stellate ganglion and the thoracic sympathetic chain.

5. Pulmonary resection which is generally a lobectomy (lesser resection as wedge or anatomical segmentectomy shown to have a poorer survival).

6. Mediastinal lymph node dissection.

RESULTS

The well known common complications of the surgery are; Spinal fluid leakage, Horner's syndrome and nerve deficits, hemothorax and chylothorax. Atelectasis can be frequently seen in the postoperative course due to extended chest wall resection with or without phrenic nerve sacrificing. In the treatment of atelectasis to achieve complete lung expansion is mandatory. Tools used to perform this are: adequate ventilation using mechanical support, satisfactory chest tube function, pulmonary toilet (clearing of secretions) by mobilising, coughing, chest physiotherapy, nasotracheal, orotracheal, or bronchoscopic suctioning, or a temporary tracheostomy, adequate analgesia, and increase in transpulmonary pressure with incentive spirometry or continuous positive airway pressure mask.

If the subclavian vein has been resected, the ipsilateral forearm should be kept elevated to facilitate venous drainage and correct the edema, which usually disappears within 1 to 2 months [5,9].

OTHER TREATMENT MODALITIES

Radiation therapy(Radiotherapy) can be used as a single therapy and the results are poor. Radiotherapy prior to surgery has been proven to improve resectability, decreasing tumour seeding at surgery, blocking lymphatic channels(thus limiting potential metastases) and maximising local control [4]. The dose used per patient is between 30-45 Gy. Modern radiotherapy techniques have better results in multimodality therapy [4]. Also, alternative forms of radiation therapy with or without beam therapy can also be used. The techniques using brachytherapy [20] and intraoperative radiotherapy [21] have promising results in selected patients.

Chemotherapy has been used for palliation of patients with metastatic disease. Complete response rates are not high in non small cell lung cancer. The role of induction therapy prior to surgery or definitive radiation therapy [22], also in the setting with concurrent radiation therapy [23] is more clearly defined. Preoperative chemoradiotherapy has gained popularity in the recent time period [4,24].

The overall five-year survival rates after combined multimodality therapy range from 18% to 56% [9]. The best prognosis was achieved of patients without nodal involvement, T4 stage or Horner's syndrome and having a complete resection [5, 9,17, 25]. Despite the improvement in survival of patients with superior sulcus tumour treated with combined preoperative radiation and surgery there is still high incidence of local recurrence between 25% to 70%. Ginsberg and associates studied 69 patients with complete resections and with negative margins after preoperative irradiation. The first sign of recurrence was locoregional in two thirds of the cases and the incidence of distant metastases was from 40% to 80% [6,9].

CONCLUSION

For the 40 year time period despite the improvement in imaging, surgical technique, and the delivery of radiation therapy optimal management and survival continue to be major challenges [9]. The surgical approach could be adapted to the different clinical and radiological presentations in order to achieve a complete surgical resection which seems to be the most important positive prognostic factor in the survival [14]. Even recent medical tools made the diagnosis of Pancoast-Tobias syndrome easier and faster, this time period for diagnosis of the disease is still about 6 months [5]. All the diagnosed patients who do not have absolute contraindications for surgery should be evaluated for combined therapy including surgical excision. Optimal chemotherapy regimens and dose escalation in radiation therapy should be investigated more in prospective studies.

ACKNOWLEDGEMENTS

Declared none.

CONFLICT OF INTEREST

The authors confirm that this article content has no conflict of interest.

REFERENCES

[1] Pancoast HK. Importance of careful roentgen-ray investigations of apical chest tumours. JAMA 1924;83:1407–11

[2] Pancoast HK. Superior sulcus tumours. JAMA 1932;99:1391–6

[3] Kraut MJ, Vallieres E, Thomas CR Jr. Pancoast (superior sulcus) neoplasms. Curr Probl Cancer 2003;27:81-104.

[4] Archie VC, Thomas CR Jr. Superior sulcus tumours: a mini-review. Oncologist. 2004;9(5):550-5.

[5] Dartavelle P, Macchiarini P Optimal Management in the Superior Sulcus Tumours.In: L. Franco, Putnam JB Advanced Therapy In Thoracic Surgery London B.C. Decker Inc. Hamilton 1998:106-116

[6] Ginsberg RJ, Martini N, Zaman M, *et al.* Influence of surgical resection and brachytherapy in the management of superior sulcus tumour. Ann Thorac Surg 1994; 57:1440–1445

[7] Chardack WM, MacCallum JD. Pancoast tumour: five-year survival without recurrence or metastases following radical resection and postoperative irradiation. J Thorac Surg 1956;31:535-542.

[8] Paulson DL. The survival rate in superior sulcus tumours treated by presurgical irradiation. JAMA 1966;196:342

[9] Dartevelle P, Macchiarini P. Surgical management of superior sulcus tumours. Oncologist. 1999;4(5):398-407.

[10] Cavanaugh DG, Barry MJ, Knight JA *et al.* Diagnosis of superior sulcus tumours: a further use of the thoracoscope. MilMed 1993;158:577-578.

[11] Rusch VW, Parekh KR, Leon L *et al.* Factors determining outcome after surgical resection of T3 and T4 lung cancers of the superior sulcus. J Thorac Cardiovasc Surg 2000;119:1147-1153.

[12] Paulson DL. Technical considerations in stage III disease: the"superior sulcus" lesion. In: Delarue NC, Eschapasse H, eds. International Trends in General Thoracic Surgery, Volume I. Philadelphia: W.B. Saunders, 1985:121-133.

[13] Dartavelle P,Mussot S Anterior Approach to Superior Sulcus Lesion In: Shields TW, LoCicero J, Ponn RB, eds. General Thoracic Surgery, 6th ed. Philadelphia: Lippincott Williams & Wilkins, 2005:545-553

[14] Shaw RR, Paulson DL, Kee JL Jr. Treatment of the superior sulcus tumour by irradiation followed by resection. Ann Surg 1961;154:29–36

[15] Shamji F, Ginsberg RJ,Urschel H.C. Superior Sulcus Tumour In:. Pearson, FG, Deslauriers J, Ginsberg RJ, Hiebert CA, McKneally MF, Urschel HC (eds). Thoracic Surgery 2nd edition Churchill Livingstone, New York, 1999:1027-36

[16] Alifano M, D'Aiuto M, Magdeleinat P, Poupardin E, Chafik A, Strano S, Regnard JF. Surgical treatment of superior sulcus tumours: results and prognostic factors. Chest. 2003 Sep;124(3):996-1003.

[17] Bains MS, Ginsberg RJ, Jones WG *et al.* The clamshell incision: an improved approach to bilateral pulmonary and mediastinal tumours. Ann Thorac Surg 1994;58:30-33

[18] Masoaka A, Ito Y, Yasumitsu T. Anterior approach for tumours of the superior sulcus. J Thorac Cardiovasc Surg 1979;78:413–5.

[19] Tatsamura T, Sato H,Mori A, *et al.* A new surgical approachto apical segment lung diseases, including carcinomas and inflammatory diseases. J Thorac Cardiovasc Surg 1994;107:32–36.

[20] Hilaris BS, Nori D. The role of external radiation and brachytherapy in unresectable non-small cell lung cancer. Surg Clin North Am 1987;67:1061-1071

[21] Martinez-Monge R, Herreros J, Aristu JJ *et al.* Combined treatment in superior sulcus tumours. Am J Clin Oncol 1994;17:317-322.

[22] Dillman RO, Herndon J, Seagren SL *et al.* Improved survival in stage III non-small-cell lung cancer: seven-year follow-up of cancer and leukemia group B (CALGB) 8433 trial. J Natl Cancer Inst 1996;88:1210-1215.

[23] Curran W, Scott C, Langer D *et al.* Phase III comparison of sequential *vs.* concurrent chemo-radiation for pts with unresected stage III non-small cell lung cancer (NSCLC): report of Radiation Therapy Oncology Group (RTOG) 9410. Lung Cancer 2000;29(suppl 1):93.

[24] Rusch V, Kraut M, Hazuka M *et al.* Induction chemotherapy followed by surgical resection for non-small cell lung cancer involving the superior sulcus (Pancoast tumours): a phase II intergroup trial. Study protocol SWOG 9416 1995.

[25] Hagan MP, Choi NC, Mathisen DJ *et al.* Superior sulcus tumours: impact of local control on survival. J Thorac Cardiovasc Surg 1999;117:1086-1094.

Send Orders of Reprints at reprints@benthamscience.net
Lung Cancer: Clinical and Surgical Specifications, 2013, 311-322

CHAPTER 10

Part H: Interventional Bronchoscopy

Sedat Altin*

Erzincan University, Faculty of Medicine, Department of Chest Diseases, Turkey

Abstract: The field of interventional bronchoscopy includes several endobronchial treatment techniques that are used to relieve obstruction of the trachea and large bronchi secondary to either benign or malignant process. Balloon dilatation, endobronchial laser therapy, electrocautery, argon plasma coagulation, cryotherapy, photodynamic therapy, brachytherapy and stent application are all frequently used in the management of these disorders. Each technique has a unique set of characteristics that may make it the more or less appropriate modality to use for a specific patient and condition.

These procedures are performed using either rigid or flexible bronchoscopy depending on the particular patient and disease process involved, as well as the bronchoscopist's experience. Indications of interventional bronchoscopy are [1] malignant airway obstruction, [2] troubleshooting of benign airway obstruction, [3] foreign body aspiration, [4] hemoptysis, and [5] rarely the other applications.

Keywords: Interventional bronchoscopy, endobronchial treatment, malignant obstruction.

Interventional pulmonology can be defined as 'standard pulmonology added diagnostic and invasive therapeutic scientific applications'. To take in consider disease processes are; complex airway strategy problems, benign and malign central airway obstructions, pleural diseases and pulmonary vascular procedures [1,2].

Diagnostic and therapeutic procedures are rigid bronchoscopy, transbronchial needle aspiration, autofluorescence bronchoscopy, endobronchial ultrasound, transthoracic needle aspiration biopsy, laser bronchoscopy, endobronchial electrosurgery, argon-plasma coagulation, cryotherapy, airway stent applications, balon bronchoplasty and dilatation techniques, endobronchial radiation (brachitherapy), photodynamic therapy, percutaneous dialatation tracheotomy,

***Address correspondence to Sedat Altin:** Erzincan University, Faculty of Medicine, Department of Chest Diseases, Turkey; Fax: +90 212 5472233; E-mail: sedataltin@yahoo.com transtracheal oxygen catheter application, medical thoracoscopy and X-ray assisted procedures [1,2]. İnterventional brochoscopy, however, includes the part of those done with bronchoscope.

The history of interventional bronchoscopy is as old as the invention of rigid bronchoscope. Gustav Killian, otolaryngologist, had removed the first foreign body *via* translaryngeal way in 1897. Since then by this method applied to two patients, he published the method as direct bronchoscopy in 1898.

Killian had developed methal and silastic stent which would be used in state of stenosis as dilatation for foreign body which could not be removed because of granulation tissue. In 1914 using mesotorium he defined endoluminal brachytherapy in larynx cancer [3].

In 1962 while Ikeda had invented fiberoptic bronchoscope, he had inserted fiber illumunation channel into rigid tube by this way could be reached to distal airway. Ikeda had inserted lock system into the proximal tip of rigid bronchoscope and from here by passing fiberoptic bronchoscope he combined two systems [4,5].

In 1980's and 1990's, expectation in paliation of malignant airway obstruction with the incidence of inoperable lung cancer had increased. In this term JF Dumon and French pulmonologs seriously contributed to the use of rigid bronchoscope by airway dilatation, laser and stent insertion. Dumon also improved bronchoscopy systems, stents and stents applications used commonly around the world. He developed the rules of modern therapeutic bronchoscopy [4,5]. The main stone of interventional pulmonology is the rigid bronchoscopy. Rigid bronchoscopy supplies convenience for the extraction of foreign body, dilatation of tracheobronchial stenosis, ablation of tumour obstruction, treatment of massive hemorrhage and insertion of stent. Recently parallel to the increased interest in interventional pulmonology also brings the increase in rigid bronchoscopy [4]. For interventional bronchoscopy rigid bronchoscope is usually used for advantages in safe airway supply, large diameter operation opportunity.

Recent fiberoptics equipped with digital imaging and electricity isolation technology, intrabronchial applications -like laser, electrocauter, cryotherapy, argon plasma coagulation- supply also fiberoptic bronchoscopy, but rigid bronchoscopy has more advantages in therapeutic applications and well known by interventional bronchoscopist. Bronchoscopist should have experience to choose the most suitable method planned [5].

Even though bronchoscopy is mostly used in diagnostic purpose, recently interventional bronchoscopy applications are used for therapeutic purpose gradually increased rates. Also in Turkey endobronchial treatment units have been started in last 5 years, and this has provided benefit to Turkish medicine.

The most utilised application is endobronchial treatment methods, as mentioned it is also used for therapeutic purposes like extraction of foreign body, cleaning mucus plugs, controlling hemoptysis, therapeutic lavage application for pulmoner alveolar proteinosis, and sealing bronchial fistulas [6].

Selection of the method of endobronchial treatment changes according to the type of lesion, general, pulmonary and cardiac state of patient, emergency in the referred time, the stage of the disease and experience of the physician [7]. There are no randomised studies comparing each treatment method due to ethical values [8].

Histological type of the tumour, expectancy of life and answer to improve other treatment methods determine treatment of endobronchial malignities [9]. Stage of disease and performance status of patient are also the other indicatives in selection of treatment [10,11].

Interventional bronchoscopy is usually palliative which decreases or improves the symptoms for malignant lesions. Rarely in cases of early stage localised bronchial tumours or like typical carcinoid, lipoma can also show curative effect [11,12]. The cure of early lung cancer is still improving, but definite guideline is not yet available [8].

BASIC INSTRUMENTS

Rigid Bronchoscope: Owing to new modifications of rigid bronchoscope, it has become an ideal instrument in taking out large tumours in main airways, dilatation of tracheobronchial stenosis, laser bronchoscopy, inserting stents to airways and extraction of foreign bodies [13].

Fiberoptic Bronchoscope: By the help of flexible bronchoscopes which have larger working channel, bronchoscopists can take larger and more qualified biopsy specimens from airways by using larger biopsy forceps, balloon catheters, laser fibers and other instruments [6].

Equipment & Personnel

Only bronchoscopist is not enough. This team must contain at least two nurses, anesthesiologist, technician, and coorperation with pathology, chest surgeon and oncology is necessary. At least two bronchoscopes (one rigid, the other videobronchoscope), various forceps, brush, TBNA needles, different diameter stents are needed. Laser and/or electrocautery/argon plasma coagulation and cryotherapy devices are the parts for hot-cold applications. In advanced units, for evaluating the patient better, C-armed scopy, fluorescence bronchoscopy system and endobronchial ultrasound are also required systems.

The factors decreasing the complications are sufficient equipment and sterilisation, educated personnel, choise of proper patient, adequate sedation, premedication, anesthesia, and further monitoring and treatment after bronchoscopy. Interventional procedures should not begin without adequate equipment and experienced team, and patients must be sent to the reference centers.

INDICATIONS

I. Malignant Central Airway Obstructions

In principle, there are three kinds of malignant central airway obstruction [endoluminal, extraluminal and mixed obstruction]. The tumour expanding into airway lumen causes endoluminal obstruction; external compression extraluminal obstruction, and together mixed obstruction. The fourth one of central airway obstruction is usually tracheomalasia which is seen in benign diseases and consisted in the lack of cartilage support.

Endobronchial Treatment Methods

Endobronchial treatment methods which are still in practice are indexed in Table **1**. These methods, usually used separately, but in some cases some of them are used together.

Table 1: Endobronchial therapy methods:

■	Mechanic wash out with rijid bronchoscope,
■	Balloon dilatation,
■	Laser [Nd-YAG],
■	Criyotherapy,
■	Stent application,
■	Photodynamic treatment,
■	Brachitherapy
■	Argon plasma coagulation
■	Electrocautery

A. Dilatation of Airway

In proximal airways, using telescopes with gradually increasing diameters of rigid bronchoscope can be done. In fibrotic structures of distal airways, dilatation can be provided by fiberoptic bronchoscope which passed through balloon catheter blown up gradually with the help of syringe externally. The procedure should be done under fluoroscope. However, it gives quick recovery. Because of temporary benefit, it needs to be repeated. The success of balloon dilatation depends on the cause of stenosis, due to tumour of stenosis, effect is lots more. The main complications are chest pain during operation, bronchospasm after operation, atelectasis, airway laserasion or rupture of bronchus, acute hemorrhage and mucosal oedema.

B. Laser Therapy

The commonly used method in the treatment of endobronchial obstruction is laser application which is used in medicine for more than 40 years. In selected patients, laser therapy improves quality of life and functional status, also in some of them prolongs the survey. For protection of airway patency, it can be used electively or in emergency situations. According to the source of energy, CO_2, argon, diode, Nd-YAG and YAP type lasers are available commercially. The most commonly used one is Nd-YAG type. While low power Nd-YAG laser is used for tissue coagulation, the one with high power is for evaporation of tissue. Nd-YAG laser photoresection is very effective in relieving symptoms of cough, dyspnea and hemoptysis as well as in achieving endoscopic, radiologic, spirometric and quality of life parameters. This method prevents or delays improvement of respiratory insufficiency in patients with breathlessness. Due to the experience of user and factors of patients, laser is more applicable than rigid or fiberoptic bronchoscope.

C. Endobronchial Electrocautery

It is an electrical flow application which is used for coagulation or evaporation of tissues in tracheobronchial three. Electrocautery became an alternative to laser in treatment of lung cancer due to improvement of beter bronchoscopes, probes, electrodes and high freguency electrical generators. Because, the cost of equipment and maintenance is lower than Nd-YAG laser.

Complications in electrocautery are hemorrhage, temporary desaturation, cough, mucosal burnt and bronchoscope damage, but when applied by experienced bronchoscopists, the risks are lower.

D. Argon Plasma Coagulation [APC]

Between electrode and tissue, ionised argon gas is used as conducter. This method is ideal for superficial hemorrhagic tumours, unreached bronchial tumour in upper lobe segmentals and lower lob superior segmental bronchus. With isolated probes high frequency electrical generator is needed. There are many kinds of probes according to their shapes and polarite [monopolar *vs.* bipolar]. For the security of the patient and the team adequate isolation precautions should be taken. Isolated flexible equipments are also available. For APC, a special catheter is needed permitting argon gas and electrical flow pass. This catheter is not used in electrocautery with direct tissue touch. Indications are same as laser. This method is safer and has less side effects than laser in obstructive endobronchial lesions causing pneumonia and symptoms like dyspnea and cough.

E. Cryotherapy

Cryotherapy when applied in extremely low temperatures (-20 to -40 ^{o}C) causes local tissue destruction. It has four different efficacy mechanisms: 1.Intracellular dehydratation 2. Mechanic cellular destruction, occurs fast refregerations and slow dissolution 3. Intracellular ice crystals, besides protein and enzymes, Forming intracellular ice crystals damage mitochondria and endoplasmic reticulum which are intracellular organelles. 4. In slow flowing venule vasoconstruction and formation of micro thrombosis hence devascularization causes cell death.

Cryo apparatus consists of one panel, one cryo probe and nitrogen tube. Special designed and sometimes rigid, semi-rigid or flexible cryoprobe liquid cryogen or refrigerant gas [usually nitric oxide or nitrogen]is given. While rigid or semi-rigid cryoprobes are used only with rigid bronchoscope, flexible ones can be used either fiber or rigid. Generally area frozen by rigid probe is wider, and removing probe from tissue is easier. The gas frequently used in cryotherapy and commercial availabe is nitric oxide.

F. Brachytherapy

Endobronchial brachytherapy is a local with radiation treatment method which temporarily applied to the tumour or near radioactive source with capsule. Brachytherapy needs cooperation with radiation oncology and pulmonology.

G. Photodynamic Treatment [PDT]

PDT is a two phase procedure which sensitizes the substance, known as dihematoporfirin eter/ester [DHE: Photofrin II], applied intravenously and used as laser beam. It is a treatment option depending on the chemical photosensitizer to stimulate tumour tissue with appropriate light corresponding to the absorption band of the 630 nm wavelength. Photodynamic reaction which causes cell necrosis, free oxygen radicals and forming cytotoxic agent performes cell death.

DHE is administered to the tumour and then kept waited for six hours. Because DHE is purified from lung, reticuloendothelial tissues and skin cells in 6 hours, after that the tumour is expose to laser beam which has 630 nm wavelength with a flexible bronchoscope. DHE when directly stimulated with this wavelength, released superoxide and hydoxide radicals destroy the tumour. Usually 2-4 days after operation application zone is cleaned by bronchoscope.

For the lung cancer bronchoscopic PDT performes a two stage procedures, respectively name photosensitization and illumination.

Precondition for bronchoscopic PDT is bronchoscopically reach malignant endobronchial lesion which is corrected by cytologically for illumination. While patients with superficial bronchus, cancer is used for curative, in late staged patients who haven't had the choice of operation or external radiotherapy as paliation. It is contraindicated in patients who have photosensitive allergy.

H. Tracheobronchial Stents

If we make a general definition, stent is a tube shaped device that consists of methal wire, plastic rubber [usually silicone] or combination of two [hybrid or combined stent], and that is used for opening airway obstructed partially or strictured, supporting weak cartilage [tracheomalasia] or sealing the fistula. Especially they are mechanical support devices that provide airway integrity due to barrier effect of stent in the situations that decrease or remove the patency of airway as external compress. They are in polymer, methal or hybrid character, with straight, J and Y shaped, various diameter and length prepared according to airway. They can be inserted according to the type of stent by rigid and fiberoptic bronchoscope. Enhanced download and guidance systems are available for convenient insertion. Airway stents or tracheobronchial prothesis are used to treat obstructive lesions in trachea, main bronchus and lober bronchi. You must keep in mind that the application is not therapeutic, it is a mechanic paliation.

In USA more than 500.000 bronchoscopies are made per year and 15000 tracheobronchial stent are inserted over the world. In our country it has been known that about 45.000 bronchoscopic operations are made and about 400 stents are inserted.

Occasions of stent application:

1. Extrensic bronchial compression or submucosal disease.
2. Endobronchial obstruction > 50 % after bronchoscopic laser treatment.
3. Recurrence although repeated laser therapy and aggresive endobronchial tumour growth.
4. Lacking of cartilage tissue due to tumour destruction.
5. Sealing oesophageal and tracheobronchial fistula.

II. Troubleshooting of Benign Airway Obstruction

Postentubational tracheal stenosis is the most common type of tracheal stenosis, and gradually increases. Excluding PDT, the other endobronchial techniques can be used for treating benign tumour, obstructive granuloma and airway obstruction due to stenosis. Laser and electrocautery are often used to treat benign endobronchial lesions like hemongioma, lipoma, myoblastoma, chondroma, leiomyoma, histiocytoma and hamartoma. Intervention with laser, APC, electrocautery and criyotherapy can be easily done to endotracheal entubation, foreign body, tracheostomy tube, transtracheal oxygen catheter, suture material and symptomatic obstructive granuloma due to inflamatory diseases like Wegener granulomatosis or sarcoidosis [5,6].

Treatment of subglottic and tracheal stenosis still is an argued subject between pulmonologists and chest surgeons. Non-surgical interventional procedures like bougie dilatation, electrocautery, cryotherapy and laser can cause mucosal trauma, repeat stenosis and prolonge recovery duration.

Although done successfully laryngotracheal resection or reconstruction, can cause damage in vocal cords. Because of this, in treatment of subglottic tracheal stenosis, our approach is dilatation of region with angioplasty balloon catheter in proper diameter and together laser or electrocautery which removes damaged tissue from mucosa. With careful patient choice and meticulous patient care, success of the operations increases. If stenosis is refractory although repetition of the treatment at least three times, surgical intervention is suitable.

III. Foreign Body Aspiration [FBA]

Foreign body aspiration constitutes an essential subject of therapeutic bronchoscopy. Foreign body aspiration in airway, especially seen in childhood and fateful problem. The most common one is vegetable food aspiration especially peanut aspiration. Except this, pieces of toys are frequent aspirated bodies. FBA relatively rarely seen in adults. Adults often aspirate pin, hairpin, nail, denthal protesis and piece of food. The main goal in FBA is to prevent the body from going more peripherally.

Obstruction of bronchus due to FBA leads to more complications like asphyxia, haemoptysis, postobstructive pneumonia. They may cause granulation tissue.

Extraction of FBA usually depends on bronchoscopic techniques. Although no controlled studies comparing fiberoptic and rigid bronchoscope, rigid one is preferred. If fiberoptic brochoscope will be used for diagnostic or therapeutic purpose, it should be done under conditions of rigid bronchoscopy system. Because rigid bronchoscope has wider working channel and ventilation facilities, it provides the usage of more stronger hand instrument by patient safety. During operation you need to take care not to push the foreign body to distal airways and break it up.

In situation that foreign body is larger than the diameter of rigid scope, foreign body strongly held with forceps can be extracted with bronchoscope. Body must be extracted orally. In intubated patients if body cannot be immobilized, removing can be done together with the tube.

IV. Hemoptysis

Hemopytsis is a serious problem that has the potential to cause quick death. The most important factors determine the result are hemorrhage velocity and patient's cardiopulmonary state. Bronchoscope can be used either for diagnose and evaluation or therapy. Fiberoptic bronchoscopy is feasible as main diagnostic tool in minimal hemoptysis, but it must kept in mind that there is a possibility of hemorrhage during the operation. Because massive hemoptysis tends to give vital results, one must, as soon as possible, pass to rigid bronchoscopy. When it is thought that only 150 ml hemorrhage is enough for filling up trachea, right and left main bronchus, in severe hemorrhage fiberoptic bronchoscope profits only to decrease this volume [4].

Rigid bronchoscope, on the one hand maintaines guarantee of airway patency, on the other hand prevents easily fill up the airway due to larger aspiration possibility. Vision loss is possible in rigid bronchoscopy due to optic use but telescope can easily be cleaned. Although rigid tube itself facilitates to tamponade bleeding airway, it makes it possible to apply like adrenalin immersed gas, sponge from present patency. Although aspiration with bronchoscope, lavage with icy and adrenalin added serum physiologic, acute bleeding which occurs after interventional bronchoscopy or identifiable source by occluding the related segment bronchus orifice with tip of bronchoscope or Fogarty catheter for a short time [4-5 minutes] can control the hemoptysis, for local bleedings caused by endobronchial tumours electrocautery, ND-YAG laser or APC can be used.

V. The Other Applications

The most common use of bronchoscopy for therapy is to clear mucous plugged and secretions due to respiratory muscle weakness [postoperative period, neuromuscular disease] and/or some patients of ventilator bundle. Bronchoscopic toilet must be done in patients not excreted secretions and improved athelectasis through respiratory physiotherapy. In cases with pulmonary alveolar proteinosis for washing proteins and lipids collected in lungs mechanically, each lung is washed with 20-30 litre serum physiologic by inserting double-lumen tracheal tube under general anesthesia. Therapeutic lavage can be done for washing tenacious secretions in patients with ABPA and cyctic fibrosis, hence by inserting catheter for therapy of lung abcess. By using fiberoptic bronchoscope bronchoplevral fistula diagnose and seal can be done. Fibrin adhesives like gelform, tissue adhesive, autolog blood clot, cryoprecipitate, thrombin injections are materials used for fistula sealing. Bronchoscopic methods are successful in fistulas smaller than 3 mm while surgical intervention is needed in fistulas bigger than 8 mm [5].

CONCLUSION

Bronchoscopic techniques like laser, electrocautery, argon plasma, cryotherapy, photodynamic therapy, brachytherapy and stents are effective tools in the palliation and local control of lung cancer. Therapeutic bronchoscopy is not only effective in relieving dyspnea, controlling hemoptysis, and improving the quality of life, importantly it also avoids the need for mechanic ventilation in patients with respiratory distress, facilitates weaning from mechanic ventilation and allows time for the institution of radiotherapy and chemotherapy.

ACKNOWLEDGEMENTS

Declared none.

CONFLICT OF INTEREST

The author confirms that this article content has no conflict of interest.

REFERENCES

[1] Seijo LM, Sterman DH. Interventional pulmonology. N Engl J Med 344:740–749; 2001.
[2] 2.Wahidi MM, Herth FJF, Ernst A. State of the art: interventional pulmonology.Chest; 131:261–274, 2007.
[3] Prakash UBS. Advances in bronchoscopic procedures. Chest 116: 1403-8; 1999.
[4] Gorden JA, Wood DE. Rigid bronchoscopy. In Thoracic Endoscopy: Advances in Interventional Pulmonology.In.Simoff MJ, Sterman DH, Ernst A. Blackwell.Massachusets. 121-133; 2006
[5] Miyazawa T, Miyazu Y, Iwamato Y. Interventional Flexible Bronchoscopy. In Interventional Pulmonary Medicine.Lung Biology in health and disease. Ed. Beamis JF, Mathur P, Mehta AC.Markel Deccer.Newyork Basel, 33-48; 2004.
[6] Lee P, Mehta AC. Theurapeutic Flexible Bronchoscopy: Overview. In Interventional Pulmonary Medicine.Lung Biology in health and disease. Ed. Beamis JF, Mathur P, Mehta AC.Markel Deccer.Newyork Basel, 49-88, 2004.
[7] Ernst A, Simoff M, Ost D, *et al.* Prospective risk-adjusted morbidity and mortality outcome analysis after therapeutic bronchoscopic procedures:results of a multiinstitutional outcomes database. Chest; 134:514–519, 2008.
[8] Levine DJ, Angel LF. Role of the interventional pulmonologist. Clin Pulm Med 13[2]; 128-141, 2006.
[9] Sohrab S, Mathur PN. Management of central airway obstruction. Clin Lung Canc; 8:305–312,2007.
[10] Bolliger CT, Mathur PM, Beamis JF, *et al.* ERS/ATS statement on interventional pulmonology. Eur Respir J; 19: 356-373, 2002.
[11] Ernst A, Silvestri GA, Johnstone D. Interventional pulmonary procedures:guidelines from the American College of Chest Physicians. Chest; 123:1693-171, 2003.
[12] Unger M. Endobronchial therapy of neoplasms. Chest Surg Clin N Am;13:129–147, 2003.
[13] Lamb C., Beamis JF. Rigid bronchoscopy: An interventional tool with a history and a future. In Interventional Pulmonary Medicine.Lung Biology in health and disease. Ed. Beamis JF, Mathur P, Mehta AC.Markel Deccer.Newyork Basel.13-32; 2004.
[14] Altın S. Bronchoskopy unit and patient monitorisation-report systems. In Bronkoskopi Ed. Metintas M.Poyraz Yayıncılık, Ankara, 35-45, 2008

CHAPTER 10

Part I: Carcinoid Tumours of the Lung

Altuğ Koşar[1,*], Alpay Orki[2], Tülay Kayacan Örki[3] and Bülent Arman[2]

[1]Dr. Lütfi Kirdar Research and Training Hospital, Department of Thoracic Surgery, Istanbul; [2]Maltepe University School of Medicine, Department of Thoracic Surgery, Istanbul and [3]Kartal Koşuyolu Cardiovascular Surgery Research and Training Hospital, Department of Anesthesiology, Istanbul, Turkey

Abstract: Bronchial carcinoid tumours were in the past defined as benign and classified as "bronchial adenomas". Currently bronchial carcinoid tumours are considered to be part of a spectrum of malignant neoplasms with neuroendocrine differentiation. Bronchial carcinoid tumours are classified by pathologic features as typical carcinoid tumours or atypical carcinoid tumours with different clinical course prognosis. The most common symptoms are cough, hemoptysis and recurrent pulmoner infection. Paraneoplastic syndromes are uncommon and include Carcinoid syndrome, Cushing's syndrome, and ectopic growth hormone-releasing hormone secretion. Bronchial carcinoid tumours are generally central location for this reason being visible by bronchoscopy. Endobronchial biopsy *via* bronchoscopy is safe, with a very low risk of bleeding. Atypical carcinoid tumours affected preferentially patients older than typical carcinoid tumours and demonstrated a more aggressive oncological behaviour with a high percentage of nodal involvement and distant metastases. The primary treatment is complete surgical resection (especially parenchyma-sparing procedures for typical carcinoid tumours) and formal mediastinal lymph node dissection. Long term prognosis is excellent in typical carcinoid tumours, although it is worse in atypical carcinoid tumours.

Keywords: Bronchial carcinoid, Neuroendocrine lung tumours, Bronchoplastic procedures.

HISTORY

Bronchial carcinoid tumours which were once considered as benign and classified as "bronchial adenomas" are now accepted as malign tumours. Earliest records of bronchial carcinoid tumours were reported by Heschl in 1877 and Mullen in 1882.

***Address correspondence to Altuğ Koşar:** Dr. Lütfi Kirdar Research and Training Hospital, Department of Thoracic Surgery, Istanbul, Turkey; Tel: +90 216 4413900/2480; Fax: +90 216 3520083; E-mail: altugkosar@yahoo.com

Initially, detailed pathological studies of these tumours were conducted by Lubarsch in 1888 [1]. In 1907, Oberndorfel highlighted similarity of bronchial carcinoid tumours lung cancer and therefore suggested the name "Carcinoid", which means similar to carcinoma [1,2]. Contemporary information traces back to Hamperl's typical and well-differentiated definition of 1937. Additionally, Hamperl also determined similarities between bronchial carcinoid tumour and its equivalents in the gastrointestinal system [1,3]. In 1944, Englebreth-Holm and in 1951, Von Albertini depicted a group of bronchial carcinoid tumours having malignant histological structure and displaying aggressive prognosis [4]. Further, in 1972 Arrigoni for the first time defined a group of carcinoid tumours that displayed extremely aggressive behaviour and had worse prognosis than other carcinoid tumours as "atypical carcinoid tumour" [5].

CLINICAL MANIFESTATION

Over 80% of carcinoid tumours stem from the gastrointestinal system. Furthermore, they might be present in the lung, thymus, parotid gland, liver, bile ducts, pancreas, ovarium and testicles. Bronchial carcinoid tumours are malignant tumours with an annual incidence of approximately 2.3 to 2.8 cases per 1 million population. They comprise 25 % of all carcinoid tumours, but account for 2% to 5% of all primary lung cancers. While bronchial carcinoid tumour is rare during the childhood period, it is the most common one among the primary pulmonary tumours during childhood [6,7]. Bronchial carcinoid tumours do not show a strict correlation with tobacco use, and the survival rate does not show any difference between smokers and nonsmokers. However, some authors indicate a possible association between atypical carcinoid and smoking [8].

Despite the gender distribution being equal, publications in which it is dominant for both genders have been reported. Even though the age limit includes a wide range varying from young people to the old (range, 4 to 86), generally the age in which 90% of the cases are seen is below 50. Median age is between 30 and 40 [9,10].

PATHOPHYSIOLOGY

Etiology of the bronchial carcinoid tumours is still ambiguous and difficult to prove. No relationship has been found between the environmental factors and being exposed to known carcinogens. Possible etiologic cells are shown in Table **1** [11].

Table 1: Possible Etiologic Cells

1	Amine Precursor Uptake and Decarboxylate (APUD) cells migrating from neural crest.
2	Kulchitsky cells.
3	Argentaffin cells in bronchial mucus glands.
4	Neuroendocrine undifferentiated epithelial stem cells originating from the bronchial layer.

Recently, the bronchial carcinoid tumours that stem from the undifferentiated epithelial stem cells originating from the bronchial layer have gained importance.

All classification systems prepared for bronchial carcinoid tumours consider the spectrum of this disease and include the evolution of a more normal histological process over a transition phase to a higher undifferentiated cell group. The classification of bronchial carcinoid tumours can be seen in Table **2** [11-13].

Table 2: Classification of Neuroendocrine Tumours

New Classifications	**Old Classifications**	
Typical carcinoid	Bronchial	KCC-I
Atypical carcinoid	Well-differentiated Neuroendocrine Carcinoma	KCC-II
Large-Cell Neuroendocrine Carcinoma	Intermediate Type Neuroendocrine Carcinoma	KCC-III
Small-Cell Lung Cancer	Small Cell Type Neuroendocrine Carcinoma	

KCC: Kulchitsky cell carcinoma

Large cell neuroendocrine carcinoma (intermediate type neuroendocrine carcinoma), which has been recently defined, displays behaviour in between being atypical carcinoid and small cell carcinoma.

Despite the fact that sub-groups of all bronchial carcinoid tumours are comprised of the same type of cell, the definition of the progression remained considerably vague. Paladugu reported that progression of KCC-II's (atypical carcinoid) to KCC-III (small cell carcinoma of the lung) is manifested in 10% of the cases [13].

Typical Carcinoid Tumours: This type of tumours mostly emerge in younger age group (median age:45). Most of them are centrally localised. 20% being in the main bronchi, approximately 60 % in lobe bronchus or segment bronchus and 20% located in the periphery. Location in carina and trachea is infrequent and finding multiple or multicentric typical carcinoid tumour is rare [8].

While a few typical carcinoid tumours display bulky structure, most of them are non pedunculated and attached to the tissue below. Most of the tumour bulk grows along the outside of the lumen of the bronchus, towards the inside of the lung parenchyma and lymph node. This type of carcinoid tumours are named as "*iceberg tumour*" [14,15].

Typical carcinoid tumours have well-differentiated, significantly eosinophilic organised cells with clear cytoplasm and granular chromatin, which are round, arranged as bird's nest, bow tie or trabecular way, made up of an organic pattern composed of frozen cell. These rounds and bow-ties are separated from each other by a connective tissue stroma comprising rich capillary mesh. There is no increased mitotic activity and they are rich in vessels. They are seen closely packed with desmoid cells, being small in order. Fragile fibrovascular stroma of the typical carcinoid tumours might be exposed to intense hyalinisation and sometimes bone metaplasia. Grossly, these are the reddish tumours with multi-vessels covered with intact epithelium [1,16,17].

Lymph node metastasis is only seen in 10-15% of the patients with typical carcinoid tumour [8,18,19].

Atypical Carcinoid Tumours: This group of tumours displaying malignant histological appearance and aggressive behaviour emerges in old age group on the contrary to the typical carcinoid tumours (median age:55). Several studies evaluating smoking history have found that approximately a third of patients present with typical carcinoid tumours, whereas 60 to 80% of patients with atypical carcinoid tumours. Again on the contrary to typical carcinoid tumours, 50% of these tumours are peripherally localised. Approximately 10% of the carcinoid tumours are comprised of atypical carcinoid tumours [3,20-22].

Atypical carcinoid tumours have some of the structural characteristics of typical carcinoid tumours. However these are high grade tumours with higher degree of nuclear and cytological polymorphism, increased mitotic activity, even comprising haemorrhage and necrosis areas. It might be difficult to differentiate them from small cell carcinoma [10,11].

Lymph node metastasis or distant metastasis between 50 to 75 % is seen in patients with atypical carcinoid tumour [3].

Both typical carcinoid tumours and atypical carcinoid tumours include support cells as seen in paragangliomas. These cells (stained by S-100 protein, glial fibrils acidic protein and nerve growth factor receptors) are rich in number in typical carcinoid tumours [16,23].

The distinction between typical and atypical carcinoid tumours was first described by Engelbreth-Holm. The histological criteria for this distinction were later established by Arrigoni *et al.* The initial classification of these tumours produced by the World Health Organisation (WHO) in 1982 has been amended various times. As a result of clinical and prognostic disputes, new histological criteria proposed by Travis *et al.* to separate typical and atypical carcinoid tumours have recently been considered and accepted by the WHO and IASLC in the 1999 classification of lung tumours. The acceptance of these classification criteria allows us better to clarify patients' prognosis. These criteria can be seen in Table **3**. In older series, about 10% of carcinoids are atypical carcinoids, but subsequent to the revision in the criteria for diagnosis, many typical carcinoids have been reclassified as atypical carcinoids (25%) [4,5,10,11,18,24].

Melanocytic Carcinoid: The rare pigmented carcinoid was initially reported by Cebelin and Grazer in the 1980s. The presentation and treatment are generally similar to those of atypical carcinoids [25,26].

Oncocytic Carcinoid: Oncocytic carcinoid is a rare subtype of the typical carcinoid tumour. It is composed of a variable mixture of eosinophilic oncocytes and cells that are more typical of carcinoid tumour. Ghadially has described this tumour and its differentiation as a true oncocytic tumour [27].

Tumourlets: Tumourlets, lexical meaning being small tumours, are isolated foci of atypical hyperplastic bronchial epithelium that are histologically similar to neuroendocrine tissue. Despite they were first defined in 1926, they were named as tumourlets in 1995 by Whitewell. They are usually incidental findings in lung that have been resected for infection, tumour, or they may be found at autopsy. Miller described them especially common in those with emphysema or restrictive lung disease. Tumourlets are more common in older patients, and the vast majority occurs in women. Immune staining and electron microscope displayed the difference of the secretory products between the tumourlets and typical carcinoid tumours. Even through metastasis from the tumourlets to the lymph nodes are reported, these are very rare [28-30].

Table 3: Histopathologic and Molecular Features of Pulmonary Neuroendocrine Tumours

	Typical Carcinoid	**Atypical Carcinoid**	**Large Cell Neuroendocrine Carcinoma**	**Small Cell Lung Cancer**
Morphology				
N/C ratio	Moderate	Moderate	Moderate	High
Mitoses	<1/10 HPF	1-10/10 HPF	>10/10 HPF	>20/10 HPF
Necrosis	Absent	Present	Present	Present
Nuclear pleomorphism	Absent/rare	Present	Present	Present
DNA encrustation vessel walls	Rare	Mild		Moderate
Vascular invasion	Absent	Present	Present	Present
Chemical analysis reactivity				
Chromogranin A	Positive	Positive	Positive	Positive
CEA	Positive/negative	Positive/negative	Positive	Positive
Synaptophysin	Positive/negative	Positive/negative	Positive	Positive
TTF-1	94% positive	100% positive	44% positive	92% positive
Molecular analysis: loss of heterozygosity (%)				
3p	40	50	83	85
5q	0	25	41	86
p53 mutation	10	45	72	90
Rb	20	22	62	71
11q13 (MEN-1)	44	50	71	67

CEA, carcinoembryonic antigen; HPF, high-power field; N/C, nuclear/cytoplasmic; NSE; neuron-specific enolase; TTF-1, thyroid transcription factor 1.

FINDINGS AND SYMPTOMS

Symptoms and physical examination findings determined in bronchial carcinoid tumours are related with the localisation of the tumours. 85 % of the bronchial carcinoid tumours are centrally localised. Remaining 15% display peripherial location. Carcinoid tumours displaying central location are in the major bronchi. 10% of them are in the primary bronchus and 75 % of them are in sub-bronchus [18,31].

Tumour with central location grows in the bronchus in a way to block the bronchus lumen partially or completely. Vascularity of the tumour reveals the symptoms together with the result of full or partial endobronchial obstruction. Cough, recurrent infections, mucus, wheezing, dyspnea, stridor, fever, chest pain, pleural effusion and hemoptysis, depending on the vascularity of the tumour, are the symptoms that might be observed.

Hemoptysis is seen in at least 50% of the cases and this reflects the vascular nature of the tumour. Cough, hemoptysis and recurrent infections form the "*classic symptom triad* ". Stridor is a symptom seen in trachea or main bronchus tumours. This upper airway obstruction sometimes might threaten life. Peripheric atelectasia and obstructive pneumonia are seen under complete endobronchial obstruction situations. Massive collapse due to atelectasia is very common however collateral air flow might prevent the complete obstruction in the bronchus as it prevents the atelectasia. Bronchiectasis and chronic lung abscess are inevitable due to long term obstruction and recurring infections [9,14,18,32].

Peripherically localised carcinoid tumours are asymptomatic and might be determined by chance during radiological examinations conducted due to the other reasons. Clinical findings of 2135 patients are given in Table **4** [33].

Wheezing in childhood period bronchial carcinoid tumours has been added to the cough, hemoptysis and recurrent infection (classical symptom triad) which are the most frequent symptoms seen in adults [7].

The fact that the mass of these tumours is small and the progress is slow, symptoms might continue for years until the patient is diagnosed. Symptoms in centrally localised carcinoid tumours emerge 10 years earlier than those of the peripherically localised. Often the symptoms between the emergence of the symptoms and the diagnosis are postponed by the patients. Accordingly, waiting period for the cases before contacting the doctor is 7 months on average and the delay period between the final diagnosis and the treatment is 13 months on average. In some cases, the period between the emergence of the symptoms and the start of the treatment might take years. During this delay period, patients might be treated with the diagnosis of asthma bronchial, chronic bronchial and bronchiectasis [9,18].

Table 4: Clinical Presentation of 2.135 Patients with Carcinoid Tumours

Symptom	**Percent of all Patients(a)**
Asymptomatic	30
Recurrent pneumonia	21
Cough	21
Hemoptysis	19
Pain	5
Dyspnea	3
Wheezing	2

a: Patients may have more than one symptom.

While carcinoid tumours cause symptoms related to its location, they also result in various endocrinologic symptoms and disease because of the neuroendocrine proteins produced due to being originated from neuroendocrine cells. Neuroendocrine proteins produced by carcinoid tumours are given in Table **5** [24,34-38].

Table 5: Neuroendocrine Proteins Produced by Bronchial Carcinoid Tumours.

***Peptides**
Amylase
Bombesin
Calcitonin
Corticotropin
Corticotropin Releasing Hormone
Gastrin
Glucagon
Growth Hormone Releasing Factor

Table 5: contd...

Human Chorionic Gonadotropin
Insulin
Melanocyte Stimulating Hormone
Motilin
Neurotensin
Pancreatic Polypeptide
Secretin
Somatostatin
Substance K
Substance P
Vasoactive Intestinal Polypeptide
Vasopressin
Vasoactive Amines
Catecholamines
Histamine
Kinines
Bradykinin
Tachykinin (Neurokinin A)
Endorphins vs. Enkephalins
Beta Endorphin
Leu – Enkephalin
Met – Enkephalin
Pan – Opioid
Other
Kallikrein
Prostaglandins

Endocrinopathies that might occur as a result of the neuroendocrine protein (peptides, kinins, prostaglandins, vasoactive amines *etc.*) produced by bronchial carcinoid tumours are seen in Table **6** [18,37-39].

Carcinoid Syndrome: Carcinoid syndrome, defined for the first time in 1956, is observed more in the carcinoid tumours stemming from the gastrointestinal system. Rarely do bronchial carcinoid tumours produce serotonin and cause carcinoid syndrome [4,40].

Table 6: Endocrinopathies Caused by Bronchial Carcinoid Tumours

* Carcinoid Syndrome.
* Cushing syndrome due to excess ACTH release.
* Hyperparatroid like situation together with hypercalcemia.
* Hyponatremia due to improper ADH secretion.
* Hypoglycemia due to insulin like secretion.
* Gynecomastia due to excess gonadotropin secretion.
* Hyperpigmentation on skin due to excess MSH secretion.
* Acromegaly. It might be independent of excess GHRH secretion.

The incidence of carcinoid syndrome with bronchial carcinoid tumour is reported as 2%. It emerges especially when the tumour has large or widespread liver metastasis (approximately 90% of cases). Carcinoid tumours with pulmonary origin might cause carcinoid syndrome without causing metastasis since they directly release the substances secreted in the blood [18,34,41].

Carcinoid syndrome is a well defined clinical entity with **Cutaneous;* rashes such as paroxysmal flushing (redness that emerges on the skin from time to time by itself or due to the effect of predisposing factors such as stress, exercise, alcohol or some foods), demography, pellagra. **cardiovascular;* endocardial fibrosis, valve diseases, and hypotension. **gastrointestinal;* throw up, abdominal pain, and diarrhea (sometimes steatorrhea) **respiratory;* wheezing, asthma attacks, and cyanosis symptoms [1,9,18].

On the contrary to the gastrointestinal system, carcinoid tumours causing liver metastasis and holding right cardiac valve, bronchial carcinoid tumours are related with the left cardiac valve. Valve lesions reaching the deposits in the fibrosis tissue might cause narrowing of valve orifice [18,31].

Rare observance of the syndrome in carcinoid tumours with pulmonary origin might be related with the issue that each gram of tissue includes serotonin less than the intestinal carcinoid tumours. It is possible to determine low levels of serotonin, since lung includes high level of monoamine oxidase (MAO) enzyme that detoxicates serotonin [18,42].

Cushing Syndrome: Cushing syndrome occurs in 2% of bronchial carcinoid tumours. Approximately 80% of patients with Cushing syndrome have localised disease. Most of these tumours are peripheral, with about 80% being typical carcinoids, and about 60% having node involvement. Dimensions of these tumours are very small. Classically average dimension is between 0.3 - 1.3. Therefore, computerized chest tomography or magnetic resonance imaging should be examined carefully for their diagnosis. Sometimes, they might be so small that they cannot be diagnosed before they grow up to screenable dimensions [18,36].

Bronchial carcinoid tumours might release adrenocorticotropic hormone (ACTH) in an amount to cause cushing syndrome which cannot be clinically separated from cushing disease due to pituitary. This syndrome develops in most of the cases depending on the formation of ectopic ACTH originating from inside the thorax [34,36].

Patients with carcinoid tumours including cushing syndrome display clinical symptoms of severe hypercortisolism. However, hypercorticolism might be the only finding in occult bronchial carcinoid tumour. Widely seen findings and symptoms are; myolysis, exhaustion, weight loss, striae, hypertension, acne and moon face [38,42].

Bronchial carcinoid tumours presenting with cushing syndrome are clinically much more aggressive. Accordingly, a more aggressive surgical treatment is needed when compared to typical carcinoid tumours [2,36].

DIAGNOSIS METHODS

Some important clues concerning diagnosis might be obtained in patients with bronchial carcinoid tumour through a careful anamnesis and physical examination. The purpose of imaging methods for diagnosis and invasive diagnostic methods is to obtain a certain histological diagnosis to apply the most appropriate treatment and to determine the stage of the tumour. Most of the time it is possible to localise and accurately determine the tumour through radiologic screenings and bronchoscopy. However histological examination of the tumour tissue is the only dependable method for diagnosis.

Radiologic Examination Methods

Standard chest radiographs might display lung parenchyma changes due to tumoural mass or tracheobronchial obstruction. A standard radiograph may detect no abnormality in just a little less than half of the patients [18,41].

Segmental or lobar atelectasia are the most common findings in centrally localised tumours. Obstructive pneumonia or distal consolidation might be seen with atelectasia. Atelectasia and obstructive pneumonia might periodically increase or decrease depending on the opening intervals of the obstruction occurring in the bronchus. 25% of the tumour is seen as hilar mass in central lesion. Rarely, can a tumour cause single-sided lung hypoperfusion secondary to check-valve mechanism and related increased shininess and obstructive emphysema. Again hypertension might be seen depending on the collateral air flow in the distal of the blocked bronchus. The most frequent radiologic symptom during childhood period is atelectasia [7,9,12,18,43].

Solitary pulmonary nodule in peripherically localised bronchial carcinoid tumours is the most frequent symptom. Generally, they are seen as sharp edged, round or elliptic masses with homogenous density and with no calcification and they are rarely seen as lobule masses in the radiograph. They are 4 cm. in diameter on average (between 1-10 cm) and often formed in the upper right, mid lobes and lingual [42].

Oblique images might be used for unrealised central lesions and might reveal the endobronchial component of the tumour which is not seen in routine screenings of the tumour [37].

Computed Tomography (CT) might display intrabronchial tumour as well as lober or segmental atelectasia or consolidation. CT gives the exact dimensions and location of the mass especially when there is a hilus and mediastinal extraluminal spread.

They are seen in CT screening of centrally localised lesions as a mass with well-defined borders, narrowing, deforming or blocking the adjacent airway. It is generally adjacent to an airway in peripheric lesions. There is calcification as diffuse or spots in approximately 30% of the lesions and this symptom indicates that the tumour is a carcinoid [18,37].

CT is also helpful in staging of bronchial carcinoid tumours. Node enlargement by CT has a false-positive rate of 20% to 40%, whereas the false-negative rate is lower.

Common characteristic symptom of the bronchial carcinoid tumour in CT is the hypervascular appearance formed following the IV contrast agent. This appearance is an important finding for diagnosis [18,37,42].

Positron Emission Tomography (PET), The role of PET scanning is not well defined for pulmonary carcinoids, with widely disparate sensitivity (14% to 100%). Erasmus and colleagues indicated that pulmonary carcinoids are generally hypometabolic on PET scan and have a low standardized uptake ratio, with a range of 1.6 to 2.4. Although some studies have found lesions smaller than 3 cm to be hypermetabolic and thus positive on PET scan. PET should not be used routinely for mediastinal or systemic staging in pulmonary carcinoids because the reliability of a positive or negative result is unknown [44,45].

Bronchoscopy: If the tumour is centrally localised, bronchoscopy is the gold standard for diagnosis and provides material for histological examination. Bronchoscopy is not successful in the determination of the tumours located in the proximal segment orifice. A diagnosis of bronchial carcinoid tumour was achieved in only 70% to 80% of patients in whom adequate biopsy specimens were obtained [18,42].

Carcinoid tumours are in varying colours from pink to purple (blackberry colour) macroscopically and in lobule appearance in bronchoscopy. They are covered by intact mucosa and display vascularisation [9,19].

Since carcinoid tumours are located in submucosa, deeper biopsy when compared to other malign bronchial tumours is required. Bleeding might occur during biopsy due to connective tissue stroma of the tumour comprised of rich capillary. Some authors reported that massive bleedings occurred after carcinoid tumour biopsies however there was no need for blood transfusion or thoracotomy. Actually, all severe postbronchoscopic bleedings occur during the excision efforts to remove the tumour partially or completely even though this tumour is excessively vascular and has the tendency to bleed. Today, safe biopsy might be performed by using diluted epinephrine before and after the biopsy for flexible bronchoscopy and vasoconstruction. However, there are authors recommending rigid bronchoscopy through general anesthesia to secure the airways since uncontrollable bleedings might occur during flexible bronchoscopy. Furthermore, larger biopsy materials can be taken by rigid bronchoscopy and the possibility of confusion between atypical carcinoids and carcinoma with smaller chance might be decreased. An erroneous diagnosis (typically SCLC or squamous carcinoma) is made in about 10% of patients [9,19,46,47].

Cytological examination of transbronchial fine needle aspiration biopsy might be helpful in diagnosing carcinoid tumours due to the fact that biopsy will not be safe or useful and it is a routine part of bronchoscopy during submucosal tumour research. Moreover, it is shown that bronchial brushing displays cytological findings to enable differentiation of carcinoid tumour during determination of bronchial carcinoid tumour cells. Bronchoscopy should be often redone intraoperatively to better define precise extent of bronchial resection in cases of central tumours [14,48].

Biochemical Studies: Unless there is a suspicion of carcinoid syndrome, there is no use of searching degradation products such as serotonin and 5 hydroxyindole acetic acid in the blood and urine of the patients to have bronchial carcinoid tumour. However, some authors determined that elevated levels were a contradictory prognostic variable [39].

Immunohistochemical Examinations: Today, immunohistochemical examinations might differentiate the tumours in carcinoid pattern especially from small cell carcinoma and lymphoproliferative diseases. Studies have shown that chromogranine A and neuron specific enolase (NSE) for the tumours in neuroendocrine character have distinctive characteristics when compared to the other tumours. However, they are not helpful in accurate distinction of the sub-groups. Moreover, neurofilament proteins (NF), (especially NF-70) and desmoplakin are useful in the determination of Carcinoid tumours. Blondal *et al.*. displayed that argyrophil staining method is helpful in the separation of small cell carcinoma and carcinoid tumours. Immunohistochemical staining characteristics between carcinoid tumours, small cell carcinoma and lymphoproliferative diseases can be seen in Table **7** [3,16,40].

Table 7: Immunohistochemical Staining Patterns of Pulmonary Tumours

	Kulchitsky Cell Cancers	**Non-Small Cell Cancers**	**Lympho proliferative Diseases**
Cytokeratins	+	+	-
Neurofilaments	+ [a]	-	-
Immunoglobulins	-	-	+
Neuron Specific Enolase	+	-	-
Chromogranines	+	-	-
Leu - 7	+	-	+ [b]

a: changeable and b: on natural killer cells.

Mucus Cytology: Cytological examination of the mucus is negative since carcinoid tumours are covered with intact bronchial epithelium unless they are ulcerated [48].

Fine Needle Aspiration Biopsy: It has been reported that cytological examination of fine needle aspiration biopsy especially in periphericaly localised carcinoid tumours is helpful in carcinoid tumour diagnosis (approximately 40 %). The ability to accurately distinguish the carcinoid subtype is 10% to 20% lower [17,49].

Radionuclide Examinations: These are especially helpful in determining the location of occult bronchial carcinoid tumours and during the situations when other examinations are negative and the patients are asymptomatic. Carcinoid tumours have somatostatine receptors. This technique is based on the overexpression of somatostatin receptors on carcinoids. Thus, they might be screened through a sensitive somatostatin analogue (for example octreotide, lanreotide, and pentetreotide). Octreotide scanning of carcinoid tumours has a sensitivity of 86% to 96%. Although octreotide scanning is also positive in many tumours, granulomas, and autoimmune diseases, bronchial carcinoid tumours might be displayed through adequate amount of accumulation of Iodine-123 N-isopropyl-p-iodoamphetamine, which is also a radionuclide [18,38].

Mediastinoscopy: Mediastinoscopy does not have a value in carcinoid tumour diagnosis and preoperative nodal staging. However, it might be useful in rare cases which are diagnosed with atypical carcinoid and which are suspected to be unresectable with mediastinal spread during the imaging studies. Mediastinoscopy might be applied to carcinoid tumours unintentionally in order to stage the tumours for the cases in which another lung tumour diagnosis is made pathologically due to the collection of small biopsy materials crushed with bronchoscopy [8,15,18].

STAGING

Due to negative prognostic effects of lymph node metastasis on bronchial carcinoid tumours and in accordance with the treatment results reported it is appropriate to use American Joint Committee on Cancer (AJCC) Lung Cancer Staging criteria for carcinoid tumours. According to the studies performed, no correlation is determined for the prognosis due to histology, size of the tumour, localisation of the tumour, lymph node retention (positive or negative) and whether the distant metastasis is present when the tumour is determined or not. Systematic mediastinal lymph node dissection should be performed without keeping in mind the width of the resection in order to conduct adequate treatment of the tumour and accurate staging [3,18].

Most of typical carcinoid tumours are evaluated as stage I lesions and 50% of the atypical carcinoid tumours together with hilar or mediastinal lymph node retention are evaluated as stage II or stage III [18].

TREATMENT

Nowadays, the accepted treatment method of carcinoid tumours is to completely resect the primary lesion by preserving the maximum possible lung tissue.

Bronchoplastic procedures and procedures preserving the lung tissue such as bronchotomy or sleeve resection have been applied frequently during the last ten years considering that typical carcinoid tumours have low malign potential. However, in practice, lung resection is frequently required. Resection is mandatory in 88 % of the cases of ineffective changes in the distal of the tumour or spread of the tumour in the lung parenchyma (iceberg tumour). Minor resections to protect the lung tissue should not be performed in the cases which are not pathologically defined for sure and in atypical carcinoid tumours in which malignant potential is high [14,15,18,42,50].

Endoscopic Resection

Endoscopic renewal of carcinoid tumours was a frequently used treatment method before the modern surgical techniques allowing resection of the lung tissue with low morbidity and mortality, anesthesia and postoperative developments. This method was defined by Fraser in 1957 for the first time [33,42].

Tumours having connective tissue with excessive vessel structure and trying to remove it with forceps make this treatment method dangerous including the drowning of the patient due to bleeding. Some authors report that development of Neodymium-Yttrium-Aluminum-Garnet (Nd-YAG) laser decreases the bleeding risk during photocoagulation of carcinoid tumours endoscopically. Recurrence in carcinoid tumours is frequent as a result of not being removed entirely since most of them are extramural and only a small part can be seen intraluminally during bronchoscopy. Endoscopic Resection with Nd-YAG laser might be performed in rare pedunculated polypoid carcinoid tumours which are intraluminal and have no invasion. Sutedja *et al.*. examined the postoperative resection material of the patients to whom preoperative Nd- YAG laser treatment was applied in typical and intraluminal carcinoid tumours and displayed that there was no residual tumour left. Luckraz *et al.* informed their experience over a 26-year period with the management of endobronchial, proximal, polypoid, typical carcinoid tumours using bronchoscopic resection and reported the long-term outcome [15,18,39,46,47].

Surgical Resection

The purpose of the surgical treatment is to remove primary lesion completely by preserving maximum possible lung tissue unless there is a distant metastasis by keeping the local invasive characteristics of the carcinoid tumours in mind. Level of the resection is not only dependent on the location of the tumour but also related with the distal parenchyma and the condition of respiration reserves. Therefore, damaged and nonfunctioning lung tissue in the distal of the lesion should be removed. Preferred method of treatment in carcinoid tumours with metastasis in mediastinal lymph nodes is to remove the entire tumour with mediastinal lymph curage because the prognosis of both typical and atypical carcinoid tumours is good in the long term [8,14,15,18,42,51,52].

It is necessary to conduct surgical stating in each thoracotomy. Biopsies of the lymph nodules with bronchopulmonary segment, lobar areas, hilus and mediastinal localisation should be performed. Accordingly, frozen section analyses are required. Larger tumour surgery in addition to complete lymph node dissection including mediastinal nodules is required for the patients with nodal metastasis. Types of surgeries applied in carcinoid tumours can be seen in Table **8** [8,18,53,54].

Table 8: Frequency of Surgical Resections for Carcinoid Tumours

Surgical Procedures	**Frequency**
Lobectomy (including bronchoplastic procedures)	51-58%
Bilobectomy	9-15%
Segmentectomy or wedge resections	2-15%
Bronchoplastic procedures	5-18%
Pneumonectomy	6-16%

Pneumonectomy is rarely performed in carcinoid tumours since the development of bronchoplastic procedures. It might only be considered when all the lobes in the distal of the tumour are damaged, which is very rare. Accordingly preoperative endoscopic resection of the tumour is helpful in understanding whether the destruction in the distal lung parenchyma could be restored or not [15,18,42,55,56].

Lobectomy is performed in the tumours starting in the lob bronchus and cause destruction in the lobe for which bronchoplastic procedures could be performed. Moreover, lobectomy is the accepted operation type in peripheric carcinoid tumours [18,30,35].

Segmentectomy and Wedge resection is recommended for peripheric bronchial carcinoid tumours due to low local recurrence of the tumour. In order to perform wedge or segment resection for peripheric bronchial carcinoid tumours there should be no mediastinal lymph adenopathy in thorax CT, no invasion in the regional lymph nodules in the frozen section analysis, no benign tumour characteristics and no medical and pulmonary risk factors in the patient when a large scale operation is performed [2,15,18].

VATS has recently completely changed the treatments of some pulmonary and mediastinal anomalies and has also started to be used in carcinoid tumours by some researchers. Researchers conducted sampling from mediastinal and hilar lymph nodes during the resections conducted *via* VATS and reported that VATS is better for the patient comfort in terms of standard thoracotomy. VATS resection might be preferred especially in bronchial carcinoid tumours causing cushing syndrome since cushing syndrome generally causes debility and myolysis and resection with standard thoracotomy might increase morbidity and mortality incidence during pre and postoperative periods for these patients [2,55,57].

Sleeve resection was used by Price Thomas in 1947 for the first time during a bronchus adenoma. The benefit of sleeve resections is that it prevents pneumonectomy in order to remove centrally located pathologic lesions. Carcinoid tumours located in the primary bronchus or sometimes in intermediary bronchus might be removed by sleeve resection of the bronchus by preserving the entire lung tissue. 0.5 cm. is adequate for frozen section border in sleeve resection. This technique is preferred to pneumonectomy and bilobectomy [18,35,58].

Sometimes, *bronchotomy* and wedge resection of the bronchus wall might be applied to polypoid tumours. On the contrary to endoscopic removal, polypoid tumours might completely be resected through bronchotomy together with the bronchial wall they are attached to. Unfortunately, the application of this simple bronchotomy approach is rarely possible [59,60].

Radiotherapy

Since bronchial carcinoid tumours are resistant to radiation. Radiation treatment therefore, should not be preferred as a primary therapy instead of surgical resection. However, some researchers reported that some inoperable cases or cases with metastatic lesion basis respond to radiation treatment. Again in this study average life span is reported for the following patients through radiation treatment; 39 months for primary carcinoid tumour in the lung, 33 months for the patients with brain metastasis, and 32 months for the patients with hepatic metastasis. Postoperative radiotherapy is recommended for the patients with atypical carcinoid tumour and lymph node who did not undergo complete surgical resection [18,41,61].

Chemotherapy

Even though it is thought as the ancillary therapy for atypical carcinoid tumours, it does not have significant contribution in treatment. Use of chemotherapy for Stage I and II atypical carcinoid tumours is still debatable due to unproved benefits for increasing life expectancy and life threatening side effects. Additionally, use of chemotherapy for the control of stage III atypical carcinoid tumours seems correct. 67 % response is received in atypical carcinoid tumours with etoposide and cisplatin [3,62,63].

PROGNOSIS AND LIFE EXPECTANCY

It is shown that carcinoid tumours have slow growing and extended life history. Thus they have perfect long-term prognosis. Life span depends on the increasing age, whether the tumour size is bigger than 3.5 cm., the grade, type of the carcinoid tumour, tumour and nodal stage (T, N stage) during resection and whether it is distant metastasis (M stage) [15,18,64].

Lymph node metastasis is seen in 10-15 % of the typical carcinoid tumour patients and distant metastasis is seen in less than this percentage [8,15,18,30,62,64]. Lymph node metastasis or distant metastasis is seen in 50- 75 % of the patients with atypical carcinoid tumour [18,20,60,64]. Distant metastasis is mostly seen in liver, bone and adrenal glands as in others. Metastasis in the brain and orbit is rarely reported. Perkins *et al.*. think that genetic tendency affects the metastatic potential of some carcinoid tumours [1,65,66].

Metastasis rate on the patients with paediatric bronchial carcinoid tumour is similar to the metastasis rate reported in the adult patients. Despite the fact that the total number of paediatric patients with bronchial carcinoid tumour is very few metastasis rate seen upon diagnosis is reported between 5- 27 % [6,7].

In typical carcinoid tumours 5 year disease free survival rate is 97-100% when there is no lymph node retention. 5 year disease free survival rate for stage I is 94 % and 25 year disease free survival rate is 66 %. Once the lymph node metastases have occurred with typical carcinoids, complete excision with lymph node dissection still allows an excellent prognosis. 5 year disease free survival rate for typical carcinoid tumours with lymph node retention is 71%. 5 year disease free survival rate for atypical carcinoid tumours with lymph node and distant metastasis is lower being not more than 69%. In Table **9**, postoperative 5-10-15 year disease free survival periods reported by several researches in bronchial carcinoid tumours are given [18,22-24,39,58,60,64,67,68].

Table 9: Survival of Resected Patients with Typical and Atypical Carcinoid Tumours

Study	**Typical Carcinoid (%)**			**Atypical Carcinoid (%)**		
	5y	**10y**	**15y**	**5y**	**10y**	**15y**
Garcia-Yuste *et al.* (2007)	97	92	-	78	67	-
Rea *et al.* (2007)	97	93	87	78	64	53
Cardillo *et al.* (2004)	99	-	-	70	-	-
Terzi *et al.* (2004)	100	95	90	70	55	55
Filosso *et al.* (2002)	97	93	84	77	53	53
Thomas *et al.* (2001)	95	95	-	54	54	-
Travis *et al.* (1998)	87	87	-	56	35	-
Akiba *et al.* (1992)	100	91	-	25	25	-
Harpole *et al.* (1992)	96	92	-	40	31	-

y: Years.

ACKNOWLEDGEMENTS

Declared none.

CONFLICT OF INTEREST

The authors confirm that this article content has no conflict of interest.

REFERENCES

[1] Nida TY, Hall WA, Glantz MJ, *et al*: Metastatic Carcinoid Tumour to the Orbit and Brain. Neurosurgery November 1992; 31(5): 949-52.

[2] Gharagozloo F, Dausmann MJ, Whitaker MD, *et al*: Thoracoscopic Excision of a Peripheral Corticotropin - Secreting Pulmonary Carcinoid Tumour. Mayo Clin Proc 1994; 69: 594-6.
[3] Marty-Ane CH, Costes V, Pujol JL, *et al*: Carcinoid Tumours of the Lung: Do Atypical Features Require Aggressive Management ? Ann Thorac Surg 1995; 59: 78-83.
[4] Engelbreth-Holm J. Benign Bronchial Adenomas. Acta Chir Scand 1944; 90: 383-409.
[5] Arrigoni MG, Woolner LB, Bernatz PE: Atypical Carcinoid Tumours of the Lung. J Thorac Cardiovasc Surg 1972; 64: 413-21
[6] Lack EE, Harris GBC, Eraklis AJ, Vawter GF: Primary Bronchial Tumours in Childhood. A Clinicopathologic Study of Six Cases. Cancer, 1983; 51: 492-7
[7] Wang LT, Wilkins EW, Bode HH: Bronchial Carcinoid Tumours in Pediatric Patients. Chest, 1993; 103: 1426-8
[8] .Marty-Ane CH, Costes V, Pujol JL, *et al*: Carcinoid Tumours of the Lung: Do Atypical Features Require Aggressive Management ? Ann Thorac Surg 1995; 59: 78-83.
[9] Rozenman J, Pausner R, Lieberman Y, *et al*: Bronchial Adenoma. Chest 1987; 92(1): 145-7
[10] World Health Organization/International Association for the Study of Lung Cancer classification, 3rd ed. Berlin: Springer-Verlag, 1999.
[11] The World Health Organization Histological Typing of Lung Tumours. Second Edition. Am J Clin Pathol 1982; 77: 123-36.
[12] Warren WH, Faber LP, Gould VE: Neuroendocrin Neoplasm of the Lung. J Thorac Cardiovasc Surg 1989; 98: 321-32.
[13] Paladugu RR, Benfield RJ, Pak HY, *et al*: Bronchopulmonary Kulchitsky Cell Carcinomas. A New Classification Scheme for Typical and atypical Carcinoids. Cancer 1985; 55: 1303-11.
[14] Hurt R, Bates M: Carcinoid Tumours of the Bronchus: A 33 Year Experience. Thorax, 1984; 39: 617-23.
[15] Schreurs AdJM, Westermann CeesJJ, Van Den Bosch JMM, *et al*: A Twenty-five-year Follow-up of Ninety-three Resected Typical Carcinoid Tumours of the Lung. J Thorac Cardiovasc Surg, 1992; 104(5): 1470- 5.
[16] Mitchell ML, Parker FP: Capillaries: A Cytologic Feature of Pulmonary Carcinoid Tumours. Acta Cytologica 1991; 35(2): 183-5.
[17] Collins CT, Cramer HM: Fine Needle Aspiration Cytology of Carcinoid Tumours. Acta Cytologica, 1996; 40(4): 695-707.
[18] Escalon J, Detterbeck F. Carcinoid Tumours. In: Shields T, LoCicero JI, Reed C, Feins R (eds). General Thoracic Surgery. 7th ed. Philadelphia: Lippincott Williams & Wilkins; 2009:1539-54
[19] Pelosi G, Rodriguez J, Viale G, *et al*: Typical and Atypical Pulmonary Carcinoid Tumour Overdiagnosed as Small-cell Carcinoma on Biopsy Specimens: A Major Pitfall in the Management of Lung Cancer Patients. Am J Surg Path 2005; 29: 179-87.
[20] Beasley MB, Thunnissen FB, Brambilla E, *et al.* Pulmonary Atypical Carcinoid: Predictors of Survival in 106 Cases. Hum Pathol 2000; 31:1255-65.
[21] Grote TH, Macon WR, Davis B, *et al*: Atypical Carcinoids of the Lung. Chest, 1988; 93: 370-5.
[22] Thomas CF, Tazelaar HD, Jett JR. Typical and Atypical Pulmonary Carcinoids: Outcome in Patients Presenting with Regional Lymph Node Involvement. Chest 2001; 119: 1143-50.
[23] Akiba T, Naruke T, Kondo H, *et al*: Carcinoid Tumour of the Lung: Clinicopathological Study of 32 Cases. Jpn J Clin Oncol 1992; 22: 92-5.
[24] Travis WD, Rush W, Flieder DB, *et al.* Survival Analysis of 200 Pulmonary Neuroendocrine Tumours with Clarification of Criteria for Atypical Carcinoid and Its Separation from Typical Carcinoid. Am J Surg Pathol 1998; 22: 934-44.

[25] Cebelin MS: Malenocytic Bronchial Carcinoid Tumour. Cancer, 1980; 46: 1843.
[26] Grazer R: Melanin-containing Peripheral Carcinoid of the Lung. Am J Surg Pathol, 1982; 6: 73.
[27] Ghadially FN, Block HJ: Oncocytic Carcinoid of the Lung. J Submicrose Cytol Pathol, 1985; 17: 435
[28] Whitwell F: Tumourlets of the Lung. J Pathol Bacteriol, 1955; 70: 529-41.
[29] Aubry MC, Thomas CF Jr, Jett JR, *et al.* Signaficance of Multiple Carcinoid Tumours and Tumourlets in Surgical Lung Specimens: Analysis of 28 Patients. Chest 2007; 131: 1635-43
[30] Ferolla P, Daddi N, Urbani M, *et al*: Tumourlets, Multicentric Carcinoids, Lymph-Nodal Metastases, and Long-Term Behaviour in Bronchial Carcinoids. J Thorac Oncol 2009; 4: 383-7
[31] Detterbeck FC. Management of Carcinoid Tumours. Ann Thorac Surg 2010; 89: 998-1005.
[32] Okike N, Bernatz PE, Woolner LB: Carcinoid Tumours of the Lung. Ann Thorac Surg, 1976; 22: 270-7
[33] McCaughan BC, Martini N, Bains MJ: Bronchial Carcinoids: Review of 124 Cases. J Thorac Cardiovasc Surg 1985; 89: 8-13.
[34] Shrager JB, Wright CD, Wain JC, *et al*: Bronchopulmonary Carcinoid Tumours Associated with Cushing's Syndrome: A More Aggressive Variant of Typical Carcinoid. J Thorac Cardiovasc Surg, 1997; 114(3): 367-75.
[35] Daddi N, Ferolla P, Urbani M, *et al*: Surgical Treatment of Neuroendocrine Tumours of the Lung. Eur J Cardiothorac Surg 2004; 26: 813-7.
[36] Dusmet ME, McKneally MF: Pulmonary and Thymic Carcinoid Tumours. World J Surg, 1996; 20(2): 189-95.
[37] Forster BB, Muller NL, Miller RR, Nelems B, Evans KG: Neuroendocrine Carcinomas of the Lung: Clinical, Radiologic and Pathologic Correlation. Radiology, 1989; 170: 441-5.
[38] Phlipponneau M, Nocaudie M, Epelbaum J, *et al*: Somatostatin Analogs for the Localization and Preoperative Treatment of An Adrenocorticotropin Secreting Bronchial Carcinoid Tumour. J Clin Endocrinol Metab, 1994; 78: 20-4
[39] Harpole DH Jr, Feldman JM, Buchanan S, *et al*: Bronchial Carcinoid Tumours: A Retrospective Analysis of 126 Patients. Ann Thorac Surg, 1992; 54: 50-5
[40] Blondal T, Grimelius L, Nou E, *et al*: Argyrophil Carcinoid Tumours of the Lung. Incidence, Clinical Study, and Follow-Up of 46 Patients. Chest, 1980; 78(6): 840-4.
[41] Bernstein C, McGoey J, Lertzman M: Recurrent Bronchial Carcinoid Tumour. Chest, 1989; 95(3): 693-4.
[42] Smith RA: Bronchial Carcinoid Tumours. Thorax, 1969; 24: 43-50
[43] Miller M, Mark G, Kanarek D: Multiple Peripheral Pulmonary Carcinoid and Tumourlets of Carcinoid Type with Restrictive and Obstructive Lung Disease. Am J Med 1978; 65: 373-8.
[44] Daniels CE, Lowe VJ, Aubry M-C, *et al*: The Utility of Fluorodeoxyglucose Positron Emission Tomography in the Evaluation of Carcinoid Tumours Presenting as Pulmonary Nodules. Chest 2007; 131: 255-60.
[45] Marom EM, Sarvis S, Herndon II JE, *et al*: T1 Lung Cancers: Sensitivity of Diagnosis with Fluorodeoxyglucose PET. Radiology 2002; 223: 453-9.
[46] Luckraz H, Amer K, Thomas L, *et al*: Long-term Outcome of Bronchoscopically Resected Endobronchial Typical Carcinoid Tumours. J Thorac Cardiovasc Surg 2006; 132: 113-5
[47] Sutedja TG, Schreurs AJ, Vanderschueren RG, *et al*: Bronchoscopic Therapy in Patients with Intraluminal Typical Bronchial Carcinoid. Chest, 1995; 107(2): 556-8
[48] Nguyen GK: Cytopathology of Pulmonary Carcinoid Tumours in Sputum and Bronchial Brushings. Acta Cytol, 1995; 39(6): 1152-60

[49] Anderson C, Ludwig ME, O'Donnell M, *et al*: Fine Needle Aspiration Cytology of Pulmonary Carcinoid Tumours. Acta Cytologica 1990; 34: 505-10

[50] Ferguson MK, Landreneau RJ, Hazelrigg SR, *et al*: Long-term Outcome After Resection for Bronchial Carcinoid Tumours. Eur J Cardiothorac Surg 2000; 18: 156-61.

[51] Fink G, Krelbaum T, Yellin A, *et al.* Pulmonary Carcinoid: Presentation, Diagnosis, and Outcome in 142 Cases in Israel and Review of 640 Cases from Literature. Chest 2001; 119: 1647-51

[52] Fischer S, Kruger M, McRae K, *et al*: Giant Bronchial Carcinoid Tumours: A Multidisciplinary Approach. Ann Thorac Surg 2001; 71: 386-93.

[53] Kurul IC, Topcu S, Tastepe I, *et al*: Surgery in Bronchial Carcinoids: Experience with 83 Patients. Eur J Cardiothorac Surg 2002; 21: 883-7

[54] Modlin IM, Sandor A: An Analysis of 8305 Cases of Carcinoid Tumours. Cancer 1997; 79: 813-29.

[55] Craig SR, Hamzah M, Walker WS: Video-Assisted Thoracoscopic Pneumonectomy for Bronchial Carcinoid Tumour in A 14-Year-Old Girl. J Pediatr Surg, 1996; 31(12): 1724-6

[56] El Jamal M, Nicholson AG, Goldstraw P. The Feasibility of Conservative Resection for Carcinoid Tumours: Is Pneumonectomy Ever Necessary for Uncomplicated Cases? Eur J Cardiothorac Surg 2001; 18: 301-6.

[57] Watanabe M, Ono K, Sato M, *et al*: Lobectomy by Video-Assisted Thoracic Surgery for A Hilar Bronchial Carcinoid Tumour. Surg Laparosc Endosc, 1996; 6: 476-9

[58] Garcia-Yuste M, Matilla JM, Cueto A, *et al*: Typical and Atypical Carcinoid Tumours: Analysis of the Experience of the Spanish Multi-centric Study of Neuroendocrine Tumours of the Lung. Eur J Cardiothorac Surg 2007; 31: 192-7.

[59] Alp M, Uçanok K, Doğan R, *et al*: Surgical Treatment of Bronchial Adenomas. Thorac Cardiovasc Surgeon 1987; 35: 290-4.

[60] Filosso PL, Rena O, Donati G, *et al*: Bronchial Carcinoid Tumours: Surgical Management and Long-Term Outcome. J Thorac Cardiovasc Surg 2002; 123: 303-9.

[61] Chakravarthy A, Abrams RA: Radiation Therapy in the Management of Patients with Malignant Carcinoid Tumours. Cancer, 1995; 75(6): 1388-90.

[62] Hage R, De la Riviere AB, Seldenrijk CA, *et al*: Update in Pulmonary Carcinoid Tumours: A Review Article. Ann Surg Oncol 2003; 10: 697-704.

[63] Pinchot SN, Holen K, Sippel RS, *et al*: Carcinoid Tumours. The Oncologist 2008; 13: 1255-69.

[64] Cardillo G, Sera F, Di Martino M, *et al*: Bronchial Carcinoid Tumours: Nodal Status and Long-Term Survival After Resection. Ann Thorac Surg 2004; 77: 1781-85.

[65] Perkins P, Lee JR, Kemp BL, *et al*: Carcinoid Tumours of the Lung and Family History of Cancer. J Clin Epidemiol, 1997; 50(6): 705-9.

[66] Onuki N, Wistuba II, Travis WD, *et al.* Genetic Changes in the Spectrum of Neuroendocrine Lung Tumours. Cancer 1999; 85: 600-7.

[67] Rea F, Rizzardi G, Zuin A, *et al*: Outcome and Surgical Strategy in Bronchial Carcinoid Tumours: Single Institution Experience with 252 Patients. Eur J Cardiothorac Surg 2007; 31: 186-91.

[68] Terzi A, Lonardoni A, Fiel B, *et al.* Bronchoplastic Procedures for Central Carcinoid Tumours: Clinical Experience. Eur J Cardiothorac Surg 2004; 26: 1196-9

Send Orders of Reprints at reprints@benthamscience.net
Lung Cancer: Clinical and Surgical Specifications, 2013, 347-354

CHAPTER 10

Part J: Bronchoplasty

Kamil Kaynak*, Ahmet Demirkaya and Burcu Kilic

Istanbul University Cerrahpasa Medical Faculty, Department of Thoracic Surgery, Kocamustafapasa/Fatih Istanbul, Turkey

Abstract: Although bronchoplasty for malignant lung lesions is common, bronchoplasty for benign lung lesions is relatively rare. Bronchoplasty is a parenchyma–saving operation in which a segment of main bronchus is removed in continuity with a lobe. Bronchoplastic procedures can be achieved by both two main bronchus and five major lobe bronchus. In all reported series, lesions in the hilum of the right upper lobe represent the most common indication for sleeve lobectomy. High-dose corticosteroid therapy, active bronchial inflammation, and prior high-dose irradiation are principal relative contraindications. Occasionally, sleeve resections can be indicated for patients with low respiratory capacity, a condition that contraindicates pneumonectomy. Local recurrence is low as long as the margins are free of disease. Sleeve lobectomy was strongly favored over pneumonectomy.

Keywords: Lung cancer, Bronchoplastic procedures, Bronchoplasty.

HISTORY

Sleeve lobectomy was first introduced by Price-Thomas in 1947 for an adenoma protruding out of the origin of the right upper lobe bronchus and occluding the main bronchus [1]. Allison reported the first case of bronchogenic carcinoma treated by right upper lobectomy, sleeve resection of the right main bronchus, in addition to partial elliptical resection of the right main pulmonary artery in 1956 [2]. In 1955, Paulson and Shaw published their first report entitled 'Bronchial anastomosis and bronchoplastic procedures in the interest of preservation of lung

***Address correspondence to Kamil Kaynak:** Istanbul University Cerrahpasa Medical Faculty, Department of Thoracic Surgery, Kocamustafapasa/Fatih Istanbul, Turkey; Tel: +90 212 4143590; Fax: +90 212 6328474; E-mail: kamil@istanbul.edu.tr tissue" [3]. The last historically significant series popularizing sleeve lobectomy was published by Vogt-Moykopf and colleagues in 1986 [4].

Although bronchoplastic procedures for malignant lung lesions are common, bronchoplasty for benign pulmonary lesions is performed relatively rarely. Bronchoplasty is a parenchyma –saving operation in which a segment of main bronchus is removed in continuity with a lobe. Good knowledge of the surgical anatomy of the tracheobronchial tree and of its vein and arterial tributaries is necessary to reduce postoperative morbidity. Bronchoplasty can be achieved with low operative mortality and morbidity even after inducting chemo/radio therapies. The major aim of bronchoplastic procedures is to preserve viable lung tissue to ensure a better functional result [5,6]. Bronchoplastic procedures can be performed for two main bronchus and five major lobe bronchus.

INDICATIONS

The main indication for bronchoplasty is an anatomically suitable lesion confined to a bronchus or a lobe [7]. Indications are twofold; 1) benign or malignant tumours 2) posttraumatic, non neoplastic bronchial stenosis which originates from inflammatory or infectious conditions. The ideal circumstance is a benign or low-grade lesion anatomically situated in the main bronchus or at the origin of a lobar bronchus [7,8]. Anatomically suitable malignant neoplasms are also suitable for bronchoplastic procedures [5,9]. Lesions involving hilum of the right upper lobe are the most common indication for sleeve lobectomy. Left upper lobe is the next most common site of sleeve resection. The sleeve resection is ideal for tumours of low or intermediate grade such as a typical carcinoids and bronchial strictures developed because of benign disease such as tuberculosis or thoracic trauma, causing bronchial rupture or stenosis.

CONTRAINDICATIONS

High-dose corticosteroid therapy, active, infective bronchial inflammation, and prior high-dose irradiation are relative contraindications. Low dose steroids can be safe but anastomosis should be buttressed with adjacent tissues such as omentum and intercostal muscle. Determining the underlying pathology of inflammation is important. When bronchoplasty is achieved in such patients, it is recommended to wrap the anastomosis with pedicled omentum [10,11]. Omentum appears to be the most reliable anastomotic buttress in high-risk patients [8]. Occasionally sleeve resections can be indicated for patients with low pulmonary capacity and contraindicating pneumonectomy. The incidence of both anastomotic dehiscences and operative mortality increase in patients with inflammatory diseases after the operation.

PREOPERATIVE ASSESSMENT

Standard pulmonary function tests and quantitative ventilation-perfusion scan (if needed) must be performed for surgery planning.

During surgical strategy planning, a detailed bronchoscopy must be performed before surgery. Endobronchial lesion involving lobar or main bronchus, suspicious mucosal abnormalities attributable to submucosal invasion, bronchial extrinsic compression caused by metastatic lymph nodes, should be sought.

CT imaging is useful for defining tumour location and size. Lung cancer patients with mediastinal adenopathy of greater than 1.0 cm can be identified and must undergo mediastinoscopy prior to thoracotomy. Magnetic resonance imaging was reported to be useful for delineating vascular components [12]. However, the practicability of this modality needs confirmation. Selective pulmonary arteriography may be performed to accurately delineate the pulmonary arterial anatomy at the lobar level [12], however, double lumen endobronchial tube is necessary.

SURGICAL TECHNIQUES

Certain principles are common to all bronchoplastic techniques. Sleeve resections are generally performed through a standard posterolateral or muscle-sparing anterolateral thoracotomy. However, it should be noted that, the most appropriate approach is posterolateral because of the good exposure and easy handling of bronchial and arterial structures. During thoracotomy, a pedicled intercostal muscle flap can be mobilized for later use as a buttressing the anastomosis [12]. The thorax preooperative findings such as the location of tumour and lymphatic spread must be confirmed. The surgeon first dissects the the anterior hilum then completely remove out the main pulmonary artery. Left-sided resections are more challenging because of the aortic arch and heart, limiting exposure and handling. The lobe to be removed is then mobilized.

The next step is a careful dissection of bronchus which is planned to be resected. Unnecessary dissection that may devascularize the bronchial blood supply must be avoided. Nodal dissection is recommended before anastomosis. Frozen section analysis of resection margins must be done intraoperatively. Mild bleeding from bronchial surface incision is considered to be a successful anastomosis. A positive margin must be resected. The distal bronchus should be divided close to its segmental subdivisions in order to obtain the most robust pulmonary collateral circulation [13]. The distal lung must be mobilized for a tension free anastomosis. Firstly, the mobilization involves the release of the inferior pulmonary ligament. Anastomosis is usually performed as an end-to-end manner. During anastomosis 4/0 or 5/0 monofilament absorbable sutures are preferable. If there is a huge difference between bronchi to be anastomosed, telescoping can be performed. Sutures must be placed transmurally and knots tied outside in order to reduce the tension. Most surgeons recommend the use of absorbable sutures because of lower chance of intraluminal granuloma, anastomotic narrowing [12]. After the last step of the sewing, the field is flooded with saline and the lung is inflated to check for air leaks. The anastomosis should be airtight despite an airway pressure of 35 to 40 cm of water. Most authors recommend a pedicled flap of pleura or pericardial encircled fat around the anastomosis as a buttress and for isolation of suture line from nearby vascular structures (usually pulmonary artery). The anastomosis should be inspected with a flexible bronchoscope postoperatively to detect problem (if any) and to aspirate residual secretion and blood from the distal lobe. Patients should undergo bronchoscopy before being discharged in order to evaluate the anastomosis.

SPECIFIC BRONCHOPLASTIES

Right Upper Sleeve Lobectomy

Right upper lobe sleeve resection is the most common of all bronchoplasties. The hilum of the right upper lobe is first dissected and divided in a standard fashion.

The bronchus is encircled by a surgical tape at the levels of the right mainstem bronchus and bronchus intermedius. The bronchotomy to main bronchus is made to the right upper lobe take off and the intermediate bronchus is divided just before the orifice of the middle lobe (Fig. **1**). A right upper lobe tumour which involves the middle lobe parenchyma and not the intermedial bronchus is best managed by removal of the middle and upper lobes. Middle lobectomy with sleeve resections of the bronchus intermedius is an infrequently performed operation.

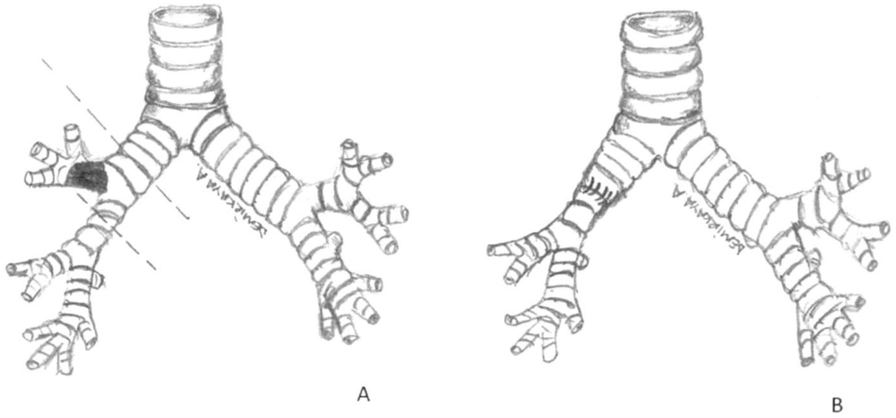

Figure 1: Right upper lobe sleeve lobectomies.

Segmental Bronchoplasty, Wedge Bronchoplasty

In this procedure, very precise anastomosis of smaller segmental bronchi is required. In some patients, in which excision of the carina between the upper and lower divisions of the left upper lobe bronchus for a tiny carcinoid tumour without pulmonary resection, is necessary the exposure becomes difficult since all segmental vessels must be preserved. With careful dissection and meticulous reconstruction, results have been good in these cases [14].

Wedge resections of the main bronchus have been reported infrequently as an alternative technique for parenchyma conservation [12]. Wedge resection is performed longitudinally along the bronchus and the bronchial defect is approximated transversely. Postoperative complications such as bronchostenosis, bronchial deformity and pneumonia are common especially after wedge bronchoplasties [12].

POSTOPERATIVE CARE

Additional measures must be taken in patients who underwent bronchoplastic resection. Patient must be extubated as early as possible with bronchoscopic control. Respiratory exercises should be taught during the preoperative period the patients must receive mucolytics, bronchodilator and intensive pulmonary rehabilitation. When these maneuvers are inadequate, a bed-side flexible bronchoscopy should be performed in order to aspirate mucus plugs under direct vision. The use of corticosteroids postoperatively can be given for anti-edema effect that can reduce secretion retention, atelectasis and granuloma formation at the level of anastomosis [12]. However, more studies are needed for confirmation of the usage of corticosteroids in these patients.

OUTCOME

Atelectasis occurs in approximately 6.7% and 5.4% of patients [12]. Atelectasis can be developed due to secretion retention secondary to inability to cough, edema at the level of the anastomosis and loss of ciliary function. Bronchoscopy should be performed in these circumstances.

Major complications following sleeve resection include:anastomotic dehiscence, empyema and bronchovascular fistula. The rate of these complications is fortunately low. A complete dehiscence can be caused by anastomotic tension. If dehiscence is greater than 10 mm requires completion pneumonectomy. An empyema may occur with or without bronchopleural fistula. Empyema can be managed with chest-tube drainage, empirical wide spectrum antibiotics and prevention and/or obliteration of remaining space. If there is a bronchopleural fistula, pneumonectomy is required and infection control must be initiated. Bronchoscopy fistula may be present with massive hemoptysis due to erosion of the adjacent pulmonary artery into the bronchial tree across the anastomosis. Immediate bronchoscopy must be performed to examine the anastomosis and bleeding area. Immediate completion pneumonectomy (if the patient is not in a septic condition) is usually required.

Local recurrence is low as long as the margins are free of disease. Local control of disease after bronchoplastic lobectomies is 22.5% and patients sometimes developed a locoregional recurrence after sleeve lobectomy [12].

Sleeve lobectomy is strongly favored over pneumonectomy. Schirren [15] reported a 51% survival at 5 years in patients with stage 1 disease, a 41% survival at 5 years in patients with stage II disease, and a 25% survival at 5 years in patients with stage IIIA disease. In 300 sleeve lobectomies, Deslauriers [16] reported a 5 year survival rate of 54%.

Table 1: Benign indications for bronchoplastic resections

Posttraumatic stenosis, histoplasmosis, granulomatous and idiopathic, post-surgical
Neoplasms, hamartoma, mucus gland cystic adenoma, inflammatory pseudotumour, lymphoid aggregates.

Table 2: Malign indications for bronchoplastic resections

Low grade malignancy	Bronchogenic carcinomas
Carcinoid	Squamous cell carcinoma
Mucoepidermoid carcinoma	Adenocarcinoma
Fibrous histiocytoma	Large cell carcinoma
Adenoid cystic carcinoma	Adenosquamous carcinoma
Granular cell tumour	
Hemangiopericytoma	

ACKNOWLEDGEMENTS

Declared none.

CONFLICT OF INTEREST

The authors confirm that this article content has no conflict of interest.

REFERENCES

[1] Price-Thomas C. Conservative resection of the bronchial tree.JR Coll Surg Edinb 1956,1:169-186.

[2] Allison PR Personal communicaiton, quoted by Johnston JB,Jones PH: The treatment of bronchial carcinoma by lobectomy and sleeve resection of the main bronchus.Thorax 14:49,1959.

[3] Paulson DL,Shaw RR Preservation of lung tissue by means of bronchoplastic procedure. Am J Surg 89:347-355,1955.

[4] Vogt-Moykopff I,Fritz TH,Meyer G, et al: Bronchoplastic and angioplastic operation in bronchial carcinoma:Long term results of a retrospective analysis from 1973 to 1983.Int Surg 7:211-220,1986.

[5] Gaissert HA, Mathisen DJ, Moncure AC, *et al.* Survival and function after sleeve lobectomy for lung cancer. Thorac Cardiovasc Surg 1996;111:948–53.

[6] Deslauriers J, Gaulin P, Beaulieu M, *et al.* Long-term clinicaland functional results of sleeve lobectomy for primary lung cancer. J Thorac Cardiovasc Surg 1986; 92:871–9.

[7] Bueno R,Wain JC,Wright CD, *et al.* Bronchoplasty in the Main and Lobar Bronchoplasty management of low-grade airway neoplasms and benign bronchial stenoses. Ann Thorac Surg 1996; 62:824–9.

[8] Newton JR, Grillo HC, Mathisen DJ. Main bronchial sleeve resection with pulmonary conservation. Ann Thorac Surg 1991;52:1272–80

[9] Faber LP, Jensik RJ, Kittle CF. Results of sleeve lobectomy for bronchogenic carcinoma in 101 patients. Anz Thorac Surg 1984;37:279–85.

[10] Mathisen DJ, Grillo HC, Vlahakes G, Daggett WM. The omentum in the management of complicated cardiothoracic problems. J Thorac Cardiovasc Surg 1988; 95:677–84.

[11] Muehrcke DD, Grillo HC, Mathisen DJ. Reconstructive airway surgery after irradiation. Ann Thorac Surg 1995;59:14–8.

[12] Francoise Tronc,Joceln Gregorie and Jean Deslauriers.Bronchoplasthy in Pearsons Thoracic And Cardiovascular Surgery.Churchil Livingstone Elsevier,Philadelphia.2008 894-908.

[13] Takeda SI, Maeda H,Koma M, et al Comparison of surgical results afeter pneumonectomy and sleeve lobectomy for non small cell lung cancer:trends over time and 20 year institutional experience.Eur J Cardiothorac Surg 2006;29;276-280.

[14] Douglas J.Mathisen, Main and Lobar Bronchoplasty in Grillo Hermes J. Surgery of the Trachea and Bronchi. London BC Decker Inc,2004 620-629.

[15] 15.Schirren J,et al In Shields TW,ed General Thoracic Surgery,5th ed. Vol 1.Malvern, PA: Williams & Wilkins, 1999:399.

[16] Deslaures J.Pneumonectomy *versus* sleeve resections for the management of resectable lung cancer.J Thorac Oncol 2007:2 (8 suppl):S169-S170.

Send Orders of Reprints at reprints@benthamscience.net
Lung Cancer: Clinical and Surgical Specifications, **2013, 355-364**

CHAPTER 10

Part K: Intraoperative Mediastinal Lymph Node Examination Techniques in Non-Small Cell Lung Cancer

Mehmet Ali Bedirhan*

Yedikule Hospital for Chest Disease, Istanbul, Turkey

Abstract: Nodal status at the time of staging is a critical determinant of survival in non-small cell lung cancer [NSCLC]. Despite the fact that the use of positron emission tomography [PET] scan and cervical mediastinoscopy–whether in combination or not—in staging has shown an acceptable accuracy rate, the extent of dissection still remains a problem. To date, there has been no consensus among either thoracic surgeons or oncologists regarding the optimal dissection of mediastinal lymph nodes [MLNs] in the early stages of NSCLC. Mediastinal lymph node dissection [MLND] is one of the techniques for MLN assessment and is not dependent on the location of the tumour or the lobe. All mediastinal fatty tissue containing lymphatics and lymph nodes is dissected from surrounding anatomical landmarks by either sharp or blunt dissection. Another technique is mediastinal lymph node sampling [MLNS], in which all mediastinal fatty tissue that potentially contains lymph nodes is not removed. The lymph nodes to be resected are determined preoperatively or intraoperatively. Because of the aggressiveness of MLND and the relative subjectivity of MLNS, some surgeons prefer dissection of the lymphatic pool and do no further dissection if that pool is negative. It is also important to consider N1 disease, and fixed lymph nodes to the bronchus usually necessitate more extensive surgery than lobectomy alone. In brief, questions still remain regarding the extent of lymph node removal. In patients undergoing resection for stage I and stage II NSCLC, it is recommended that intraoperative systematic MLNS or MLND be performed for accurate pathologic staging. Grade of recommendation: 1B.

Keywords: Lymph nodes, mediastinum, intraoperative staging, NSCLC, MLN, MLND, MLNS.

INTRODUCTION

Nodal status at the time of staging is a critical determinant of survival in non-small cell lung cancer [NSCLC] [1, 2]. However, the accurate delineation of

***Address correspondence to Mehmet Ali Bedirhan:** Yedikule Hospital for Chest Disease, Istanbul, Turkey; Tel: +90 212 6641700/1162; Fax: +90 212 5472233; E-mails: bedirhans@superonline.com and bedirhans@gmail.com mediastinal lymph nodes [MLNs] is still controversial. Even though lobectomy and pneumonectomy with mediastinal lymph node dissection [MLND] have been recommended as the standard curative operation for NSCLC cases, some believe that the incidence of postoperative complications are much higher in patients undergoing MLND [3].

Despite the fact that the use of positron emission tomography [PET] scan and cervical mediastinoscopy—-whether in combination or not—in staging has shown an acceptable accuracy rate, the extent of dissection still remains a problem. To date there has been no consensus among either thoracic surgeons or oncologists regarding the optimal dissection of MLNs in the early stages of NSCLC [4]. The difference in practice patterns could be explained by inadequate training, lag in communication, [5] or nononcologic surgery.

DISSECTION TECHNIQUES

It is first necessary to mention the types of dissection techniques. MLND is not dependent on the location of the tumour or the lobe. All mediastinal fatty tissue containing lymphatics and lymph nodes is dissected from the surrounding anatomical landmarks by either sharp or blunt dissection. This approach involves dissection of the upper mediastinal nodes [ATS 2 and 3], subcarinal nodes [ATS 7], and the lower mediastinal nodes [ATS 8 and 9] on the right side. All fatty tissue around these stations is also resected. Subcarinal nodes and fatty tissue along the left main bronchus to the extent of 3–4 cm are also resected. Lymph nodes located at stations 2 and 4 are usually dissected *en bloc* between the superior caval vein and the trachea, and sometimes lymph nodes located at station 10 are also resected *en bloc* with them by dissection beneath the azygos vein.

On the left side, MLND includes the resection of the paraaortic [ATS 6] and subaortic [ATS 5] lymph nodes and ATS 7, 8, and 9, and dissection of all surrounding fatty tissue around the paraaortic and subaortic area, subcarinal fatty tissue, and tissue around the inferior pulmonary ligament and esophagus.

Some authors mention the necessity of more extended dissection techniques for left-sided tumours to get more accurate staging, such as division of the ductus

Botalli to mobilize the aortic arch to access the left paratracheal nodes [6] and dissection by the use of median sternotomy to dissect all mediastinal tissue [7]. This author's personal opinion is that it is not necessary today, because any combination of PET scanning, cervical mediastinoscopy, or endobronchial ultrasound (EBUS) helps to evaluate this area with an acceptable accuracy rate or lowers the rate of false negativity to very acceptable levels.

Another technique is mediastinal lymph node sampling (MLNS), in which all mediastinal fatty tissue that potentially contains lymph nodes is not removed. The lymph nodes to be resected are determined preoperatively or intraoperatively. In MLNS, the number of lymph nodes to be resected is determined both by the surgeon and the pathologist; in MLND, this is determined by the pathologist alone. It is clear that MLNS is a subjective technique, because the selection of lymph nodes to be resected either preoperatively or postoperatively depends on the surgical team.

Because of the aggressiveness of MLND and the relative subjectivity of MLNS, another procedure is presented by Okada *et al.* [4]. Okada's study procedure reported the validation and utility of selective MLND (SMLND) [8]. In this technique, dissection of the upper mediastinal or subcarinal lymph nodes is performed if the tumour is located in the upper lobe. Dissection of the lower mediastinal lymph nodes is not performed if previous nodes are negative by frozen section. Moreover, in lower lobe tumours, upper mediastinal dissection is not performed if lower mediastinal nodes are negative by frozen section.

To date, there has been no consensus among thoracic surgeons and oncologists regarding the optimal extent of dissection of MLNs [4]. The aim of all surgeons and oncologists treating NSCLC is to perform superior surgical procedures, to have more appropriate mediastinal staging and more accurate treatment, shorter operating times, and fewer postoperative complications. Several studies researching the best procedure for MLN resection techniques will possibly provide surgeons with indications that allow the selection of a personal preference based on the criteria of the quality of radiological assistance, the spectrum of patients' stages, and surgical experience.

MORBIDITY RELATED TO MLND AND MLNS

The arguments in favor of MLND are the improved accuracy of intraoperative staging and better locoregional control because of extensive dissection. It is clear that extensive dissection collects more lymph nodes and lowers the rate of skip metastasis [6]. Arguments against routine MLND are increased morbidity when compared to MLNS, with a possible lack of evidence of improved staging or survival [6]. A more accurate evaluation of these two dissection procedures is the morbidity related to the techniques of each procedure.

Okada *et al.* [4] compared the morbidity rates of a prospective cohort of 377 patients who underwent MLNS and 358 patients who underwent MLND. The overall complication rate was 10.1% for the MLNS group and 17.3% for the MLND group. The rate of dysrhythmia, pulmonary complications, chylothorax, and persistent air leak was higher in the MLND group, but not significantly. However, several other studies have reported that there are no differences between mortality or morbidity rates with either technique [4,6]. In the American College of Surgeons Oncology Groups (ACOSOG) Z0030 trial, morbidity rate after MLND and MLNS did not differ significantly, but the MLND group had a greater median operative time than did the MLNS group, by 15 minutes [$p<0.0001$] [9].

To what extent does nodal evaluation affect survival? A retrospective cohort study involving 442 patients with clinical stage I NSCLC showed that those who underwent random sampling had a significantly lower survival rate compared to those who underwent MLNS (51% *vs.* 80%, $p<0.001$) [9]. Another study presented by Lardinois, comparing overall survival among different tumour stages and nodal involvement, [6] determined that there was no significant difference between the MLND group (51.7 months) and MLNS group (50.9 months) [$p=0.4$].

In Okada's study, [4] the MLND group was compared with a SMLND group. There was no significant difference in disease-free survival [$p=0.376$] or in overall survival [$p=0.06$] between the two groups.

MLND was associated with more favorable overall survival rates in the Eastern Cooperative Oncology Group (ECOG) 3590 study [10]. Patients with N1 disease,

N2 disease, and right-sided tumours had a higher overall survival rate after MLND. However, MLND did not confer a survival advantage to patients with left-sided tumours [10]. The ECOG 3590 researchers speculated that the lack of survival benefit for left-sided tumours might be due to the difficulty in accessing the paratracheal, perivascular, and subcarinal lymph nodes, or because MLND carries a higher benefit for right-sided tumours due to more complicated lymphatic pathways and a shorter right main bronchus.

In a prospective randomized study, 532 patients with operable clinical stage I to stage IIIA disease underwent either MLND or MLNS. MLND was statistically associated with a significantly higher survival rate in patients with stage I disease and stage IIIA disease when compared to MLNS [82% *vs.* 57% and 27% *vs.* 6%, respectively]. Even in stage II disease, MLND had a marginally significant survival advantage against MLNS [32% and 26.9%, p=0.0523] [10].

It is known that several studies [6,11] have discussed this subject extensively. However, it seems that some factors have strong correlation not only with overall prognosis, but also with the risk of recurrence. These factors are sex [male], age [older], size [larger tumour], and pN factor [positive lymph nodes]. The type of dissection performed did not significantly affect either disease-free survival [p=0.636] or overall survival [p=0.119] [4].

RECURRENCE RATES AND MORTALITY RATES

After the models of dissection techniques, their morbidity, and their effect on survival, the next step in the discussion is the extent of recurrence. In the Lardinois study, [6] all patients were in clinical stages T 1-3 and N0-1. During follow up, the overall local and distal recurrences for pathological stages I, II, and IIIA were 59%, 82%, and 90%, respectively, for the MLDS group and 38%, 75%, and 62%, respectively, for the MLND group. What was more interesting was that local recurrence was 40% after MLNS and 16% after MLND. During follow up, local recurrence in patients with a pathological nodal negative mediastinum [N0-1 disease] was observed in 46% after MLNS and 13% after MLND [p=0.004].

However, in another study, MLND did not confer local recurrence rates or lower patients' survival rates. Nonetheless, subgroup analysis shows significantly lower local recurrence rates after MLND as against MLNS in patients with pathologic stage I disease [12.5% 45%, $p=0.002$]. Disease-free survival was also higher in the MLND group patients with pathologic stage I disease [60.2 months *vs.* 44.8 months, $p<0.03$] [13].

In the ACOSOG Z0030 trial, [9] MLND diagnosed 3.8% more patients with N2 disease than did MLNS, or MLNS missed 3.8% more patients with N2 disease than did MLND. In this case, it is clear that when the mediastinum is clearly and accurately detected, those patients will be upstaged and will have appropriate adjuvant therapy. Several other studies report relevant findings [11-14].

Another matter in operative mediastinal lymphatic procedures is skip metastasis. A tumour can metastasize anywhere in the mediastinum *via* lymphatic pathways. Generally, a single-level N2 disease confers more favorable survival rates than multilevel N2 disease [15]. It seems that MLND is more accurate than MLNS at collecting more lymph nodes and prevents the possibility of skip metastasis.

Accurate preoperative staging is the gold standard of NSCLC surgery. This is proven by postoperative pathologic examination, but no data were achieved during operations. The more accurate the staging for a patient, the more appropriate the adjuvant therapy the patient receives. Since all mediastinal fatty tissue and lymph nodes are dissected in the MLND technique, the number of lymph nodes to be resected is important in MLNS cases. The aim of the surgery is to achieve good surveillance and to improve the disease-free interval with low morbidity and mortality. Here, the question is how many lymph nodes should be resected and how many stations should be dissected to get an accurate staging. The optimal number of lymph nodes that should be evaluated is contentious [16,17].

In a review of the surveillance, epidemiology, and end-results database, the mortality rates of 16,800 patients were enrolled in a study. The patients had no adjuvant therapy. The mortality rates were correlated with the number of lymph nodes resected. The number of lymph nodes were grouped in the following manner: 1–4, 5–8, 9–12,13–16, and more than 16. The highest survival rate was noted in the group of 13–16 nodes and the more-than-16 lymph nodes group did not confer an improvement in survival [4,6,18].

The number of stations to be resected is also open to question, as mentioned above. It seems to be important when surgeons prefer MLNS or SMLND. The answer probably depends on the least number of lymphatic pathways of the lobe to be resected. Doddoli and colleagues [6] demonstrated that MLND provides a survival advantage against MLNS, and concluded that at least 2 MLN stations must necessarily be evaluated to get an accurate MLN staging. Also, a retrospective study by Gajra and colleagues [12] reported that patients were found to have statistically significant higher survival rates when three or more stations were examined than when two or fewer stations were examined. Based on the results of these studies, the National Comprehensive Cancer Network Practice Guidelines recommend examining at least three mediastinal lymphatic stations.

EVALUATION OF TECHNIQUES

Briefly, questions still remain regarding the extent of lymph node removal [sampling *vs.* dissection] or the minimum number of lymph node stations or nodes sampled. At present, there is insufficient information to recommend one technique as superior. In patients undergoing resection for stages I and II NSCLC, it is recommended that intraoperative systematic MLNS or MLND be performed for accurate pathologic staging. Grade of recommendation: 1B [19].

The next step in NSCLC cases is the possibility of N1 disease after excluding N2 disease by frozen section. The question is what action should be taken when N1 positivity is found intraoperatively. As discussed above, full evaluation of lymph nodes gives more accurate staging and therefore more appropriate treatment.

As is known, it is usually not possible to make an accurate preoperative assessment of N1 disease by computed tomography [CT]. PET scanning may help in this matter, but has a high false-positive rate. The only definitive way is surgical staging. There are several well-designed studies related to N1 disease. They demonstrate that multiple N1 disease has a worse prognosis than single N1 disease, and that the negative prognostic effect for stations 10 and 11 is worse than for stations 12, 13, and 14 [2, 0].

It is obvious that lobectomy should always be preferred over pneumonectomy, because of the high morbidity and mortality associated with the latter. Station 10 usually does not change the operative strategy unless fixed to the main bronchus or the main pulmonary artery. In case of fixation, sleeve bronchial or arterial resections should also be considered. Pneumonectomy may be preferred to achieve complete surgery with tumour-free margins.

In cases of station 11 positivity, lobectomy is still the preferred option, with adjuvant therapy. When capsule invasion is found or when the positive node is fixed to the bronchus, bronchial sleeve lobectomy is the treatment of choice [21-23].

CONCLUSION

This paper has evaluated the description, the importance, the types of intraoperative mediastinal lymphatic staging and morbidity during elective cancer surgery of NSCLC cases, as well as the disease-free period and effects on survival of each method. It is obvious that the ideal treatment of a properly staged cancer case is dependent on a properly staged mediasten, regardless of the T stage. Currently, multislice tomography PET scanning and EBUS and final evaluation by mediatinoscopy are reliable tools for mediastinal examination. Surgery is not accepted as curative in a case without mediastinal assessment.

The surgeon may be influenced by his nature, training, experience, and oncological approach when selecting a staging procedure completing non-invasive mediasten techniques performed preoperatively. However, MLND is the clear requirement in selected cases such as small-cell cancer surgery and operations following neoadjuvant therapy.

Today the increasing frequency of advanced-age tumours, minimal invasive resections, and more frequent early-stage tumours emphasizes the importance of mediastinal lymphatic evaluation and reiterates the question of how frequently such evaluations should be done.

ACKNOWLEDGEMENTS

Declared none.

CONFLICT OF INTEREST

The author confirms that this article content has no conflict of interest.

REFERENCES

[1] Mountain CF. Revisions in the International System for Staging Lung Cancer. Chest 1997;111:1710 –7.

[2] Naruke T, Goya T, Tsuchiya R, Suemasu K. Prognosis and survival in resected lung carcinoma based on the new international staging system. J Thorac Cardiovasc Surg 1988; 96:440 –7.

[3] Tanita T, Hoshikawa Y, Tabata T, Noda M, Handa M, Kubo H, Chida M, Suzuki S, Ono S, Fujimura S. Functional evaluation for pulmonary resection for lung cancer in octogenarians. Investigation from postoperative complications. Jpn J Thorac Cardiovasc Surg 1999;47:253–61.

[4] Okada M, Sakamoto T, Yuki T, Mimura T, Miyoshi K, Tsubota N. Selective Mediastinal Lymphadenectomy for Clinico-Surgical Stage I Non-Small Cell Lung Cancer. Ann Thorac Surg 2006;81:1028–32.

[5] Doddoli C, Aragon A, Barlesi F, *et al.* Does the extent of lymph node dissection influence outcome in patients with stage I non-small-cell lung cancer? Eur J Cardiothorac Surg 2005;27:680–5.

[6] Lardinois D, Suter H, Hakki H, Rousson V, Betticher D, Ris HB. Morbidity, survival, and site of recurrence after dissection *versus* systematic sampling after complete resection for non-small cell lung cancer. Ann Thorac Surg 2005;80:268-75.

[7] Watanabe Y, Shimizu J, Oda M, Hayashi Y, Tatsuzawa Y, Watanabe S, Yoshida M, Iwa T. Improved survival in left non-small-cell N2 lung cancer after more extensive operative procedure. Thorac Cardiovasc Surg. 1991 Apr;39[2]:89–94.

[8] Okada M, Tsubota N, Yoshimura M, Miyamoto Y. Proposal for reasonable mediastinal lymphadenectomy in bronchogenic carcinomasrole of subcarinal nodes in selective dissection. J Thorac Cardiovasc Surg 1998;116:949–53.

[9] Allen MS, Darling GE, Pechet TT, *et al.* Morbidity and mortality of major pulmonary resections in patients with early-stage lung cancer: initial results of the randomized, prospective ACOSOG Z0030 trial. Ann Thorac Surg 2006;81: 1013–19; discussion 1019–20.

[10] Wu Y, Huang ZF, Wang SY, Yang XN, Ou W. A randomized trial of systematic nodal dissection in resectable non-small cell lung cancer. Lung Cancer 2002;36:1–6.

[11] 11.Izbicki JR, Thetter O, Habekost M. et.al. Radical systhematic mediastinal lymphdenectomy in non-small cell lung cancer: a randomised controlled trial. Br J Surg 1994;81;22935

[12] Gajra A, Newman N, Gamble GP, Kohman LJ, Graziano SL. Effect of number of lymph nodes sampled on outcome in patients with stage I non-small-cell lung cancer. J Clin Oncol 2003;21:1029–34.

[13] Misthos P, Sepsas E, Athanassiadi K, Kakaris S, Skottis I. Skip metastases: analysis of their clinical significance and prognosis in the IIIA stage of non-small cell lung cancer. Eur J Cardiothorac Surg 2004;25:502–8.

[14] Prenzel KL, Monig SP, Sinning JM, *et al.* Role of skip metastasis to mediastinal lymph nodes in non-small cell lung cancer. J Surg Oncol 2003;82:256–60.

[15] Yoshino I, Yokoyama H, Yano T, *et al.* Skip metastasis to the mediastinal lymph nodes in non-small cell lung cancer. Ann Thorac Surg 1996;62:1021–5.

[16] Watanabe A, Koyanagi T, Obama T, *et al.* Assessment of node dissection for clinical stage I primary lung cancer by VATS. Eur J Cardiothorac Surg 2005;27:745–52.

[17] Asamura H, Nakayama H, Kondo H, Tsuchiya R, Naruke T. Lobe-specific extent of systematic lymph node dissection for non-small cell lung carcinomas according to a retrospective study of metastasis and prognosis. J Thorac Cardiovasc Surg 1999;117:1102–11.

[18] Oda M, Watanabe Y, Shimizu J, *et al.* Extent of mediastinal node metastasis in clinical stage I non-small-cell lung cancer: the role of systematic nodal dissection. Lung Cancer 1998;22:23–30.

[19] Ginsberg RJ. Resection of non-small cell lung cancer: how much and by what route. Chest 1997;112:203S–5S.

[20] Keller SM, Adak S, Wagner H, *et al.* A randomized trial of postoperative adjuvant therapy in patients with completely resected stage II or IIIA non-small-cell lung cancer. Eastern Cooperative Oncology Group. N Engl J Med 2000;343: 1217–22.

[21] Scott WJ, Howington J, Feigenberg S, Movsas B, Pisters K. Clinical Practice Guidelines [2nd Edition] Stage I and Stage II *: ACCP Evidence-Based Treatment of Non-Small Cell Lung Cancer. Chest 2007;132;234S–42S.

[22] Sayar A, Turna A, Kiliçgün A, Solak O, Urer N, Gürses A. Prognostic significance of surgical-pathologic multiple-station N1 disease in non-small cell carcinoma of the lung. Eur J Cardiothorac Surg. 2004 Mar;25[3]:434–8.

[23] Aydogmus U, Cansever L, Sonmezoglu Y, Karapinar K, Kocaturk CI, Bedirhan MA. The impact of the type of resection on survival in patients with N1 non-small-cell lung cancers. Eur J Cardiothorac Surg. 2010 Feb;37[2]:446–50.

CHAPTER 11

Oncologic Treatment of Non-Small Cell Lung Cancer

Part A: Neoadjuvant Chemotherapy Options for Non-Small Cell Lung Carcinoma

Ahmet Taner Sumbul and Ozgur Ozyilkan*

Division of Medical Oncology, Baskent University, Research and Treatment Center, Adana, Turkey

Abstract: Lung cancer remains the most common malignancy and the most common cause of cancer mortality worldwide for both men and women. In 2008, an estimated 1.6 million new cases of lung cancer were diagnosed and an estimated 1.4 million deaths from lung cancer occurred. Nearly 85 % of lung cancers are diagnosed as Non-Small Cell Lung Cancer. The mortality from advanced stage Non-Small lung cancer is still high even with new therapeutic agents. The chemotherapy and palliative radiotherapy are the only treatment options at the advanced stage of the disease. Surgical resection and adjuvant chemotherapy is the mainstay of treatment at early stage disease and concomitant curative chemoradiotherapy is the recommended treatment modality in locally advanced stage. The neoadjuvant chemotherapy is shown to be useful for various types of cancer. The benefit of neoadjuvant chemotherapy in Non-Small cell lung cancer is being investigated in ongoing phase II and III trials.

Keywords: Neoadjuvant Chemotherapy, lung cancer.

MAIN BODY

Lung cancer is the leading cause of cancer related mortality in both sexes. Non-Small cell lung cancer (NSCLC) accounts for about nearly 80-85% of all lung cancers. Surgical resection is the mainstay of treatment in early stage NSCLC. Unfortunately, approximately 55-60% of NSCLCs are diagnosed at advanced stage when the cure is nearly impossible. The prognosis of the patients after resection is mostly related to stage of the disease and the lymph node involvement. The 5 year survival rates vary from 70 % for stage I to 15 % for stage IIIB disease. The mortality after complete resection is usually related to

***Address correspondence to Ozgur Ozyilkan:** Division of Medical Oncology, Baskent University, Research and Treatment Center, Adana, Turkey; Tel: +90 322 3444444/1258; Fax: +90 322 3444452; E-mail: ozyilkano@hotmail.com occult micro metastasis of tumour to distant tissues. This problem may be solved by initiation of chemotherapy either in neoadjuvant or in adjuvant setting. It has been shown that adjuvant chemotherapy is useful in treatment of early stage NSCLC (stages IB-IIIA) [1, 2].

Neoadjuvant chemotherapy was first defined by Frei. The aim was to improve progression free and overall survival by the administration of therapeutic agents before the main treatment [3]. Neoadjuvant therapy has some advantages and disadvantages. The treatment response can be assessed early and down staging of the disease could be achieved which may increase the possibility of surgical resection of the primary disease. There are also well known disadvantages. The neoadjuvant chemotherapy may increase the perioperative mortality. The time required for the administration of neoadjuvant chemotherapy may result in exclusion or delay of curative local treatment modalities.

There are several studies designed to compare neoadjuvant chemotherapy *versus* surgery in patients with early stage and locally advanced NSCLC.

Main Phase III Trials Conducted in Early Stage NSCLC are as follows:

SWOG 9900 trial was designed to investigate neoadjuvant chemotherapy followed by surgery *versus* immediate surgery in patients with early stage NSCLC [4]. A total of 354 patients were randomly enrolled for 3 cycles of paclitaxel plus carboplatin followed by surgery *versus* immediate surgery. There was a difference in progression free and overall survival rates (33 *versus* 21 months respectively) and also in five year survival rates (50% *versus* 40%) but all these results did not reach statistically significant level.

Multicenter European LU 22/EORTC 08012 trial was the largest randomized trial which compared platinum doublet neoadjuvant chemotherapy protocols with surgery alone [5]. Most of the patients' enrolled for this study had clinical stages I and II disease. Patients were prescribed to use 3 cycles of cisplatin plus vinorlbine or gemcitabine. Approximately, 75% of patients completed three cycles of therapy and response rate was reported to be 47% in chemotherapy group (44% partial, 3% complete response). No improvement was observed either in the terms of progression or in overall survival rate. The important factor for the negative results was the presence of high percentage of patients with stage I disease.

NATCH trial was another trial designed to evaluate the effect of carboplatin and paclitaxel in early stage NSCLC patients [6]. A total of 624 patients with stages IA, IB, II or III (T3N1) NSCLC were randomly assigned to surgery alone or neoadjuvant chemotherapy, followed by surgery or surgery followed by adjuvant chemotherapy. Paclitaxel plus carboplatin combination was used as chemotherapy regimen and 90% of patients in neoadjuvant arm and 60% of patients in adjuvant arm that completed the chemotherapy course. The primary objective of the study was the comparison of disease free survival times of the arms. Results of this study was published recently and there were no statistically significant differences found in both disease free survival (34-38-37% respectively for surgery alone, neoadjuvant chemotherapy followed by surgery and surgery followed by adjuvant chemotherapy) and overall survival rates (44-47-46% respectively for surgery alone, neoadjuvant chemotherapy followed by surgery and surgery followed by adjuvant chemotherapy).

In conclusion, as compare to the immediate surgery, current studies do not support initiation of neoadjuvant chemotherapy in patients with early stage NSCLC but further studies with newer chemotherapeutic regimens effecting disease free survival, progression free survival or overall survival may change these recommendations.

Neoadjuvant chemotherapy is another important issue in patients with stage IIIA-N2 NSCLC because this group represents a heterogeneous group of patients which is ranging between minimal N2 diseases (incidentally found) to multistation bulky N2 disease. Five year survival rates between these groups are very different; it changes between 5% to 35% related with nodal status of patients. There are several studies conducted to investigate the role of neoadjuvant chemotherapy in patients with stage IIIA-N2 NSCLC.

Mattson *et al.* investigated three cycles of preoperative chemotherapy with Docetaxel 100 mg/m2 followed by surgery or radiotherapy *versus* surgery or radiotherapy alone [7]. Objective response rate and complete response rate in patients treated with docetaxel was 28% and 3%, respectively. Median survival rate was much better than surgery or radiotherapy alone (14.8 *versus* 12.6 months) but this difference was not statistically significant.

Intergroup 0139 trial was conducted to investigate the role of neoadjuvant chemotherapy in 429 patients with stage IIIAN2 NSCLC [8]. Patients were randomly assigned to two arms. First arm received cisplatin plus etoposide concurrent with thoracic radiotherapy (45Gy) followed by surgery, and the second arm received the same chemotherapy concurrent with definitive radiotherapy (61 Gy). Both arms received consolidation chemotherapy with two cycles of cisplatin plus etoposide. Progression free survival was significantly better in surgery group but treatment related mortality was higher and there was no statistically significant difference found in overall survival between two groups.

EORTC 08941 trial was another important trial designed to investigate treatment modalities in patients with locally advanced NSCLC over five hundred patients with stage IIIAN2 disease who underwent platinum based induction therapy (Cisplatin 80 mg/m2 or Carboplatin AUC $\geq$ 5) in conjunction with at least one of the following drugs paclitaxel, docetaxel or gemcitabine [9-10]. After completion of 3 cycles of chemotherapy, patients responses were screened by computed tomography and responsive patients were randomized to surgery or radiotherapy up to 60 Gy and no adjuvant chemotherapy was given to both groups. The primary endpoint was progression free survival rates and overall survival and there was no statistically significant difference found between the two groups.

German Lung Cancer Cooperative Group investigated the role of induction chemotherapy and concomitant radiotherapy in patients with stage IIIA N2 disease [9-11]. Patients were randomly assigned to three cycles of cisplatin plus etoposide with or without twice daily chemoradiation up to 45 Gy and they all patients underwent surgery. Radiotherapy up to 54 Gy was performed to the group which did not receive radiotherapy as induction. No statistically significant difference was found in progression free survival and overall survival rates between two groups.

All of these results showed that chemotherapy conjunction with radiotherapy are seem to be the standard treatment for stage IIIA N2 NSCLC.

In conclusion, the recent studies did not reveal statistically significant benefit in progression free survival and overall survival rates with neoadjuvant chemotherapy. The role of neoadjuvant chemotherapy in both early stage and locally advanced NSCLC needs to be clarified further. The studies involving new chemotherapeutic agents in large patient groups are required prior to developing recommendations for neoadjuvant chemotherapy in early stage and locally advanced NSCLC.

ACKNOWLEDGEMENTS

Declared none.

CONFLICT OF INTEREST

The authors confirm that this article content has no conflict of interest.

REFERENCES

[1] Arriagada, R; Bergman, B; Dunant, A; *et al.* International Adjuvant Lung Cancer Trial Collaborative Group. Cisplatin-based adjuvant chemotherapy in patients with completely resected non-small-cell lung cancer. N Engl J Med., 2004, 350,351-60.

[2] Douillard, JY; Rosell, R; De Lena, M *et al.* Adjuvant vinorelbine plus cisplatin *versus* observation in patients with completely resected stage IB-IIIA non-small-cell lung cancer (Adjuvant Navelbine International Trialist Association [ANITA]): a randomised controlled trial. Lancet Oncol., 2006,7,719-27.

[3] Frei, E. 3rd. Clinical cancer research: an embattled species. Cancer.,1982,50,1979-92.

[4] Pisters, K; Vallieres, E; Bunn, PA; *et al.* Presentation: S9900: Surgery alone or surgery plus induction (ind) paclitaxel/carboplatin (PC) chemotherapy in early stage non-small cell lung cancer (NSCLC): Follow-up on a phase III trial. J Clin Oncol., 2007, 25,389

[5] Gilligan, D; Nicolson, M; Smith, I; *et al.* Preoperative chemotherapy in patients with resectable non-small cell lung cancer: results of the MRC LU22/NVALT 2/EORTC 08012 multicentre randomised trial and update of systematic review. Lancet., 2007,369,1929-37.

[6] Felip, E; Vilar, E; The expanding role of systemic treatment in non-small cell lung cancer neo-adjuvant therapy. Ann Oncol., 2006,17,108-12.

[7] Mattson, KV; Abratt, RP; Ten, Velde, G; *et al.* Docetaxel as neoadjuvant therapy for radically treatable stage III non-small-cell lung cancer: a multinational randomised phase III study. Ann Oncol., 2003,14,116-22.

[8] Albain, KS; Swann, RS; Rusch, VW; *et al.* Radiotherapy plus chemotherapy with or without surgical resection for stage III non-small-cell lung cancer: a phase III randomised controlled trial. Lancet., 2009,374,379-86.

[9] De, Pauw, R; Van, Meerbeeck, JP; Neoadjuvant chemotherapy in the treatment of nonsmall-cell lung cancer. Curr Opin Oncol., 2007,19,92-7.

[10] Van, Meerbeeck, JP; Kramer, GW; Van, Schil, PE; *et al.* European Organisation for Research and Treatment of Cancer-Lung Cancer Group. Randomized controlled trial of

resection *versus* radiotherapy after induction chemotherapy in stage IIIA-N2 non-small-cell lung cancer. J Natl Cancer Inst., 2007 21,99,442-50.

[11] Thomas, M; Rübe, C; Hoffknecht, P; German Lung Cancer Cooperative Group. Effect of preoperative chemoradiation in addition to preoperative chemotherapy: a randomised trial in stage III non-small-cell lung cancer. Lancet Oncol., 2008,9,636-48.

Send Orders of Reprints at reprints@benthamscience.net
Lung Cancer: Clinical and Surgical Specifications, 2013, 371-376

CHAPTER 11

Part B: Adjuvant Chemotherapy for Resected Non-Small Cell Lung Carcinoma

Fatih Kose and Ozgur Ozyilkan*

Division of Medical Oncology, Baskent University, Research and Treatment Center, Adana, Turkey

Abstract: Lung cancer is the primary reason for cancer related mortality in the world. Although initial treatment for early stage Non-small Cell Lung Cancer (NSCLC) is a complete surgical resection, the recurrence rate of NSCLC in its early stages remains high. Even after a complete resection, the 5-year survival rates range from 67% to 23% for Stage IA to Stage IIIA disease, respectively. Recurrences, which are the primary factor for reduced survival rates, generally occur at distant, extra thoracic sites. As a result, even within its early stages, NSCLC is considered as a systemic disease at diagnosis and further improvement in survival rate can only be achieved with the eradication of micrometastatic disease to reduce the risk of distant recurrences.

Several recent phase III trials provide robust evidence for chemotherapy in adjuvant settings. In the meta-analysis of these trials, pooled analysis of LACE, cisplatin based adjuvant chemotherapy showed 5.4% of absolute benefit in 5-year survival rates. The effectiveness of the chemotherapy strongly depends upon the stage of the disease as well as the performance status of the patient. While patients with performance scale 0-1 gain significant overall survival (OS) benefit from chemotherapy, one should be very careful about patients with performance scale of 2 or greater. There were significant OS benefits for stage II and III disease, while chemotherapy may have detrimental effects on OS in Stage IA patients. Based on the subgroup analysis of CALGB 9633 trial, adjuvant chemotherapy may be offered to Stage IB patients with a big tumour.

Further improvements can be achieved by defining reliable and clinically approved predictive and prognostic factors and tailor treatment by using these parameters. RAS, p53 ERCC1, and gene expression profiles are all seemed to be reliable predictive and prognostic factors, but to the best of the authors' knowledge, there are no prospective data to support routine their clinical use.

Keywords: Adjuvant chemotherapy, lung cancer.

***Address correspondence to Ozgur Ozyilkan:** Division of Medical Oncology, Baskent University, Research and Treatment Center, Adana, Turkey; Tel: +90 322 3444444/1258; Fax: +90 322 3444452; E -mail: ozyilkano@hotmail.com

MAIN BODY

According to Globacan 2000, lung cancer is the most common and lethal cancer type in the world. Worldwide prevalence of the lung cancer was 1.2 million, and it caused 1.1 million losses in the year of the 2000 [1]. Though relatively effective chemotherapy and targeted agents are used for lung cancer in the last two decades, all of the trials that used these agents failed to report median overall survival(OS) more than 13 months at advanced stages. Even for early stage non-small cell lung cancer (NSCLC) patients who were completely resected with no additional treatment, 5-year survival rates range from 67% to 23% for Stage IA to Stage IIIA disease, respectively [2, 3]. Most of the deaths in early stage NSCLC are directly related with tumour relapse, and these relapses typically occur at distant extrathoracic sites [4]. These results strongly suggest that NSCLC is a systemic disease at diagnosis. Therefore, while surgery is a standard initial treatment for early stage NSCLC, effective systemic chemotherapy aiming the eradication of micro-metastatic disease will further decrease the rate of distant recurrences, and improve OS.

After the identification of the primary reason for lower survival in early stage NSCLC, many adjuvant chemotherapy trials were conducted to decrease distant recurrences to gain absolute benefit in disease free survival (DFS) and OS. In 1991, Holmes EC *et al.* reported a consensus report that adjuvant chemotherapy for early stage NSCLC does not have a proven benefit although this report used more than 50 randomized clinical trials including more than 10.000 cases [2,5]. In 1995, another meta-analysis to investigate the role of adjuvant chemotherapy was published [6]. This meta-analysis also failed to demonstrate the statistically significant benefits of the adjuvant chemotherapy. But interestingly, though five trials using alkylating based regimen as adjuvant regimen seemed to be have detrimental effects on OS, eight trials using cisplatin-based regimen showed a five percent improvement in OS among those who received chemotherapy (HR, 0.87; 95% CI, 0.74-1.02; p=0.08) without reaching a statistically significant level. The results of this meta-analysis strongly suggest that cisplatin-based regimen could have beneficial effects on OS which could reach a statistically significant level.

The International Adjuvant Lung Cancer Trial (IALT) was the first phase III randomized trial to demonstrate the survival benefits of adjuvant chemotherapy in an early stage NSCLC. 1867 patients with stage I, II, III NSCLC were included in this trial [7]. Patients were categorized randomly into 3 or 4 cycles of cisplatin based chemotherapy (adjuvant radiotherapy and accompanying drug to cisplatin were at discretion of participating center) *vs.* observation. After median follow-up of 56 months, OS was observed to be significantly better for chemotherapy arm as compared to the observation (HR, 0.86; 95% CI, 0.76-0.98; $p<0.03$). National Cancer Institute of Canada Clinical Trial Group Trial (JBR10) conducted adjuvant phase III randomized trial using adjuvant cisplatin plus vinorelbine *versus* observation in resected stage IB and stage II NSCLC patients [4]. The first results of JBR10 trial was published in 2005, OS was significantly prolonged in the chemotherapy arm compared with the observation group (94 *vs.* 73 months; HR, 0.69; $p=0.04$), as was relapse-free survival (not reached *vs.* 46.7 months;HR,0.60;$p<0.001$). IALT and BJR 10 studies were pivotal studies and after results of these trials adjuvant cisplatin doublet treatment was accepted as a standard treatment for completely resected Stage IB-III NSCLC patients.

The possible role of chemotherapy (mitomycin, vindesine, and cisplatin) after complete resection of stage I,II, and IIIA lung cancer patients are investigated in the Adjuvant Lung Project Italy (ALPI) trial [8]. Adjuvant thoracic radiotherapy was at the discretion of participating site. In this trial, chemotherapy failed to yield statistically significant DFS and OS gain over observation. Another negative study was The Big Lung Trial (BLT) which searched the role of cisplatin based regimen in stage I-III NSCLC after complete surgical resection. After a median follow-up of 34.6 months, HR for OS among those assigned to chemotherapy as compared to those assigned to observation alone was 1.02 (95% CI, 0.77-1.35; $p=0.90$) [9].

In CALGB 9633 trial completely resected only stage IB NSCLC patients were categorized randomly to chemotherapy (carboplatin-paclitaxel) or observation. OS was not statistically different (HR, 0.83; CI,0.64 to 1.08; $p=0.12$) between these groups. However, subgroup analysis revealed statistically significant survival advantage for tumours ≥ 4 cm in diameter for chemotherapy arm [10].

In Adjuvant Navelbine International Trialist Association (ANITA) trial [11], 840 patients with stage IB-IIIA NSCLC were randomly assigned to chemotherapy (cisplatin plus vinorelbine) or observation. After median follow-up of median 76 months (range 43-116), OS was observed to be 65.7 months (95% CI, 47.9-88.5) in the chemotherapy arm and 43.7 months(95% CI,35.7-52.3) in the observation arm. In this trial, disease specific mortality was significantly reduced in the chemotherapy arm as compared to the observation arm (HR 0.80[95% CI 0.66-0.96]; p=0.017).

After these conflicting results observed in recent trials, Lung Adjuvant Cisplatin Evaluation (LACE) collaborative group published pooled analysis using individual patient data from five large, recently randomized phase III studies which used cisplatin doublet as adjuvant regimen in early stage NSCLC [12]. Five trials and 4,584 patient were eligible for LACE meta-analysis. The primary objective of this meta-analysis was to describe most effective adjuvant regimen or to answer which particular group of patients would have benefited from adjuvant chemotherapy. A statistically significant benefit was observed on OS and DFS which favored chemotherapy with absolute benefits of 5.4% and 5.8% at 5 years, respectively. The rate of grade 3-4 toxicities – which was neutropenia in most of the cases -- was 66%. At the time of analysis, 2,390 deaths were observed. 342 of them were considered non lung cancer death and 103 of these 342 patients died within the first 6 months. Therefore, it can be stated that chemotherapy significantly increases the non-lung cancer death (HR=1.36; 95% CI, 1.10 to 1.69;p=0.004) while decreasing the cancer related deaths with an absolute benefit of 6.9% at 5 years. A significant proportion of the non-cancer related deaths were related to pulmonary/cardiovascular problems and later deaths related with chemotherapy toxicity. Although, the effect of vinorelbine as a second drug was marginally better than other drugs like etoposide, vinka alkaloids, and mitomycin, due to the total dose of cisplatin used in each trial varied significantly between trials, the independent efficacy of the second drug could not be evaluated by further analysis. LACE meta-analysis provided significant interaction between chemotherapy effect and stage. Biological age should not be used as a sole criteria for adjuvant chemotherapy with the possible wrong assumption of its efficacy for the more advanced stages [13]. For Stage IA NSCLC, there was no clear evidence demonstrating that chemotherapy could yield benefit for these patients. For stage IB patients, adjuvant chemotherapy also failed to show significant benefits on OS

(HR=0.92;95% CI, 0.78 to 1.10). The LACE meta-analyses revealed similar results with CALGB 9633 trial [10]. In the LACE analysis, however, there was no subgroup analysis to depict the possible beneficial effect of chemotherapy in tumours (>4 cm) as CALGB 9633 trial. For stage II and III patients, LACE analysis clearly showed that chemotherapy performs significantly better than observation in terms of both OS and DFS. Additionally, LACE meta-analysis strongly suggested that chemotherapy may be detrimental for the patients with performance score of 2.

To conclude, adjuvant chemotherapy should be offered for the patients with stage II and III completely resected NSCLC with performance score between 0 and 1. Based on the subgroup analysis of CALGB 9633 trial, adjuvant chemotherapy may also have beneficial effects for stage IB tumours greater than 4 cm.

ACKNOWLEDGEMENTS

Declared none.

CONFLICT OF INTEREST

The authors confirm that this article content has no conflict of interest.

REFERENCES

[1] Ferlay, J; Bray, F; Pisani, P; Parkin DM. GLOBOCAN 2000: cancer incidence, mortality and prevalence worldwide, version 1.0. Lyons, France: international agency for research on cancer, 2001(software)

[2] Chhatwani, L; Cabebe, E; Wakelee, A,H. Adjuvant treatment of resected lung cancer. Proc Am Thorac Soc. 2009; 6: 194-200

[3] Mountain, CF; Revisions in the international system for staging lung cancer. Chest., 1997.111, 1710-1717

[4] Winton, T; Livingston,R; Johnson, D, *et al.* Vinorelbine plus cisplatin *vs.* observation in resected non-small-cell Lung cancer. N Engl J Med., 2005, 352, 2589-2597

[5] Holmes, E,C; Bleehen,N,M; Le Chevalier, T; *et al.* Postoperative adjuvant treatments for non-small cell Lung cancers: a consensus report. Lung cancer., 1991, 7,11-13

[6] Non-small cell lung collaborative group. Chemotherapy in non-small cell lung cancer: a meta analysis using updated data on individual patients from 52 randomized clinical trials. BMJ., 1995,311,899-909

[7] Arrigada, R; Bergman, B; Dunant, A; *et al.* Cisplatin-based adjuvant chemotherapy in patients with completely resected non-small-cell lung cancer. N Engl J Med., 2004,350,351-360.

[8] Scagliotti, G, V; Fossati,R; Torri,V; *et al.* Randomized study of adjuvant chemotherapy for completely resected stage I,II, or IIIa non-small-cell lung cancer. J Natl Cancer Inst.,2003, 95,1453-1461.

[9] Waller, D; Peake M,D; Stephens,R,J; *et al.,* Chemotherapy for patients with non-small cell lung cancer: the surgical setting of the big lung trial. Eur J Cardio-thorac Surg., 2004,26,173-182.

[10] Adjuvant paclitaxel plus carboplatin compared with observation in stage IB non-small-cell lung cancer: CALGB 9633 with the cancer and leukemia group B, radiation therapy oncology group, and north central cancer treatment study groups. Strauss, G,M; Herndon II,J,E; Maddaus,M,A; *et al.* J Clin Oncol.,2008,26,5043-5051.

[11] Adjuvant vinorelbine plus cisplatin *versus* observation in patients with completely resected stage IB-IIIA non-small-cell lung cancer (Adjuvant Navelbine International Trialist Association[ANITA]): a randomized controlled trial. Douillard, J-Y; Rosell,R; Lena,DM; *et al.* Lancet Oncol.,2006,7,719-727.

[12] Pignon, J,P; Tribodet,H; Scagliotti,G,V; *et al.* Lung adjuvant cisplatin evaluation: a pooled analysis by the LACE Collaborative Group. J Clin Oncol.,2008, 26,3552-3559.

[13] Yildirim, Y; Ozyilkan, O; Calikusu, Z; Akcali, Z; Akcay, Y; Demirhan, B; Management of elderly patients with advanced non-small cell lung cancer in Turkey. Asian Pac J Cancer Prev.,2009,10,699-700

Send Orders of Reprints at reprints@benthamscience.net
Lung Cancer: Clinical and Surgical Specifications, **2013, 377-411** **377**

CHAPTER 11

Part C: Radiation Therapy for Non-Small Cell Lung Cancer

Cem Önal*

Baskent University Faculty of Medicine, Adana Research and Treatment Center, Department of Radiation Oncology, Yuregir/Adana, Turkey

Abstract: Radiotherapy is an important component of non-small cell lung cancer (NSCLC) treatment for both curative and palliative purposes. Regarding the curative intent, radiotherapy of inoperable tumours can be performed preoperatively, postoperatively, or definitively. For patients with early-stage NSCLC that is unsuitable for resection, local high-dose radiotherapy is the treatment of choice. Stereotactic radiotherapy has been demonstrated to be an effective treatment approach for early-stage tumours, combining the accurate focal dose delivery of stereotactic techniques with the biological advantages of dose-escalated hypofractionated radiotherapy, achieving local control rates of up to 90% and favorable results, especially for patients with a good performance status. Postoperative radiotherapy should not be used for stage I or II NSCLC, and its use remains controversial for resected stage IIIA (N2) disease. To increase the efficacy of radiotherapy, chemotherapy can be used concurrently, resulting in better results as well as increased toxicity. Concurrent chemoradiotherapy is presently the standard treatment for stage III inoperable NSCLC. Within this treatment framework, conventional fractionated radiotherapy at a total dose of 60–66 Gy has proven effective. The chemotherapy should be performed using a cisplatin-based regimen or, if contraindicated, a carboplatin-based regimen. For metastatic disease, short-course palliative treatment with hypofractionated schemas is preferred, and prolonged palliation effects (6–12 months) can be achieved in many cases. There is a close relationship between dose escalation and efficacy; that is, a better outcome is achieved with higher doses. New drug combinations with better radiotherapy techniques will result in better local control and overall survival without increasing toxicity.

Keywords: Non-small cell lung cancer, radiotherapy, chemoradiotherapy, definitive treatment, palliative treatment.

PRINCIPLES OF RADIOTHERAPY (RT)

Non-small cell lung cancers (NSCLCs) account for more than 85% of all cases. The most common presenting symptoms include dyspnea, cough, and weight loss.

***Address correspondence to Cem Önal:** Baskent University Faculty of Medicine, Adana Research and Treatment Center, Department of Radiation Oncology, Yuregir/Adana, Turkey; Tel: +90-322-3444444/1305; Fax: +90 322 3444452; E-mail: hcemonal@hotmail.com

Akın Eraslan Balcı (Ed)

RT plays a key role in treatment of NSCLC, both for curative intent for patients with non-metastatic disease and for symptom palliation in patients with metastatic disease. For early-stage lung cancer, lobectomy is the standard of care, although stereotactic body radiation therapy (SBRT) is a good option for patients with medically inoperable tumours. The role of postoperative radiotherapy (PORT) in treating NSCLC is controversial. It is indicated only for positive-margin disease and perhaps for pathologic N2 disease. Neoadjuvant or adjuvant curative therapy is recommended for most patients with stage II or III disease. Patients with stage IV disease require short-course palliative RT or chemotherapy alone.

In this chapter, the current role of RT is discussed in detail in the neoadjuvant, adjuvant, and definitive settings. Additionally, the efficacy of the combination of chemotherapy and RT is discussed briefly.

THE ROLE OF RT IN EARLY-STAGE NSCLC

Surgical resection with lobectomy is preferred for patients with early-stage NSCLC based on the findings of randomized trials. For complete sterilization of small tumours of the lung, a radiation dose of at least 85–90 Gy is required. With conventional techniques, it is difficult to deliver such high doses to tumours without complications, as with conventional methods, larger RT fields are used and the close proximity of critical organs and tissues such as the heart, great vessels, and spinal cord limit the dose that can be delivered to the tumour. With new technologies such as intensity-modulated RT (IMRT), image-guided RT (IGRT), or Cyberknife® RT, higher doses can be delivered easily using hypofractionation. Medical inoperable candidates with T1–T2a (<5 cm) N0M0 tumours could be amendable for SBRT. Randomized trials comparing surgery with SBRT for patients with resectable tumours are still underway.

In a single-institution phase I/II study, 45 patients with stage I NSCLC received 48 Gy of RT in four fractions, using 6–10 non-coplanar beams prescribed to the isocenter. With a median follow-up of 30 months, local control was observed in 98% of patients, and the 3-year overall survival (OS) rates were 83% for stage IA and 72% for stage IB [1].

In another single-institution retrospective review with a larger number of patients, a total of 257 patients with stage I NSCLC received 18–75 Gy in 1–22 fractions, with a median biological equivalent dose (BED) of 111 Gy (range: 57–180 Gy; $\alpha/\beta=10$) [2]. With a median follow-up of 38 months, the local control rates were 92% for BED ≥ 100 Gy and 57% for BED<100 Gy. A survival benefit was also demonstrated with BED ≥ 100 compared to BED<100 (5-year OS: 71% *vs.* 30%).

In a phase II cooperative trial, 55 patients with T1–3N0 (up to 5 cm) lesions, excluding central lesions (T3 tumours invading the mediastinum or those <2 cm from the carina), were treated with SBRT at a dose of 20 Gy in three fractions. With a median follow-up of 34 months, the 3-year local control rate was 98%, and the median OS was 48 months.

The optimal dose and fractionation of SBRT remain unclear. However, the accepted consensus for SBRT is administering a dose of at least BED=100 Gy and minimizing the volume of critical structures receiving a high BED (>80 Gy). Additionally, only peripherally localized disease should be recommended for SBRT. In addition to these studies, there are numerous ongoing studies evaluating the role of SBRT for early-stage NSCLC (Table **1**), which will standardize the current use of SBRT for early-stage NSCLC.

Table 1: Ongoing trials evaluating the role of SBRT for early-stage NSCLC

Study	Details
RTOG 0618	Phase II Operable stage I/II NSCLC Accrual goal: 33 patients 18 Gy × 3 fractions
JCOG 0403	Phase II T1N0M0 NSCLC operable (65) and inoperable (100) Accrual goal: 165 patients 12 Gy × 4 fractions
ROSEL (Dutch trial)	Phase III SBRT *versus* surgery for operable stage I Radiation therapy (RT): 20 Gy × 3 for T1; 12 Gy × 5 for T2; 7.5 Gy × 8 for central tumours
Accuray/MD Anderson	Phase III SBRT (CyberKnife®) *versus* surgery in operable stage I patients RT: 12.5 Gy × 4 for central lesion and 16.7 Gy × 3 fractions for peripheral lesion
RTOG 0915	Randomized phase II trial All inoperable stage I peripheral NSCLC Accrual goal: 88 patients Comparing two SBRT schedules (34 Gy × 1 *vs.* 12 Gy × 4)

The incidence of severe toxicity is reported to be <5% after SBRT, provided that appropriate patient selection is performed and risk-adapted fractionation schemes are applied [3, 4]. However, the real risk of late toxicity may be underestimated, as long-term follow-up has been limited, owing to the relatively high non-cancer-related mortality in patients with medically inoperable tumours. The most commonly observed toxicities after SBRT are radiation pneumonitis and rib fractures near the sites of irradiation. SBRT does not have adverse effects on pulmonary function. Late chest wall toxicity, including chest wall pain, fibrosis, and rib fractures, has been observed in up to 10% of patients with peripheral tumours [4-7]. The incidence of grade ≥3 radiation-induced pneumonitis is reported to be 0–5%, which is not different from that described after conventional high-dose RT [2, 4, 8-10].

THE ROLE OF RT IN LOCALLY ADVANCED NSCLC

The optimal management of locally advanced NSCLC patients remains unclear. Primary surgery for patients with resectable stage IIIA tumours followed by postoperative radiation therapy is controversial, but it may be indicated for patients with pathologic N2 disease, any T4 disease excluding separate nodules in the same lobe, close or positive margins, and gross residual disease. However, adding concurrent chemotherapy to PORT has no value.

NEOADJUVANT TREATMENT

The goal of neoadjuvant treatment is to improve local control and to permit previously unresectable tumours to be resected. However, it is difficult to perform surgery after RT, as specialized equipment is required and the risk of impaired healing is high after RT. Moreover, the morbidity and mortality rates after preoperative RT remain elevated. For this reason, only certain patients should be selected for neoadjuvant treatment.

Preoperative RT

Preoperative RT has been previously used, and some recent studies evaluated the role of preoperative RT. However, in current practice, the use of preoperative RT is not widely accepted.

In a cooperative study by Trakhtenberg *et al.*, the efficacy of combination treatment and preoperative RT in 478 patients with lung cancer was analyzed [11]. Intensive fractionated RT was given at doses of 4 Gy for 5 days in 218 patients, and 260 patients only underwent surgery. The 5-year survival rates of patients with stage I and II disease did not reveal any advantage of the utilized therapeutic modality. However, in subgroup analysis, the survival rates of patients with stage III disease had been improved by preoperative RT. The 3- and 5-year survival rates were 49.4% and 29.2%, respectively, for the preoperative RT group, compared with 28.1% and 15.8%, respectively, for patients treated only with surgery. In all patients with regional metastases, the effectiveness of the treatment was higher when the combination method was employed.

In a more recent phase II trial conducted by the Lung Cancer Study Group (LCSG 881), patients with pathologically proven stage IIIA disease received either preoperative RT (44 Gy in 22 fractions), delivered to the primary tumour and mediastinum, or preoperative cisplatin, mitomycin, and vinblastine [12]. All patients underwent surgical staging of the mediastinum and had either unresectable N2 disease or T4 disease with proximal extension of disease along the pulmonary artery. However, the median survival time was only 12 months, with a 27% actuarial survival rate at 4 years, and a pathologic complete response (CR) was observed in only 2 of 57 patients (one patient in each arm).

Randomized trials and phase II trials have failed to demonstrate a survival benefit of preoperative RT compared to surgery alone; however, many of the trials are fairly old, and modern noninvasive and intraoperative staging techniques were not used [13]. Even in studies using more modern methods, preoperative RT does not appear to increase survival, and thus, this procedure is not accepted as a standard treatment for patients with NSCLC.

Preoperative Chemoradiotherapy

The survival benefit of reducing distant failure by adding chemotherapy to RT, as demonstrated in randomized phase III trials for inoperable NSCLC, increased interest in preoperative treatment with RT and chemotherapy instead of either RT or chemotherapy alone, particularly for patients with stage III disease. The objective of these trials was to use RT together with chemotherapy to achieve radiosensitization, shrink the size of the primary tumour and bulky N2 disease, and sterilize distant micrometastases. The role of surgery is to optimize local control by removing the residual tumour. Numerous phase I/II and retrospective studies have investigated different neoadjuvant chemotherapy and RT combinations [14-20]. These studies have demonstrated that this approach is safe and feasible, although operative morbidity and mortality are higher with the neoadjuvant treatment. Outcomes are variably reported, and the studies tend to focus on patients with resectable tumours, with less information regarding the outcomes of patients with unresectable disease. In these studies, response rates to induction therapy varied from 40% to 90%. The median survival times ranged from 11 to 52 months, and long-term OS rates ranged from 10% to 55%. Good responses to neoadjuvant treatment were associated with a significantly better outcome with a median survival of 30–36 months and long-term OS rates of 48–54%, compared to poor responders with a median survival of 11–14 months and long-term survival rates of 9–24%.

The feasibility of neoadjuvant therapy in the setting of stage IIIB NSCLC was assessed in a prospective multi-institutional trial conducted by the Southwest Oncology Group (SWOG) [21]. In this study, 51 patients with stage IIIB disease received cisplatin and etoposide with concurrent RT (45 Gy), and surgery was performed 3–5 weeks after initial therapy. In total, 32 of 51 patients (63%) underwent surgical resection with a 5.2% rate of operative mortality. For all 51 patients, the 2-year survival rate was 39%, and most of the recurrences were distant. This study firstly demonstrated the feasibility of this approach in more advanced stages.

Another SWOG phase II study (SWOG 8805) established the feasibility of surgery after two cycles of preoperative cisplatin and etoposide in combination with RT (45 Gy) in 126 patients with stage IIIA NSCLC [22]. Induction chemotherapy consisted of two cycles of cisplatin and etoposide with concurrent RT, which began on day 1 of chemotherapy. The objective response and resectability rates were 59% and 85%, respectively, and the 3-year survival rate was 26%. The strongest predictor of survival was a pathological CR in the mediastinal lymph nodes (median survival: 30 *vs.* 10 months; 5-year OS: 33% *vs.*

11%). The authors concluded that this trimodality approach was feasible, with an encouraging 26% 3-year survival rate.

On the basis of these findings, the National Cancer Institute (NCI) [23] conducted a phase III multicenter trial for patients with biopsy-proven N2 disease and potentially resectable NSCLC (NCI Protocol INT 0139) [24]. A total of 429 patients were randomized to receive two cycles of cisplatin/etoposide given concurrently with 45 Gy RT followed by either surgery or continued RT to 61 Gy. Although the trial accrued slowly, it was closed with sufficient events. Surgery was associated with higher morbidity and mortality but with longer survival. There was no significant difference in survival between the surgery and chemoradiotherapy arms (median survival: 23.6 *vs.* 22.2 months; p=0.24). Progression-free survival (PFS) was better in the surgery arm than chemoradiotherapy arm (median PFS: 12.8 months *vs.* 10.5 months; p=0.017). More deaths occurred during treatment in the surgery arm (16 *vs.* 3). Fourteen of fifteen deaths occurred in patients who had a pneumonectomy, with most being right pneumonectomies. In subgroup analysis, OS was improved among patients who underwent lobectomy, but not pneumonectomy, *versus* chemotherapy plus RT. The authors concluded that chemotherapy plus RT with or without resection (preferably lobectomy) is an option for patients with stage IIIA (N2) NSCLC.

In another phase III study (German Study), 558 patients with stage IIIA/B NSCLC were randomized to receive either three cycles of cisplatin and etoposide, followed by twice-daily RT (45 Gy; 2×1.5 Gy day^{-1}) with concurrent carboplatin and vindesine and then surgical resection (those with positive resection margins or unresectable disease were offered further twice-daily RT) or three cycles of cisplatin and etoposide followed by surgery [25]. After surgery, patients in the induction concurrent chemoradiotherapy arm received postoperative RT only if they had microscopic or gross residual disease, whereas all patients in the induction chemotherapy alone arm received postoperative RT. There were no differences in survival between the two arms (3-year survival rates: 24% *vs.* 23%; p=0.89). However, as all patients received RT, either preoperatively or postoperatively, this study did not actually address the role of RT in the surgical setting. Moreover, there was no difference in the response or resectability rates between the two arms. Thus, it appears that preoperative chemoradiotherapy increases pathological response rates and mediastinal downstaging, but does not improve survival. In addition, the authors mentioned that pneumonectomy should be avoided after induction with chemoradiotherapy.

Because treatment-related deaths were common with combined modality treatment, it is possible that operative morbidity and mortality could be reduced with better surgical techniques in centers with more experience. All deaths in the operative arm occurred in patients who underwent pneumonectomy after induction chemoradiotherapy, but patients who underwent lobectomy tolerated this treatment regimen with less toxicity. Therefore, in the neoadjuvant setting, lobectomy is the preferred surgical procedure rather than pneumonectomy. Neoadjuvant therapy has become an accepted treatment strategy for stage IIIA NSCLC but not for stage IIIB NSCLC, which is usually considered incurable and treated non-surgically.

ADJUVANT TREATMENT

The treatment of choice for early-stage (stage I and IIIA) NSCLC is surgery. However, the average 5-year survival rates remain around 65%, with a range of 55–90% [26, 27]. To achieve better local control, adjuvant therapy is required, and its use should be reflected in further improvements in OS. There have been attempts to reduce the risk of relapse and death from lung cancer by administering adjuvant chemotherapy to patients following surgical resection. However, the role of adjuvant RT remains unsettled.

The benefits of PORT have been investigated for patients in select risk groups. However, recent studies with considerable controversies regarding the RT equipment, dose regimens, and methods of radiation delivery have reported conflicting results. Given the advances in the field, it would not be wise to base our conclusions regarding the clinical benefit of PORT on studies that used interventions that were substantially different from what would be considered current standards of care in radiation oncology.

PORT

PORT after potentially curative resection of NSCLC has long been discussed, but the use of this modality remains controversial. The ability of PORT in moderate doses (45–55 Gy) to eradicate microscopic residual disease and reduce the incidence of local recurrence was strongly suggested in several early single-institution trials [28, 29]. What has remained controversial is whether the reduction in locoregional recurrence also leads to an improvement in OS. Although the nonrandomized single institution trials suggested that this PORT may be beneficial, data from the prospective trials have been less supportive [30, 31]. However, the side effects of PORT can have negative effects on several outcome parameters and can even be lethal due to the potential worsening of pulmonary and cardiac functioning. Because the rates of distant metastasis are relatively high, especially in locally advanced stages of NSCLC, the potential impact of adjuvant irradiation on survival *via* reductions in the risk of locoregionally recurrent disease can only be marginal. Given these findings, RT may have potentially detrimental effects on patients treated postoperatively [32]. However, 70–80% of patients received PORT in the early 1990s, and even after the PORT meta-analysis, 40–50% of patients continued to receive PORT [33].

In a phase III trial conducted by the LCSG, 210 patients with stage II-IIIA resected squamous cell carcinoma of the lung were randomized to receive either mediastinal irradiation (50 Gy over 5 weeks) or continued observation [30]. The majority of patients had hilar lymph node metastasis (N1), but smaller proportions had mediastinal lymph node metastasis (N2) or T3N0 disease. Although no survival difference was detected, PORT reduced local recurrence, especially in patients with N2 disease (3% *vs.* 41%). The main limitations of the LCSG study were its small sample size, the inclusion of patients with only squamous cell carcinoma, the mixture of patients with N1 and N2 tumours, the reliance on data for the site of first failure, and the lack of quality assurance. Additionally, only 74% of patients in the RT arm received the prescribed 50-Gy RT doses. Although the results demonstrated that better local control was achieved with RT, this good local control did not translate into better survival rates.

The role of PORT was evaluated in another phase III trial conducted by the British Medical Research Council (MRC) [31]. A total of 308 patients with T1-2 N1-2 tumours were randomized to receive postoperative 40 Gy in 15 fractions starting 4–6 weeks after surgery or observation. Overall, there was no advantage in either group in terms of survival, although definite local recurrence and bony metastases appeared less frequently and later in the PORT group. In a subgroup analysis of the N1 group, no differences between the treatment arms were observed, but in the N2 group, patients who received PORT had a 1-month survival advantage and delays in the times to local recurrence and to the development of bone metastases. The authors concluded that there is no clear indication for PORT for N1 disease, but the question remains unresolved for N2 disease.

A meta-analysis conducted by the PORT Meta-analysis Trialist Group evaluated 2128 patients included in nine randomized trials (six previously published series and three unpublished series) of PORT. The authors concluded that PORT was associated with a highly significant increase in the risk of death, with a risk ratio (RR) of 1.21 ($p<0.001$) [32]. The detrimental effect of RT was significant among patients with stage I disease and nearly significant among patients with stage II disease. As there are several significant differences between the treatment strategies in the trials included in this meta-analysis and current practice patterns, the results of this meta-analysis should be cautiously interpreted. First, a substantial portion of the patients (26%) included in this analysis had stage I disease without demonstrated nodal metastases, for which PORT is not beneficial. Second, the preoperative staging procedures, surgical techniques, and RT doses and techniques differed substantially from those employed in current practice. Higher daily RT doses would be expected to increase acute and late complications compared to conventional fractionation. In current practice, because of prominent radiation dose heterogeneity and poor depth-dose characteristics, treatment using ^{60}Cobalt teletherapy devices is contraindicated. Seven of the nine trials in this meta-analysis also allowed the use of ^{60}Cobalt treatment beams, and only one study included CT scan-based treatment planning, which is accepted as standard of care. Therefore, compared with present standards of treatment, the studies included in the PORT meta-analysis used outdated RT techniques and planning that would lead to excessive deaths from cardiac and pulmonary damage, resulting in detrimental PORT-related effects.

In an analysis of the SEER database, Lally and coworkers found no evidence of an OS benefit with use of PORT in 7465 stage II-III NSCLC patients treated between 1988 and 2002, that is, a period in which more modern RT techniques were used compared to those investigated in the PORT meta-analysis [33]. This analysis also revealed a survival detriment with the use of PORT in patients with N0-N1 disease. However, the SEER analysis revealed a survival benefit (hazard ratio=0.85) with the use of PORT in patients with N2 disease.

A review by the Lung Cancer Disease Site Group of Cancer Care Ontario Program of Evidence-Based Care developed an evidence-based clinical practice guideline for postoperative RT in patients with completely resected pathologic stage II or IIIA NSCLC [34]. After their review of the literature including meta-analyses, they concluded that PORT following complete resection of stage II NSCLC is not recommended, and no definitive recommendation can be made for stage IIIA disease. They therefore recommended that the decision regarding PORT be made on an individual patient basis.

To avoid the errors of previous studies, it is very important to specify the surgical procedure (most particularly lymph node exploration) as well as the RT technique. In a retrospective series reported by Matsuguma *et al.*, PORT using modern techniques reduced local recurrence and improved OS, particularly for patients with multistation N2 disease [35]. The only randomized trial evaluating the benefit of PORT was conducted by the Cancer and Leukemia Group B (CALGB), which planned to evaluate the effect of adding PORT to surgery followed by postoperative adjuvant chemotherapy [36]. However, the trial was abandoned prematurely because of poor accrual, as only 44 patients participated in this trial. Failure-free survival and OS were favorable in the PORT arm (31 and 38.8 months, respectively) compared to those in the observation arm (14 and 30.5 months, respectively). The results were not statistically significant because of the small trial size. In an unplanned analysis of patients in the Adjuvant Navelbine International Trialist Association trial, which examined the value of adjuvant chemotherapy, 52% of patients with N2 disease received PORT, and these patients exhibited higher 5-year survival rates than patients who did not receive PORT (21% *vs.* 17% in the surgery arm; 47% *vs.* 34% in the adjuvant chemotherapy arm) [37]. However, an adverse effect on survival with use of this combination was observed among patients with N0-N1 disease. A study conducted by the Eastern Cooperative Oncology Group (ECOG E3590) demonstrated that the risk of death from intercurrent disease in patients with resected stage II or IIIA NSCLC was not increased by the use of PORT alone or the use of concurrent chemotherapy and PORT.

Based on these findings, a randomized controlled trial is necessary to better assess the role of PORT in patients with resected NSCLC using better surgical techniques and RT planning strategies. A new large, multi-institution European phase III trial, the Lung Adjuvant Radiotherapy Trial, will shortly commence. This study will compare three-dimensional (3D) conformal PORT to no PORT and include patients who have proven N2 disease and undergo a complete resection irrespective of whether adjuvant or neoadjuvant chemotherapy was used.

Currently, PORT is indicated for patients with incomplete resection (either close or positive margins) and mediastinal lymph node metastasis (N2). In cases of positive or close margins, an RT dose of 50 Gy is delivered to eradicate potential microscopic disease, and 60–66 Gy is delivered to the positive or close margin. In cases of complete lymphadenectomy with positive margins, small-field RT without lymphatic region may be performed.

Postoperative Chemoradiotherapy

Patient prognosis following surgery for stage II and III NSCLC remains a significant concern, and when lymph node metastasis is observed after resection, survival dramatically falls to 29–72% for patients with N1 disease and 26–67% for those with N2 disease [38]. The sites of failure in these patients are mainly locoregional and distant. Although randomized trials investigating PORT revealed improved locoregional control and disease-free survival for stage III patients, the trials addressing the value of PORT include patients with both stage II and III disease and thus have limited statistical power in subgroup analyses [30, 31]. Chemotherapy and RT can be administered concurrently to improve local control and reduce the prevalence of distant metastasis. For this purpose, large trials have investigated adjuvant chemotherapy and RT [39-42].

The LCSG previously demonstrated that PORT with chemotherapy improved local control and disease-free survival but not OS [30]. In a randomized study conducted by the ECOG, the benefit of adding chemotherapy to RT was evaluated against RT alone [39]. A total of 488 patients with resected stage II-IIIA disease were randomly assigned to receive either four 28-day cycles of cisplatin (60 mg m^{-2}) and etoposide (120 mg m^{-2}) administered concurrently with RT (50.4 Gy in 28 daily fractions) or RT alone. No benefit was observed in the adjuvant RT and chemotherapy arm regarding OS and intrathoracic recurrence compared to RT alone. The median survival was 39 months in the RT arm, compared to 38 months in the chemotherapy and RT arm (p=0.56). The rates of in-field recurrence were 13% in the RT arm and 12% in the chemotherapy and RT alone arm (p=0.84), and the toxicity was higher in the combination arm than in the RT alone arm.

Another study by the Radiation Therapy Oncology Group (RTOG 97-05) demonstrated the benefit of adjuvant paclitaxel, carboplatin, and RT for 88 patients with resected stage II or IIIA NSCLC [39]. Concurrent thoracic RT (50.4 Gy in 28 daily fractions) was given during cycles 1 and 2, and an additional boost of 10.8 Gy (six fractions) was given for extracapsular nodal extension or T3 lesions. The median OS was 56.3 months, with 1-, 2-, and 3-year survival rates of 86%, 70%, and 61%, respectively, and the 1-, 2-, and 3-year PFS rates were 70%, 57%, and 50%, respectively. The results of this trial suggested improvements in OS and PFS in this group of patients with resected NSCLC compared with those in the previously reported ECOG trial.

The NSCLC Meta-analyses Collaborative Group demonstrated that the effect of chemotherapy is similar irrespective of the locoregional treatment employed (surgery alone or surgery plus PORT); however, the study was not designed to evaluate the effectiveness of PORT, and randomized trials are needed to assess whether modern RT is effective as an adjuvant treatment [43]. However, similarly as PORT trials, the trials evaluating the efficacy of postoperative chemoradiotherapy included patients with both stage II and III disease, further limiting the ability to detect a benefit for smaller patient subsets.

DEFINITIVE TREATMENT

For many years, RT alone was considered the treatment of choice for patients with stage IIIA or IIIB disease despite a median survival of only 9–11 months and 5-year survival rates of only 3–10% [44-46]. The lower survival rates were the result of disease progression at distant sites, reflecting the presence of systemic micrometastases at the time of initial therapy [47, 48]. Another problematic issue is disease progression within the RT fields, which may reflect the inability of RT to eliminate all macroscopic disease. Efforts to increase cure rates have therefore attempted to increase both locoregional and systemic control. For this reason, sequential chemoradiotherapy and concomitant chemoradiotherapy have been widely studied. Chemotherapy may play a cytotoxic role by eradicating distant micrometastases, a radiosensitizing role by improving local control, or both. A number of randomized clinical trials and meta-analyses support the conclusion that combined modality approaches using cisplatin-based chemotherapy improve survival compared with RT alone in patients with unresectable stage III disease. It has been demonstrated that chemoradiotherapy is more efficient than either chemotherapy alone or RT alone in the treatment of localized unresectable NSCLC [49].

Definitive RT

Patients who cannot undergo surgery because of co-morbidity, that is, medically inoperable patients, and those who refuse surgery should be treated with definitive RT. As there is co-morbid disease in these patients, the intercurrent death rates are high. For this reason, cause-specific survival is a good parameter to reflect the efficacy of such definitive treatment modalities.

In most previous studies, which administered RT (60–66 Gy) in daily doses of 1.8–2 Gy, the reported 5-year local control and OS rates ranged from 30 to 50% and from 10 to 30%, respectively [50, 51]. However, several studies demonstrated the benefit of dose escalation, suggesting that better local control and survival can be achieved with higher radiation doses [50-52]. With better treatment modalities such as 3D-conformal RT (3DCRT), IMRT, or stereotactic body RT (SBRT), which have been increasingly used in recent years, higher tumour doses can be delivered without increasing toxicity. SBRT is an alternative method for delivering higher, biologically effective doses. SBRT for lung cancers considers tumour movement with respiration and decreases setup uncertainties by using IGRT techniques.

Definitive Chemoradiotherapy

The median OS for patients with unresectable stage III treated with RT alone is only 10 months, with a 5-year overall survival rate of 5%. These results necessitate more effort to improve local control and decrease distant metastasis by using chemotherapy and RT together. Currently, the American Society of Clinical Oncology guidelines recommend definitive cisplatin-based chemoradiotherapy for treating unresectable stage III NSCLC [53]. However, the timing of chemotherapy RT remains controversial (either sequentially after chemotherapy or concurrently with chemotherapy) [54].

Sequential Chemoradiotherapy

Sequential administration of platinum-based chemotherapy and RT may improve outcome by reducing distant failure rates. Moreover, in sequential treatment modalities, if the post-chemotherapy volume is irradiated, a smaller irradiation volume may result in less toxicity. Several randomized trials demonstrated the benefit of induction chemotherapy before RT in stage III NSCLC (CALGB 8433) [55], which was subsequently verified by the RTOG 8808 randomized phase III study [56, 57].

The CALGB 8433 trial compared standard 60-Gy RT with two sequential cycles of cisplatin (100 mg m^{-2} on days 1 and 29) plus vinblastine (5 mg m^{-2} weekly for 5 weeks) followed by 60 Gy of RT given in 30 fractions beginning on day 50 [55]. A total of 155 patients were evaluated with more than 7 years of follow-up. The sequential chemotherapy and RT arm exhibited significantly improved median survival compared to that in the RT alone arm (13.8 *vs.* 9.7 months; p=0.01) and a doubling of the 3-year survival rate (25% *vs.* 12%). Although the tumour response rate was 56% for the chemoradiotherapy and RT arm and 43% for the RT arm, the difference was not statistically significant (p=0.09). A retrospective control of this study demonstrated that approximately 23% of cases failed to completely encompass the tumour [58]. However, the authors concluded that as many as 80–85% of patients still die within 5 years because of treatment failure occurring both in-field and at distant sites in patients receiving either sequential chemotherapy and RT or RT alone.

In the RTOG 8808 trial, 458 patients with clinical stage II-IIIB disease were prospectively randomized to receive 2 months of cisplatin and vinblastine chemotherapy followed by 60 Gy of RT at 1.2 Gy per fraction delivered twice daily to a total dose of 69.6 Gy or 2.0 Gy per fraction delivered once daily to a total dose of 60 Gy [56, 57]. In this study, OS was statistically superior for the patients receiving chemotherapy and RT compared to that in the other two RT-only arms of the study (p=0.04). The median survival times after 5 years were 11.4, 13.2, and 12 months with standard irradiation, chemoradiotherapy, and hyperfractionated irradiation, respectively. The respective 5-year survival was 5%, 8%, and 6% for standard radiation therapy, chemotherapy followed by RT, and hyperfractionated irradiation, respectively. The survival of the twice-daily RT arm, although better, was not statistically superior to that of the conventional RT arm.

Although these two multicenter randomized trials demonstrated a survival benefit of sequential chemotherapy and RT, some trials failed to demonstrate this benefit [59]. However, these studies used less intensive chemotherapy and a smaller cohort of patients. However, the survival advantage of induction chemotherapy was confirmed by a recent meta-analysis [60].

Concurrent Chemoradiotherapy

By contrast, concurrent chemoradiotherapy using low-dose cisplatin was reported to improve survival by reducing local recurrence without affecting distant metastases. In view of these observations, concurrent chemoradiotherapeutic approaches integrating both radiosensitizing agents and dose levels of chemotherapy with proven efficacy against micrometastases have been the most studied strategies.

The first approach tested as a concurrent chemoradiotherapy regimen was the combination of RT with radiosensitizing low-dose chemotherapy, and this approach was evaluated by the European Organization for Research and Treatment of Cancer (EORTC) trial 08844, which compared RT alone with RT and concomitant (daily 6 mg m^{-2} or weekly 30 mg m^{-2}) cisplatin in 331 patients with non-metastatic NSCLC [61]. RT was delivered in a split-course fashion for 2 weeks (3 Gy given 10 times in five fractions per week), followed by a 2-week rest period and 2 more weeks of RT (2.5 Gy given 10 times in five fractions per week). This study demonstrated a significant survival advantage for daily cisplatin and RT compared with RT alone (3-year survival rates: 16% *vs.* 2%; p=0.009); the weekly cisplatin/radiation therapy arm produced intermediate results (3-year survival rate: 13%). However, cisplatin induced nausea and vomiting in 86% of patients in the weekly arm and 78% of patients in the daily arm. This study demonstrated a gain in local control with concurrent chemoradiotherapy, which have been translated into a survival benefit with substantial side effects.

Numerous phase III trials have evaluated concurrent chemoradiotherapy *versus* sequential chemotherapy and RT. The West Japan Lung Cancer Group randomized 314 evaluable patients with unresectable stage III NSCLC into concurrent and sequential arms [62]. Chemotherapy consisted of cisplatin (80 mg m^{-2} on days 1 and 29), vindesine (3 mg m^{-2} on days 1, 8, 29, and 36), and mitomycin (8 mg m^{-2} on days 1 and 29), and 54 Gy of RT were delivered in a split course (2 Gy per fraction and five fractions per week for a total of 14 fractions followed by a rest period of 10 days, after which the course was repeated). In the concurrent arm, RT began on day 2, and in the sequential arm, RT was initiated after completing chemotherapy. A 3.2-month median survival advantage (median survival: 16.5 *vs.* 13.3 months; 5-year survival rates: 15.8% *vs.* 8.9%; p=0.04) was observed in the concurrent arm. However, myelosuppression was significantly greater among patients in the concurrent arm than among those in the sequential arm (p=0.0001). Despite the disadvantages of split-course techniques, which permit both the repair of normal tissues and proliferation of tumour clones during the break, the 5-year survival rate significantly favored the concurrent approach. The authors also reported the patterns of failure, which demonstrated a benefit of concurrent chemoradiotherapy in improving the local relapse-free survival (p=0.04), but the distant relapse rates were similar (~60% in each arm).

The largest randomized trial conducted by the RTOG (RTOG 94-10) evaluated both concurrent *versus* sequential treatment and also the value of hyperfractionated RT with concurrent chemotherapy [63]. A total of 595 patients were randomized into the following three treatment arms: once-daily RT (total dose of 60 Gy) after induction cisplatin (100 mg m^{-2}) and vinblastine (5 mg m^{-2}), once-daily RT (total dose of 60 Gy) with concurrent cisplatin (100 mg m^{-2}) and vinblastine (5 mg m^{-2}), and hyperfractionated RT (total dose of 69.6 Gy) with concurrent cisplatin (50 mg m^{-2}) and oral etoposide (50 mg twice daily). The median survival times for these three treatment groups were 14.6, 17.0 and 15.6 months, respectively. The 4-year survival rate was significantly better in the concurrent chemotherapy and once-daily RT arms than in the sequential arm (21% *vs.* 12%; p=0.04). The 4-year survival rate in the concurrent chemotherapy and hyperfractionated RT arm was 17%. The locoregional relapse rate was lower in the hyperfractionated arm than in the sequential arm and once-daily RT arms (34% *vs.* 50% *vs.* 43%). There was no significant difference in survival between the once-daily and hyperfractionated RT arms. Although acute grade 3–4 non-hematological toxicities were more frequent in the concurrent arm than in the sequential arm, no significant difference was observed regarding late toxicities. The high rates of toxicity may be related to the conventional 2D planning. These data strongly favor concurrent chemoradiotherapy with standard RT over sequential and hyperfractionated treatment.

A similar experience was reported by the Groupe Lyon-Saint-Etienne d'Oncologie Thoracique – Groupe Français de Pneumo-Cancérologie study NPC 95-01, which randomly assigned 212 patients to receive sequential *versus* concurrent chemoradiotherapy [64]. In the sequential arm, patients received two cycles of induction chemotherapy with cisplatin (120 mg m^{-2}) and vinorelbine (30 mg m^{-2} wk^{-1}) followed by RT at a dose of 66 Gy delivered in 33 fractions. In the concurrent arm, the same RT protocol was started on day 1 with two concurrent cycles of cisplatin (20 mg m^{-2} day^{-1}) and etoposide (50 mg m^{-2} day^{-1}); patients then received consolidation therapy with cisplatin (80 mg m^{-2}) and vinorelbine (30 mg m^{-2} wk^{-1}). The median survival was 14.5 months in the sequential arm and 16.3 months in the concurrent arm (p=0.24). The 2-, 3-, and 4-year survival rates were better in the concurrent arm (39%, 25%, and 21%, respectively) than in the sequential arm (26%, 19%, and 14%, respectively). The benefit was maintained long-term, as the difference in OS between the two strategies (6.2% at 3 years and 6.5% at 4 years) was apparently constant. The local control rate was improved in the concurrent arm compared to that in the sequential arm (40% *vs.* 24%). The concurrent arm had higher rates of grade 3/4 esophagitis (26.1% *vs.* 0%) and dysphagia (19.3% *vs.* 1%). The lack of a significant survival difference between sequential and concurrent therapy in this study might be related to the lack of statistical power, or alternatively, to the excessive number of early deaths in the concurrent arm (25 *vs.* 17), particularly toxic deaths (10 *vs.* 6) [65].

These phase III trials consistently reported longer survival in concurrent arm, and the difference was significant in two of the trials [63]. After 2001, the concurrent chemoradiotherapy regimen was accepted as the standard of care for patients with inoperable stage III NSCLC who have a good performance status and no significant weight loss. However, the rates of acute non-hematological toxicities were higher in the concurrent arm, but the rates of late toxicities were similar. To improve outcomes, different techniques with newer drug regimens have been assessed in numerous studies.

In a phase III Czech Republic study, 102 patients with stage III NSCLC were randomly assigned to a concurrent chemoradiotherapy arm (with RT started on the fourth day of the second cycle of chemotherapy) or a sequential chemoradiotherapy arm (started 2 weeks after the completion of chemotherapy) [66]. The chemotherapy schedule consisted of up to four cycles of cisplatin (80 mg m^{-2} on day 1) and vinorelbine (25 mg m^{-2} in the first and fourth cycles on days 1, 8, and 15, of a 28-day cycle). RT was prescribed at a dose of 60 Gy (total of 30 fractions given in five fractions per week for 6 weeks). The concurrent treatment was superior ($p<0.023$) with a better median survival (16.6 *vs.* 12.9 months) and 3-year survival (18.6% *vs.* 9.5%). Although more toxicity was observed in the concomitant arm, there were no treatment-related deaths.

The most recent randomized phase III study conducted by the EORTC (EORTC 08972-22973) compared sequential and concurrent chemoradiotherapy in 158 patients with NSCLC. In this study, the efficacy of gemcitabine together with higher daily RT doses of 2.75 Gy was assessed. Patients were randomized to receive two courses of gemcitabine (1250 mg m^{-2}) and cisplatin (75 mg m^{-2}) prior to RT or daily low-dose cisplatin (6 mg m^{-2}) concurrently with RT; in both arms, RT consisted of 24 fractions of 2.75 Gy over 32 days, with a total dose of 66 Gy delivered using a 3D conformal technique [67]. For the sequential and concurrent arms, the median survival was 16.2 and 16.5 months, respectively; the 2-year overall survival was 34% and 39%, respectively; and the 3-year overall survival was 22% and 34%, respectively. However, acute hematological toxicity was more frequent in the sequential arm (21% *vs.* 5%), but grade 3/4 esophagitis was more frequent in the concurrent arm (14% *vs.* 5%). The authors concluded that 66 Gy of RT with concurrent daily low-dose cisplatin or after two courses of gemcitabine/cisplatin was well tolerated. However, due to early closure of this study, no conclusions can be drawn regarding the relative merits of the two strategies, although good survival was observed in both arms.

In a meta-analysis, the Rowell's Cochrane review [14] evaluated 14 randomized studies with 2393 patients comparing concurrent chemoradiotherapy *versus* RT alone [68]. There was a reduction in the risk of death at 2 years (RR=0.93; p=0.01) and improvements in the 2-year locoregional PFS (RR=0.84; p=0.03) and PFS at any site (RR=0.90; p=0.005) in the concurrent chemoradiotherapy arm. The authors concluded that there were 14% and 7% reductions in the risk of death at 2 years with concurrent chemoradiotherapy compared to those with sequential chemoradiotherapy and RT alone, respectively. However, in both cases, there was an increase in the incidence of acute esophagitis.

In a recent meta-analysis of six trials of 1205 patients, Aupérin *et al.* reported that the addition of concurrent chemoradiotherapy improved survival compared to that observed with sequential chemotherapy and RT in patients with locally advanced NSCLC [69]. The absolute benefits of concurrent chemoradiotherapy were 5.7% and 4.5% at 3 and 5 years, respectively. However, concurrent treatment increased the acute esophageal toxicity rate from 4% to 18%, but there was no significant effect on pulmonary toxicity.

CRANIAL PROPHYLAXIS

Regarding SCLC, prophylactic cranial irradiation (PCI) is accepted as a standard component of treatment, as randomized trials and meta-analyses have demonstrated a survival benefit for PCI [70-73]. However, unlike SCLC, few randomized and retrospective studies have addressed the efficacy of PCI against locally advanced NSCLC [74]. A Cochrane review identified four published randomized trials [75]. In these studies, a significant reduction in the cumulative incidence of brain metastases of 50– 90% was observed, but none of these studies individually demonstrated any effect of PCI on OS. In a recent SWOG study, a relative reduction in the incidence of brain metastases was demonstrated with PCI, but an unexpected shortening of survival was observed for patients who received PCI, with a median survival of 8 and 11 months, respectively (p=0.004). However, these studies are old and heterogeneous in terms of patient selection.

A modern multicenter randomized trial of 112 patients with operable stage IIIA NSCLC compared two different therapeutic strategies, one of which included PCI as a treatment component [76]. Patients were randomized to receive either adjuvant thoracic RT after surgery or preoperative chemotherapy followed by concurrent chemoradiotherapy and definitive surgery with PCI (30 Gy in 15 fractions). After more than 5 years of follow-up, the incidence of brain metastases as the first site of failure was significantly reduced from 34.7% to 7.8% (p=0.02), and the overall brain relapse rate was significantly reduced from 27.2% to 9.1% (p=0.04) in the preoperative CRT/PCI arm. Although this trial was not designed to investigate the efficacy of PCI against NSCLC, the incidence of brain metastases could have been influenced by a more aggressive locoregional trimodality treatment.

In a randomized phase III trial (RTOG 0214), the efficacy of PCI against locally advanced NSCLC was investigated [77]. This trial was initially powered to illustrate a survival benefit in favor of PCI, which would require 1058 participants, but unfortunately, this trial was closed early due to slow accrual after the inclusion of 356 patients (340 evaluable patients). Patients who received completed definitive locoregional therapy for stage IIIA or IIIB NSCLC were randomized to receive PCI (2 Gy per fraction up to 30 Gy) or observation. The results revealed a significant reduction in the incidence of brain metastases from 18% to 7.7% in the PCI group at 1 year (p=0.004) and a non-significant trend toward an increase in the relapse-free survival at 1 year (51.2% and 56.4% for the observation and PCI arms, respectively, p=0.11). There was no difference in OS between the two groups (p=0.86), which could be either due to a non-significant effect of PCI on OS in NSCLC or to the low power achieved by this study after early closure.

It appears clear that the administration of PCI to patients with NSCLC reduces the incidence of brain metastasis by 50%. However, the translation of this effect into an improved OS remains an open question that other ongoing randomized phase III trials may help to solve.

Even if there are strong data indicating that PCI reduces the incidence of brain metastases in both SCLC and NSCLC and improves OS in SCLC, the potential neurotoxicity of this procedure remains problematic. Although acute toxicity is generally manageable, consisting primarily of alopecia, headache, fatigue, nausea, and vomiting, the long-term toxicity is of concern, as sequelae such as severe memory loss, intellectual impairment or even dementia, ataxia, and seizures have been reported in retrospective studies. However, most of these studies were small, and their methodology was questionable. In previous retrospective studies, controversial findings have been reported [70, 71, 78-80]. Arriagada *et al.* reported no significant differences in neurocognitive function between patients receiving PCI (24 Gy in eight fractions) and those in the observation group [81]. Additionally, no significant differences were detected in the patient cohort receiving PCI in comparison with those without PCI despite a detailed neurocognitive investigation of long-term survivors more than 4 years after treatment. Based on the current evidence from SCLC and NSCLC studies, it is reasonable to assume that PCI regimens consisting of 20–30 Gy given in 2–3-Gy fractions, as used in the current cohort, will produce little toxicity on brain tissue within the first 1–2 years after PCI.

RT TECHNIQUES

3DCRT

The aim of RT in NSCLC is to deliver higher doses to the tumour while sparing normal surrounding tissues. It is difficult to accomplish this aim with traditional conventional techniques. With the development of 3DCRT and the assistance of computerized tomography (CT)-based treatment planning, it is easy to calculate the tumour doses and surrounding organ at risk (OAR) doses. The advantages of 3DCRT are tumour and OAR delineation, accurate dose calculation, and the ability to manipulate beam geometry to achieve a homogenous dose distribution (Fig. **1**). In addition, with the assistance of dose-volume histograms, the OAR doses can easily be evaluated (Fig. **2**).

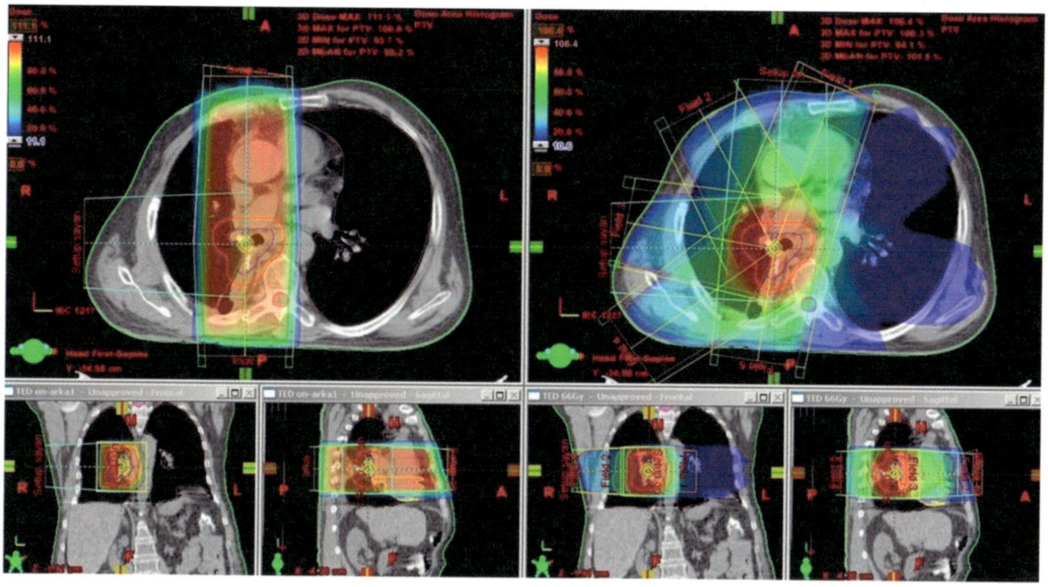

Figure 1: The dose distribution of the classical AP-PA conventional plan (left) and five-field conformal plan (right). In the AP-PA plan, the high-dose region (orange) completely encompasses the target volume as well as normal lung, mediastinal, and heart tissue. In the five-field conformal plan, the high-dose region only encompasses the target volume; however, the volume of the lungs receiving low doses (blue-green) increases.

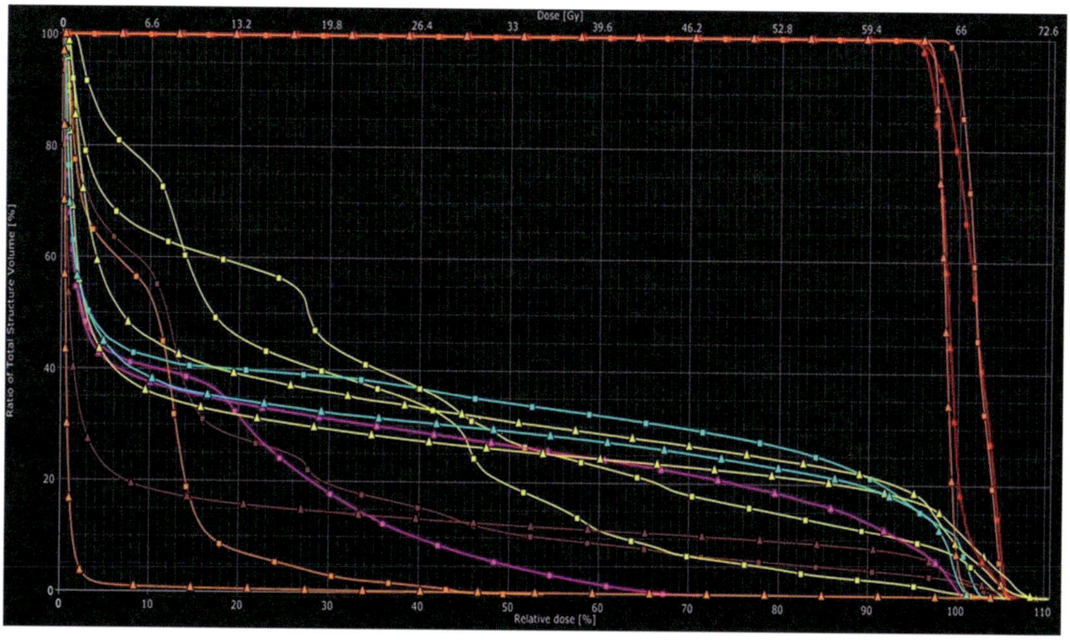

Figure 2: Dose-volume histogram of the AP-PA conventional plan and five-field conformal plan demonstrating the target volume doses and OAR doses.

With the integration of new diagnostic techniques such as magnetic resonance imaging and positron-emission tomography-CT (PET-CT), better delineation of tumours can be established, which will minimize the likelihood of geographic miss. PET scanning may be useful in treatment planning, but this has not been formally evaluated in clinical trials. The integration of PET and CT will increase the accuracy of the procedure *via* tumour delineation. The main advantage of PET-CT is its capability of distinguishing atelectasis from the tumour (Fig. **3**). However, significant changes in the definition of target volumes have been reported in 30–60% of patients with NSCLC [82]. Nevertheless, the false-positive rates of PET scans for detecting the involvement of mediastinal nodes can be as high as 39% depending on the patient population studied. Consequently, histological confirmation is preferred, and this can be achieved using endoscopic ultrasound-guided fine needle aspiration (EUS-FNA) in up to 70% of patients in whom FDG-PET scans indicated nodal metastases [83]. The combination of PET and EUS-FNA qualifies as a minimally invasive staging strategy for defining the involved fields for RT planning.

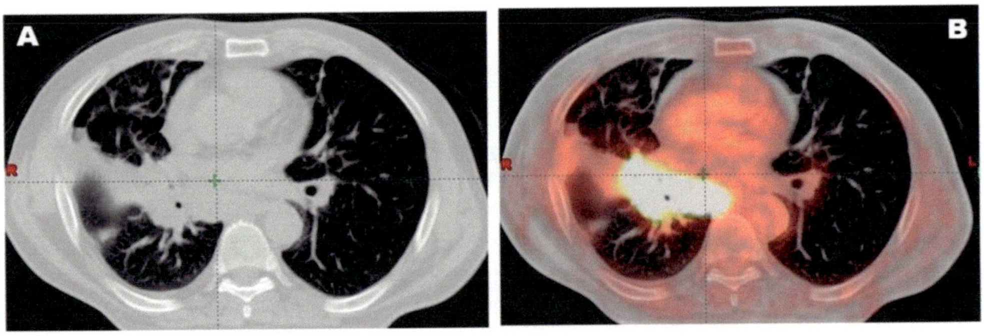

Figure 3: (**A**) A mass located in the hilum extending to the mediastinum and causing atelectasis. However, a clear margin between the tumour and the atelectasis cannot be established. (**B**) Better delineation of the tumour was obtained using integrated PET-CT.

While evaluating tumour movement during respiration *via* the technique of 4D, or respiration-correlated, CT scanning, the use of individualized margins for treatment planning and the safe delivery of respiration-gated RT can be established [84, 85]. In this technique, irradiation is limited to a predetermined window in the respiratory cycle in which the tumour is relatively immobile. Gating permits the use of smaller treatment portals, which in turn reduces the risk of radiation-induced toxicity.

IMRT

IMRT is based on the use of optimized non-uniform radiation beam intensities. Although the benefit of dose escalation without causing toxic effects was established for patients with prostate and head and neck cancers, the application of IMRT to lung cancer has been delayed because of low doses to a larger volume of the normal lung tissue. Treatment planning studies suggest that IMRT can be beneficial for patients with N2 disease and those with centrally located tumours [86]. IMRT is characterized by steep dose gradients, and both geographical misses and unexpected toxicity can arise in the presence of patient setup errors or organ mobility. Therefore, high levels of precision in dose delivery and tumour localization are required. Although it was demonstrated that IMRT might be more suitable than 3DCRT for advanced stage NSCLC, it is still considered as investigational in lung cancer in view of the complexity of tumour and normal organ mobility in the thorax, as well as the limitations of commonly used dose-calculation algorithms [87, 88]. Moreover, omission of elective nodal irradiation can achieve significant reduction in normal tissue irradiation without the need for IMRT [86].

SBRT

Stereotactic radiotherapy (SRT) was originally developed for the treatment of small intracranial lesions. Improvements in treatment planning and delivery have led to the application of SRT to extracranial sites, including the thorax and abdomen, in a procedure termed SBRT. SBRT represents a form of high-precision RT delivery characterized by advanced measures to account for tumour mobility and accurate patient setup prior to treatment. The use of multiple non-coplanar radiation beams or arcs results in highly conformal dose distributions, with rapid dose falloff in surrounding normal tissues (Fig. **4**).

The hypofractionation of SBRT (generally three to eight fractions) will lead to a decrease in an overall treatment time of less than two weeks, improving both patient compliance and resource utilization. However, the treatment time of hypofractionated SBRT is longer than that of other conventional RT techniques. Reported median delivery times range from 22 to 100 min, depending on the doses administered and delivery techniques used [89, 90]. The other limitation of

SBRT for lung cancers is the availability of this technique for smaller and peripherally located tumours (Fig. **5**).

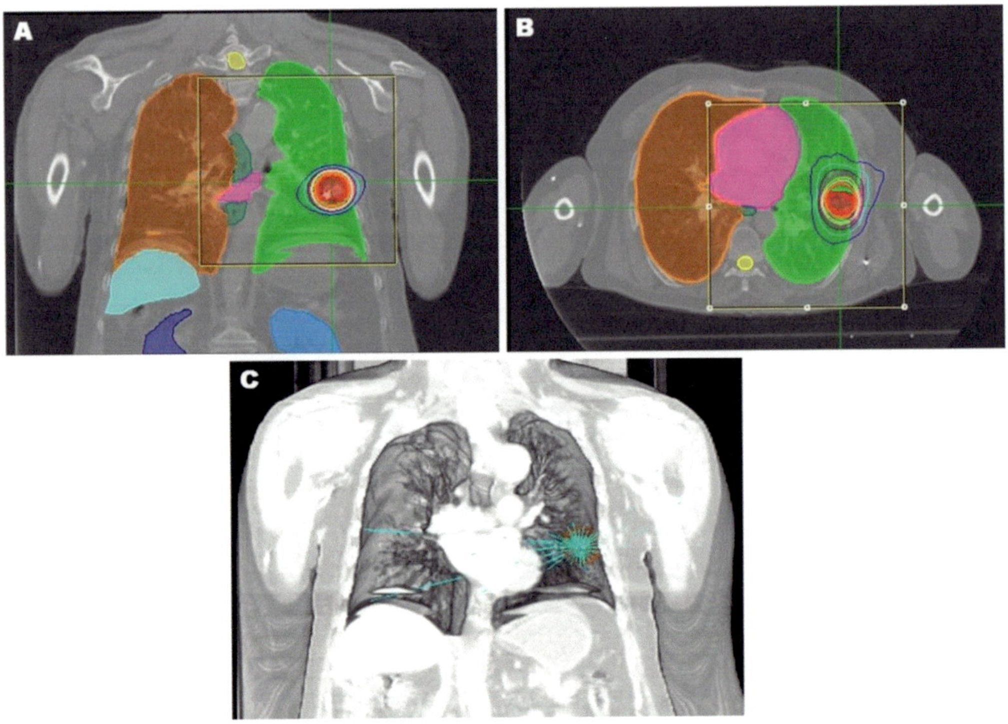

Figure 4: Treatment planning of a patient with a T1N0 peripherally located tumour in the left lung treated with SBRT. In the first step of treatment planning, CT scans (2.5–3 mm slice thickness) were taken of the treatment position, and images were transferred to the treatment planning system. All target volumes including the gross tumour volume and critical target volume were delineated. Additionally, the lungs (left and right lungs are green and orange, respectively), spinal cord (yellow), heart (pink), liver (light blue), and esophagus (dark green) were also delineated in coronal (**A**) and axial sections (**B**). A treatment planning strategy using multiple non-coplanar beams (**C**) established a homogenous dose distribution to the tumour and lower doses to OARs.

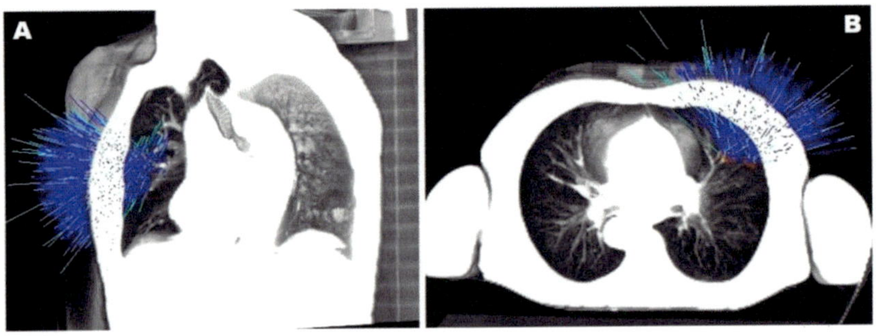

Figure 5: Multiple beam arrangement (blue lines) for a peripherally located tumour.

PALLIATIVE RT

The role of RT has been demonstrated not only for the curative treatment of non-metastatic NSCLC, but also for symptom palliation for metastatic NSCLC. The symptoms may be due to distant metastasis, such as headache, nausea, vomiting due to brain metastasis, bone pain, fracture due to bone metastasis, dyspnea, hemoptysis, or chest pain due to primary tumour progression [91-93]. Short courses of external-beam RT (between 2 and 10 fractions) offer a quick and effective means to palliate symptoms such as hemoptysis (in 72–86% of patients), chest pain (59–80%), cough (48–65%), and breathlessness (41–57%) [94].

A series of randomized studies has been performed to determine the optimal regimens of palliative RT in NSCLC, with various response rates being reported. In an RTOG study, no differences in survival and symptom palliation were observed between patients given 30 Gy of continuous irradiation, 40 Gy of continuous irradiation, and 40 Gy of split-course irradiation [23]. In another randomized study, there was no survival difference between patients who received 45 Gy in 18 fractions over 4.5 weeks and those who received 31.2 Gy in four fractions over 4 weeks; however, palliation was more effective with the higher dose [95]. Two MRC studies demonstrated that hypofractionated regimens were safe and well tolerated [96]. Moreover, follow-up study demonstrated that conventional RT (36–39 Gy given in 12 or 13 fractions) is associated with longer survival than the two-fraction regimen of 17 Gy [97]. Symptomatic relief occurred more rapidly and more durably in the hypofractionated arm compared to that observed with longer conventional fractionation. Thereafter, short schemes with one to five fractions have gained popularity regarding palliation among patients with NSCLC, as such schemes can achieve quicker palliation than that observed in patients who received five fractions [97]. A recent randomized clinical trial demonstrated a 2-month survival benefit ($p=0.03$) among patients who received five fractions compared to those who received one fraction [43]. However, this finding remains to be confirmed by other trials, particularly in patient populations that are eligible to receive this treatment. A recent Cochrane review of 14 randomized trials did not find any strong evidence that any regimen provides greater palliation. Higher dose regimens result in a higher incidence of acute toxicity, particularly esophagitis [44]. It was stated that the majority of patients should be treated with short courses of palliative RT (one or two fractions), whereas the use of high-dose palliative regimens should be considered for and discussed with selected patients with a good performance status.

Brain metastasis is a rapid neurological process that results in a survival of only 1–2 months [93]. Whole-brain RT (WBRT) with high-dose corticosteroids is the standard treatment for brain metastases in NSCLC, but it results in a median survival of only 3–6 months [91, 92]. The dose and fractionation schedule for WBRT remains controversial despite numerous studies designed to determine the optimum delivery (Fig. **6**).

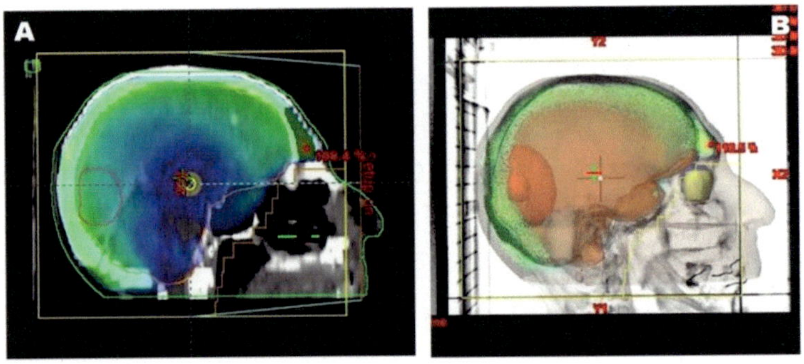

Figure 6: (A) Treatment planning for WBRT demonstrating the dose distribution (blue-green). (B) Simulation graphic of WBRT demonstrating the treatment field.

However, RT (a total of 30 Gy delivered in 10 fractions) continues to be the standard treatment for most patients. Typically, the radiographic and clinical response rates range from 50% to 75%. In the absence of systemic tumour activity, surgical excision of a solitary metastasis followed by WBRT can result in good local control, and long-term survival is possible [98]. In patients with a single non-resectable brain metastasis, the combination of WBRT and conformal boost to the tumour or stereotactic RT improves functional autonomy and survival in comparison with WBRT alone [99].

In patients with up to three metastases, the addition of stereotactic radiosurgery (SRS) to WBRT also results in a significant improvement in the performance score and decreased steroid use at 6 months [99]. Although no randomized trials have compared surgery with SRS, the latter appears to provide similar local control rates (in the order of 80–90% when combined with WBRT) [100].

Bone metastases are painful and frequently observed in advanced NSCLC. There are two important problems to be solved regarding bone metastases; one is pain, and second is the risk of fractures in weight-bearing bones, especially the vertebrae and pelvic bones. RT has been reported to be effective in palliating painful bone metastases, with partial pain relief observed in 80–90% of patients and complete pain relief observed in 50% of patients. Similarly as for brain metastasis, the current dose regimen for bone metastases is not yet standardized, but a commonly used regimen consists of a total of 30 Gy delivered in 10 fractions. For patients with a poor performance status, difficulty in making multiple trips for treatment, extensive non-osseous metastases, and/or a short life expectancy, the most appropriate treatment is a single fraction of 8 Gy. The use of bisphosphonates with external-beam RT may further improve the outcome in terms of both pain and bone healing.

ACKNOWLEDGEMENTS

Declared none.

CONFLICT OF INTEREST

The author confirms that this article content has no conflict of interest.

REFERENCES

[1] Onishi, H., *et al.*, Stereotactic hypofractionated high-dose irradiation for stage I nonsmall cell lung carcinoma: clinical outcomes in 245 subjects in a Japanese multiinstitutional study. Cancer, 2004. 101(7): p. 1623-31.

[2] Onishi, H., *et al.*, Hypofractionated stereotactic radiotherapy (HypoFXSRT) for stage I non-small cell lung cancer: updated results of 257 patients in a Japanese multi-institutional study. J Thorac Oncol, 2007. 2(7 Suppl 3): p. S94-100.

[3] Nguyen, N.P., *et al.*, Can stereotactic fractionated radiation therapy become the standard of care for early stage non-small cell lung carcinoma. Cancer Treat Rev, 2008. 34(8): p. 719-27.

[4] Lagerwaard, F.J., *et al.*, Outcomes of risk-adapted fractionated stereotactic radiotherapy for stage I non-small-cell lung cancer. Int J Radiat Oncol Biol Phys, 2008. 70(3): p. 685-92.

[5] Hoppe, B.S., *et al.*, Acute skin toxicity following stereotactic body radiation therapy for stage I non-small-cell lung cancer: who's at risk? Int J Radiat Oncol Biol Phys, 2008. 72(5): p. 1283-6.

[6] Kawase, T., *et al.*, Extrapulmonary soft-tissue fibrosis resulting from hypofractionated stereotactic body radiotherapy for pulmonary nodular lesions. Int J Radiat Oncol Biol Phys, 2009. 74(2): p. 349-54.

[7] Stephans, K.L., *et al.*, Comprehensive analysis of pulmonary function Test (PFT) changes after stereotactic body radiotherapy (SBRT) for stage I lung cancer in medically inoperable patients. J Thorac Oncol, 2009. 4(7): p. 838-44.

[8] Baumann, P., *et al.*, Outcome in a prospective phase II trial of medically inoperable stage I non-small-cell lung cancer patients treated with stereotactic body radiotherapy. J Clin Oncol, 2009. 27(20): p. 3290-6.

[9] Inoue, T., *et al.*, Clinical outcomes of stereotactic body radiotherapy for small lung lesions clinically diagnosed as primary lung cancer on radiologic examination. Int J Radiat Oncol Biol Phys, 2009. 75(3): p. 683-7.

[10] Takeda, A., *et al.*, Possible misinterpretation of demarcated solid patterns of radiation fibrosis on CT scans as tumour recurrence in patients receiving hypofractionated stereotactic radiotherapy for lung cancer. Int J Radiat Oncol Biol Phys, 2008. 70(4): p. 1057-65.

[11] Trakhtenberg, A., *et al.*, Preoperative radiotherapy in the combined treatment of lung cancer patients. Neoplasma, 1988. 35(4): p. 459-65.

[12] Wagner, H., Jr., *et al.*, Randomized phase 2 evaluation of preoperative radiation therapy and preoperative chemotherapy with mitomycin, vinblastine, and cisplatin in patients with technically unresectable stage IIIA and IIIB non-small cell cancer of the lung. LCSG 881. Chest, 1994. 106(6 Suppl): p. 348S-354S.

[13] Shields, T.W., Preoperative radiation therapy in the treatment of bronchial carcinoma. Cancer, 1972. 30(5): p. 1388-94.

[14] Green, M.R., *et al.*, Induction therapy for stage III NSCLC: a consensus report. Lung Cancer, 1994. 11 Suppl 3: p. S9-10.

[15] Gralla, R.J., New directions in non-small cell lung cancer. Semin Oncol, 1990. 17(4 Suppl 7): p. 14-9.

[16] Holmes, E.C., Preoperative neoadjuvant therapy in non-small-cell lung cancer: open season? J Natl Cancer Inst, 1991. 83(4): p. 228-9.

[17] Albain, K.S., Induction therapy followed by definitive local control for stage III non-small-cell lung cancer. A review, with a focus on recent trimodality trials. Chest, 1993. 103(1 Suppl): p. 43S-50S.

[18] Strauss, G.M., *et al.*, Multimodality treatment of stage IIIA non-small-cell lung carcinoma: a critical review of the literature and strategies for future research. J Clin Oncol, 1992. 10(5): p. 829-38.

[19] Bleehen, N.M., *et al.*, Combined radiation and chemotherapy for unresectable non-small cell lung carcinoma. Lung Cancer, 1994. 10 Suppl 1: p. S19-23.

[20] Johnson, D.H., Challenges of preoperative chemotherapy in non-small cell lung cancer. Lung Cancer, 1994. 10 Suppl 1: p. S195-203.

[21] Rusch, V.W., *et al.*, Neoadjuvant therapy: a novel and effective treatment for stage IIIb non-small cell lung cancer. Southwest Oncology Group. Ann Thorac Surg, 1994. 58(2): p. 290-4; discussion 294-5.

[22] Albain, K.S., *et al.*, Concurrent cisplatin/etoposide plus chest radiotherapy followed by surgery for stages IIIA (N2) and IIIB non-small-cell lung cancer: mature results of Southwest Oncology Group phase II study 8805. J Clin Oncol, 1995. 13(8): p. 1880-92.

[23] Simpson, J.R., *et al.*, Palliative radiotherapy for inoperable carcinoma of the lung: final report of a RTOG multi-institutional trial. Int J Radiat Oncol Biol Phys, 1985. 11(4): p. 751-8.

[24] Albain, K.S., *et al.*, Radiotherapy plus chemotherapy with or without surgical resection for stage III non-small-cell lung cancer: a phase III randomised controlled trial. Lancet, 2009. 374(9687): p. 379-86.

[25] Thomas, M., *et al.*, Effect of preoperative chemoradiation in addition to preoperative chemotherapy: a randomised trial in stage III non-small-cell lung cancer. Lancet Oncol, 2008. 9(7): p. 636-48.

[26] Arriagada, R., *et al.*, Cisplatin-based adjuvant chemotherapy in patients with completely resected non-small-cell lung cancer. N Engl J Med, 2004. 350(4): p. 351-60.

[27] Scagliotti, G.V., *et al.*, Randomized study of adjuvant chemotherapy for completely resected stage I, II, or IIIA non-small-cell Lung cancer. J Natl Cancer Inst, 2003. 95(19): p. 1453-61.

[28] Choi, N.C., *et al.*, Basis for new strategies in postoperative radiotherapy of bronchogenic carcinoma. Int J Radiat Oncol Biol Phys, 1980. 6(1): p. 31-5.

[29] Rudnick, S.A., *et al.*, Randomized phase II comparison of methotrexate with or without L-asparaginase in non-small cell cancer of the lung. Cancer Treat Rep, 1982. 66(3): p. 541-4.

[30] Effects of postoperative mediastinal radiation on completely resected stage II and stage III epidermoid cancer of the lung. The Lung Cancer Study Group. N Engl J Med, 1986. 315(22): p. 1377-81.

[31] Stephens, R.J., *et al.*, The role of post-operative radiotherapy in non-small-cell lung cancer: a multicentre randomised trial in patients with pathologically staged T1-2, N1-2, M0 disease. Medical Research Council Lung Cancer Working Party. Br J Cancer, 1996. 74(4): p. 632-9.

[32] PORT Meta-Analysis Trialists Group: Postoperative radiotherapy for non-small cell lung cancer. Cochrane Database Syst Rev, 2005(2): p. CD002142.

[33] Lally, B.E., *et al.*, Postoperative radiotherapy for stage II or III non-small-cell lung cancer using the surveillance, epidemiology, and end results database. J Clin Oncol, 2006. 24(19): p. 2998-3006.

[34] Okawara, G., *et al.*, Postoperative radiotherapy in stage II or IIIA completely resected non-small cell lung cancer: a systematic review and practice guideline. Lung Cancer, 2004. 44(1): p. 1-11.

[35] Matsuguma, H., *et al.*, Postoperative radiotherapy for patients with completely resected pathological stage IIIA-N2 non-small cell lung cancer: focusing on an effect of the number of mediastinal lymph node stations involved. Interact Cardiovasc Thorac Surg, 2008. 7(4): p. 573-7.

[36] Wakelee, H.A., *et al.*, Post-operative radiotherapy (PORT) or chemoradiotherapy (CPORT) following resection of stages II and IIIA non-small cell lung cancer (NSCLC) does not increase the expected risk of death from intercurrent disease (DID) in Eastern Cooperative Oncology Group (ECOG) trial E3590. Lung Cancer, 2005. 48(3): p. 389-97.

[37] Douillard, J.Y., Impact of radiation on survival after complete resection of non-small cell lung cancer: descriptive analysis in the randomized adjuvant chemotherapy trial ANITA 1(abstract). Int J Radiat Oncol Biol Phys, 2006. 66(Suppl.): p. 52.

[38] Mountain, C.F., Prognostic implications of the International Staging System for Lung Cancer. Semin Oncol, 1988. 15(3): p. 236-45.

[39] Keller, S.M., *et al.*, A randomized trial of postoperative adjuvant therapy in patients with completely resected stage II or IIIA non-small-cell lung cancer. Eastern Cooperative Oncology Group. N Engl J Med, 2000. 343(17): p. 1217-22.

[40] Dautzenberg, B., *et al.*, Adjuvant radiotherapy *versus* combined sequential chemotherapy followed by radiotherapy in the treatment of resected nonsmall cell lung carcinoma. A

randomized trial of 267 patients. GETCB (Groupe d'Etude et de Traitement des Cancers Bronchiques). Cancer, 1995. 76(5): p. 779-86.

[41] Bradley, J.D., *et al.*, Phase II trial of postoperative adjuvant paclitaxel/carboplatin and thoracic radiotherapy in resected stage II and IIIA non-small-cell lung cancer: promising long-term results of the Radiation Therapy Oncology Group--RTOG 9705. J Clin Oncol, 2005. 23(15): p. 3480-7.

[42] Arriagada, R., *et al.*, Long-term results of the international adjuvant lung cancer trial evaluating adjuvant Cisplatin-based chemotherapy in resected lung cancer. J Clin Oncol, 2010. 28(1): p. 35-42.

[43] Arriagada, R., *et al.*, Adjuvant chemotherapy, with or without postoperative radiotherapy, in operable non-small-cell lung cancer: two meta-analyses of individual patient data. Lancet, 2010. 375(9722): p. 1267-77.

[44] Johnson, D.H., *et al.*, Thoracic radiotherapy does not prolong survival in patients with locally advanced, unresectable non-small cell lung cancer. Ann Intern Med, 1990. 113(1): p. 33-8.

[45] Dillman, R.O., *et al.*, Recent outcomes for patients with carcinoma of the lung. Cancer Invest, 1991. 9(1): p. 9-17.

[46] Payne, D.G., Non-small-cell lung cancer: should unresectable stage III patients routinely receive high-dose radiation therapy? J Clin Oncol, 1988. 6(3): p. 552-8.

[47] Rosell, R., The integration of newer agents into neoadjuvant therapy. Semin Oncol, 1998. 25(3 Suppl 8): p. 24-7.

[48] Gandara, D.R., *et al.*, Neoadjuvant therapy for non-small cell lung cancer. Anticancer Drugs, 2001. 12 Suppl 1: p. S5-9.

[49] Group, N.-S.C.L.C.C., Chemotherapy in non-small cell lung cancer: a meta-analysis using updated data on individual patients from 52 randomised clinical trials. Non-small Cell Lung Cancer Collaborative Group. BMJ, 1995. 311(7010): p. 899-909.

[50] Dosoretz, D.E., *et al.*, Local control in medically inoperable lung cancer: an analysis of its importance in outcome and factors determining the probability of tumour eradication. Int J Radiat Oncol Biol Phys, 1993. 27(3): p. 507-16.

[51] Kaskowitz, L., *et al.*, Radiation therapy alone for stage I non-small cell lung cancer. Int J Radiat Oncol Biol Phys, 1993. 27(3): p. 517-23.

[52] Sibley, G.S., *et al.*, Radiotherapy alone for medically inoperable stage I non-small-cell lung cancer: the Duke experience. Int J Radiat Oncol Biol Phys, 1998. 40(1): p. 149-54.

[53] Pfister, D.G., *et al.*, American Society of Clinical Oncology treatment of unresectable non-small-cell lung cancer guideline: update 2003. J Clin Oncol, 2004. 22(2): p. 330-53.

[54] Akyurek, S., *et al.*, Mid-course thoracic radiotherapy with cisplatin-etoposide chemotherapy in limited-stage small-cell lung cancer. Med Oncol, 2006. 23(4): p. 499-505.

[55] Dillman, R.O., *et al.*, Improved survival in stage III non-small-cell lung cancer: seven-year follow-up of cancer and leukemia group B (CALGB) 8433 trial. J Natl Cancer Inst, 1996. 88(17): p. 1210-5.

[56] Sause, W., *et al.*, Final results of phase III trial in regionally advanced unresectable non-small cell lung cancer: Radiation Therapy Oncology Group, Eastern Cooperative Oncology Group, and Southwest Oncology Group. Chest, 2000. 117(2): p. 358-64.

[57] Sause, W.T., *et al.*, Radiation Therapy Oncology Group (RTOG) 88-08 and Eastern Cooperative Oncology Group (ECOG) 4588: preliminary results of a phase III trial in

regionally advanced, unresectable non-small-cell lung cancer. J Natl Cancer Inst, 1995. 87(3): p. 198-205.

[58] Donaldson, N., *et al.*, Sequential re-analysis of a phase-III clinical trial in non-small cell lung cancer. Eur Respir J, 2000. 15(5): p. 821-7.

[59] Morton, R.F., *et al.*, Thoracic radiation therapy alone compared with combined chemoradiotherapy for locally unresectable non-small cell lung cancer. A randomized, phase III trial. Ann Intern Med, 1991. 115(9): p. 681-6.

[60] Marino, P., A. Preatoni, and A. Cantoni, Randomized trials of radiotherapy alone *versus* combined chemotherapy and radiotherapy in stages IIIa and IIIb nonsmall cell lung cancer. A meta-analysis. Cancer, 1995. 76(4): p. 593-601.

[61] Schaake-Koning, C., *et al.*, Effects of concomitant cisplatin and radiotherapy on inoperable non-small-cell lung cancer. N Engl J Med, 1992. 326(8): p. 524-30.

[62] Furuse, K., *et al.*, Phase III study of concurrent *versus* sequential thoracic radiotherapy in combination with mitomycin, vindesine, and cisplatin in unresectable stage III non-small-cell lung cancer. J Clin Oncol, 1999. 17(9): p. 2692-9.

[63] Curran, W.J., C.B. Scott, and C.J. Langer, Long-term benefit is observed in a phase III comparison of sequential *vs.* concurrent chemo-radiaton for patients with unresectable stage III NSCLC: RTOG 9410. Proc Am Soc Clin Oncol, 2003 (abstr 2499). 22: p. 621.

[64] Fournel, P., *et al.*, Randomized phase III trial of sequential chemoradiotherapy compared with concurrent chemoradiotherapy in locally advanced non-small-cell lung cancer: Groupe Lyon-Saint-Etienne d'Oncologie Thoracique-Groupe Francais de Pneumo-Cancerologie NPC 95-01 Study. J Clin Oncol, 2005. 23(25): p. 5910-7.

[65] Movsas, B., Will future progress in non-small-cell lung cancer be step by step. or by leaps and bounds? J Clin Oncol, 2005. 23(25): p. 5859-61.

[66] Zatloukal, P., *et al.*, Concurrent *versus* sequential chemoradiotherapy with cisplatin and vinorelbine in locally advanced non-small cell lung cancer: a randomized study. Lung Cancer, 2004. 46(1): p. 87-98.

[67] Belderbos, J., *et al.*, Randomised trial of sequential *versus* concurrent chemo-radiotherapy in patients with inoperable non-small cell lung cancer (EORTC 08972-22973). Eur J Cancer, 2007. 43(1): p. 114-21.

[68] Rowell, N.P. and P. O'Rourke N, Concurrent chemoradiotherapy in non-small cell lung cancer. Cochrane Database Syst Rev, 2004(4): p. CD002140.

[69] Auperin, A., *et al.*, Meta-analysis of concomitant *versus* sequential radiochemotherapy in locally advanced non-small-cell lung cancer. J Clin Oncol, 2010. 28(13): p. 2181-90.

[70] Auperin, A., *et al.*, Prophylactic cranial irradiation for patients with small-cell lung cancer in complete remission. Prophylactic Cranial Irradiation Overview Collaborative Group. N Engl J Med, 1999. 341(7): p. 476-84.

[71] Gregor, A., *et al.*, Prophylactic cranial irradiation is indicated following complete response to induction therapy in small cell lung cancer: results of a multicentre randomised trial. United Kingdom Coordinating Committee for Cancer Research (UKCCCR) and the European Organization for Research and Treatment of Cancer (EORTC). Eur J Cancer, 1997. 33(11): p. 1752-8.

[72] Patel, S., O.K. Macdonald, and M. Suntharalingam, Evaluation of the use of prophylactic cranial irradiation in small cell lung cancer. Cancer, 2009. 115(4): p. 842-50.

[73] Le Pechoux, C., *et al.*, Standard-dose *versus* higher-dose prophylactic cranial irradiation (PCI) in patients with limited-stage small-cell lung cancer in complete remission after

chemotherapy and thoracic radiotherapy (PCI 99-01, EORTC 22003-08004, RTOG 0212, and IFCT 99-01): a randomised clinical trial. Lancet Oncol, 2009. 10(5): p. 467-74.

[74] Yavuz, A.A., *et al.*, Prophylactic cranial irradiation in locally advanced non-small cell lung cancer: outcome of recursive partitioning analysis group 1 patients. J Exp Clin Cancer Res, 2008. 27: p. 80.

[75] Lester, J.F., B. Coles, and F.R. Macbeth, Prophylactic cranial irradiation for preventing brain metastases in patients undergoing radical treatment for non-small cell lung cancer. Cochrane Database Syst Rev, 2005(2): p. CD005221.

[76] Pottgen, C., *et al.*, Prophylactic cranial irradiation in operable stage IIIA non small-cell lung cancer treated with neoadjuvant chemoradiotherapy: results from a German multicenter randomized trial. J Clin Oncol, 2007. 25(31): p. 4987-92.

[77] Gore, M., *et al.*, A phase III comparison of prophylactic cranial irradiation *versus* observation in patients with locally advanced non-small cell lung cancer: Initial analysis of Radiation Therapy Oncology Group 0214 [abstract #7506]. J Clin Oncol, 2009. 27 (Suppl).

[78] Cull, A., *et al.*, Neurological and cognitive impairment in long-term survivors of small cell lung cancer. Eur J Cancer, 1994. 30A(8): p. 1067-74.

[79] Johnson, B.E., *et al.*, Neurologic, computed cranial tomographic, and magnetic resonance imaging abnormalities in patients with small-cell lung cancer: further follow-up of 6- to 13-year survivors. J Clin Oncol, 1990. 8(1): p. 48-56.

[80] van Oosterhout, A.G., *et al.*, Neurologic disorders in 203 consecutive patients with small cell lung cancer. Results of a longitudinal study. Cancer, 1996. 77(8): p. 1434-41.

[81] Arriagada, R., *et al.*, Patterns of failure after prophylactic cranial irradiation in small-cell lung cancer: analysis of 505 randomized patients. Ann Oncol, 2002. 13(5): p. 748-54.

[82] Bradley, J., *et al.*, Impact of FDG-PET on radiation therapy volume delineation in non-small-cell lung cancer. Int J Radiat Oncol Biol Phys, 2004. 59(1): p. 78-86.

[83] Annema, J.T., *et al.*, Towards a minimally invasive staging strategy in NSCLC: analysis of PET positive mediastinal lesions by EUS-FNA. Lung Cancer, 2004. 44(1): p. 53-60.

[84] Underberg, R.W., *et al.*, Four-dimensional CT scans for treatment planning in stereotactic radiotherapy for stage I lung cancer. Int J Radiat Oncol Biol Phys, 2004. 60(4): p. 1283-90.

[85] Underberg, R.W., *et al.*, Benefit of respiration-gated stereotactic radiotherapy for stage I lung cancer: an analysis of 4DCT datasets. Int J Radiat Oncol Biol Phys, 2005. 62(2): p. 554-60.

[86] Grills, I.S., *et al.*, Potential for reduced toxicity and dose escalation in the treatment of inoperable non-small-cell lung cancer: a comparison of intensity-modulated radiation therapy (IMRT), 3D conformal radiation, and elective nodal irradiation. Int J Radiat Oncol Biol Phys, 2003. 57(3): p. 875-90.

[87] Liu, H.H., *et al.*, Feasibility of sparing lung and other thoracic structures with intensity-modulated radiotherapy for non-small-cell lung cancer. Int J Radiat Oncol Biol Phys, 2004. 58(4): p. 1268-79.

[88] Murshed, H., *et al.*, Dose and volume reduction for normal lung using intensity-modulated radiotherapy for advanced-stage non-small-cell lung cancer. Int J Radiat Oncol Biol Phys, 2004. 58(4): p. 1258-67.

[89] Hodge, W., *et al.*, Feasibility report of image guided stereotactic body radiotherapy (IG-SBRT) with tomotherapy for early stage medically inoperable lung cancer using extreme hypofractionation. Acta Oncol, 2006. 45(7): p. 890-6.

[90] van der Voort van Zyp, N.C., *et al.*, Stereotactic radiotherapy with real-time tumour tracking for non-small cell lung cancer: clinical outcome. Radiother Oncol, 2009. 91(3): p. 296-300.

[91] Gaspar, L., *et al.*, Recursive partitioning analysis (RPA) of prognostic factors in three Radiation Therapy Oncology Group (RTOG) brain metastases trials. Int J Radiat Oncol Biol Phys, 1997. 37(4): p. 745-51.

[92] Lagerwaard, F.J., *et al.*, Identification of prognostic factors in patients with brain metastases: a review of 1292 patients. Int J Radiat Oncol Biol Phys, 1999. 43(4): p. 795-803.

[93] Onal, C. and E. Ozyar, Intracranial metastasis and increased intracranial pressure. Turkiye Klinikleri J Surg Med Sci, 2006. 2(33): p. 6-10.

[94] Bleehen, N.M., *et al.*, A Medical Research Council phase II trial of alternating chemotherapy and radiotherapy in small-cell lung cancer. The Medical Research Council Lung Cancer Working Party. Br J Cancer, 1991. 64(4): p. 775-9.

[95] Teo, P., *et al.*, A randomized study on palliative radiation therapy for inoperable non small cell carcinoma of the lung. Int J Radiat Oncol Biol Phys, 1988. 14(5): p. 867-71.

[96] Inoperable non-small-cell lung cancer (NSCLC): a Medical Research Council randomised trial of palliative radiotherapy with two fractions or ten fractions. Report to the Medical Research Council by its Lung Cancer Working Party. Br J Cancer, 1991. 63(2): p. 265-70.

[97] Macbeth, F.R., *et al.*, Randomized trial of palliative two-fraction *versus* more intensive 13-fraction radiotherapy for patients with inoperable non-small cell lung cancer and good performance status. Medical Research Council Lung Cancer Working Party. Clin Oncol (R Coll Radiol), 1996. 8(3): p. 167-75.

[98] Noordijk, E.M., *et al.*, The choice of treatment of single brain metastasis should be based on extracranial tumour activity and age. Int J Radiat Oncol Biol Phys, 1994. 29(4): p. 711-7.

[99] Andrews, D.W., *et al.*, Whole brain radiation therapy with or without stereotactic radiosurgery boost for patients with one to three brain metastases: phase III results of the RTOG 9508 randomised trial. Lancet, 2004. 363(9422): p. 1665-72.

[100] Rades, D., *et al.*, Comparison of stereotactic radiosurgery (SRS) alone and whole brain radiotherapy (WBRT) plus a stereotactic boost (WBRT+SRS) for one to three brain metastases. Strahlenther Onkol, 2008. 184(12): p. 655-62.

Send Orders of Reprints at reprints@benthamscience.net

CHAPTER 12

Alternatives to Surgical Resection for Non–Small Cell Lung Cancer

Akın Eraslan Balcı*

Euphrates University School of Medicine, Department of Thoracic Surgery, Elazig, Turkey

Abstract: Surgical resection for lung cancer remains the mainstay of therapy for early-stage non–small cell lung cancer (NSCLC) and provides the best opportunity for cure. Every patient with locoregional NSCLC should be approached as a potential candidate for resection. For stage 1A, 1B, 2A and 2B NSCLC, an operation is the treatment of choice [1-5].

Patients with clinical stage I non-small cell lung cancer (NSCLC) can be considered falling into three treatment groups: (1) good-risk patients, who are usually treated with lobectomy; (2) high-risk patients, who are usually treated with sublobar (segmental or wedge) resection; and (3) medically inoperable patients, who traditionally have been treated with external beam radiation therapy [6]. Stereotactic body radiation therapy (SBRT) and radiofrequency ablation (RFA) are two nonoperative approaches that are gaining increasing popularity for the treatment of NSCLC. Radiofrequency ablation (RFA) therapy is a minimally invasive technique that can be used in the management of inoperable non-small-cell lung cancer and for palliation in selected patients with pulmonary metastases. Surgical resection remains the gold standard of treatment; however, many patients are ineligible due to comorbidities or poor cardiopulmonary reserve. Some have claimed that SBRT is superior to sublobar resection and may even be equivalent to lobectomy. This assumption is incorrect. At best, stereotactic body radiation therapy and radiofrequency ablation can only approximate a wedge resection if it is assumed that 100% tumour destruction has occurred. Lymph node dissection and sampling can also be undertaken at the time of sublobar resection, potentially improving outcomes and allowing identification of unsuspected nodal disease. Despite this, stereotactic body radiation therapy and radiofrequency ablation may be clinically equivalent to sublobar resection for the high-risk patient because of lower procedural morbidity and more rapid return to normal function [6, 7].

Keywords: Radiofrequency, radiosurgery, stereotactic, microwave, ablation, cyberknife, lung cancer.

***Address correspondence to Akın Eraslan Balcı:** Euphrates University School of Medicine, Department of Thoracic Surgery, Elazig, Turkey; Tel: +90 424 2333555/2134; Fax: +90 424 2388096; E-mail: akineraslan.balci@hotmail.com

Akın Eraslan Balcı (Ed)

INTRODUCTION

Most patients with stage II and a subset of patients with stage Ib are offered adjuvant chemotherapy. Adjuvant treatment should be considered for patients after resection for stage 2 lung cancer. For incidental finding of mediastinal lymph node involvement from surgical specimens (unexpected), adjuvant therapy can be considered. Selected patients with stage 3A and 3B may be candidates after neoadjuvant treatment. An operation is most effective for stage 1 cancer and less than 25% of patients are found to have lung cancer at an early stage. On the other hand tumour recurrence occurs in approximately half of patients who undergo surgery [1, 5, 8, 9]. When recurrence is limited to the lung, surgical intervention is considered the best treatment to provide longer survival.

Unfortunately, many patients present with advanced disease. The lungs are one of the most common locations for metastases, yet the pathophysiology of pulmonary metastases is complex [10]. Pulmonary metastases have primary tumours of many varied origins, and, unlike primary tumours, they are usually asymptomatic. Although lung metastases from a solid malignant tumour are usually associated with distant and hematogenous disease indicating widespread disease, in certain circumstances, metastatic lung disease is isolated, slowly evolving and requires local treatment. Stage 3A or 3B should not be resected primarily but they considered for multimodality therapy. Stage 3 patients are generally not surgical candidates, although patients with technically resectable stage 3A (N2 disease) can be surgical candidates after neoadjuvant treatment. Patients with T3N0 (stage 2B) NSCLC due to chest wall invasion or carinal proximity are candidates for initial complete resection. Stage 4 patients are rarely candidates for resection. Only under exceptional circumstances should patients with stage 4 be considered for resection. Despite aggressive multimodality therapy, 5-year survival in patients with advanced stage NSCLC was very poor and limited to small pathological subsets. Patients with advanced stage NSCLC who did not belong to one of these subsets had a small chance of long-term survival [8, 9, 11]. Operation in cases of T4 cancer due to malignant pleural effusion offers no survival advantage over less invasive therapies. Resection of tumours with satelllite lesions in the same lobe is acceptable. The presence of multiple extrathoracic metastases is almost always an absolute contrindication to pulmonary resection. If a patient has a solitary brain or solitary adrenal metastasis and otherwise a stage 1 lung cancer, then both sites can be resected. Resection can be done only after thorough imaging and invasive assessment. Clinically proven lymph node dissemination is also nonsurgical. N3 disease remains out of bounds for resection. Patients discovered to have N2 disease, particularly single-station N2 disease, at thoracotomy following an appropriate negative invasive evaluation should undergo resection at that time.

On the other hand many of those with resectable early-stage disease are unable to tolerate pulmonary resection because of compromised cardiopulmonary function. It has been estimated that more than 20% of patients diagnosed with stage I or II NSCLC do not undergo operation [12]. The usual mechanism for an MI in the nonpostoperative setting is the coronary artery plaque rupture resulting in obstruction of a vessel causing myocardial damage due to this abrupt change in supply. Treatment for acute coronary syndromes (plaque ruptures) include antithrombotic regimens, therapies designed to decrease myocardial oxygen demand and myocardial revascularisation. In patients who are candidates for resection, evidence for plaque rupture must be sought after adequate control of blood pressure, heart rate, volume status and anemia has been achieved. Such evidence may include recurrent chest pain, electrocardiographic changes, ventricular arrhythimias or refractory heart failure. Abnormally elevated pulmonary vascular resistance or pulmonary artery pressure at rest or during the exercise has been associated with a high rate of operative mortality after major lung resection. Postoperative predicted FEV1 < 800-1000 ml precludes resection. Patients who are candidates for pneumonectomy but who have a preoperative FEV1 < 2 L should undergo quantitative radionuclide lung perfusion scanning to assess relative distribution of function between two lungs. Patients who are candidates for major lung resection for cancer are increasingly likely to undergo induction chemotherapy prior to surgery. High-dose chemotherapy has been shown to cause a 40% to 50% reduction in DL_{CO}.

Approximately 15% to 20% of patients with stage 1 or 2 NSCLC are unable to undergo any operation owing to existing comorbid diseases. The standard therapy for these high-risk patients has been external beam radiation therapy (EBRT). Adjuvant EBRT is an option that has been reported to decrease local recurrence after wedge resection. Although the results with radiation have been better than with no treatment, treatment results with EBRT are still inferior when compared with resection and the chance for cure is small. In a study of 71 node-negative patients who received at least 60 Gy to their cancers, the 3- and 5-year survival rates were 19% and 12%, respectively [5]. A more recent report described results after radiation therapy in 60 patients with stage I or II NSCLC.[6] Local progression occurred in 53% of the patients, with a median progression-free survival time of 18.5 months and an overall median survival time of 20 months. Another concern with EBRT is the issue of radiation injury to surrounding tissues because it is difficult to deliver a precise area of radiation to a target area due to lung movement with respiration. This unwanted exposure of normal tissue (*i.e.*, normal lung parenchyma, heart, spine, and esophagus) is a limiting factor. Radiation pneumonitis is a potentially life-threatening problem, particularly for a patient with severely impaired pulmonary function who is not a candidate for resection (the type of patient usually referred for nonoperative therapy). In the series described earlier [6], radiation pneumonitis occurred in 8.3% of patients treated with definitive radiotherapy [8, 9].

An alternative to EBRT is the use of intraoperative adjuvant brachytherapy. The term brachytherapy, meaning "short," signifies both the distance of the radiation source from the tissue being treated and the duration of therapy. Brachytherapy typically is performed with the radiation source remaining within the airway. The most commonly used source of radiation is iridium-192 (^{192}Ir), which is delivered *via* a catheter. On the other hand suture techniques has also been described for brachytherapy: Paired sutures adjacent to staple lines are placed. These contain iodine-125 and deliver the radiation. A second method is the placement of the same sutures into a Vicryl mesh. Then this mesh is placed over the staple line. The advantage of bracyhtherapy is that this provides a means of delivering radiation in a more uniform manner, with 100% patient compliance and in the same setting as the lung resection. The local recurrence rate after the brachytherapy was 6.1%, which was similar to the 6.4% reported after lobectomy in the Lung Cancer Study Group.

New alternatives to resection or standard EBRT are now entering clinical practice for the treatment of lung cancer or limited pulmonary metastases. The two principal modalities that are being offered by many centers around the world are radiofrequency ablation (RFA) and stereotactic radiosurgery (SRS). Another ablative modality, microwave ablation (MWA), also is being introduced into practice, although currently the clinical experience is very small. This chapter reviews these therapies and their roles in clinical practice.

RADIOFREQUENCY ABLATION

Systems and Mechanism of Action

Radiofrequency ablation (RFA) is gaining popularity for the treatment of lung cancer, because it is technically simple and safe, providing good local control [13]. RFA has proven to be a suitable option for high-risk patients with metastases as well as those who have previously undergone metastatectomy. Therefore, RFA is especially suitable for patients with limited pulmonary reserve because this technique minimizes damage to lung parenchyma. RFA could be complementary to chemotherapy. Central hypoxic cells, which can be resistant to chemotherapy, may be more sensitive to RFA because of increased cell sensitivity to heat in the hypoxic state and decreased heat dissipation due to poor tumour perfusion. In fact, the clinical course of patients after RFA was relatively good, with the ablated lesion becoming completely necrotic after 3–4 months after RFA if complete ablation was performed on the lung mass. RFA has several advantages as follows: minimal invasiveness with fewer complications, well tolerated by outpatients, repeatable treatment of residual or recurrent nodules, relatively short treatment time, and rapid recovery of physical performance.

Radiofrequency energy consists of an alternating current that moves from an active electrode placed within a tumour to disperse electrodes placed on the patient. RFA systems therefore have three components: a generator, an active electrode, and a dispersive electrode. RFA involves the application of high-frequency electric current to heat and coagulate target tissue. In RF ablation, an alternating electrical current (approximately 500 KHz) with 10 to 200 W of power is applied to the target tissue *via* an interstitial electrode. Once the position of the needle electrode is confirmed, multiple times or hooks are deployed within the tumour. The needle systems are designed to offer maximal distribution of energy, producing a spherical ablation zone. The application of an alternating current causes ionic agitation, resulting in tissue heating. This rise in temperature results in coagulative necrosis and tissue destruction in the vicinity of the probe [1]. Two to four grounding pads on the skin surface complete the electrical circuit through the body. Current conducted through tissue adjacent to the electrode leads to ion agitation, which is converted by means of friction into heat. Heat generation is proportional to the current density and is attenuated exponentially with increasing distance from the electrode. As tissue is heated, predictable changes occur based on time and temperature. At temperatures between 42°C and 45°C, cells become susceptible to damage by outside agents like radiation and chemotherapy. Temperatures maintained above 46°C for a prolonged period of time (on the order of 30 to 60 minutes) cause irreversible cell damage. Between 50°C and 52°C, the time to cytotoxicity is reduced to 4 to 6 minutes. The goal of RF ablation is to achieve temperatures between 60°C and 100°C, where there is near instantaneous induction of protein coagulation with damage to cytosolic and mitochondrial enzymes and DNA–histone complexes leading to coagulative necrosis. Conversely, temperatures above 105°C cause boiling, desiccation, vaporisation, and carbonisation of tissues. The resulting impedance rise limits electrical current flow, leading to reduced coagulative necrosis volumes. Thus, the therapeutic temperature range for RF ablation is narrow (60°C to 100°C) [1, 14]. As the radiofrequency energy moves from the active electrode to the dispersive electrode and then back to the active electrode, ions within the tissue oscillate in an attempt to follow the change in the direction of alternating current. This results in frictional heating of the tissue; as the temperature within the tissue rises to more than 60°C, instantaneous cell death begins due to protein denaturation and coagulation necrosis. Typically when RFA is performed, the local temperature in the ablated tumour rises to the range of 90°C to 100°C. Subsequent to the RF procedure, the tumour diameter increases in size due to edematous and hemorrhagic alterations in the surrounding lung parenchyma. For up to 3 months, the ablated area decreases in size; at 6 months, it is of the same size or smaller than before RFA. Later, it becomes stable or shrinks [15]. The ablation zone may start to decrease in size as early as 2 to 3 weeks following ablation as tissue repair progresses.

Cavitation has been reported in up to 30% of patients following ablation and is associated with effective ablation and further complicates interpretation of postablation imaging. Pulmonary function may decrease after RFA. RFA-induced severe pleuritis and ablation of a large volume of marginal parenchyma are associated with impaired pulmonary function. Recovery time of the pulmonary function is about 3 months [13]. Pneumothorax is the most common complication following all modalities of thermal ablation. A median pneumothorax rate of 28% (range 4.5 to 61.1%) was reported for RF ablation in a recent meta-analysis with approximately 11% (range 3.3 to 38.9%) of these requiring chest tube placement. In RF ablation, the risk of pneumothorax has been shown to be greater in patients in whom multiple lesions are treated, in patients without history of previous lung surgery, and in patients with a longer pleura-to-lesion distance [16, 17]. Hemoptysis is a common occurrence after pulmonary ablation, but is usually low volume and self-limited. Large and fatal events may be occured. Brachial nerve injuries have been reported in patients who underwent percutaneous radiofrequency ablation of apical lung cancer, as long as 7 days afterward [18].

According to reports on pulmonary function after surgical resection, FEV1 at 1 and 3 months after lobectomy was 79.5 and 84% of the baseline value, respectively, and FEV_1 at 1 and 3 months after pneumonectomy was 65 and 66% of baseline, respectively. Forced VC and FEV_1 at 2 months after segmentectomy were 89.6 and 90.5% of baseline, respectively, and those at 2 months after lobectomy were 84 and 83.2% of baseline, respectively. RFA seems to affect pulmonary function less than the pulmonary surgeries. Nevertheless, pulmonary function may decrease by up to 30% if the patients suffer from severe pleuritis or the ablated parenchymal volume is ≥20 cm [3]. This relatively new modality is widely used for the treatment of liver tumours. It is being used either as an adjunct to resection or as a primary therapy, and because of its lower rate of complications, it has largely replaced other, less invasive modalities [9]. A large international, multicenter study of 2320 patients who received percutaneous RFA for liver malignancies reported a periprocedural mortality rate of 0.3% and an overall complication rate of 7.1% [19]. Midterm survival after this treatment seems promising: 68% at 2 years, 75% at 2 years, and 74% at 3 years for patients with clinical stage I non-small cell lung cancer; and 66% at 2 years and 46–48% at 3 years for patients with metastatic colorectal cancer [13]. Several reports primarily demonstrate the safety and feasibility of this technique for lung tumours [1, 13, 20, 21]. Lung RFA has the possibility to provide nonsurgical candidates with survival benefit. Good local tumour control seems to contribute to prolonged survival.

There are multiple US Food and Drug Administration (FDA)-approved RF ablation devices on the market with different performance characteristics. Examples include: the Angiodynamics 1500X RF generator with the StarBurst and Uniblate electrodes (Latham, NY, USA), the Boston Scientific RF3000 with LaVeen electrodes (Natick, MA, USA) (both of which use multitined, expandable electrodes) and the Covidien Cool-tip system (Boulder, CO, USA), which uses either a single straight electrode, cluster of three electrodes, or up to three independent, switched straight electrodes that are actively cooled during ablation. Importantly, these systems were all developed for use in liver, and have been applied in lung without modification. Currently, there are no devices available for clinical use optimised for treating tumours in the lung [14].

The most common method used for pulmonary RFA is a percutaneous CT-guided approach. This has the advantage of being truly minimally invasive, an important factor for the higher-risk patients who are treated with this modality. Either general or local anesthesia can be used when performing CT-guided RFA. Previously, RFA techniques performed *via* open thoracotomy. Although the video-assisted thoracic surgery (VATS) approach may be attractive because of its minimally invasive nature, in practice the RFA technique is not easily compatible with VATS. The main reason is that it is important to obtain optimal needle deployment within the tumour. When VATS is performed, the lung is collapsed to allow visualisation within the pleural space, and the tumour (particularly if it is deep to the visceral pleural surface) may not be seen. In an open thoracotomy, the tumour can easily be palpated to place the active electrode; this is not the case with VATS [9, 10]. The alternative of anaesthesia by thoracic epidural could offer an answer to the problem of the patient who requires RFA but has poor lung function [22].

The Boston Scientific (BOS) (Natick, MA), RITA Medical (Fremont, CA), and Valley Lab (VL) (Boulder, CO) systems. With the impedance-based BOS device, the end point of treatment is determined by a significant rise in impedance, which indicates that the tumour has been ablated, resulting in cell necrosis that prevents further conduction. Thermal ablation is achieved with an impedance-based feedback generator delivering an output frequency of 460 kHz (RF3000; Boston Scientific, Natick, MA), with LeVeen CoAccess multitined expandable 14-gauge electrodes (Boston Scientific), and with a 15 cm-long, 14-gauge, insulated, diamond-tip guiding needle. Prone, supine, or lateral positions are used to obtain the shortest access route to the tumour and to give access to all metastases in both lungs. Repositioning of the patient is possible if the first position did not give a direct route to the metastases [6]. The RITA and VL systems are temperature-based devices that rely on raising the tumour temperature to high levels for specified periods of time, depending on the device used and the size of tumour being ablated. The BOS and RITA active probes both consist of an expandable needle system, whereas the VL system uses either a single needle or three parallel needles placed into the tumour. The VL electrode consists of a proximal insulated portion and a distal noninsulated active tip. The electrode is irrigated with a continuous infusion of ice water, and for this reason it is sometimes referred to as a so-called cool-tip electrode [4, 5].

RFA is principally employed for either prolonging survival in nonsurgical candidates or palliation of symptoms. The technique is used to target both primary and metastatic disease. Pulmonary tumours can be extensive, causing chest pain, dyspnea, cough, and hemoptysis. Although tumours that are large in size are unlikely to be completely eradicated, the technique may be employed for debulking, particularly of lesions involving the pleura or chest wall that are typically more painful. Lung RFA is also a safe and effective treatment in patients with recurrent NSCLC and can be the alternative therapeutic methods to surgery in non-surgical candidates. Additionally this technique have an advantage of re-use in the setting of local tumour progression after the first RFA treatment. Five-year survival rates have been reported as being 23–42% after repeat surgery in such patients [1, 23]. Kodama and colleagues performed curative lung RF ablation for 51 recurrent NSCLC (mean diameter 1.7 ± 0.9 cm, range 0.6 to 4.0) after surgical intervention. Patient was not candidate for a second surgery. In these patients the technical success rate of RF ablation was 82.4% (42 of 51). Local tumour progression rate was found 11.4% (5 of 44 patients)1. The 1-, 3- and 5-year primary local tumour progression rates were 5.4%, 14.2%, and 42.8%, respectively. Local tumour progression was ablated again by repeat RF ablation in 4 of the 5 patients (80.0%). Ablated tumours were controlled after the second RF ablation in 3 of the 4 patients. The 1-, 3-, and 5-year overall survival rates were 97.7%, 72.9%, and 55.7%, respectively. Recurrences were found in 19 patients (43.2%, 19 of 44) in total. Of 5 patients with local tumour progression, new lung tumours emerged in the nontreated lung parenchyma in 3 patients. New lung tumours developed in another 12 patients. Of them, 2 patients had metastases other than lung: There were liver metastases in 1 patient and brain, lymph node, and liver metastases in 1 patient. Nodal metastases were found in the 18th patient, and bone metastasis and carcinomatous pleuritis were fund in the 19th patient. The 1- and 3-year recurrence-free survival rates were 76.7 and 41.1%, respectively. Tumour size and sex were independent significant predictors in the multivariate analysis. Prognostic factors identified in the this study are almost identical to those reported for surgical intervention. The larger the tumour becomes, the greater the incidence of nodal or vessel invasion, which leads to local tumour progression and/or distant metastasis The 5-year survival rates were 73.3% in 18 women and 60.5% in 38 patients who had small tumours measuring $\leq$ 3 cm. In this study pneumothorax was the only major complication.

For lung metastases this treatment is reserved for those patients who have a limited number of metastases, disease localised to the chest, and a primary cancer that is either controlled or controllable. RFA offers the advantage of potentially treating bilateral metastases in a single session. Palussière [10] and coworkers treated 27 patients with bilateral lung metastases in the same session. Sixty-six metastases were treated by RFA: 55 were intraparenchymatous, 9 with less than 50% pleural contact, and 2 with more than 50% pleural contact. Mean size was 14 (range, 4–43) mm. All metastases (range, 2–4) were treated for all patients. Three patients had previously received a thoracotomy for metastases. Median time per ablation per patient was 41 (range, 25–72) min. During the single session procedure, pneumothoraces were the most frequent complication, occurring in 18 cases (66.7%, 14 unilateral and 4 bilateral). Among the 14 patients with unilateral pneumothoraces, unilateral chest tube drainage was needed in 8 patients. Among the four patients with bilateral pneumothoraces, unilateral chest tube drainage was performed for two and bilateral for two. The median follow-up time was 21.3

months. Median survival time was 26 (19–33) months. Four recurrences in four patients were depicted on a RFA site during follow-up, all on tumours <3 cm in diameter. Twelve patients had new lung metastases and seven of them were retreated by RFA with two treated again for bilateral metastases in the same session. Median time to tumour progression was 9.5 (4.2–23.5) months. They concluded that single-session treatment of bilateral metastases is possible and effective, with low morbidity and short hospitalisation durations if strict patient inclusion criteria are respected. Pennatur [24] and colleagues performed RFA in 22 patients with pulmonary metasteses. A percutaneous CT-guided approach was used in 17 patients (with 1 open conversion) and RFA was performed as an adjunct to surgical resection in 5 patients. Thoracic surgeons performed all procedures. The primary cancer was colorectal in 9 (41%), renal in 2 (9%), sarcoma in 4 (18%), and other in 7 (32%). CT-guided RFA was the sole treatment in 17 patients (77%) and combined with surgical resection in 5 (23%). No procedurally related deaths occurred. At a mean follow-up of 27 months (range, 13.3 to 53.6 months), 9 patients are alive. The median survival was 29 months (95% confidence interval, 9.1 to 33.8). Lesion size was an important prognostic variable associated with overall and disease-free survival. Size (< 3 cm *vs.* > 3 cm) was a significant factor in both overall and disease-free survival. The median survival for patients with lesion diameter of 3 cm or less was 39.1 months *vs.* 7.9 months for patients with lesion size exceeding 3 cm. Survival rates in patients treated by RFA for lung metastasis similar to those obtained by surgery. Several factors have already been shown to influence efficacy, such as tumour size larger than 2 cm, size of ground glass opacities at first posttreatment checkups (48 h). Contact between the tumour and a large vessel (heat sink effect), and location close to the heart are predictive of lower complete local ablation rates. The use of multi line expandable electrodes also has been reported as more effective than single electrodes, but single internally cooled electrodes often were used in more difficult situations (tumours close to the hilum) [25-29]. Thermal conductivity of the tissue being ablated is an important factor influencing the effectivity of thermal ablation. Thermal conductivity is lower in lung than in other tissues such as bone, liver and kidney due to its high percentage of air by volume [30]. Low tissue conductivity can be overcome by infusion of sodium chloride solutions into the targeted ablation zone. Infusion during treatment also prevents charring and keeps the ablated tissue hydrated, resulting in a larger zone of ablation. This method is not routinely performed because it can produce irregular effect and may leads to serious complications.

Lee [31] and coworkers compared the survival rate in patients with non-small-cell lung cancer (NSCLC) treated with radiofrequency ablation (RFA), surgery, or chemotherapy according to lung cancer staging. In the RFA group, 40 patients with inoperable NSCLC underwent RFA under computed tomography (CT) guidance. These included 16 patients with stage I to II cancer and 24 patients with stage III to IV cancer who underwent RFA in an adjuvant setting. In the comparison group (n = 37), 13 patients with stage I to II cancer underwent surgery; 18 patients with stage III to IV cancer underwent chemotherapy; and 6 patients with stage III to IV cancer were not actively treated. Median survival times for patients treated with (1) surgery alone and (2) RFA alone for stage I to II lung cancer were 33.8 and 28.2 months, respectively. Median survival times for patients treated with (1) chemotherapy alone and (2) RFA with chemotherapy for stage III to IV cancer were 29 and 42 months, respectively. Conclusion RFA can be used as an alternative treatment to surgery for older NSCLC patients with stage I to II inoperable cancer and can play a role as adjuvant therapy with chemotherapy for patients with stage III to IV lung cancer. Thirty-four patients (85%) who underwent RFA were able to go home within 24–72 h after the procedure because there were no major complications. Six patients who had major complications were able to go home within 7–10 days after they completely recovered from their complications. Twelve patients (92.3%) who underwent surgery in the comparison group were able to go home on 14–21 days after surgery because there were no complications. However, one patient died early due to acute respiratory distress syndrome after surgery. All patients treated by RFA did not result in any loss of pulmonary function tests at follow-up, but 11 of 13 (84.6%) patients who underwent surgery had decreased pulmonary function at follow-up (ratio of mean presurgical to postsurgical FEV1 2.27–1.9 l).

The efficacy of RFA falls when nodules greater than 5 cm in diameter are treated. Tumour diameter larger than 4 cm and less from 1 cm to the hilum carry an important risk of incomplete treatment and the possible damage of surrounding organs [6, 14]. Additionally, a massive hemoptysis after ablation of a central lung nodule may develope [19]. On the other hand, contact with permeable vessels larger than 3 mm in diameter will cool the tumour down (heat-sink effect) and will prevent complete coagulation necrosis of the nodule. In NSCLC, RFA can be used for patients with stage I disease who are believed to be at increased risk for any kind of pulmonary resection or who refuse surgery. For those patients who are believed to be at increased operative risk, RFA is a good alternative. Other patients who may be considered for treatment with RFA include those with advanced-stage disease who have responded to definitive irradiation and chemotherapy but have a persistent solitary peripheral focus of cancer and those who present with a recurrent isolated cancer after previous lung resection. A major obstacle for all thermal ablation techniques is the heat sink effect, which describes how bloodflow or airflow through or adjacent to the target tissue can offset the applied cooling or heating, thus limiting intended tissue damage [14].

STEREOTACTIC RADIOSURGERY

The advent of technology allowing improved tumour localisation and the precise delivery of high doses of radiotherapy has allowed for stereotactic body radiation therapy (SBRT) to become an effective treatment for patients with medically inoperable lung cancers. For medically inoperable patients and those patients who are unwilling to undergo surgery, external beam radiotherapy to cumulative doses of 60 Gy or greater delivered in daily fractions over 6 or more weeks has historically been the standard treatment option. However, the efficacy of conventional radiation therapy is poor with high crude local failure rates of 19-70% and a five-year survival rate of only about 15%. When compared to observation alone, radiation therapy improves median overall survival from 14 to 21 months [32, 33, 42]. More recently, substantial improvements in radiation therapy technology have allowed for dose-intensification, which has led to promising treatment outcomes. Stereotactic radiotherapy has been widely used in clinical practice. Radiation therapy is also commonly used when resection for NSCLC is not possible. SBRT regimens generally deliver high doses of daily radiotherapy (≥8 Gy) with a small number of overall fractions (≤5). The improved accuracy is achieved by precise spatial localisation of the tumour and the delivery of multiple cross-fired beams of radiation to converge upon the tumour. SBRT regimens are in contrast to conventional treatments for lung cancer that generally span 6–8 weeks with individual fractions of 180–200 cGy. Patients are generally treated with three fractions of 10–20 Gy for a total dose of 30–60 Gy in SBRT. On the other hand 5-year survival rates of radiation therapy are usually poor and have been reported to range from 10% to 30% [7-9]. Radiosurgical procedures are generally performed over a 2-week period with a minimum of 48 h between treatment fractions. Respiratory motion creates difficulties in the delivery of precise radiation to lung tumours. These respiratory displacements are greatest near the diaphragm and less significant near the lung apex and adjacent to the carina [34]. Several techniques have been developed for the integration of breathing motion into the radiotherapy workflow. The need for patient's compliance is the lowest for treatment delivery in freebreathing: breathing motion is either compensated by adding safety margins using geometrical or preferably dosimetric approaches or by continuous tracking of the target with a dynamic multileaf-collimator or a dynamic treatment couch. Alternatively, one can reduce the effective target motion by irradiation in breath-hold technique or gated beam delivery in only specific phases of the breathing cycle: the reduction of the effective target motion is then associated with prolonged total treatment times [35]. Breath holding and/or abdominal compression can limit the respiratory movements.

Patient selection is virtually identical to that for RFA. However, an advantage of SRS is that centrally based tumours can be treated.

Complications may be severe emphysema, massive local tumour progression, and severe atelectasis from bronchial collapse, respectively. Rib fracture and chest wall pain may be occurred. Adequate tumour coverage remains the primary objective when treating lung or liver lesions with SBRT. To minimize toxicity when treating lesions in close proximity to the CW, Dmax of the CW and/or ribs should remain <50 Gy, and <5 cc of CW should receive ≥ 40 Gy [36]. Recurrences may be risen after SBRT. Neri [37] and coworkers treated seven of the patients who received SBRT with salvage surgery for local recurrence and they suggested that SBRT may not be the cause of difficulties encountered during the surgical process, and surgery is a good alternative treatment for local recurrence after SBRT. Chen [38] and coworkers rewiewed their patients who were initially operable, but chosing SBRT. After SBRT, the tumours shrank initially in all patients, but increased in size within 18 months of SBRT in the case of 4 patients. During surgical extirpation, they did not find any significant SBRT-related adhesions in any of the patients.

The reported risk of toxicity after pulmonary SBRT is low, regardless of the technique of treatment planning and delivery. Nevertheless, a dose–response relationship has been demonstrated for radiation induced pneumonitis. Higher radiation doses appear to enhance local tumour control but dose escalation is limited because increased doses of radiation result in increased toxicity and damage to surrounding pulmonary parenchyma. The major toxicity encountered in treatment of lung tumours is pulmonary toxicity. Fibrotic changes observed following pulmonary SBRT are due to intermediate radiation doses in the range of 18 Gy [7, 35]. The maximal tolerable doses ara under investigation for safe and effective tumour treatment. A new study from Brown [39] and coworkers emphasised that it is feasible to treat peripheral NSCLC with individualised maximal tolerable doses ranging from 67 Gy to 75 Gy in five fractions chosen on the basis of location, histopathological type, grade of histopathological differentiation, tumour diameter/volume, and normal tissue constraints.

Yu [40] and colleagues reported 15 patients with non-small cell lung cancer and solitary metastatic lung cancer were treated with hypofraction stereotactic radiotherapy. The short-term results showed that the complete response (CR) rate, the partial response (PR) rate, the overall response (CR+PR) rate, the one-year local control rate, the one-year survival rate was 60%, 20%, 80%, 100% and 86.67% respectively. Two patients had radiation pneumonitis of 0 grade. Acute radiation pneumonitis of grade I occurred in 9 patients, 4 patients had radiation pneumonitis of grade II and no patient developed serious (grade III) radiation pneumonitis.

Champeaux [41] and colleagues reported 33 patients with stage I and II non small cell lung cancer were treated by stereotactic body radiation therapy. Breathing control was obtained by passive diaphragm control. Two CT-scans were performed 1 week apart to determine the accuracy of patient repositioning and define target volumes. Five or six fields were set up to achieve a conformal dose distribution. According to tumour size, a total of 50 or 40 Gy was delivered in 10 fractions. Ten patients with a complete response are still alive. Eight patients have died from local progression, eight from metastasis, and six from comorbidity. Median disease-free survival was 22.6 months. No acute toxicity up to grade II (CTC AE 3.0) was observed. None of the patients still alive has developed any complications. However, Qiao [42] and associates summarised results from 18 studies reporting on radiotherapy for stage I NSCLC. The mean 3- and 5-year survival rates were 34% and 21%, respectively. Futamura [43] and associates used stereotactic radiotherapy for the treatment of small lung tumours in 31 patients (stage IA, n=13; stage IB, n=5; stage IIIA, n=1; stage IIIB, n=1; recurrence, n=11). In one patient who had radiation pneumonitis before SRT, a progression of pulmonary fibrosis was observed, and treated with steroid therapy. Invaluable 29 tumours of 27 patients, the recurrence rates are 11/29 (37.9%). Median progression free survival time was 8 months. The recurrence rate and median progression free survival time of stage IA and IB subgroups were 4/17 (23.5%) and 12 months, respectively. High uptake of (18)F-fluoro-2-deoxy-d-glucose (FDG) in a primary tumour had been found the significant unfavorable factor for local control after stereotactic body radiotherapy in stage I non-small-cell lung cancer [44].

It has been known that patients with early stage but medically inoperable lung cancer have a poor rate of primary tumour control (30%-40%) and a high rate of mortality (3-year survival, 20%-35%) with current management. Timmerman [45] and colleagues evaluated the toxicity and efficacy of stereotactic body radiation therapy in a high-risk population of patients with early stage but medically inoperable lung cancer. In this phase 2 multicenter study, there were 55 patients (44 patients with T1 tumours and 11 patients with T2 tumours) aged 18 years or older with biopsy-proven peripheral T1-T2N0M0 non-small cell tumours (measuring <5 cm in diameter) and medical conditions precluding surgical treatment. The prescription dose was 18 Gy per fraction x 3 fractions (54 Gy total) with entire treatment lasting between 1(1/2) and 2 weeks. the estimated 3-year primary tumour control rate was 97.6%. Three patients had recurrence within the involved lobe; the 3-year primary tumour and involved lobe (local) control rate was 90.6%. Two patients experienced regional failure; the local-regional control rate was 87.2%. Eleven patients experienced disseminated recurrence; the 3-year rate of disseminated failure was 22.1%. The rates for disease-free survival and overall survival at 3 years were 48.3% and 55.8%, respectively. The median overall survival was 48.1 months. Protocol-specified treatment-related grade 3 adverse events were reported in 7 patients; grade 4 adverse events were reported in 2 patients. No grade 5 adverse events were reported. They conluded that patients with inoperable non-small cell lung cancer who received stereotactic body radiation therapy had a survival rate of 55.8% at 3 years, high rates of local tumour control, and moderate treatment-related morbidity.

The Cyberknife Stereotactic Radiosurgery System is a frameless SRS system and has unique characteristics that make it well suited for SABR of lung tumours. The system integrates a compact robotically positioned linear accelerator (linac) with image-guided stereotactic localisation, eliminating the need for invasive anatomic fixation while maintaining precise and accurate radiation delivery [33]. Its unique ability to dynamically track targets that move with breathing is a key feature that differentiates the CyberKnife from other commercially available image-guided platforms, which typically use either respiratory manipulation or respiratory gating in order to manage breathing-induced motion.

Whyte [46] and colleagues published the first results of SRS for the lung using the Cyberknife system. This study included 23 patients from two institutions. Respiratory gating was used in 14 patients and breath-holding in 9. A single fraction of 15 Gy was used. Three patients developed a pneumothorax after fiducial placement. At a mean follow-up of 7 months, 2 patients (8.6%) had a complete response, 15 (65.2%) had a partial response, 4 (17.4%) had stable disease, and 2 (8.7%) had evidence of progression. Brown [47] and colleagues reviewed of treatment details and outcomes for 59 patients with 61 tumours, treated by image-guided robotic stereotactic radiosurgery (CyberKnife). Target localisation and respiratory movement compensation were accomplished using a single fiducial marker placed within the tumour, and the X-Sight and Synchrony systems. Total doses ranged from 15 Gy to 67.5 Gy delivered in 1-5 fractions with an equivalent dose range of 24-110 Gy normalised treatment dose in 2 Gy fractions (alpha/beta = 20 Gy). Four patients with stage 1A NSCLC and 2 patients with stage 1B NSCLC had persistent or recurrent disease. All patients tolerated the radiosurgery well, fatigue being the main side effect. Of the 59 patients treated, 51 (86%) were still alive at 1-33-month follow-up. Eight patients have died, 2 of diseases other than cancer progression. The results indicate that the delivery of precisely targeted ablative radiation doses with surgical precision to limited treatment volumes of lung tumours in a hypofractionated fashion is feasible and safe. Image-guided robotic stereotactic radiosurgery of lung tumours with CyberKnife(R) achieves excellent rates of local disease control with limited toxicity to surrounding tissues and, in many cases, might be curative for patients for whom surgery is not an option.

Stereotactic body radiotherapy (SBRT) is the treatment of choice for patients with early stage non-small cell lung cancer (NSCLC), who are inoperable because of medical co-morbidities or who refuse surgical resection. Prospective trials report excellent local control rates, which appear significantly higher compared to control rates achieved with conventionally fractionated radiotherapy. The survival in inoperable patients is usually limited by their co-morbidities and as a consequence these high local control rates have not yet convincingly translated into improved survival. However, survival for patients with good performance status and limited co-morbidity approaches the survival results following surgery. In patients with stage I NSCLC who do not undergo surgery, SBRT achieves superior survival as compared to treatment using conventionally fractionated radiotherapy. In stage I tumours measuring up to 5 cm in diameter, SBRT can achieve local tumour control rates of up to 97% [48]. In patients identified to be at high risk for surgical complications, SBRT appears to provide an effective alternative with low risks of hospitalisation and 30-day mortality. Future treatment algorithms should include individualised assessment of surgical risks, and the consideration of SBRT for high-risk patients, in order to develop a personalised treatment approach.

RADIOFREQUENCY ABLATION AND STEREOTACTIC RADIOSURGERY: COMBINATION THERAPY

Both RFA and SRS have benefits and limitations. The larger lesions have less desirable responses with either of these techniques. When radiation therapy is a viable treatment option, RF ablation and external beam radiation appear to be synergistic. RF ablation is most effective in the center of relatively avascular tumours, while external beam radiation and stereotactic radiosurgery are most effective at the periphery of the tumour where there is high oxygen content and a hyperthermic rim around the ablation zone. Combining the two therapies has been shown to increase survival, at no additional toxicity, as compared with radiation therapy alone, and this technique should be considered for larger tumours [14, 49-51].

MICROWAVE ABLATION

MWA is the most recent development in the approaches to tumour ablation. Percutaneous microwave ablation may be used in the treatment of intraparenchymal pulmonary malignancies and may offer beneficial survival rates and local tumour control in patients who are unsuitable for surgery [1, 55, 56]. The mechanism of MWA is dielectric heating (frictional heating of water molecules in tissue). Microwave radiation is in the 900 to 2450 MHz wavelength of the electromagnetic spectrum. Because microwave radiation interacts with water molecules, the polarity of these molecules changes, resulting in heating and eventually leading to cell death. The theoretic advantages of microwave over other heatbased modalities, such as RF or laser, are the larger and faster volume of tissue heating with a given applicator. In addition, because microwave ablation does not rely on an electrical circuit as does RF ablation, multiple applicators can be applied simultaneously. One of the weaknesses of thermal-based ablation devices in the treatment of solid tumours is marginal recurrences. These are higher in anatomic areas adjacent to heat sinks, such as larger blood vessels or airways. Given the higher heat potential with microwave energy, one may be able to reduce effects of adjacent blood flow or airflow on the size and shape of the ablation zone. Unlike RFA, MWA is not limited by tissue boiling and charring of the tissue. This may allow intratumoural temperatures to be driven higher, resulting in a larger ablation zone in a shorter time [52]. RFA or MWA of tumours in liver, kidney, bone and lung can be performed safely in patients with permanent intra-cardiac devices, but careful planning between radiology and cardiology is essential to avoid adverse outcomes [53].

Santos [54] and colleagues performed an experimental study on swins to detect the effect of MWA on lung tissue. In their study, 20 microwave ablation procedures were performed in the lungs of 10 swine. Bilateral thoracotomy using a clamshell approach was used. In one lung, ablation was performed with continuous ventilation. In the contralateral lung, single-lung ventilation was achieved by clamping the bronchus before ablation. The ablation zone was clearly demarcated on gross examination, and in all cases 100% ablation occurred, without skip areas of viability. The ablation zones were elliptical with the long axis parallel to the axis of the ablation probes (active tip, 3.7 cm). Ablation diameters and volume were compared between the ventilated and nonventilated lungs. Ablation volume was superior in nonventilated lungs (10.74 cm^3 *versus* 7.35 cm^3) primarily because of differences in the short axis of the ablation zone. They concluded that microwave energy can effectively ablate normal pulmonary parenchyma without skip areas of viable tissue within the gross ablation field. The volume of necrosis is increased in nonventilated lungs, suggesting that ablation results can be improved in patients by using general anesthesia with single-lung ventilation.

Clinical Experience

Wolf and colleagues [1] performed microwave ablation in 50 patients with intraparenchymal pulmonary malignancies. Eighty-two masses (mean, 1.42 per patient) in 50 patients (28 men, 22 women; mean age, 70 years) were percutaneously treated in 66 microwave ablation sessions. Each tumour was ablated with computed tomographic (CT) guidance. Tumours that were smaller than 2 cm in maximal diameter were treated with a single applicator, and tumours that were 2 cm or larger were treated with multiple antennae or a multiprobe array. During treatment sessions, applicators were placed directly contiguous to segmental branches of the pulmonary artery and aorta if necessary. During treatment sessions, patients underwent multiple applications, resulting in a mean number of applications per tumour of 2 ± 1, with each application lasting 7–10 minutes. Antennae were repositioned between applications, thus assuring full coverage of the tumour. Initial technical success (no detectable enhancement on the initial postablation CT scan) was achieved in 95% of ablations. Follow-up contrast material-enhanced CT and positron emission tomographic (PET) scans were reviewed. An actuarial survival of 65% at 1 year, 55% at 2 years, and 45% at 3 years from ablation. Cancer-specific mortality yielded a 1-year survival of 83%, a 2-year survival of 73%, and a 3-year survival of 61%; these values were not significantly affected by index size of larger than 3 cm or 3 cm or smaller or presence of residual disease. Cavitation (43% [35 of 82] of treated tumours) was associated with reduced cancer-specific mortality. Immediate complications included pneumothorax. Pneumothorax occurred after 39% (26 of 66) of ablation sessions, and 69% (18 of 26) of these occurrences of pneumothorax were classified as mild and did not require chest tube placement.

Feng and coworkers [55] reported on MWA of 28 tumours in 20 patients. A response of 50% or greater was noted in 13 nodules (46.4%), and a complete response in 3 (10.7%). No significant complications were noted. An ablate and resect study was performed by Simon and colleagues [56]. Patients undergoing elective lung resection had MWA before their resection. The mean tumour diameter was 3 cm (range, 2-5.5 cm), with an average tumour volume of 7.1 cm^3. The maximum ablation achieved was 4 cm (range, 3-5 cm), with a tumour volume of 23.4 cm^3. Carrafiello [57] and coworkers reported nine patients who underwent percutaneous MWA of ten intraparenchymal pulmonary masses (mean 1.1 lesions per patient) in ten ablation sessions. treatments were performed with a microwave generator with 45 W and 915 MHz connected to a 14.5-gauge antenna for 10 min. Antenna placement was performed with computed tomography (CT) fluoroscopy guidance. Technical success was obtained in all cases; mortality at 30 days was 0%.

ACKNOWLEDGEMENTS

Declared none.

CONFLICT OF INTEREST

The author confirms that this article content has no conflict of interest.

REFERENCES

[1] Wolf FJ, Grand DJ, Machan JT, Dipetrillo TA, Mayo-Smith WW, Dupuy DE. Microwave ablation of lung malignancies: effectiveness, CT findings, and safety in 50 patients. Radiology. 2008;247:871-9.

[2] Roy AM, Bent C, Fotheringham T. Radiofrequency ablation of lung lesions: practical applications and tips. Curr Probl Diagn Radiol 2009; 38: 44-52.

[3] Kodama H, Yamakado K, Takaki H, Kashima M, Uraki J, Nakatsuka A, Takao M, Taguchi O, Yamada T, Takeda K. Lung Radiofrequency Ablation for the Treatment of Unresectable Recurrent Non-Small-Cell Lung Cancer After Surgical Intervention. Cardiovasc Intervent Radiol 2011. DOI 10.1007/s00270-011-0220-0

[4] Youlden DR, Cramb SM, Baade PD. The international epidemiology of lung cancer: geographical distribution and secular trends. J Thorac Oncol 2008; 3: 819–831

[5] Moldvay J, Scheid P, Wild P. Predictive survival markers in patients with surgically resected non-small cell lung carcinoma. Clin Cancer Res 2000; 6:1125–1134

[6] Fernando HC, Schuchert M, Landreneau R, Daly BT. Approaching the high-risk patient: sublobar resection, stereotactic body radiation therapy, or radiofrequency ablation. Ann Thorac Surg. 2010;89:S2123-7

[7] Prendergast BM, Bonner JA, Popple RA, Spencer SA, Fiveash JB, Keene KS, Cerfolio RJ, Minnich DJ, Dobelbower MC. Dosimetric analysis of imaging changes following pulmonary stereotactic body radiation therapy. J Med Imaging Radiat Oncol. 2011; 55: 90-6.

[8] Fernando HC, Abbas G. Alternatives to surgical resection for non-small cell lung cancer. In: Patterson GA, Cooper JD, Deslauriers J, Lerut EMR, Luketich JD, Rice TW, eds. Pearson's Thoracic & Esophageal surgery. 3rd edition. Philadelphia, PA: Churchill Livingstone; 2008: 796-803.

[9] Santos RS, Khawaja F, Fernando HC. Emerging technologies and techniques for the management of non-small cell lung cancer. In: Shields TW, LoCicero III J, Reed CE, Feins RH, eds. General Thoracic Surgery. 7th edition. Philadelphia, PA: Lippincott Williams & Wilkins; 2009: 1513-1518.

[10] Palussière J, Gómez F, Cannella M, Ferron S, Descat E, Fonck M, Brouste V, Avril A. Single-Session Radiofrequency Ablation of Bilateral Lung Metastases. Cardiovasc Intervent Radiol. 2011. DOI 10.1007/s00270-011-0191-1.

[11] Wang T, Nelson RA, Bogardus A, Grannis FW Jr. Five-year lung cancer survival: which advanced stage nonsmall cell lung cancer patients attain long-term survival? Cancer. 2010; 116:1518-25.

[12] Bach PB, Cramer LD, Warren JL, et al: Racial differences in the treatment of early stage non-small cell lung cancer. N Engl J Med 1999; 341:1198-1205.

[13] Tada A, Hiraki T, Iguchi T, Gobara H, Mimura H, Toyooka S, Kiura K, Tsuda T, Mitsuhashi T, Kanazawa S. Influence of Radiofrequency Ablation of Lung Cancer on Pulmonary Function. Cardiovasc Intervent Radiol. 2011. DOI 10.1007/s00270-011-0221-z

[14] Sonntag PD, Hinshaw JL, Lubner MG, Brace CL, Lee FT Jr. Thermal ablation of lung tumours. Surg Oncol Clin N Am. 2011; 20: 369-87

[15] Schneider T, Reuss D, Warth A, Schnabel PA, von Deimling A, Herth FJ, Dienemann H, Hoffmann H. The efficacy of bipolar and multipolar radiofrequency ablation of lung neoplasms - results of an ablate and resect study. Eur J Cardiothorac Surg. 2011; 39: 968-73.

[16] Zhu JC, Yan TD, Morris DL. A systematic review of radiofrequency ablation for lung tumours. Ann Surg Oncol. 2008; 15:1765–74.

[17] Hiraki T, Tajiri N, Mimura H, *et al.* Pneumothorax, pleural effusion, and chest tube placement after radiofrequency ablation of lung tumours: incidence and risk factors. Radiology. 2006; 241:275–83.

[18] Hiraki T, Gobara H, Mimura H, Sano Y, Toyooka S, Shibamoto K, Kishi R, Uka M, Kanazawa S. Brachial nerve injury caused by percutaneous radiofrequency ablation of apical lung cancer: a report of four cases. J Vasc Interv Radiol. 2010;21:1129-33.

[19] Livraghi T, Solbiati L, Meloni MF, et al: Treatment of focal liver tumours with percutaneous radio-frequency ablation: Complications encountered in a multicenter study. *Radiology* 2003; 226:441-451.

[20] DE, Zagoria RJ, Akerley W, et al: Percutaneous radiofrequency ablation of malignancies in the lung. *AJR Am J Roentgenol* 2000; 174:57-59.

[21] Schaefer O, Lohrman C, Langer M: CT guided radiofrequency ablation of a bronchogenic carcinoma. *Br J Radiol* 2003; 76:268-270.

[22] Pouliquen C, Kabbani Y, Saignac P, Gékière JP, Palussière J. Radiofrequency ablation of lung tumours with the patient under thoracic epidural anaesthesia. Cardiovasc Intervent Radiol. 2011 Feb;34 Suppl 2:S178-81

[23] Asaph JW, Keppel JF, Handy JR Jr *et al.* Surgery for second lung cancers. Chest 2000; 118: 1621–1625

[24] Pennatur A, Abbas G, Qureshi I, Schuchert MJ, Wang Y, Gilbert S, Landreneau RJ, Luketich JD. Radiofrequency Ablation for the Treatment of Pulmonary Metastases. Ann Thorac Surg 2009;87:1030 –9.

[25] de Baere T. Lung tumour radiofrequency ablation: where do we stand? Cardiovasc Intervent Radiol 2011; 34:241–251

[26] Anderson EM, Lees WR, Gillams AR. Early indicators of treatment success after percutaneous radiofrequency of pulmonary tumours. Cardiovasc Intervent Radiol 2009; 32:478–483

[27] Gillams AR, Lees WR. Radiofrequency ablation of lung metastases: factors influencing success. Eur Radiol 2008; 18:672–677.

[28] Iguchi T, Hiraki T, Gobara H *et al.* Percutaneous radiofrequency ablation of lung tumours close to the heart or aorta: evaluation of safety and effectiveness. J Vasc Interv Radiol 2007; 18: 733–740.

[29] Hiraki T, Sakurai J, Tsuda T *et al.* Risk factors for local progression after percutaneous radiofrequency ablation of lung tumours: evaluation based on a preliminary review of 342 tumours. Cancer 2006; 107:2873–2880

[30] Solazzo SA, Liu Z, Lobo SM, *et al.* Radiofrequency ablation: importance of background tissue electrical conductivity–an agar phantom and computer modeling study. Radiology. 2005; 236:495–502.

[31] Lee H, Jin GY, Han YM, Chung GH, Lee YC, Kwon KS, Lynch D. Comparison of Survival Rate in Primary Non-Small-Cell Lung Cancer Among Elderly Patients Treated With Radiofrequency Ablation, Surgery, or Chemotherapy. Cardiovasc Intervent Radiol. 2011. DOI 10.1007/s00270-011-0194-y

[32] Wisnivesky, J. P., Bonomi, M., Henschke, C., Iannuzzi, M., McGinn, T. Radiation therapy for the treatment of unresected stage I-II non-small cell lung cancer. Chest 2005; 128, 1461-1467.

[33] Gibbs IC, Loo BW Jr. CyberKnife stereotactic ablative radiotherapy for lung tumours. Technol Cancer Res Treat. 2010; 9: 589-96

[34] Liu HH, Balter P, Tutt T, Choi B, Zhang J, Wang C, Chi M, Luo D, Pan T. Assessing respiration-induced tumour motion and internal target volume using four-dimensional

computed tomography for radiotherapy of lung cancer. Int J Radiat Oncol Biol Phys. 2007; 68: 531-40.

[35] Guckenberger M, Kavanagh A, Webb S, Brada M. A novel respiratory motion compensation strategy combining gated beam delivery and mean target position concept --a compromise between small safety margins and long duty cycles. Radiother Oncol. 201; 98: 317-22.

[36] Andolino DL, Forquer JA, Henderson MA, Barriger RB, Shapiro RH, Brabham JG, Johnstone PA, Cardenes HR, Fakiris AJ. Chest wall toxicity after stereotactic body radiotherapy for malignant lesions of the lung and liver. Int J Radiat Oncol Biol Phys. 2011; 80: 692-7.

[37] Neri S, Takahashi Y, Terashi T, Hamakawa H, Tomii K, Katakami N, Kokubo M. Surgical treatment of local recurrence after stereotactic body radiotherapy for primary and metastatic lung cancers. J Thorac Oncol. 2010; 5: 2003-7

[38] Chen F, Matsuo Y, Yoshizawa A, Sato T, Sakai H, Bando T, Okubo K, Shibuya K, Date H. Salvage lung resection for non-small cell lung cancer after stereotactic body radiotherapy in initially operable patients. J Thorac Oncol. 2010;5:1999-2002

[39] Brown WT, Fayad F, Hevezi J, Fowler J, Monterroso MI, Garcia S, Medina A, Schwade J. Individualised higher dose of 70-75 Gy using five-fraction robotic stereotactic radiotherapy for non-small-cell lung cancer: a feasibility study. Comput Aided Surg. 2011;16:1-10.

[40] Yu R, Li Y, Zhu G. Stereotactic body radiaton therapy for 15 patients with small lung neoplasms. Zhongguo Fei Ai Za Zhi. 201;14:266-70.

[41] Champeaux-Orange E, Wachter T, Bouscayrol H, Barillot I. Stereotactic radiotherapy for stage I and II lung cancer: a study of 33 patients. Cancer Radiother. 2011; 15: 192-6.

[42] Qiao X, Tullgren O, Lax I, Sirzén F, Lewensohn R. The role of radiotherapy in treatment of stage I non-small cell lung cancer. Lung Cancer. 2003; 41:1-11

[43] Futamura Y, Sawa T, Horiba A, Ishiguro T, Yoshida T, Iida T, Marui T. The efficacy and safety of stereotactic radiotherapy for non-resectable non-small cell lung cancer. Gan To Kagaku Ryoho. 2010; 37: 2744-6

[44] Hamamoto Y, Sugawara Y, Inoue T, Kataoka M, Ochi T, Takahashi T, Sakai S. Relationship between pretreatment FDG uptake and local control after stereotactic body radiotherapy in stage I non-small-cell lung cancer: the preliminary results. Jpn J Clin Oncol. 2011; 41: 543-7.

[45] Timmerman R, Paulus R, Galvin J, Michalski J, Straube W, Bradley J, Fakiris A, Bezjak A, Videtic G, Johnstone D, Fowler J, Gore E, Choy H. Stereotactic body radiation therapy for inoperable early stage lung cancer. JAMA. 2010 Mar 17;303:1070-6

[46] Whyte RI, Crownover R, Murphy MJ, Martin DP, Rice TW, DeCamp MM Jr, Rodebaugh R, Weinhous MS, Le QT. Stereotactic radiosurgery for lung tumours: preliminary report of a phase I trial. Ann Thorac Surg. 2003; 75: 1097-101.

[47] Brown WT, Wu X, Fayad F, Fowler JF, Amendola BE, García S, Han H, de la Zerda A, Bossart E, Huang Z, Schwade JG. CyberKnife radiosurgery for stage I lung cancer: results at 36 months. Clin Lung Cancer. 2007; 8: 488-92.

[48] Palma D, Senan S. Stereotactic radiation therapy: changing treatment paradigms for stage I nonsmall cell lung cancer. Curr Opin Oncol. 2011;23:133-9

[49] Yasui K, Kanazawa S, Sano Y, *et al.* Thoracic tumours treated with CT-guided radiofrequency ablation: initial experience. Radiology. 2004; 231:850–7.

[50] Horkan C, Dalal K, Coderre JA, *et al.* Reduced tumour growth with combined radiofrequency ablation and radiation therapy in a rat breast tumour model. Radiology. 2005; 235:81–8.

[51] Dupuy DE, DiPetrillo T, Gandhi S, *et al.* Radiofrequency ablation followed by conventional radiotherapy for medically inoperable stage I non-small cell lung cancer. Chest. 2006; 129:738–45.

[52] Dupuy DE. Microwave ablation compared with radiofrequency ablation in lung tissue-is microwave not just for popcorn anymore? Radiology. 2009; 251: 617-8.

[53] Skonieczki BD, Wells C, Wasser EJ, Dupuy DE. Radiofrequency and microwave tumour ablation in patients with implanted cardiac devices: Is it safe? Eur J Radiol. 2010. doi:10.1016/j.ejrad.2010.04.004

[54] Santos RS, Gan J, Ohara CJ, Daly B, Ebright MI, Desimone M, Fernando HC. Microwave ablation of lung tissue: impact of single-lung ventilation on ablation size. Ann Thorac Surg. 2010; 90: 1116-9.

[55] Feng W, Liu W, Liu C, et al: Percutaneous microwave coagulation therapy for lung cancer. *Zhonghua Zhong Liu Za Zhi* 2002; 24:388-390.

[56] Simon CS, Dupuy DE, Mayo-Smith WW: Microwave ablation: Principles and applications. *Radiographics* 2005; 25:S69-S83.

[57] Carrafiello G, Mangini M, De Bernardi I, Fontana F, Dionigi G, Cuffari S, Imperatori A, Laganà D, Fugazzola C. Microwave ablation therapy for treating primary and secondary lung tumours: technical note. Radiol Med. 2010; 115: 962-74.

CHAPTER 13

Immunological Approach to Lung Cancer

Part A: Immunology of Lung Cancer

Fulya Ilhan*

Euphrates University, Faculty of Medicine, Department of Immunology, 23119, Elazig, Turkey

Abstract: Immune system direct or indirectly can be effective in the movement of cancer.A lot of moleculer study was made for explaining immune mechanism of lung cancer. Different immune mechanisms and tumour factors relating the existence mechanism of the disease are examined in this manuscript.

Keywords: Lung cancer, immunology, immune mechanism, CTLA-4, PD-1.

INTRODUCTION

Nowadays lung cancer is one of the most important death reasons in the world and unfortunately there was no enough data about both early diagnosis and effective therapy. The world of science and medical is continuing to search the disease according to its immunology and genetics and the studies of molecules which can be an indicator or constitute aims for antiserum or immunology, are quickly continuing especially for early diagnosis. The results of various studies and aimed molecules which can direct on this matter as the activities are not proven yet will be examined in this section. Immune mechanisms and tumour factors relating the existence mechanism of the disease are shown on the Table **1**.

Immunity originating from T cells plays a main role in immunological destroying of lung tumours and all solid tumours. All thing effects the immune system direct or indirectly can be effective in the movement of cancer. Various paraneoplastic syndromes, especially in small-cell bronchial carcinoma and in non-paraneoplastic syndrome antibodies were shown against the tumour suppressor genes p53, presence of some autoantibodies was detected [1]. If the proportion of

***Address correspondence to Fulya Ilhan:** Euphrates University, Faculty of Medicine, Department of Immunology, 23119, Elazig, Turkey; Tel: +90 2333555/2166; Fax: +90 424 2388096; E-mail: fulhan23@yahoo.com

CD4+/CD8+ T cell is low, death risk was found more than 34% independent of genus, age and phase in Small Cell Lung Cancer [2]. It was shown that CD8+ T cells and the development of lung cancer is associated with tumour progression and monitored in the amount of lymphocytes infiltrating high number of tumour especially in squamous cell carcinoma [3]. In the opposite of this, the increased CD4+CD25+ T regulatory (Treg) cells activity in cancer patients may suppress the response against autologous tumour cells [4]. It was determined that Tregs, suppressed antitumoural immune response in experimental tumour models and had found highest number in peripheral blood of a variety of cancer patients. Moreover, these cells also suppress the proliferative and cytolytic function of the tumour infiltrating lymphocytes (TIL) and natural killer (NK) cells infiltrating tumour [5]. Also due to suppressing tumour output of Treg cells and obstruction of cytotoxicity *via* NK, it is seen that they present CTLA+4 in regulator in CD4+CD25+ T levels which inhibits to T cell activation in familiar lung cancer tissues. Strength of vaccine-based therapy may be increased in cancer patients by reducing or modifying the Treg cells [6].

Table 1: Mechanisms of Impaired Immune Response Against Cancer

Lymphocyte Factors
• The absence of T cell support
• Incompetence of differentiation, or lack of number for antitumour T cells
• Insufficient avidity of T cells against tumours
• Tolerized T cells
• Reduction of T cell receptor signal transmission
• Apoptosis of T cells when compared with tumours
• Lack of T cell cytokine synthesis and lysis functions
• Cannot entering T cells into tumour stroma
Tumour Factors
• Tumours cannot activate silent predecessors.
• Lack of tumour antigen representation or little difference from self-antigens
• The absence of MHC1 representation of tumour and escape from CD8 response
• Producing the local immunosuppressive factors such as TGF-β's of tumour
• Rapid proliferation of tumour cells or insufficient other cell damage and apoptotic pathways

IL-10 is the most important inhibitory cytokine which produce from Treg cells and suppress T cell activity, inflammation *etc.* It was found that the levels of IL-10 in the LPS stimulated cultures were statistically greater from the cancer biopsies compared to the normal adjacent tissue. An environment is described in cancer patients who is characterized by increased cytokine production and decreased proliferative potential likely under the influence of a significant population of Tregs. Taken together, these results are discussed as they relate to the potential implications in lung cancer patients immune response to their disease [7]. Metastatic potential was also increased in IL-10-expressing lung tumour cells, leading to a greater number of tumour cells in lymph nodes draining the primary tumour site. In one *in vitro* research it was shown that applied exogen IL-10 on Lewis lung tumour cells were increased dramatically to resistance of these cells to the UV-induced apoptosis. These results indicate that a primary effect of IL-10 on lung cancer cells may be to increase their metastatic potential by promoting angiogenesis and resistance to apoptosis [8].

Some receptor activity researched in different studies but it remains unknown whether the inhibitory immunoreceptor programmed death-1 (PD-1) plays a role in conditions of human non-small cell lung cancer (NSCLC). Results showed that tumour-infiltrating CD8(+) T cells had increased PD-1 expression and impaired immune function, including reducing cytokine production capability and impairing capacity to proliferate. These data, provide direct evidence that the PD-1/PD-L1 pathway is involved in CD8(+) T-cell dysfunction in NSCLC patients [9].

Nuclear factor kappa B (NF-κB) is a classic mediator of inflammation and there is a strong connection between chronic inflammation with NF-κB and cancer. Synergistic interaction was shown between the NF-κB and classic tumour suppressant gen p53. p53 is playing an inhibitor role in the transcription and many promoter gen dependent of NF-κB and monitored extreme macrophage activation and cytokine increasing in the absence of p53. It was thought that the NF-κB activation and inflammation growing through it were extreme since there is p53 mutation in smokers, in patients with COPD and in lung cancer. Uncontrolled cell proliferation, absence of cellular apoptosis, skin invasion and angiogenesis has primary importance in cancer. Apoptosis, matrix degradation, inflammation, local and systemic immune responses are dominant in COPD. Transactivation of genes associated with NF-κB activation and inflammation may play a fundamental role both in COPD and cancer [10]. Moreover, it was observed that tumour supernatants increase apoptosis in active T cells by a mechanism depending on inhibitory kappa B (IκB) [11]. Cytotoxic T lymphocyte-associated antigen (CTLA-4), which inhibits T lymphocyte response, may inhibit T cell response and is associated with tolerance to self antigens. Cancer regression was detected in patients with metastatic melanoma by CTLA-4 blockade [12]. It was determined that the antitumour immune response against lung tumours were increased by blocking the communication of CTLA-4 and B7 in mice which have severe combined immunodeficiency (SCID) [13].

CD28 is an important costimulatory signal molecule but it's expression of CD28 mRNA and it's protein is reduced in the elderly. The reduced expression of CD28 mRNA and it's protein in the elderly may lead to impaired immunosurveillance and possible spread of tumour cells. The increased risk for lung cancer was closely associated with age, down-regulation of CD28 mRNA and up-regulation of CD95 mRNA, and an inverse correlation between CD28 mRNA expression and CD95 mRNA expression was found. In the elderly, and that up-regulation of CD28 mRNA or down-regulation of CD95 mRNA in peripheral blood T cells may play an important role in inhibiting oncogenesis and development of primary NSCLC in the elderly [14]. The presence of metastases correlated with the downregulation of T cell receptor (TCR) zeta, especially CD8(+) T cells. The most striking feature was the reduction in the number of myeloid CD11c(+) dendritic cells in the lymph node of patients with lymph node metastases. This could be a reflection of the immunodeficient state observed in lung cancer patients [15].

Toll-like receptors (TLRs) are the important molecules of innate immune response which express on the macrophage. TLR agonists are considered adjuvants in clinical trials of cancer immunotherapy. In one study researchers indicated that TLR3 or TLR7 ligand stimulation of tumour cells enhances the cytotoxic activity of expanded gammadelta T cells of cancer patients *in vitro* [16]. Gal-3 is a molecule which expressed at a relatively higher level in CD133(+) lung adenocarcinoma cells and could induce CD8(+) T cell apoptosis *in vitro*. In this study indicated that Gal-3 may play an important role during oncogenesis, implying a potential therapeutic target for pulmonary adenocarcinoma [17].

Immunogenic cancer testis antigen NY-ESO-1 is highly immunogenic and patients with NY-ESO-1-expressing tumours frequently show a spontaneous immune response to the NY-ESO-1 antigen. Most patients who showed an antibody response also showed CD4+ and CD8+ T cell responses. Such strong immunogenicity indicates the NY-ESO-1 antigen to be a very promising candidate target molecule for a cancer vaccine. The strong immunogenicity of these peptide epitopes may have contributed to the rather high frequency of NY-ESO-1-specific CD4 and CD8 T cells in this patient [18].

Mitogen-active protein kinase (MAPK)/activator protein-1 (AP-1) may activate with various signals and may play a critic role in cell proliferation and specialization. It was shown that many enzymes are active on the way of MAPK by smoking. Smoking cause extreme representation of cell cycle proteins dependent of AP-1, cycline D1 and prolifered nuclear antigen PCNA. These findings was shown the illness such as lung cancer related with smoking on the way of pathogenesis the route of MAPK/AP-1 is playing an important role [19]. Actine dependent proliferation and the life characteristic on dependence of NF-κB is a reason underlying harmful effect of smoking for the cancer in cancer patients [20].

Mitsudomi *et al.* were determined p53 mutations in the 75% of lung cancer patients unless looking at their histology. Plus, it was shown that these mutant p53 proteins are immunogenic and the patients have p53 autoantigens. Although there are some papers reporting that there was no correlation between clinical admission and p53 antigens [21], there were also opposite resulted studies reported that these autoantigens are correlated with long life period in lung cancers [22]. Normally, immunologic proteins presented in testis and over and presented in cancer cells temporarily were isolated and is named *cancer/testisantigens* (CTA) [23]. Among these CTA's, MAGE (melanoma antigen) and NYSEO1, which were isolated nowadays are being potential target in lung cancer immunotherapy were defined. MAGE genes close to 50 were defined nowadays and the most studied ones were *MAGEA1, MAGEA2, MAGEA3 and MAGEA6*. It was determined that 30-50% of these in non-small cell lung, 60-80% of these in small cell cancer is representing. It was shown that MAGE proteins control the advance of cell cycles, drug sensitivity in cancer cells and apoptosis unless together main role is not known very much [24, 25]. It was shown that presentation of MAGE3 is together with life period decreasing in cancer with pulmonary flat cell. It was reported that MAGE3 is not very widespread and NYSEO1 was determined in a proportion of 25% in non-small very cell lung cancer [26].

Secondary immune cells and some soluble factors which produce by these cells can play a role on T cells function, tumour growth, metastasis, pathological angiogenesis *etc.* Endothelial cells are potent regulators of immune cell functions and in one study demonstrated that tumour-derived VEGF induces endothelial cells to upregulate production of PGE_2 which, in turn, leads to suppression of T-cell functions. PGE_2 is a multifunctional ligand whose biological actions are determined in part by the type of E prostanoid receptors (EP) it binds. In many transformed cells, PGE_2 engagement initiates signals that block apoptosis, promote angiogenesis and stimulate tumour growth. As a result endothelial cells have role in tumour-induced immune suppression [27].

Inflammation and immunosuppression: Chronic inflammation is important risk factor for epithelial carcinogenesis. Prostaglandins (PG) are increased assistance of COX-2 induction originating from cytokine in the regions presence of chronic inflammation. It was thought that this situation is one of the reasons which increase cancer risk in chronic inflammation. Typically, the growing of tumour is associated with immunosuppression [28]. It was shown that the increased PGI2 production prevent the lung cancer and PGE_2 receptor subtype 2 (EP_2) defective mice have resistance against the lung cancer. PGE_2 enhances tumour growth in lung effecting through EP_2, independence of proinflammatory activity. EP_2 may be a target in the point of view of chemoprevention strategies [29]. Meshotelin antibody mesothelioma is known to be sensitive and specific indicators. Moreover, proteins associated with mesotheline can be positive in the serum of patients with lung adenocarcinoma [30]. Colony stimulatory factors secreted from tumour cells stimulate prostaglandin E2 (PGE_2) synthesis in monosit and macrophages. PGE_2 inhibits production of immunregulatuar lymphochins, proliferation of T and B cell, cytotoxic activities of natural murder cells. PGE2 inhibits tumour necrosis factor, interlocking 10, which has immunosuppression effect at the same time [31]. It was shown that growing transcription factor SOX-4 was presented as important and characteristic as in lung carcinoma with primer small cell. Moreover, SOX4 may have a potential of usage as vaccine in lung cancer. It was observed that mRNA of SOX-4 represented also in flat and big cell tumour specimen in primer adenocarcinoma of the lung behind in type with small cell. Plus, obtained T cell and Ab epitops has advantageous in the improvement of peptide based vaccination strategies and monitoring of responses of vaccinated person against SOX-4 [32].

Expression of neuroectodermal markers is a key feature of small cell lung carcinoma (SCLC). Anti-neuroectodermal antibodies were found in most patients with SCLC have. The authors investigated the frequency of IgG autoantibodies against Sry-like high-mobility group box (SOX)1, 2, 3 and Zinc-finger gene of the cerebellum (ZIC)2 proteins Antibodies to SOX1 were present in 28% of patients and another 28% had anti-ZIC2 antibodies, classifying these as some of the most frequent antibody responses observed in SCLC. The frequent and stable presence of SOX Group B and/or ZIC2 antibodies in SCLC, but not in healthy individuals examined, indicates they are serological markers of SCLC. However, the correlation between known clinical parameters of less aggressive disease and seroreactivity suggests that these antibodies are indicators of better prognosis in SCLC and warrants further studies to clarify the nature of the underlying immune responses [33].

It was shown that IL-27 suppresses expression of COX-2 and PGE(2) decreases the levels of vimentin and the abilities of cellular migration and invasion. Furthermore, inoculation of LLC/scIL-27 into immunodeficient NOD/SCID mice also exhibited reduced tumour growth [34].

The presence of various growth factors such as insulin like growth factor I and transforming growth factor-beta (TGF-beta), and some receptors was shown in Mezotelyoma (MM) cell line (18). Tumour specific immunity was seen 32% of the patient and observed stability in the illness but not observed an important tumour regression during the application of autolog malign mezotelyoma tumour cell lysate with GM-CSF together [35].

Somatic mutation was determined in the kinase domain of epidermal growth factor receptor tyrosine kinase (EGFR) gen in non-small cell lung cancer. It was found that this mutation is correlated with the response of tyrosine kinase inhibitors [36].

Hypoxia-inductive factor (HIF)-1 is produced as a response for hypoxia and is a factor which increases either cell life or apoptosis under different conditions. Extreme representation of HIF-1 increases *in vivo* tumour growth and together with bad prognoses especially in non-small cell lung cancer. Also epidermal growth factor receptor (EGFR) increase tumour cell proliferation and angiogenesis and inhibits apoptosis. Representation of EGFR increases during the tumour genesis and represent more than 50% in non-small cell lung cancer [37].

Some researchers were sequenced the receptor tyrosine kinase genes in NSCLC and were found somatic mutations of the epidermal growth factor receptor gene EGFR. The EGFR were more frequent in adenocarcinomas. They reported that treatment with the EGFR kinase inhibitor gefitinib (Iressa) causes tumour regression in some patients with NSCLC. These results suggest that EGFR mutations may predict sensitivity to gefitinib [38]. Patients with NSCLC with EGFR mutations had better survival than wild type [39].

Chemokines, cytokines, and interleukins, which are expressed in leukocytes, endothelial cells, fibroblasts, tumour cells, and other cell types, regulate the trafficking of leukocytes and endothelial cells to sites of infection, inflammation, trauma, and malignancy. Pro-inflammatory chemokines and interleukins are present at high levels in the microenvironment of epithelial tumours. Activating mutations in K-ras occur in approximately 10% of NSCLC specimens overall and 30% of the adenocarcinoma subtype. Several lines of evidence suggest that the *in vivo* transforming activity of oncogenic K-ras is mediated in part through epithelial cell non-autonomous mechanisms. In KrasLA1 mice, lung adenocarcinomas that develop due to somatic activation of a latent oncogenic K-ras allele recruit macrophages, endothelial cells, neutrophils, and fibroblasts, a process driven in part by high expression of CXCR2 ligands. Strategies to inhibit tumour/stromal cell interactions may be useful as therapeutic approaches in NSCLC patients [40].

Activated mutation in K-ras gene is one of the most widespread genetic changes in human lung cancer. It was observed that K-ras activiation in lung stimulate inflammatuar chemokins and increase tumour [41]. It was observed that tumour NF-κB activation, arranges the growing of pleural tumour. Decreasing of pleural liquid amount and tumour bursting were observed by giving lung cancer cell submitting dominant NF-κB inhibitors although NF-κB inhibition in lung cancer cell did not influence tumour cell life [42].

The role of chemokines in the pathogenesis of lung cancer has been increasingly appreciated. Monocyte chemoattractant protein-1 (MCP-1, CCL2) is secreted from tumour cells and associated tumour stromal cells. Blockade of CCL2 mediated by neutralizing antibodies has been shown to reduce tumourigenesis of several solid tumours, but the role of CCL2 in lung cancer has been controversial, with evidence of pro- and anti-tumourigenic effects. The mechanism of CCL2 blockade were evaluated in several animal models of non-small cell lung cancer (NSCLC). CCL2 blockade significantly slowed the growth of primary tumours in all the models studied and inhibited lung metastases in a model of spontaneous lung metastases of NSCLC. In NSCLC models show that CCL2 blockade can inhibit tumour growth of primary and metastatic disease [43].

Chemokines and interactions between their receptors are strictly important for tumour growth or metastasis. For example, interactions between CXCL12 and its receptors CXCR4 or CXCR7 are involved in tumour growth and metastasis in various types of human cancer. CXCL12 was overexpressed with CXCR4 or CXCR7 in lung cancer cell lines especially in NSCLCs from females compared to non-malignant human bronchial epithelial cell lines and disruption of CXCL12 inhibits the growth and migration of lung cancer cells [44]. The CXCR4 chemokine receptor is associated with growth and the metastasis of tumour cells. Its role is uncertain in representation presented in its ligand CXCL12 and tumours and in tumoural infiltration of immune cells. CXCL12 infiltration between the T cells which infiltrate lung adenocarcinoma among the thoracic region tumours were detected in high levels and it was thought that this representation presented in chemokine may affect tumour progression [45].

In the opposite model, some findings proved that CXCR4 promotes tumour cell proliferation and metastasis when present in the cytoplasm or cell membrane, whereas localization of this molecule in the nucleus prevents it from exerting these effects [46]. Macrophage migration inhibitory factor (MIF) induces expression of angiogenic CXC chemokines by tumour-associated monocytes, and that MIF-dependent expression of angiogenic CXC chemokines is one of several major pathways by which lung cancer tumours induce an angiogenic environment. It was shown that MIF and its cell surface receptor CD74 are markedly overexpressed in lung cancer. This coexpression was associated with higher levels of angiogenic CXC chemokines and greater tumour vascularity. CD74 may be a valuable therapeutic target for anti-angiogenic therapy [47].

Macrophages are the main source of a lot of chemokines and cytokines. In particular, when macrophages are located within tumour epithelial islets, a striking improvement in patient survival is evident. This supports the view that these islet-associated macrophages contribute to cytotoxic mechanisms which limit tumour dissemination. Macrophage-recruiting chemokines within the tumour islets by either tumour cells themselves or infiltrating immune cells is likely to be a key mechanism. Therefore an improved understanding of chemoattractant pathways that are active may lead to the development of novel chemotherapeutic agents. Median expression of CXCR2, CXCR3 and CCR1 in the tumour islets is associated with increased survival in NSCLC, and expression of CXCR3 correlates with increased macrophage and mast cell infiltration in the tumour islets [48]. DC's are special antigen presenting cells and they produce a lot of chemokines and cytokines like macrophages. It was determined that β2 microglobulin representation that increase the robustness of MHC I complexes was decreased in various cancers. In DC progeny pre-cDCs are found the precursors for conventional (cDCs) in tumours. The chemokine CCL3, which is markedly upregulated in tumours, promotes pre-cDC recruitment. Both pre-cDCs and their cDC progeny actively proliferate within the tumour. cDCs that arise from pre-cDCs in tumours express lower levels of CD11c and MHC class II as compared with those in spleen. In one study it was shown that supporting role for pre-cDCs in DC development in tumours and suggesting a potential target for cancer immunotherapy [49]. Heat shock proteins (HSP) are either innovator of shaperon peptide or alert signal giving to DC. Cross stimulate capability of Hsp 70 is independent of NK but interaction with DC-hsp70 is required NK adjuvant effect and this interaction stimulate cytotoxic T cell response and make medical therapeutic influence against lung metastases. The best alternative shall be obtained by cell vaccines released hsp70 [50].

DKK1 (Dickkopf-1) is a secreted protein which encodes a negative regulator of the Wnt signalling pathway in colon cancer cells. Some studies have shown that DKK1 is overexpressed in lung cancer, elucidated and suggested that the detection of circulating DKK1 autoantibody could serve as a useful non-invasive marker for determining lung cancer status [51]. The REIC/Dkk-3 gene has been reported to be a tumour suppressor and the expression is significantly down-regulated in a broad range of cancer cell types. The protein is secretory, but the physiological function remains unclear. In one study it was demonstrated that recombinant REIC/Dkk-3 protein induced the differentiation of human CD14+ monocytes into a novel cell type (REIC/Dkk-3Mo). REIC/Dkk-3Mo resembles immature dendritic cells (DC) generated with IL-4 and GM-CSF. Both these cell populations exhibit similar proportions of CD11c+, CD40+, CD86+ and HLA-DR+ cells and endocytic capacity, but REIC/Dkk-3Mo is negative for CD1a antigen. REIC/Dkk-3 induces phosphorylation of STAT 1 and STAT 3. Furthermore, intratumoural administration of REIC/Dkk-3 protein significantly suppressed tumour growth with CD11c+ and CD8+ (dendritic and killer T cell marker, respectively) cell accumulation and enhanced anti-cancer cytolytic activity of splenocytes. These data indicated a cytokine-like role of REIC/Dkk-3 protein in monocyte differentiation that might be exploited therapeutically [52].

Efforts have been made to understand if there are cancer-related chromosome abnormalities in lymphocytes and the suitability of these abnormalities to predict cancer development or metastases. A group of researchers were reported on chromosome 3 abnormalities in lymphocytes. Since 3p abnormalities are specific for small cell lung cancer (SCLC), it is important to show that these cancer-related abnormalities can be found in blood cells [53]. Ribosomal protein L19 (RPL19) was overexpressed in the lung cancer tissue. All of the normal tissues examined expressed lower levels of RPL19 mRNA than that of the lung cancer tissue [54]. Significantly elevated GOLPH2 expression was observed in adenocarcinoma (ADC) tumour tissues. The levels of sGOLPH2 were about 30% higher in lung cancer patients compared with healthy individuals [55]. The immunohistochemical analyses revealed substantially aberrant Interferon Regulatory Factor 3(IRF3) expression specific to the cancer lesions while the morphologically normal region around the tumours exhibited only cytoplasmic staining [56].

Recently, the nuclear factor erythroid derived 2-like 2 (NFE2L2) gene mutations were identified in lung cancer. The constitutive activation of NFE2L2 in lung cancer cells promotes tumourigenicity. However, the correlation between NFE2L2 mutation status and clinicopathologic features of lung cancer has not been well characterized. NFE2L2 mutations might play a role in tumour prognosis of squamous cell carcinoma of the lung [57].

Metastasis-associated protein CD24 has been identified as a new prognostic factor and stem cell marker in the human neoplasm. However, the importance of the CD24 in non-small cell lung carcinomas (NSCLCs) has not been elucidated well. CD24 expression in NSCLC is associated with ADC histology and disease progression and cancer-related death, indicative of aggressive tumour behaviour [58].

Circulating tumour cells (CTCs) have been identified in peripheral blood of NSCLC patients. Detection of thyroid transcription factor-1 (TTF-1) and TTF-1$^{(+)}$CTCs was found to be specific to NSCLC patients. In the postsurgery period TTF-1$^{(+)}$CTCs-positive status was found to be more associated with disease progression. In this study reported that TTF-1 mRNA-expressing CTCs might be a useful surrogate predictor of disease progression before clinical manifestations are apparent, and that monitoring of TTF-1$^{(+)}$CTCs status after surgery may be useful for identifying high-risk patients among surgically resected NSCLC cases [59].

Exosomes are nanovesicles originating from late endosomal compartments and secreted by most living cells in *ex vivo* cell culture conditions. The interest in exosomes was taken in the consideration when B-cell and dendritic cell-derived exosomes were shown to mediate MHC-dependent immune responses. Despite limited understanding of exosome biogenesis and physiological relevance, accumulating evidence points to their bioactivity culminating in clinical applications in cancer. Focused on the preclinical studies exploiting the immunogenicity of dendritic cell-derived exosomes (Dex) and will elaborate on the past and future vaccination trials conducted using Dex strategy in melanoma and non-small cell lung cancer patients [60].

In clinical progress pneumonia is observed frequently in lung tumours and generally the reason of this is bronchial obstruction. The application of malignancy treatment increases the risks of malnutrition, infection of the cancer patients. Lost integrity of epithelial and tissue bleeding relating the patient to whom radiotherapy is applied, causes to delay wound healing and necrosis. Pneumonia is also one of the developed complications. The materials which are used in chemotherapy applications as intravenous catheter and extended time of stay in the hospital increase the risk of infection.

The cells of mucous epithelial tissue secrete many antimicrobial peptides as laktoferrin (iron sequestration), lysozyme (hydrolysis of peptidoglycan in gram positive bacteria), phospholipase A_2 (separation of structural phospholipid of bacteria). Defensins found in primary granules of azurophilic neutrophils are cystein rich small antimicrobial peptides and found in Paneth cells of intestinal crypts and bronchial epithelium. Neutropenia and anatomical damage of the epithelial barrier is also predisposing to the development of pneumonia. In a significant proportion of cancer patients develop pneumonia. It might be a way of further treatment strengthening the mucosal immune system to give external peptides such as defensins *etc.* When the high fever is observed with local infiltration in the lungs of neutropenic patients, the approach applied to febrile neutropenic patients would be appropriate. Gram-negative bacteria are responsible for most of the cases. Invasive diagnostic interventions may be consulted for shown after empirical antibiotic therapy was initiated and more severe progress along with diffuse lung infiltrations cases. If bronchoscopy and BAL cannot be specific diagnosed, empirical antibiotics should be added against anaerobes, gram-positive bacteria and *Legionella.* If no response is received for antibacterial treatment and if there are nodular or cavitary lesions in the lung, antifungal and antituberculosis therapy should be added. Anti tumoural immune response is generally cellular and many studies about therapeutic approach for improving the response have been done. Immune system activation has been shown in the early stages of bronchial carcinoma. However, in advanced cases of cancer, especially in the cellular response to the presence of various degrees of immune suppression has been demonstrated.

The presence of autoantibodies was detected with various paraneoplastic syndromes especially in small cell bronchial carcinomas. Moreover, non-paraneoplastic syndrome against P53 tumour suppressor gene also has been shown [61]. Paraneoplastic syndromes, which is often seen in small cell lung cancer, may be seen in other types of lung cancer. It is consists of a group of signs and symptoms which are often seen on tumour itself or from distant metastases common areas, depending on the development of cancer. Polypeptide hormones are formed by hormone-like peptides, antibodies, immune complexes, cytokines, prostaglandins, or systemic factors such as the tumour-generated products. Recognition of paraneoplastic syndrome of underlying lung cancer may allow early diagnosis and treatment.

ACKNOWLEDGEMENTS

Declared none.

CONFLICT OF INTEREST

The author confirms that this article content has no conflict of interest.

REFERENCES

[1] Meert AP, Berghmans T, Mascaux C, Sculier JP.Immune responses in broncho-pulmonary cancer Rev Mal Respir 2003;20(4):566-79.

[2] Annakkaya A. N, Yaman M, Erturan S, Aydın G, Müsellim B., Altuğ E. Cellular and Humoral Immunity in advanced stage of lung cancer Respiration 2002;4:224-228.

[3] Carretero A, Elmberger PG, Skold CM, Collins BT. A low number of CD8s may correlate with a favorable prognosis. Acta Cytol. 2006;50(4):455-459.

[4] Wolf AM, Wolf D, Steurer M, Gastl G, Gunsilius E, Grubeck-Loebenstein B. Increase of regulatory T cells in the peripheral blood of cancer patients Clin. Cancer Res 2003;9: 606.

[5] Grabenbauer GG, Lahmer G, Distel L, Niedobitek G. Tumour-infiltrating cytotoxic T cells but not regulatory T cells predict outcome in anal squamous cell carcinoma Clin. Cancer Res 2006;12(11):3355-60.

[6] Wolf D, Rumpold H, Wolf AM. Regulatory T cells in cancer biology: a possible new target for biochemical therapies Mini Rev Med Chem 2006 May;6(5):509-13.

[7] Yannelli JR, Tucker JA, Hidalgo G, Perkins S, Kryscio R, Hirschowitz EA. Characteristics of PBMC obtained from leukapheresis products and tumour biopsies of patients with non-small cell lung cancer Oncol. Rep 2009;22(6):1459-71

[8] Zeng L, O'Connor C, Zhang J, Kaplan AM, Cohen DA. IL-10 promotes resistance to apoptosis and metastatic potential in lung tumour cell lines. Cytokine. 2010;49(3):294-302

[9] Zhang Y, Huang S, Gong D, Qin Y, Shen Q. Programmed death-1 upregulation is correlated with dysfunction of tumour-infiltrating CD8(+) T lymphocytes in human non-small cell lung cancer. Cell. Mol. Immunol 2010

[10] Jerome S. Brody and Avrum Spira, Chronic Obstructive Pulmonary Disease, Inflammation, and Lung Cancer The Proceedings of the American Thoracic Society 2006;3:535-537.

[11] Batra RK, Lin Y, Sharma S, Dohadwala M, Luo J, Pold M, Dubinett SM. Non-small cell lung cancer-derived soluble mediators enhance apoptosis in activated T lymphocytes through an I kappa B kinase-dependent mechanism. Cancer Res. 2003;63(3):642-6.

[12] Maker AV, Phan GQ, Attia P, Yang JC, Sherry RM, Topalian SL, Kammula US, Royal RE, Haworth LR, Levy C, Kleiner D, Mavroukakis SA, Yellin M, Rosenberg SA. Tumour regression and autoimmunity in patients treated with cytotoxic T lymphocyte-associated antigen 4 blockade and interleukin 2: a phase I/II study. Ann. Surg Oncol. 2005;12(12):1005-16.

[13] Sabel MS, Hess SD, Egilmez NK, Conway TF, Chen FA, Bankert RB. CTLA-4 blockade augments human T lymphocyte-mediated suppression of lung tumour xenografts in SCID mice Cancer Immunol Immunother 2005;54(10):944-52.

[14] Wang L, Pan XD, Xie Y, Zhang GB, Jiang M, Zheng L, Wang JH, Shi JF, Zhang XG.Altered CD28 and CD95 mRNA expression in peripheral blood mononuclear cells from elderly patients with primary non-small cell lung cancer. Chin Med J 2010 5;123(1):51-6.

[15] Zieliński P, Dyszkiewicz W, Piwkowski CT, Dworacki G, Gasiorowski L.Can the condition of the cell microenvironment of mediastinal lymph nodes help predict the risk of metastases in non-small cell lung cancer? Cancer Epidemiol. 2009;33(5):387-90.

[16] Shojaei H, Oberg HH, Juricke M, Marischen L, Kunz M, Mundhenke C, Gieseler F, Kabelitz D, Wesch D. Toll-like receptors 3 and 7 agonists enhance tumour cell lysis by human gammadelta T cells Cancer Res. 2009: 15;69(22):8710-7.

[17] Li W, Jian-jun W, Xue-Feng Z, Feng Z. CD133(+) human pulmonary adenocarcinoma cells induce apoptosis of CD8(+) T cells by highly expressed galectin-3 Clin Invest Med. 2010;1;33(1):44-53.

[18] Isobe M, Eikawa S, Uenaka A, Nakamura Y, Kanda T, Kohno S, Kuzushima K, Nakayama E.Correlation of high and decreased NY-ESO-1 immunity to spontaneous regression and subsequent recurrence in a lung cancer patient. Cancer Immun. 2009;1;9:8.

[19] Zhong CY, Zhou YM, Douglas GC, Witschi H, Pinkerton KE. MAPK/AP-1 signal pathway in tobacco smoke-induced cell proliferation and squamous metaplasia in the lungs of rats Carcinogenesis 2005;26(12):2187-2195.

[20] Tsurutani J, Castillo SS, Brognard J, Granville CA, Zhang C, Gills JJ, Sayyah J, Dennis PA Tobacco components stimulate Akt-dependent proliferation and NFkappaB-dependent survival in lung cancer cells. Carcinogenesis. 2005;26(7):1182-95.

[21] Mitsudomi T. Molecular lesions as targets for diagnosis and therapy of lung cancer. Gan To Kagaku Ryoho. 2002;29(1):112-116.

[22] Bergqvist M, Brattstrom D, Larsson A, Holmertz J, Hesselius P, Rosenberg L, Wagenius G, Brodin O. P53 auto-antibodies in non-small cell lung cancer patients can predict increased life expectancy after radiotherapy. Anticancer Res. 1998;18(3B):1999-2002.

[23] Chada S, Mhashilkar A, Roth JA, Gabrilovich D. Development of vaccines against self-antigens: the p53 paradigm Curr Opin Drug Discov Devel 2003;6(2):169-73.

[24] Zendman AJ, Ruiter DJ, Van Muijen GN.Cancer/testis-associated genes: identification, expression profile, and putative function. J Cell Physiol 2003;194:272-288

[25] Ohman FK, Nordqvist K:Melanoma antigen genes-any clues to their functions in normal tissues? Exp Cell Res 2001;265:185-194.

[26] Scanlan MJ, Altorki NK, Gure AO, Williamson B, Jungbluth A, Chen YT, Old LJ. Expression of cancer-testis antigens in lung cancer: definition of bromodomain

testis-specific gene (BRDT) as a new CT gene, CT9 Cancer Lett 2000;150(2):155-64.

[27] Mulligan JK, Rosenzweig SA, Young MR. Tumour secretion of VEGF induces endothelial cells to suppress T cell functions through the production of PGE2. J Immunother. 2010;33(2):126-35

[28] Kambayashi T, Alexander HR, Fong M, Strassmann G. Potential involvement of IL-10 in suppressing tumour-associated macrophages. Colon-26-derived prostaglandin E2 J Immunol 1995;1;154(7):3383-90.

[29] Keith RL, Geraci MW, Nana-Sinkam SP, Breyer RM, Hudish TM, Meyer AM, Malkinson AM, Dwyer-Nield LD.Prostaglandin E2 receptor subtype 2 (EP2) null mice are protected against murine lung tumourigenesis. Anticancer Res. 2006;26(4B):2857-2861.

[30] Galloway ML, Murray D, Moffat DF.The use of the monoclonal antibody mesothelin in the diagnosis of malignant mesothelioma in pleural biopsies. Histopathology. 2006;48(6):767-769.

[31] Stolina M, Sharma S, Lin Y, Dohadwala M, Gardner B, Luo J, Zhu L, Kronenberg M, Miller PW, Portanova J, Lee JC, Dubinett SM. Specific inhibition of cyclooxygenase 2 restores antitumour reactivity by altering the balance of IL-10 and IL-12 synthesis J Immunol 2000;164(1): 361-70

[32] Friedman RS, Bangur CS, Zasloff EJ, Fan L, Wang T, Watanabe Y, Kalos M.Molecular and immunological evaluation of the transcription factor SOX-4 as a lung tumour vaccine antigen. J Immunol 2004;172(5):3319-27.

[33] Vural B, Chen LC, Saip P, Chen YT, Ustuner Z, Gonen M, Simpson AJ, Old LJ, Ozbek U, Gure AO. Frequency of SOX Group B (SOX1, 2, 3) and ZIC2 antibodies in Turkish patients with small cell lung carcinoma and their correlation with clinical parameters. Cancer 2005 15;103(12):2575-83.

[34] Ho MY, Leu SJ, Sun GH, Tao MH, Tang SJ, Sun KH. IL-27 directly restrains lung tumourigenicity by suppressing cyclooxygenase-2-mediated activities. J Immunol. 2009;15;183(10):6217-26.

[35] Powell A, Creaney J, Broomfield S, Van Bruggen I, Robinson B Recombinant GM-CSF plus autologous tumour cells as a vaccine for patients with mesothelioma Lung Cancer. 2006 May;52(2):189-97.

[36] Thomas RK, Greulich H, Yuza Y, Lee JC, Tengs T, Feng W, Chen TH, Nickerson E, Simons J, Egholm M, Rothberg JM, Sellers WR, Meyerson ML. Detection of oncogenic mutations in the EGFR gene in lung adenocarcinoma with differential sensitivity to EGFR tyrosine kinase inhibitors Cold Spring Harb Symp Quant Biol 2005;70:73-81.

[37] Swinson DE, O'Byrne KJ. Interactions between hypoxia and epidermal growth factor receptor in non-small-cell lung cancerClin Lung Cancer 2006;7(4):250-256.

[38] Paez JG, Jänne PA, Lee J.C, Tracy S,1 Greulich H,Gabriel S, Herman P,1 Kaye FJ, Lindeman N, Boggon TJ, Naoki K, Sasaki H, Fujii Y, Eck MJ, Sellers WR, Johnson BE, Meyerson M, EGFR Mutations in Lung Cancer: Correlation with Clinical Response to Gefitinib Therapy. Science 2004:304.; 5676:1497 – 1500.

[39] Liu HP, Isaac Wu HD, Chang JW, Wu YC, Yang HY, Chen YT, Hsieh WY, Chen YT, Chen YR, Huang SF. Prognostic Implications of Epidermal Growth Factor Receptor and KRAS Gene Mutations and Epidermal Growth Factor Receptor Gene Copy Numbers in Patients with Surgically Resectable Non-small Cell Lung Cancer in Taiwan. J Thorac Oncol 2010

[40] Zhong L, Roybal J, Chaerkady R, Zhang W, Choi K, Alvarez CA, Tran H, Creighton CJ, Yan S, Strieter RM, Pandey A, Kurie JM. Identification of secreted proteins that mediate cell-cell interactions in an *in vitro* model of the lung cancer microenvironment Cancer Res 2008 1;68(17):7237-45.

[41] Ji H, Houghton AM, Mariani TJ, Perera S, Kim CB, Padera R, Tonon G, McNamara K, Marconcini LA, Hezel A, El-Bardeesy N, Bronson RT, Sugarbaker D, Maser RS, Shapiro SD, Wong KK. K-ras activation generates an inflammatory response in lung tumours. Oncogene 2006;25(14):2105-12.

[42] Stathopoulos GT, Zhu Z, Everhart MB, Kalomenidis I, Lawson WE, Bilaceroglu S, Peterson TE, Mitchell D, Yull FE, Light RW, Blackwell TS. Nuclear factor-kappaB affects tumour progression in a mouse model of malignant pleural effusion. Am J Respir Cell Mol Biol. 2006;34(2):142-150.

[43] Fridlender ZG, Kapoor V, Buchlis G, Cheng G, Sun J, Wang LC, Singhal S, Snyder LA, Albelda SM. CCL2 Blockade Inhibits Lung Cancer Tumour Growth by Altering Macrophage Phenotype and Activating CD8+ Cells. Am J Respir Cell Mol Biol. 2010

[44] Imai H, Sunaga N, Shimizu Y, Kakegawa S, Shimizu K, Sano T, Ishizuka T, Oyama T, Saito R, Minna JD, Mori M. Clinicopathological and therapeutic significance of CXCL12 expression in lung cancer. Int J Immunopathol Pharmacol 2010;23(1):153-64.

[45] Wald O Izhar U, Amir G, Avniel S, Bar-Shavit Y, Wald H, Galun E, Peled A. Weiss ID J CD4+CXCR4highCD69+ T cells accumulate in lung adenocarcinoma. Immunol 2006; 15:177(10):6983-90.

[46] Wagner PL, Hyjek E, Vazquez MF, Meherally D, Liu YF, Chadwick PA, Rengifo T, Sica GL, Port JL, Lee PC, Paul S, Altorki NK, Saqi A. CXCL12 and CXCR4 in adenocarcinoma of the lung: association with metastasis and survival. J Thorac Cardiovasc Surg 2009;137(3):615-21.

[47] McClelland M, Zhao L, Carskadon S, Arenberg D. Expression of CD74, the receptor for macrophage migration inhibitory factor, in non-small cell lung cancer. Am J Pathol. 2009;174(2):638-46.

[48] Ohri CM, Shikotra A, Green RH, Waller DA, Bradding P.Chemokine receptor expression in tumour islets and stroma in non-small cell lung cancer. BMC Cancer. 2010;29;10:172.

[49] Diao J, Zhao J, Winter E, Cattral MS. Recruitment and differentiation of conventional dendritic cell precursors in tumours. J Immunol 2010:1;184(3):1261-7.

[50] Massa C, Melani C, Colombo MP. Chaperon and adjuvant activity of hsp70: different natural killer requirement for cross-priming of chaperoned and bystander antigens. Cancer Res 2005;65(17):7942-7949.

[51] Yao X, Jiang H, Zhang C, Wang H, Yang L, Yu Y, Yu J, Shi B, Shen Z, Gao H, Chen Z, Tian S, Lu S, Li Z, Gu J. Dickkopf-1 autoantibody is a novel serological biomarker for non-small cell lung cancer. Biomarkers. 2010;15(2):128-34.

[52] Watanabe M, Kashiwakura Y, Huang P, Ochiai K, Futami J, Li SA, Takaoka M, Nasu Y, Sakaguchi M, Huh NH, Kumon H. Immunological aspects of REIC/Dkk-3 in monocyte differentiation and tumour regression. Int J Oncol. 2009;34(3):657-63.

[53] Tarkan-Argüden Y, Hacihanefioglu S, Ongen G, Erk M, Cenani A. 3p abnormalities in peripheral lymphocytes in small cell lung cancer. Tumour 2009;95(4):535-7.

[54] Kuroda K, Takenoyama M, Baba T, Shigematsu Y, Shiota H, Ichiki Y, Yasuda M, Uramoto H, Hanagiri T, Yasumoto K Identification of ribosomal protein L19 as a novel tumour antigen recognized by autologous cytotoxic T lymphocytes in lung adenocarcinoma. Cancer Sci 2010;101(1):46-53.

[55] Zhang F, Gu Y, Li X, Wang W, He J, Peng T. Up-regulated Golgi phosphoprotein 2 (GOLPH2) expression in lung adenocarcinoma tissue Clin Biochem. 2010

[56] Tokunaga T, Naruke Y, Shigematsu S, Kohno T, Yasui K, Ma Y, Chua KJ, Katayama I, Nakamura T, Hishikawa Y, Koji T, Yatabe Y, Nagayasu T, Fujita T, Matsuyama T, Hayashi H Aberrant Expression of Interferon Regulatory Factor 3 in Human Lung Cancer. Biochem Biophys Res Commun. 2010

[57] Sasaki H, Hikosaka Y, Okuda K, Kawano O, Moriyama S, Yano M, Fujii Y. NFE2L2 gene mutation in male Japanese squamous cell carcinoma of the lung. J Thorac Oncol. 2010;5(6):786-9.

[58] Lee HJ, Choe G, Jheon S, Sung SW, Lee CT, Chung JH. CD24, a novel cancer biomarker, predicting disease-free survival of non-small cell lung carcinomas: a retrospective study of prognostic factor analysis from the viewpoint of forthcoming (seventh) new TNM classification. J Thorac Oncol 2010;5(5):649-57.

[59] Yoon SO, Kim YT, Jung KC, Jeon YK, Kim BH, Kim CW TTF-1 mRNA-positive circulating tumour cells in the peripheral blood predict poor prognosis in surgically resected non-small cell lung cancer patients. Lung Cancer 2010

[60] Viaud S, Théry C, Ploix S, Tursz T, Lapierre V, Lantz O, Zitvogel L, Chaput N. Dendritic cell-derived exosomes for cancer immunotherapy: what's next? Cancer Res 2010:15;70(4):1281-5.

[61] Meert AP, Berghmans T, Mascaux C, Sculier JP.Immune responses in broncho-pulmonary cancer Rev Mal Respir 2003;20(4):566-79.

Send Orders of Reprints at reprints@benthamscience.net
Lung Cancer: Clinical and Surgical Specifications, 2013, 455-465

CHAPTER 13

Part B: Immunological Therapies for Lung Cancer

Ayşegül Atak Yücel*

Gazi University, Faculty of Medicine, Department of Immunology, Beşevler, 06510 Ankara, Turkey

Abstract: Lung cancer is a disease with very high morbidity and mortality rate. In spite of aggressive treatment modalities, the long- term survival is very low, and these treatments have many toxic adverse effects. Immunological therapies or briefly "immunotherapy" is a promising new therapeutic modality for lung cancer; it can be in the form of active immunization (cancer vaccines), passive immunization (adoptive cell therapy or antibody-based treatment) or immunostimulation.

Keywords: Lung cancer, immunotherapy, vaccine, antibody-based treatment, cetuximab, bevacizumab, panitumumab, matuzumab, pertuzumab, transtuzumab, erlotinin, paclitaxel, carboplatin, gemtuzumab, GVAX, MUC1, MAGE-A3, TG4010.

MANUSCRIPT

Lung cancer is the deadliest cancer in the world causing over 1 million deaths per year worldwide and more than 160,000 deaths per year only in the United States [1] among whom 15-20,000 being "never smokers" [2]. The long-term survival for lung cancer is low although some very aggressive treatment modalities including surgery, radiation and chemotherapy have been used. The disease frequently progresses to metastatic stage even if the first diagnosis was made at "early stage". Only about 10% of all lung cancer patients will be cured with current therapies [3]. In spite of their modest therapeutic effects, current standard therapies have very significant toxicities. Therefore, new novel treatment modalities, such as immunotherapy, are under continuous investigation.

In general cancer immunotherapy includes **active immunization**, as in the use of

***Address correspondence to Ayşegül Atak Yücel:** Gazi University, Faculty of Medicine, Department of Immunology, Beşevler, 06510 Ankara, Turkey; Tel: +90-312-202 46 21; Fax: +90-312-212 47 47; E-mails: aysegula@gazi.edu.tr; aysegulatak@yahoo.com cancer vaccines, **passive immunization**, such as the use of adoptive cell therapy and antibodies that modulate tumour function, and **immunostimulation**, using antibodies and small molecules to treat malignancy by activating or blocking an endogenous immune response against tumour cells. Today, more than 100 different monoclonal antibodies (mAb) are in practice or under evaluation to be used as a therapeutic agent in various malignancies. Active stimulation of the host's immune system is promising for obtaining permanent remission in malignancies and it is a nontoxic therapy if tumour-specific effector cells can be selectively targeted [4]. Although some active immunotherapies are designed to induce antibodies as primary effector mechanism, these antibodies have been found to have limited direct cytotoxic ability against cancer. Therefore, main aim of the active immunotherapy against cancer is to induce antigen-specific T cell response [5]. Natural killer (NK) cells are very important arms of innate immune system that act independent of antigen targeting cells lacking or having mismatched MHC molecules [6]. Since cancer cells often down-regulate their MHC molecules, NK cells cannot be the primary effector cells of active immunotherapy [5].

Early Studies on Immunotherapy of Lung Cancer

Studies before 1990's were focused on non-specific immunostimulants like Bacille Calmette-Guerin (BCG) [7], thymosin [8] and *Corynebacterium parvum* [9]. BCG was mainly given in small cell lung cancer (SCLC). It was given as intrapleural or intratumoural injections [7]; however, there was no significant effect on disease-free or overall survival [10]. Now the role of BCG in immunotherapy of lung cancer is basically as an adjuvant immune stimulant with autologous tumour or antigen-specific vaccine therapies [11]. Early studies with *C. parvum* as a systemic anti-tumour agent for NSCLC revealed dose-related anti-tumour responses without any effect on overall survival [10]. In 1980's and 1990's non-specific immunotherapies with interleukin (IL)-2, tumour necrosis factor (TNF)-α [12, 13], interferon (IFN)-α [14, 15], and other pro-inflammatory cytokines or other mediators were tried. But these trials did not lead to any significant benefit on survival [5].

Passive Immunotherapy Targeting Lung Cancer

Passive immunotherapy involves any immunologically active agent prepared outside the body and does not depend on host's immune system to function. The most widely accepted passive immunotherapy applications use mAb's that block binding of hormones or growth factors to their receptors and by this way block tumourigenic cascades [16].

Antibody-Based Immunotherapy

Although production of monoclonal antibodies was a success more than 35 years ago, they have only recently been applied to human anti-tumour therapy, specifically after development of "humanized" mAb's. Up till now, more than 12 mAb's have received FDA approval and more than 400 of them are under clinical trials [17]. For the treatment of lung cancer, mAb's are primarily targeted against epidermal growth factor receptor (EGFR) (*i.e.* cetuximab: Erbitux®) [18, 19] and vascular endothelial growth factor (VEGF) (*i.e.* bevacizumab: Avastin®) [19, 20].

a. Anti-Growth Factor Monoclonal Antibodies

In many solid malignancies, different growth factors and/or their receptors are over-expressed and, they help proliferation and invasion of tumour cells leading to more aggressive disease and poor prognosis [21]. If these growth factors and their receptors can be blocked, this will sure help treatment. C-erb B-1 (HER1 or Epidermal Growth Factor Receptor: EGFR1) and c-erb B-2 (HER2) are the most extensively studied molecules in monoclonal antibody production for lung cancer treatment [22]. Cetuximab (Erbitux®) is a chimeric human: murine form of anti-EGFR (anti-c-erb B-1) mAb has demonstrated prolonged survival in patients with advanced disease in NSCLC in both the first- and second-line settings [23]; however, studies with larger number of patients are needed. Other anti-EGFR mAbs are panitumumab (ABX-EGF), matuzumab (EMD 72000), pertuzumab (2C4) and MDX214 for which clinical trials in lung carcinoma have been going on [24]. Transtuzumab (Herceptin®) is a humanized mAb against HER2. Its therapeutic use is approved by FDA for metastatic breast cancer, it has failed to show clinical efficacy for the treatment of lung cancer [25]. However, pertuzumab (2C4) that inhibits dimerization of HER2 with HER1 and other HER tyrosine kinases (independent of HER2 overexpression) is under investigation for NSCLC [26].

b. Kinase Inhibitors

Other factors related to tumour growth and cell proliferation *e.g.* VEGF, intercellular adhesion molecule-1 (ICAM-1) have been also selected as targets for mAb treatments. Bevacizumab (Avastin®) that is against VEGF is approved by FDA to be used in colorectal cancer treatment. A phase II clinical trial with this agent alone or in combination with chemotherapy gave promising results in metastatic NSCLC [27]. Bevacizumab was also tried in combination with erlotinin (Tarceva®) (an EGFR-tyrosine kinase inhibitor) or with paclitaxel and carboplatin in neoadjuvant setting [28, 29]. In the largest trial with bevacizumab in recurrent or advanced NSCLC (stages IIIB and IV), it was seen that median survival was increased about 2 months compared to chemotherapy-alone group; besides, progression-free survival also increased while significant bleeding rate was decreased [30].

c. Other Antibody-based Immunotherapies

In small cell lung carcinoma (SCLC), an anti-idiotype vaccine targeting ganglioside GD3 (BEC2) was tried. The European Organization for Research and Treatment of Cancer (EORTC) published data of phase III trial using BEC2/BCG in combination with chemoradiotherapy in limited stage SCLC, but there was no increase in survival, progression-free survival or quality of life unless patients developed a humoral response [31].

Monoclonal antibodies can be linked to cytocidal agents like toxins, chemotherapeutics or radionuclides to increase their cytocidal activities. Gemtuzumab ozogamicin (Mylotarg®) that linked CD33-specific antibody to toxin calicheamicin is approved for myelogenous leukemia treatment [32]. Similar immunoconjugates (drug-armed antibodies) to fight against cancer are defined for different types of malignancies [33]. But data for the use of such agents in lung cancer is very limited; Boghaert *et al.* [34] defined oncofetal protein 5T4 as a promising suitable target for antibody-guided anti-cancer chemotherapy with calicheamicin for lung cancer.

Therapeutic Lung Cancer Vaccines

Unlike protective vaccines against infections and against virus-associated cancers, vaccines for other cancer patients are only therapeutic. The main principle of these cancer vaccines is to incorporate a source of tumour antigens together with an adjuvant so that it will be easier for the immune system to recognize these tumour antigens. The source of tumour antigens may be whole autologous or allogeneic tumour cells, defined proteins or specific peptide epitopes. Since lung cancers have heterogenous histology, relevant immunologically dominant antigens are unknown. Therefore, it is proper to use autologous tumour cells for lung cancer vaccines, but then the induced immunity will not be confined to a single, specific antigen.

a. GVAX® and Allo-GVAX® (bystander GVAX®)

GM-CSF is a significant mediator of proliferation, maturation and migration of dendritic cells; and it is shown to enhance generation of potent and durable anti-tumour immunity. Genetic modification of autologous tumour cells to secrete GM-CSF (GVAX®) has been shown to induce the greatest anti-tumour immunity compared to other immunomodulatory cytokines in preclinical models [35]. Salgia *et al.* [36] reported that GVAX® gave promising results and very limited toxicities in preliminary studies in advanced NSCLC. In another GVAX® phase I/II trial conducted by Nemunaitis *et al.* [37] autologous tumour cells were transduced with GM-CSF through an adenoviral vector (Ad-GM), almost 80% of the patients developed antibody against allogeneic NSCLC cell lines.

Nemuniatis *et al.* [38] modified their approach by obtaining high GM-CSF secretion by the vaccine without any difficulty in producing the vaccine. The new vaccine mixed autologous tumour with allogeneic, NSCLC cell line (K562 erythroleukemia cells) engineered to express GM-CSF and thereby removed the requirement of gene modification in individual tumours. GM-CSF production was 25-folds higher than original GVAX® but there was no objective tumour response similar to one seen with GVAX®.

b. MUC1 Vaccines

Mucin-1 (MUC1) is expressed on cell surface in many adenocarcinomas including lung cancer. Since MUC1 is important in cell-to-cell interaction of malignant and endothelial cells, anti-MUC1 therapy may be helpful to prevent metastatic spread in addition to its direct anti-tumour effect. In a multicentre phase IIB study in NSCLC, L-BLP25 vaccine (Stimuvax®) targeting MUC1 gave promising results [39]. START study (Stimulating Targeted Antigenic Responses to NSCLC) is an international multicenter phase III randomized, double-blind, placebo-controlled trial and is opened to enroll since 2007. Its aim is to involve 1300 patients with unresectable stage III NSCLC that responded to first-line, platinum-based chemoradiotherapy [16]. This study will give us a detailed information about the usage of this vaccine.

c. Recombinant MAGE-A3 Protein Vaccine

A big pharmaceutical company produced a recombinant MAGE-A3 fusion protein combined with immune adjuvant AS02B (monophosphoryl lipid A and QS21) [16]. Melanoma associated antigen E-3 (MAGE-A3) is expressed in about 30-50% of lung cancers depending on the stage and histological subtype and is associated with poor prognosis [40]. Therefore, it is targeted in some vaccination strategies in NSCLC patients. This vaccine successfully induces both humoral and cellular immune responses, with and without adjuvant chemotherapy [41]. In a placebo controlled multinational phase II trial (in resected MAGE-3-positive stage IIB/II NSCLC) completed lately and presented at the 2006 ASCO meeting, showed 33% improvement in disease-free survival for operated and vaccinated patients, besides, there were no significant toxicities. Authors reported that vaccination with this recombinant protein provided both antibody and T cell response against tumour cells [42]. The international MAGRIT study (MAGE-A3 Adjuvant NSCLC Immunotherapy) opened to enroll since 2007, plans to involve 2270 MAGE-A3 positive patients with completely resected stage IB, II or IIIA NSCLC [16].

d. Allogeneic Whole Cell-Based Vaccine

By using allogeneic whole cell-based vaccine a more potent combination of target antigens may be delivered. Such vaccines can target all shared tumour-associated antigens and produce a polyvalent cytolytic T cell response for each antigen; therefore, they can help to prevent tumour evasion by antigenic modulation [43]. Raez *et al.* [44] developed an allogeneic cancer vaccine expressing costimulatory molecule B7.1 and showed that liberation of antigen during local inflammatory response attracted dendritic cells which in turn uptake the antigen and killed vaccine cells and cross-presented tumour-associated antigens *via* MHC of the patient to generate tumour-specific cytolytic T cell response. In this study, they applied allogeneic vaccination to advanced non-small cell lung cancer patients with B7.1 HLA-A gene-modified adenocarcinoma cell line.

e. TG4010 Vaccine

TG4010 vaccine uses a dual-gene-based approach to express both MUC1 antigen and interleukin (IL)-2 (MVA-MUC1-IL-2) with a recombinant vaccinia virus [16]. In two serial studies with this vaccine together with conventional chemotherapy in stage IIIB7IV NSCLC, there were statistically significant differences in clinical response, progression-free survival, and there was encouraging trend on overall survival. Results were presented at the American Society of Clinical Oncology in 2008 [45].

CONCLUSION

Lung cancer had been considered as a non-immune-sensitive malignancy for a long time. With the discovery of relevant tumour antigens of lung cancer and advances in cancer immunotherapy, the efforts have been accelerated in development of cancer vaccines and in passive immunotherapy modalities in lung cancer. There are several key points to consider. Most probably, the measurable immunological response to relevant tumour antigens will correlate with clinical benefits positively. And, a number of different agents give similar clinical benefits. Therefore, to measure and compare potency, well-standardized and – validated immunological assays should be used. Patients with advanced lung cancer, especially with bulky tumours, have not been benefited much from immunotherapy. It's considered that there are many biological elements that affect clinical efficacy beyond tumour burden. Larger and metastatic tumours gain enhanced resistance ability during progression, and immunosuppressive elements are more prominent in advanced cancer, *e.g.* number of regulatory T cells increase with tumour burden. Therefore, it is important to keep all this information in mind while preparing immunotherapy alternatives for lung cancer. Besides, most of the study has been performed in NSCLC, small cell lung cancer (SCLC) has not been widely investigated for immunotherapy. Since SCLC is mostly a non-surgical disease, tumour is not routinely available to prepare cancer vaccines.

Clinical immunotherapy testing researches should have been continued since this type of testing help gain relevant biological and therapeutic information to promote rational development of therapeutic modalities. Animal studies are also very valuable to provide insight into immunobiology and are critical before designing new immunotherapies. To determine the biological activity of immunotherapies in phase I-II studies, immunological endpoints are critical and help as important measures for potency in vaccine development. Both humoral and T-cell assays are very valuable to test the newly developed immunotherapies. Efficacy still depends on relevance of antigen. Besides, simplicity of development and cost are also important parameters in new treatments.

Immune regulation of lung cancer offers multiple options for immunomodulation, since researches on this issue continue, new targets will be found and efficacy will improve. In future, we hope that combinations of multiple immunoactive agents, conventional treatments and novel targeted therapies will provide significant improvements in the therapeutic outcome of lung cancer.

ACKNOWLEDGEMENTS

Declared none.

CONFLICT OF INTEREST

The author confirms that this article content has no conflict of interest.

REFERENCES

[1] Jemal A, Siegel R, Ward E, Hao Y, Xu J, Murray T, Thun MJ. Cancer statistics, 2008. CA Cancer J Clin 2008; 58: 71-96.
[2] Thun MJ, Henley J, Burns D, Jemal A, Shanks TG, Calle EE. Lung cancer death rates in lifelong nonsmokers. J Natl Cancer Inst 2006; 98:691-9.
[3] Krasna MJ, Reed CE, Nugent WC, Olak J, Sugarbaker DJ, Green MR, Kohman LJ. Lung cancer staging and treatment in multidisciplinary trials: Cancer and Leukemia Group B cooperative group approach. Thoracic suregeons of CALGB. Ann Thorac Surg 1999; 68: 201-7.
[4] Rüttinger D, Winter H, van den Engel NK, Hatz R, Jauch KW, Fox BA, Weber JS. Immunotherapy of cancer: key findings and commentary on the third Tegernsee conference. Oncologist 2010; 15: 112-8.
[5] Raez LE, Fein S, Podack ER. Lung cancer immunotherapy. Clin Med Res 2005; 3: 221-8.
[6] Waldhauer I, Steinle A. NK cells and cancer immunosurveillance. Oncogene 2008; 27: 5932-43.
[7] McCracken JD, Heilbrun L, White J, Reed R, Samson M, Saiers JH, Stephens R, Stuckey WJ, Bickers J, Livingston R. Combination chemotherapy, radiotherapy, and BCG

immunotherapy in extensive (metastatic) small cell carcinoma of the lung. A Southwest Oncology Group study. Cancer 1980; 46: 2335-40.

[8] Lipson SD, Chretin PB, Makuch R, Kenady DE, Cohen MH. Thymosin immunotherapy in patients with small cell carcinoma of the lung: correlation of *in vitro* studies with clinical course. Cancer 1979; 43: 863-70.

[9] Drapkin R, Bjornsson S, Naeher C, Higby D, Caracandas J, Wallens WT, Kuberka N, Suh K, Siddiqi N, Henderson ES. Doxorubicin, cisplatin, and Corynebacterium parvum in non-small cell bronchogenic carcinoma. Cancer Treat Rep. 1980; 64: 1367-9.

[10] Issel BF, Valdivieso M, Hersh EM, Richman S, Gutterman JU, Bodey GP. Combination of chemoimmunotherapy for extensive non-aot cell lung cancer. Cancer Treat Rep 1978; 62: 1059-63.

[11] Grant SC, Kris MG, Houghton AN, Chapman PB. Long survival of patients with small cell lung cancer after adjuvant treatment with the anti-idiotypic antibody BEC2 plus Bacillus Calmette-Guérin. Clin Cancer Res 1999; 5: 1319-23.

[12] Schiller JH, Morgan-Ihrig C, Levitt ML. Concomittant administration of interleukin-2 plus tumour necrosis factor in advanced non-small cell lung cancer. Am J Clin Oncol 1995; 18: 47-51.

[13] Yang SC, Owen-Schaub L, Grimm EA, Roth JA. Induction of lymphokine-activated killer cytotoxicity with interleukin-2 and tumour necrosis factor-alpha against primary lung cancer targets. Cancer Immunol Immunother 1989; 29: 193-8.

[14] Jansen RL, Slingerland R, Goey SH, Frank CR, Bolhuis RL, Stoter G. Interleukin-2 and interferon-alpha in the treatment of patients with advanced non-small-cell lung cancer. J Immunother 1992; 12: 70-3.

[15] Sarna G, Figlin R, Callaghan M. Alpha(human leukocyte)-interferon as treatment for non-small cell carcinoma of the lung: a phase II trial. J Biol Response Mod 1983; 2: 343-7.

[16] Hirschowitz EA, Yannelli JR. Immunotherapy for lung cancer. Proc Am Thora Soc, 2009; 6: 224-32.

[17] Gura T. Magic bullets hit the target. Nature 2002; 417: 584-6.

[18] Egri G, Takats A. Monoclonal antibodies in the treatment of lung cancer. Eur J Surg Oncol 2006; 32: 385-94.

[19] Gridelli C, Maione P, Ferrara ML, Rossi A. Cetuximab and other anti-epidermal growth factor receptor monoclonal antibodies in the treatment of non-small cell lung cancer. Oncologist 2009; 14: 601-11.

[20] Hsu JY, Wakelee HA. Monoclonal antibodies targeting vascular endothelial growth factor: current status and future challenges in cancer therapy. BioDrugs. 2009; 23: 289-304.

[21] Reissmann PT, Koga H, Figlin RA, Holmes EC, Slamon DJ. Amplification and overexpression of the cyclin D1 and epidermal growth factor receptor genes in non-small-cell lung cancer. Lung Cancer Study Group. J Cancer Res Clin Oncol 1999; 125: 61-70.

[22] Bianco AR. Targeting c-erbB2 and other receptors of the c-erbB family: rationale and clinical applications. J Chemother 2004; 16 Suppl 4: 52-4.

[23] Langer C, Soria JC. The role of anti-epidermal growth factor receptor and anti-vascular endothelial growth factor therapies in the treatment of non-small-cell lung cancer. Clin Lung Cancer 2010; 11: 82-90.

[24] Heymach JV, Nilsson M, Blumenschein G, Papadimitrakopoulou V, Herbst R. Epidermal growth factor receptor inhibitors in development for the treatment of non-small cell lung cancer. Clin Cancer Res 2006; 12: 4441s-45s.

[25] Clamon G, Herndon J, Kern J, Govindan R, Garst J, Watson D, Green M; Cancer and Leukemia Group B. Lack of trastuzumab activity in nonsmall cell lung carcinoma with overexpression of erb-B2: 39810: a phase II trial of Cancer and Leukemia Group B. Cancer 2005;103:1670-5.

[26] Johnson BE, Jänne PA. Rationale for a phase II trial of pertuzumab, a HER-2 dimerization inhibitor, in patients with non-small cell lung cancer. Clin Cancer Res 2006;12:4436s-40s.

[27] Johnson DH, Fehrenbacher L, Novotny WF, et al????Randomized phase II trial comparing bevacizumab plus carboplatin and paclitaxel alone in previously untreated locally advanced or metastatic non-small cell lung cancer. J Clin Oncol, 2004; 22: 2184-91.

[28] Sandler AB, Johnson DH, Herbst RS. Anti-vascular endothelial growth factor monoclonals in non-small cell lung cancer. Clin Cancer Res, 2004; 10: 4258s-62s.

[29] Herbst RS, Johnson DH, Mininberg E, *et al.* Phase I/II trial evaluating the anti-vascular endothelial the anti-vascular endothelial growth factor monoclonal antibody bevacizumab in combination with the HER-1/epidermal growth factor recetor tyrosine kinase inhibitor erlotinib for patients with recurrent non-small cell lung cancer. J clin Oncol, 2005; 23: 2544-55.

[30] Sandler A, Gray R, Perry MC, *et al.* Paclitaxel-carboplatin alone or with bevacizumab for non-small cell lung cancer.N Engl J Med, 2006; 355: 2542-50.

[31] Giaccone G, Debruyne C, Felip E, *et al.* Phase III study of adjuvant vaccination with Bec2/bacille Calmette-Guerin in responding patients with limited-disease small-cell lung cancer (European Organisation for Research and Treatment of Cancer 08971-08971B; Silva Study). J Clin Oncol, 2005; 23: 6854-64.

[32] Stasi R. Gentuzumab ozogamisin: an anti-CD33 immunoconjugate for tretament of acute myeloid leukemia. Expert Opin Biol Ther, 2008; 8: 527-40.

[33] Haeuw JF, Caussanel V, Beck A. Med Sci (Paris), 2009; 25: 1046-52.

[34] Boghaert ER, Shiridharan L, Khandke KM, Armellino D, Ryan MG, Myers K, Harrop R, Kunz A, Hamann PR, Marquette K, Dougher M, DiJoseph JF, Damle K. The oncofetal protein, 5T4, is a suitable target for antibody-guided anti-cancer cehmoterapy with calicheamicin. In J Oncol, 2008; 32: 221-34.

[35] Dranoff G, Jaffee E, Lazenbay A. Vaccination with irradiated tumour cells engineered to secrete murine granulocyte-macrophage colony-stimulating factor stimulates potent, specific, and long-lasting anti-tumour immunity. Proc Natl Acad Sci USA, 1993; 90: 3539-43.

[36] Salgia R, LynchT, Skarin A, *et al.* Vaccination with irradiated autologous tumour cells engineered to secrete Granulocyte-Macrophage Colony Stimulating Factor augments anti-tumour immunity in patients with metastatic non-small cell lung carcinoma. J Clin Oncol, 2003; 21: 624-30.

[37] Nemunaitis J, Sterman D, Jablons D, *et al.* Granulocyte-macrophage colony-stimulating factor-gene-modified autologous tumour vaccines in non-small cell lung cancer. J Natl Cancer Inst, 2004; 96: 326-31.

[38] Nemuniatis J, Jahan T, Ross H, Sterman D, Richards D, Fox B, Jablons DD, Aimi J, Lin A, Hege K. Phase1/2 trial of autologous tumour mixed with allogeneic GVAX vaccine in advanced-stage non-small-cell lung cancer. Cancer Gene Ther, 2006; 13: 555-62.

[39] Butts C, Murray N, Maksymiuk A, *et al.* Randomized Phase IIB trial of BLP25 liposome vaccine in stage IIIB and IV non-small-cell lung cancer. J Clin Oncol, 2005; 23: 6674-81.

[40] Gure AO, Chua R, Williamson B, *et al.* Cancer-testis genes are coordinately expressed anda re markers of poor outcome in non-small cell lung cancer. Clin Cancer Res, 2005; 11: 8055-62.

[41] Atanackovic D, Altorki NK, Stockert E, *et al.*Vaccine-induced CD4+ T cell responses to MAGE-3 protein in lung Cancer patients. J Immunol, 2004; 172: 3289-96.

[42] Halmos BH. Lung cancer II. ASCO Annual Meeting Summaries, 2006; 156-60.

[43] Raez LE, Fein S, Podack ER. Lung cancer immunotherapy. Clin Med Res, 2005; 3: 221-8.

[44] Raez LE, Cassileth PA, Schlesselman JJ, Sridhar K, Padmanabhan S, Fischer EZ, Podack ER. Allogeneic vaccination with a B7.1 HLA-A gene-modified adenocarcinoma cell line in advanced non-small cell lung cancer. J Clin Oncol, 2004; 22: 2800-7.

[45] Ramlau R, Quoix E, Rolski J, Piess M, Lena H, Levy E, Krazoski M, Hess D, Terlor E, Chenad MP, Limacher JM, Bizouarne N, Acres B, Halluard C, Velu T. A phase II study TG4010 (MVA-MUC1-IL2) in association with chemotherapy in patients with stage III/IV non-small cell lung cancer. J Thorac Oncol, 2008; 3: 735-44.

Send Orders of Reprints at reprints@benthamscience.net

CHAPTER 14

The Oncological and Surgical Management of Small Cell Lung Cancer

Akif Turna*

Istanbul University Cerrahpasa Medical Faculty, Department of Thoracic Surgery, Kocamustafapasa/Fatih Istanbul, 34303 Turkey

Abstract: Despite the fact that, approximately, one-seventh of all lung cancers are small cell lung carcinoma (SCLC), it is the fifth leading cause of cancer mortality. Histologically it represents small (<20 microns) cells with scanty cytoplasm with neuroendocrine properties. It is usually hilar tumour with early and multiple metastasis. The major symptoms are chest pain, dyspnea, wheezing and dysphonia. Paraneoplastic syndromes such as Cushing syndrome, secretion of Inappropriate ADH syndrome and some dramatic signs of tumours such as vena cava superior syndrome are not uncommon. Malignant pleural effusion develops in up to 35% of patients.The latest (seventh) TNM staging systems is defined to be applicable to SCLC, but they have been used very frequently in clinical practice because patients with SCLC seldom present at a stage for which surgery is appropriate and oncologists anonymously refused to stratify the patients according to these comprehensive staging systems. Nevertheless stratification by stages I–III should be used in all patients for early-stage SCLC whether treatment is surgical or not and full details of TNM staging should be reported.

Although, very small fraction of patients with T1N0 disease could be amenable to surgical resection, major treatment modalities for SCLC are chemotherapy and radiotherapy with elective cranial irradiation. Studies showed significantly superior survival for thoracic irradiation and adjuvant chemotherapy when compared with radiotherapy alone.

Patients with early-stage SCLC (T1–2 N0) may benefit from a combined modality approach that includes surgery. Neoadjuvant chemo/radiotherapy could possibly provide better survival in these patients.

As conclusion, SCLC is a very aggressive histologic type of lung cancer which develops metastasis rapidly and leads to very dismal prognosis. Challenging treatment approach is usually needed including chemotherapy, radiotherapy, surgery and new treatment modalities. Strategies for prohibition of smoking has been reduced and will reduce the incidence of SCLC.

***Address correspondence to Akif Turna:** Istanbul University Cerrahpasa Medical Faculty, Department of Thoracic Surgery, Kocamustafapasa, Fatih Istanbul, 34303 Turkey; Tel: +90 212 4143590; Fax: +90 212 6328474; E-mail: akif.turna@gmail.com

Akın Eraslan Balcı (Ed)

Keywords: Small cell lung cancer, SCLC, chemotherapy, radiotherapy, elective cranial irradiation, paraneoplastic syndromes.

INTRODUCTION

Small cell lung cancer (SCLC) represents approximately 15% of lung cancers overall, with incidence rates declining in men, but continuing to rise in women in most countries [1]. By itself, SCLC is the fifth leading cause of cancer mortality in the United States when it is considered independently from non-SCLC (NSCLC) [2]. SCLC is distinguished by its rapid growth rate, early dissemination to regional lymph nodes and distant sites. This tumour type comprises 15% to 20% of all lung cancers [1, 2].

The unique histologic properties of SCLC were first described in 1926 by Bernard who first published as 'oat cell sarcoma' [3]. At that time, the tumour was introduced as a 'mediastinal' sarcoma. These cells are typically small round cells with neuroendocrine features [4]. The incidence of SCLC is decreasing according to recent reports [1], however, the incidence is increasing in women, which reflects an increase in the prevalance of of smoking among women approximately 30 years ago. Tobacco use is strongly associated with SCLC, other agents include radon (alpha radiation), asbestos, bischloromethylether [5].

Histology

SCLC is an invasive carcinoma consist of small (<20 microns) cells with scanty cytoplasm (Fig. **1**). Histologically, these tumours are recognized by their finely granular nuclei(salt and pepper chromatin) by their small nucleoli and by the tendency for the nuclei to become easily deformed by contact with other cells and other structures (nuclear molding). The proliferation index of these tumour is high. The mitotic rate is usually 10 mitoses per 10 high-power fields. In small biopsy samples, crush artifact can prevent them to be defined.

In great majority of patients, the diagnosis of SCLC is obvious by histologic examination alone. However, immunohistochemical studies can serve to buttress the diagnosis and provide confirmation of diagnosis. Cytokeratin expression helps to distinguish SCLC from other small blue cell tumours such as lymphoma, which occasionally can mimic SCLC. The expression rate of TTF-1 is approximately 85% [6]. Where as the utility of TTF-1 in distinguishing tissue of origin of unknown primary is highly context dependent.

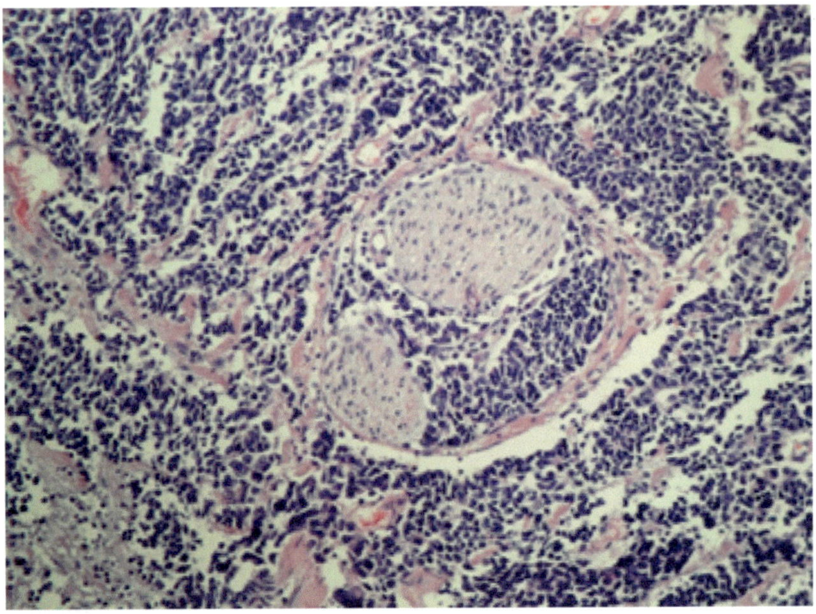

Figure 1: An hematoxylin-eosin staining of small cell lung cancer (x400).

SCLC is a neuroendocrine tumour. For this reason, neuroendocrine markers including neural cell adhesion molecule (NCAM; CD56), CD57, neuron specific enolase and synaptophysin are useful. However, approximately 50% of SCLCs express chromagranin A. Since, SCLC is a highly proliferative tumour, growth-fraction labeling protein Ki-67 is helpful in distinguishing SCLC from other neuroendocrine tumours of the lung. Epithelial Growth Factor Receptor (EGFR) is a negative marker for SCLC. It has been published that, c-kit receptor (CD117) is expressed in almost all neuroendocrine carcinomas including SCLC and large cell neuroendocrine carcinoma [7].

I. Molecular Pathology

SCLC was one of first tumours in which prominent genetic changes were defined. The 3p deletion [14-23] is one of the firstly described mutation [8]. rb1 mutation was found in 90% of SCLC. TP53 mutation was decribed in 70 % of the patients

[4]. On the other hand, k-ras, ErbB1 and p16Ink4a mutations were rarely identified.

II. Clinical Presentation

The clinical presentation of SCLC along with signs and symptoms of the disease, is of great importance in the understanding of this tumour to help make a proper diagnosis and decide on the best available therapy.

Nearly all patients with SCLC present with symptomatic disease, and less than 10% of lung cancer patients will be diagnosed prior to clinical presentation [9]. Table **1** summarizes the frequency of these signs and symptoms [10]. Chest pain is the most common symptom in SCLC. Chest pain is generally caused by chest wall involvement or local extension of disease. It can also be attributed to unrelated causes such as esophageal involvement, vascular disease or cardiac disease.

Table 1: Signs Symptoms and the Frequencies of Small Cell Lung Cancer Patients

Symptoms/Sign	**Frequency (%)**
Chest pain	20-49
Anorexia	18-33
Superior vena cava syndrome	10-15
Cough	8-75
Hemoptysis	6-35
Bone pain	6-25
Dyspnea	3-60
Hoarseness	2-18
Weight loss	0-68
Weakness	0-42
Clubbing	0-20
Dysphagia	0-2
Wheezing	0-2

Dyspnea is common but usually not a result of endotracheal obstruction. However, advanced SCLC such as obstructing tumours, lymphangitic cancer spread or central lesions can be a cause of dyspnea. SCLC patients can have wheezing attributable to main bronchial and/or tracheal obstruction. However, wheezing can be wrongly diagnosed as to have COPD.

Pericardial or atrial involvement of the tumour can induce dysrhythmias. Pericardial metastasis or effusion may also induce cardiac disturbances and should be carefully evaluated.

Locally advanced SCLC may cause esophageal compression and obstruction. These are caused by tumour and/or hilar or mediastinal enlarged lymph node.

Hoarseness can be notified due to left recurrent nerve compression or invasion by the left-sided tumour. Hoarseness or dysphonia can be partially relieved by chemoradiotherapy. However, since irreversible nerve injury occurs, it cannot be disappeared completely.

Malignant pleural effusion presents in up-to one-third of patients [11]. Pleural fluid cytology must be done in these patients. The likelihood of malignant effusion in exudative effusion is high. In patients with massive and malignant effusion, catheter drainage and pleurodesis are required to alleviate the symptoms (usually dyspnea and chest pain).

Superior vena cava syndrome (SVC syndrome) may develop because of locally advanced tumour obstructing superior vena cava or involvement of enlarged lymph nodes in the right paratracheal area. This syndrome is characterized by dyspnea, headache, swelling of the arms, neck, face and head due to venous obstruction. The patients with SVC syndrome also may have nausea, blurred vision and numerous neurologic symptoms attributable to increased intracranial venous pressure [12].

Horner syndrome, although rarely can be found in a fraction of SCLC due to the brachial plexus involvement of the tumour.

Systemic Symptoms: Generalized systemic symptoms including anorexia, weight loss and depression can be seen in patients with SCLC. These systemic symptoms becomes more prominent with more extensive disease. Attempts should be made to investigate the etiology for the cachexia associated with malignant disease, including lung cancer. Loss of appetite, increased catabolic metabolism and resulting weight loss are usually due to circulating pro-inflammatory cytokines [13].

Since SCLC can metastasize at a rapid rate, systemic symptoms due to metastases to brain, adrenal gland, contralateral lung, bone can be notified. Patients with brain metastasis may develop fatigue, weakness, complete motor function loss (*e.g.*, hemiplegia, paraplegia) localized or generalized seizures, ataxia, nausea, headache. Brain metastasis occurs in 50% of patients according to one cadaver series [14].

Bone pain due to bone metastasis is not uncommon in SCLC patients. Solitary adrenal metastasis rarely, whereas bilateral adrenal metastases usually induce hypoadrenalism [15].

SCLC patients with liver metastasis may present with jaundice or abdominal pain.

III. Paraneoplastic Syndromes

Paraneoplastic syndromes is seen in nearly half of patients with SCLC, whereas, only 10% of NSCLC patients develop paraneoplastic syndromes. The degree of symptoms from paraneoplastic syndromes may be unrelated to the size of the primary tumour or bulk of metastatic disease. However, they can be the pivotal causes of a patient to seek medical attention. On the other hand, because of the disabling effect on patients, these syndromes are clinically important. In addition, these syndromes can be useful markers of tumour activity and are proposed to carry prognostic value (Table **2**) [4].

SCLC patients usually have cachexia, weight loss and fatigue unresponsive to caloric intake. The etiology of this paraneoplastic syndrome is likely multifactorial, involving pro-inflammatory and inflammatory cytokines such as interleukin-1, TNF-alpha, interferon-gamma and hormonal factors [16]. Patients appear to have changed metabolism that results in decreased nutrient intake, increased hepatic gluconeogenesis, failure to efficiently use glucose and increased proteolysis and lipolysis [4,16]. Involved hormones include insulin, corticotropin, epinephrine, growth hormone [17].

Table 2: The paraneoplastic syndromes seen in patients with small cell lung cancer

Syndrome Category	Syndrome
General	Cachexia Depression
Endocrinologic	Cushing Syndrome Secretion of Inappropriate ADH Syndrome (SIADH)
Neurologic	Cerebellar degeneration Optic neuropathies Retinopathy Myotonia Peripheral neuropathy
Hematologic	Anemia Thrombocytosis Thrombosis
Dermatologic	Dermatomyositis Acquired tylosis Trip palms Erythema gyratum repens
Renal	Nephrotic syndrome Glomerulonephritis

SCLC cells are usually associated with the production of protein hormones or precursors to these hormones. Two proposed mechanisms can explain the production of these hormones. Firstly, mechanisms may be involved with the tumour cells producing ectopic endocrine syndromes derived from amine precursor uptake and deamination [17,18] and secondly, these hormones may not be produced ectopically, but rather represent an increased production of a normal cells influenced by tumour cells [19]. Ectopic adrenocorticotropic hormone (ACTH) can cause Cushing syndrome. This syndrome is mostly associated with SCLC [18]. SCLC cells can convert pro-ACTH to the biologically active ACTH, and in turn, cause the clinical syndrome of weakness, muscle wasting, drowsiness, confusion, edema, hypokalemic alkalosis, and hyperglycemia.

Secretion of Inappropriate ADH Syndrome (SIADH) can be found in 40% of patients with SCLC [20]. It is associated with hyponatremia, hypovolemia, increased loss of renal sodium, and inappropriately high urine osmolality. This syndrome does not lead to a worse survival and often resolves with effective treatment of SCLC [21] but it can recur with tumour progression.

Although rare, paraneoplastic syndromes of the nervous system can be caused by a systemic autoimmune reaction to an 'onconeural' antigen shared by both the tumour cells and the nervous system [22]. Lambert-Eaton myasthenic syndrome(LEMS) can be seen 3% of patients with SCLC [23]. This syndrome is associated with antibodies against voltage-gated calcium channels (VGCC) in the presynaptic neurons. Decreased calcium entry into the cell causes to decreased acetylcholine release, leading to pure motor neuropathy characterized by muscular weakness. The patients with this syndrome also present with autonomic dysfunction such as dry mouth, impotence, constipation and blurred vision.

Paraneoplastic cerebellar degeneration (PCD) can lead to ataxia, dysarthria, and dysphagia. This syndrome has been shown to result from autoantibodies against the Purkinje cells of the cerebellum [24]. In patients with PCD have been shown to have circulating anti-Hu antibodies are found [25]. Limbic encephalitis is a paraneoplastic effect consisting of memory failure, seizures, and agitation. SCLC patients may also have myotonia associated with spontaneous and continuous muscle fiber activity causing stiffness and cramping.

Cancer-related anemia is usually characterized by a normochromic or hypochromic morphology with low serum iron, but with increased bone-marrow iron stores and ferritin. It is associated with cytokines such as TNF-alpha and interleukin-1 [26]. Oncologic treatment of SCLC may reverse the anemia, but generally erthrocyte transfusion and/or recombinant erythropoietin are required due to suppressed erythropoietin levels.

Thrombocytosis can be observed in SCLC patients. Interleukin-6 has been shown to stimulate production of platelets *in vivo* and *in vitro*, and patients with cancer have been observed to have elevated serum levels of IL-6 [27]. Venous thrombosis can be seen in patients with SCLC. However, there is no clear link between thrombocytosis and the higher risk of venous thrombosis.

Digital clubbing is not a common sign of SCLC. Circulating vasodilators have been postulated as one underlying mechanism [28]. Polymyositis can be diagnosed in patients with SCLC. It is characterized by muscle pain, weakness. Polymyositis can be found a priori before the clinical manifestation of the disease.

Relatively rare paraneoplastic dermatologic findings include erythema gyratum repens, tylosis and dermatomyositis [29]. Tripe palms are tickened palms with the fingers associated with velvety texture [4]. This sign can be found in patients with acanthosis nigricans. Pruritus can be very troublesome.

Another rare renal manifestatitons of SCLC as paraneoplastic syndromes include nephrotic syndrome and glomerulonephritis [30]. Although the incidence is rare, smokers with idiopathic renal disorder should be evaluated for an underlying malignancy.

As conclusion, the clinician must be mostly aware of the diverse signs and symptoms of patients presenting with SCLC, including those related to the local tumour, regional invasion of disease to the surrounding structures, distant spread of cancer, and general symptoms or paraneoplastic syndromes that affect these patients.

IV. Staging of Small Cell Lung Cancer

Similar to other cell types, small cell lung cancer, the anatomic extent of disease or stage is second in importance only to being small cell type as histology. Accurate staging provides prognostic information and stage aids in the planning of treatment strategies for all types of lung cancer. The first staging system for SCLC was introduced in the 1950s by the Veterans' Administration Lung Study Group [31]. This simple system classifies SCLC into two disease subgroups named "Limited" and "Extensive" Disease. Limited Disease (LD) is defined by tumours confined to one hemithorax, although local extension and ipsilateral, supraclavicular nodes could also be present if they could be encompassed in the same radiation portal as the primary tumour. No extrathoracic metastases were allowed in the LD category. All other patients were classified as extensive disease (ED). Despite conterversial opinions mostly derived from thoracic surgeons, authorities have not changed this primitive staging system for SCLC [32].

Strangely enough, the tumour, node, metastasis (TNM) staging systems of the American Joint Committee on Cancer Staging (AJCC) [33] and the Union Internationale Contre le Cancer (UICC) [34] are defined to be applicable to SCLC, but they have been used very frequently in clinical practice because patients with SCLC seldom present at a stage for which surgery is appropriate and oncologists anonymously refused to stratify the patients according to these comprehensive staging systems.

The IASLC has established a database containing staging, treatment, and follow-up data for more than 100,000 patients with lung cancer from around the world, presenting between 1990 and the end of 2000. Among these are more than 12,000 cases of SCLC, including 349 cases treated by surgery [35]. The IASLC data-base was established to assess the current stage categories as defined by the AJCC [34] and the UICC, 6th edition [34] with the goal of redefining and regrouping the T, N, and M descriptors and to make recommendations for change if and where appropriate. These analyses were performed initially on the large 67,725 patient NSCLC database [36, 37] and then applied to the smaller SCLC cohort. Proposed changes for the UICC, 7th edition, for NSCLC that are relevant for SCLC are mainly those that result in changes to T categories. It has been recommended to subclassify T1 as T1a (<2cm) and T1b (>2cm but <3 cm), to subclassify T2 as T2a (3cm to 5cm or T2b by other factor and >5cm) or T2b (>=5 cm to <=7 cm) and that large sized tumours >7 cm become T3; additional nodules within the same lobe as the primary tumour also become T3; ipsilateral intrapulmonary nodules in other lobes become T4 and malignant pleural and pericardial effusions become M1 [36,37]Staging subcommittee of the IASLC Lung Cancer Staging Project38 confirms that both clinical and pathologic TNM staging are important in the evaluation and reporting of clinical and surgical stage of SCLC. The proposals made by the IASLC for the forthcoming (7th) edition of the TNM system seem to be of relevance for SCLC [35]. Stratification by stages I–III should be incorporated into all clinical trials for early-stage SCLC whether treatment is surgical or not and full details of TNM staging should be reported.

V. Treatment of Small Cell Lung Cancer

A. Chemotherapy

Older active agents including nitrogen mustard, doxorubicin, methotrexate, ifosfamide, etoposide, teniposide, vincristine, vindesine, cisplatin and carboplatin can be used as effective chemotherapeutic drugs [38]. In addition to those new agents such as paclitaxel, docetaxel, totptecan, irinotecan, vinorelbine and gemcitabine were confirmed as therapeutic agents. Table **3** summarizes single agents used for SCLC.

Table 3: Chemotherapeutic Drugs Used as Single Agent

Agent
Paclitaxel
Docetaxel
Topotecan
Irinitecan
Gemcitabine
Vinorelbine
Pemetrexed
Amirubicin

Pemetrexed, as multieffective antifolate agent, was approved for second-line treatment of advanced SCLC [39]. Median survival time (MST) for cisplatin/pemetrexed was 7.6 months, with a 1-year survivor of 33.4% and a response rate of 35%.

A metaanalysis of 36 trials concluded that regimens containing cisplatin and/or etoposide provided a significant survival advantage to patients with SCLC [40]. For this reason, etoposide+cisplatin became the preferred regimen for treating extensive-stage (Stage IV). This regimen can be combined with thoracic radiotherapy. In stage I-IIIB (limited stage) SCLC. Noda and colleagues compared cisplatin and irinotecan to cisplatin+etoposide [41]. Patients treated with cisplatin+irinotecan had a significantly better overall response rate, survival and 1-year survival compared to those treated with etoposide+cisplatin (84.4% *vs.* 67.5% 1-year survival. Irinitecan +cisplatin administration led to higher rate of grades 3 and 4 diarrhea, whereas, etopposide+cisplatin caused a higher rate of myelosuppression. A European study reported superior survival for irinotecan plus carboplatin; however, survival in both treatment groups was less than 9 months [42]. The GALES study (Global Analysis of Pemetrexed in SCLC Extensive Stage) showed the inferiority of pemetrexed (500 mg/m^2) plus carboplatin (AUC=5) to etoposide and carboplatin and was terminated prematurely [43]. In summary, platinum plus etoposide remains the standard of care for the treatment of SCLC.

Dose-escalation: Hande and colleagues [44] randomized patients with Etoposid plus doxorubicin SCLC to high dose or low dose methotrexate with leucovorin rescue in combination with cyclophosphamide, doxorubicin, and vincristine alternating with cycles of VP-16, vincristine, and hexamethylmelamine (negative study). They observed both a higher overall response rate and prolonged survival in the high-dose chemotherapy group. Long-term survivors were observed only among those patients given high-dose chemotherapy. As conclusion, the majority of trials implementing a dose intensification strategy did not produce a survival advantage over standard therapy for patients with extensive stage SCLC and were typically associated with greater toxicity. This approach should not be used in extensive disease. In limited stage-SCLC, the optimal drug doses remain unknown with several studies suggesting a possible benefit.

Alternating Non-Cross Resistant Chemotherapy

In order to obtain maximal antitumour effects using multiple active agents, they should be administered simultaneously at their optimal single-agent dose. Carboplatin (C), Adriamycin (A) and Vincristine(V) and cisplatin(P) plus etoposide(E) are found to be highly active against SCLC. However, considering published data; alternating newer and/or older cytotoxic agents to overcome drug resistance is unsuccessful and should not be pursued.

The ideal number of chemotherapy cycles in SCLC has not been clearly defined. A metaanalysis of the 14 randomized trials [45] suggests that the odds ratios for 1- and 2-year OS rates were both 0.67 ($p<0.001$) favoring prolonged treatment. Significant odds ratios for the 1- and 2-year PFS rates also support the role for consolidation and/or maintenance treatment. In general, chemotherapy after four to six cycles of a combination regimen is not necessary. Further evaluation of this strategy should based on molecularly targeted agents.

Second-Line Chemotherapy

Despite a high response rate, the majority of patients will progress or recur. The mean survival of these patients is approximately 2 months. An elegant study showed survival benefit in patients administered additional therapy [46]. A survival benefit was seen regardless of the timing of the relapse and patients receiving additional therapy. In the multivariate analyses, second-line therapy was an independent predictor of survival. Oral topotecan can be used for second-line treatment in patients with sensitive relapse based on symptom control. The most common toxicities with oral topotecan were neutropenia, thrombocytopenia and anemia. Oral topotecan was also approved by the Food and Drug Administration (FDA) for the treatment of both sensitive and resistant/refractory patients. An international phase III trial of amirubicin *versus* topotecan is ongoing despite the fact that amirubicin has produced impressive results in both sensitive and resistant/refractory patients.

Biologic Response Modifiers

Numerous studies demonstarted that, SCLC is characterized with neuropeptide autocrine growth loops [47]. As a tyrosine inhibitor against c-kit, imatinib were shown to inhibit SCLC *in vitro*. However, clinical studies failed to show a beneficial effect [48,49].

The matrix metalloproteinases (MMPs) are a family of degradative enzymes associated with tumour cell invasion of the basement membrane and stroma, blood vessel penetration, angiogenesis, and metastasis [50]. MMP expression in SCLC was found to be as high as 89% in one study and increased expression some MMPs were reported to be associated with shorter survival [51]. However, studies regarding MMP inhibitors resulted no survival advantage in survival groups.

Interferons, other immunomodulatory agents or apoptotic modulator were not shown to provide positive results in humans.

Inhibition of mTOR decreases the translation of a number of proteins regulating cell cycle [52]. CCI-779, a MTOR inhibitor was shown to increase the median survival time from 6.6 to 9.5 months without a major toxicity [53].

In a phase II study using humanized monoclonal antibody Bevacizumab in addition to carboplatin and irinotecan a 78% response rate was recorded [54]. In an another study, administering bevacizumab plus carboplatin plus radiation followed by bevacizumab maintenance showed a 2-year progression-free survival rate of 70% and 53% and a 1- and 2-year overall survival rate of 38% and 29% in 60 patients.

Other angiokinases inhibitors sorafenib (tyrosine kinase inhibitor of RAF and VEGFR), sunitinib, cediranib, vandetanib (tyrosine kinase inhibitor of VEGFR and EGFR) were found to have promising therapeutic activities. However, there is not enough evidence to advocate their use in clinical setting.

There is no evidence at this time that such therapies will replace conventional thoracic irradiation and chemotherapy. Indeed, new drugs are most likely to prosper when combined with an optimally integrated chemoradiation package. Because advances in the treatment of LSCLC over the past 20 years have largely been associated with innovations of radiotherapy, molecularly targeted therapy should focus on enhancement of radiotherapy as well as systemic therapy. Because accelerated repopulation is a major mechanism of treatment failure in cancer medicine, the molecular basis of this phenomenon must be elucidated. It seems probable that the mechanism will involve hypoxia targets, growth factors, and their receptors.

Conclusions of Chemotherapy

Chemotherapy definitely prolongs survival in patients with SCLC. Four to six cycles of a platinum doublet or an anthracycline-based combination should be offered to patients including the elderly and PS2 patient. More studies regarding new drugs such as agents for targeted therapy are needed.

B. Combination Therapies

Studies showed significantly superior survival for thoracic irradiation and adjuvant chemotherapy when compared with radiotherapy alone. The median survival for patients with LSCLC treated by radiotherapy alone was consistently about 5 to 6 months [55, 56]. Two additional randomized controlled trials [57, 58] showed some advantage for combined modality therapy, but the survival differences between the groups were not statistically significant, probably because many patients in the radiotherapy arms received chemotherapy at the time of disease progression. In an analysis of treatment factors contributing to long-term survival, it was concluded that concurrent chemotherapy and radiotherapy achieved better local tumour control than sequential therapy. These data infer that if the duration of concurrent therapy is prolonged longer than 3 weeks, the enhanced survival and local tumour effect were lost in a flood of treatment-induced toxicity.

Concurrent thoracic radiotherapy with chemotherapy containing cyclophosphamide, methotrexate, and lomustine was superior to chemotherapy given alone [59] with higher rates of remission and prolonged survival in patients with limited stage SCLC, but the benefit was offset by unacceptable pulmonary toxicity. Similarly, concurrent cyclophosphamide, etoposide, and vincristine and radiotherapy have demonstrated superiority to chemotherapy alone, but unacceptable chemotherapy attenuation from myelosuppression was associated with combined therapy [60].

In SCLC, chemotherapy must be delivered at full dose metaanalyses of randomized trials comparing early *versus* delayed thoracic irradiation in LSCLC consistently show superiority of early thoracic irradiation [61, 62].

There is no evidence at this time that such therapies will replace conventional thoracic irradiation and chemotherapy. Indeed, new drugs are most likely to prosper when combined with an optimally integrated chemoradiation package. Because advances in the treatment of limited stage SCLC over the past 20 years have largely been associated with innovations of radiotherapy, molecularly targeted therapy should focus on enhancement of radiotherapy as well as systemic therapy. Because accelerated repopulation is a major mechanism of treatment failure in cancer medicine, the molecular basis of this phenomenon must be elucidated.

C. Elective Cranial Irradiation in SCLC

SCLC the risk of early hematogenous dissemination, its marked radiosensibility and chemosensibility but also its particular propensity to disseminate in the brain. Brain metastases may occur in 50% to 80% of 2-year survivors; in patients who achieve a complete response, the incidence of cerebral metastasis as sole site of initial relapse varies between 14% and 45% at 2 years.Chemical agents have had a limited role in the treatment of cerebral metastases because of the inability of cytostatic drugs to cross the blood-brain barrier, of cerebral microvessels. However, some studies declared efficacy of chemotherapy alone, with response rates on brain metastases ranging from 40% to 76% [63,64,65]

Since brain metastases are frequent and difficult to treat, accompanied by distressing and sometimes life-threatening symptoms, prophylactic treatment seems a good alternative.

It has been shown with metaanalysis that [66, 67], elective cranial irradiation (or prophylactic cranial irradiation) should be done in patients with limited (Stage I-III) or extensive disease (stage IV).

The selection of an optimal dose for elective cranial irradiation that would lead to further decrease brain metastasis incidence with minimal toxicity is one of the challenges raised by the metaanalysis as well the ideal timing. Among patients with extensive disease, a recent EORTC trial has shown that indications of PCI should be enlarged to all responders, as the 1-year rate of symptomatic metastases is decreased from 40.4% to 14.6%, with a significant impact on survival [68].

Despite the effect of irradiation on cognitive functions, it should be considered as part of the standard treatment of SCLC patients in complete remission. For patients with extensive disease, it should be performed for all responders.

ROLE OF SURGERY

Despite the fact that, a very small fraction of patients with SCLC survived longer than 5 years compared with 15 to 25% of non-SCLC patients. The discrepancy can be explained by the biologic behaviour of SCLC, which results in dissemination to regional lymph nodes and/or distant metastatic sites in more than 90% of patients at initial presentation, thereby precluding surgery. Even patients with apparently “limited-stage” or “operable” tumours probably have micrometastatic deposits at distant sites, which have the potential to proliferate if only local therapeutic modalities, such as surgery or radiotherapy, are used.

In the 7th staging initiative undertaken by the International Association for the Study of Lung Cancer (IASLC), there were 12,620 cases of SCLC in the database [35,69] with complete tumour, node, and metastasis [TNM] staging information. Five-year survival rates for clinically staged patients with stages IA and IB tumours were 38% and 21%, respectively [69]. Interestingly, 5-year survival rates for stages IIA and IIB were similar at 38% and 18%, respectively. It has long been recognized that clinical staging does not correlate with pathologic staging. The IASLC staging project also had complete pathologic TNM staging information for 349 cases of SCLC who had undergone surgical resection [35] making this the largest SCLC surgical series reported to date. Surgically treated SCLC represented only 1.3% of all fully staged resected cases in the database and only 2.8% of all SCLC cases. Concordance between clinical and pathologic TNM staging was only 58%. Five-year survival rates for pathologically staged patients with stages IA and IB tumours were 53% and 44%, respectively, and 43% and 35%, respectively, for stages IIA and IIB.

Yu and colleagues [70] have presented the results of their analysis of 247 patients from the National Cancer Institute Surveillance Epidemiology and End Results (SEER) database who underwent surgical resection for SCLC between 1988 and 2004. Of 205 patients with stage I SCLC who required only lobectomy, the 5-year survival rate was 50.3%, virtually identical to that reported by Vallieres *et al.* [35] from the IASLC analyses. Yu and colleagues concluded that, surgery without radiotherapy reasonable survival outcomes in patients with stage I SCLC.

Table **4** shows the five-year survival rates by pathological TNM Stage for Resected Patients with SCLC.

Table 4: Five Year Survival Rates of Patients with Completely Resected Small Cell Lung Cancer in IASLC Database [35, 68]

TNM Stage	5- Year Survival Rate According to 6th Staging System (n)	5- Year Survival Rate According to 7th Staging System (n)
IA	53 (68)	56 (55)
IB	44 (91)	57 (45)
IIA	43 (37)	38 (56)
IIB	35 (34)	40 (25)
IIIA	8 (76)	12 (68)
IIIB	21 (33)	0 (12)

There are a number of reasons for why resection of SCLC is inevitable in a thoracic surgical unit.

1- A small fraction of patients undergoing wedge resection for indeterminate nodule with solitary pulmonary nodule have SCLC.

2- Some tumours with preoperative diagnosis of non-small cell lung cancer could have small cell tumour due to the heterogeneity of all solid tumours.

The average 5-year survival reported in other series for stage I SCLC after resection is 52% (range 37–76%) [70-75] which is quite comparable with the SEER data. The Veterans Administration Surgical Oncology Group reported on 148 patients who underwent a potentially "curative" resection, and noted that resection was definitely indicated in patients with T1N0 disease, with a 5-year survival rate of 59.9% [14]. A prospective multimodality trial showed a 100% local control rate in patients who had neoadjuvant chemotherapy (cisplatin/etoposide) followed by surgery in initially localized disease [21]. However, as noted previously, the only modern randomized trial that we are aware of comparing surgery followed by radiotherapy to radiotherapy after induction chemotherapy did not support the use of surgery [76]. However, in this relatively early study, authors did not report the utilized staging modalities. Also, the patient series included very early cases from non-CT era.

A number studies investigated the role of induction therapy before surgical resection [75, 77-81] (Table **5**). In all studies, complete pathological response varied between 5-37%. A complete resection could be achieved in 55-100% of patients following chemotherapy [82, 83].

Table 5: Results of Studies on Induction Chemotherapy in Resected SCLC Patients. (C: Cisplatin, A: Adriamycin, V: Vepeside, E: Etoposide)

Study	n	Chemotherapeutic Agents	Stage I	Stage II	Stage III	Resection/ Complete resection (%)	Patients with complete pathological response (%)
Prager, 1984 (78)	39	C,A,V,E x2-4	2	12	25	11/8 (88)	2(5)
Williams, 1987 (79)	38	C,A,E x 3	-	-	-	25/21 (55)	4(11)
Baker, 1987 (80)	37	C,A,E x2	-	-	-	20/20 (54)	2(5)
Shepherd, 1987 (81)	72	C,A,V x6 ± E,P	21	16	35	38/33 (36)	3(4)
Eberhart, 1999 (74)	82	E,P (IIB and upper: 2x/d XRT)	6	6	34	32/23 (50)	11(22)

Patients with early-stage SCLC (T1–2 N0 and perhaps even stage II) or "very limited" to use a phrase coined by the University of Toronto Thoracic Oncology Group may benefit from a combined modality approach that includes surgery. However, very few patients fall into this subgroup (less than 1% of all SCLC patients). Since nodal status is of pivotal importance in survival, all patients should undergo routine mediastinoscopy before resection. All studies regarding resection suggest lobectomy as maximal resection.

ACKNOWLEDGEMENTS

Declared none.

CONFLICT OF INTEREST

The author confirms that this article content has no conflict of interest.

REFERENCES

[1] Jemal A, Siegel R, Xu J, Ward E. Cancer Statistics. CA Cancer J Clin. 2010;60:277-300.

[2] Argiris A, Murren JR. Staging and clinical prognostic factors for small-cell lung cancer. Cancer J 2001;7:437– 447.

[3] Bernard WG. The nature of 'oat-celled sarcoma' of the mediastinum J Pathol 1926;29:241-44.

[4] Franklin WA, Noguchi M, Gonzalez A. Molecular and cellular pathology of lung cancer. In:Principles and Practice of Lung Cancer. eds: Pass HI, Carbone DP, Johnson DH, Minna JD, Scagliotti GV, Turrisi AT. Fourth edition.Wolters Kluwer/Lippincott Williams and Wilkins, Philadelphia, 2010,p.287-324.

[5] Steenland K. Epidemiology of occupation and coronary heart disease: research agenda. Am J Ind Med 1996;30(4):265-71.

[6] Kargi A, Gurel D, Tuna B. The diagnostic value of TTF-1, CK 5/6, and p63 immunostaining in classification of lung carcinomas. Appl Immunohistochem Mol Morphol 2007;15:415-420.

[7] Boldrini L, Ursino S, Gisfredi S, *et al.* Expression and mutational status of c-kit in small cell lung cancer: prognostic relevance. Clin Cancer Res. 2004;10:4101-4108.

[8] Whang-Peng J, Kao-Shan CS, Lee EC, et. al. Specific chromosome defect associated with human small cell lung cancer;deletion 3p (14-23). Science 1982;215;181-182.

[9] Soni MK, Cella DF, Master GA, *et al.* The validity and clinical utility of symptom monitoring in advanced lung cancer: a literature review. Clin Lung Cancer 2002;4:1-2.

[10] Chute CG, Greenber EG, Baron J, *et al.* Presenting conditions of 1539 population based lung cancer patients by cell type and stage in New Hampshire and Vermont. Cancer 1985;56:2107-2111.

[11] Lynch TJ. Management of malignant pleural effusion. Chest 1993;103(Suppl 4):S385-S389.

[12] Fincher RE. Superior vena cava syndrome: Experience in a teaching hospital. South Med J 1987;80:1243-45.

[13] Nathanson L, Puccio M. The cancer cachexia syndrome. Semin Oncol 1997;24:277-287.

[14] Pederson AG. Diagnosis of CNS metastases from SCLC. In:Hansen HH, ed. Lung Cancer: Basic and Clinical Aspects. Boston: Martinus Nijhoff, 1986:153-182.

[15] Potti A, Schel DA. Unusual presentations of thoracic tumours:case I. Acute adrenal insufficiency due to metastatic lung cancer. J Clin Oncol 2001;19:3780-82.

[16] Macdonald N. Cancer cachexia and targeting chronic inflammation: a unified approach to cancer treatment and palliative/supportive care. J Support Oncol 2007;5(4):152-62.

[17] Landstein HN, Norton JA. Mechanism of cancer cachexia. Hematol Oncol Clin North Am. 1991;5:103-123.

[18] Yellin A, Benfield JR. The pulmonary Kulchitsky cell (neuroendocrine) cancers: from carcinoid to small cell carcinomas. Curr Probl Cancer 1985;9:1-38.

[19] Odell WD. Endocrine/metabolic syndromes of cancer. Semin Oncol 1997;24:299-317.

[20] Gilby ED, Rees LH, Bondy PK. Ectopic Hormones as Markers of Response to Therapy in Cancer. Advances in Tumour Prevention, Detection and Characterization, Vol. 3. Proceedings of the 6th International Symposium on Biological Characterization of Human Tumours. New York: Elsevier, 1976:132.

[21] List AF, Hainsworth JD, Davis BW, *et al.* The syndrome of inappropriate secretion of antidiuretic hormone (SIADH) in small cell lung cancer. J Clin Oncol 1986;4:1191–1198.

[22] Dalmau JO, Posner JB. Paraneoplastic syndromes affecting the nervous system. Semin Oncol 1997;24:318–328.

[23] Erlington GM, Murray NM, Spiro SG, *et al.* Neurological paraneoplastic disorders in patients with small cell lung cancer: a prospective survey of 150 patients. J Neurol Neurosurg Psychiatr 1991;54:764–767.

[24] Lieberman FS, Schold SC. Distant effects of cancer on the nervous system. Oncolog 2002;16:1539–1548.

[25] Gultekin SH, Rosenfeld MR, Voltz R, *et al.* Paraneoplastic limbic encephalitis: neurological symptoms, immunological findings, and tumour association in 50 patients. Brain 2000;123:1481–1494.

[26] Spivak JL. Cancer-related anemia: its causes and characteristics. Semin Oncol 1994;21(Suppl 3):3–8.

[27] Gastl G, Plante M, Finstead CI, *et al.* High IL-6 levels in ascitic fluid correlate with reactive thrombocytosis with epithelial ovarian cancer. Br J Hematol 1993;83:433–441.

[28] Schneerson JM. Digital clubbing and hypertrophic osteoarthropathy: The underlying mechanisms. Br J Dis Chest 1981;75:113-131.

[29] Sigurgeirsson B, Lindelof B, Edhag O, *et al.* Risk of cancer in patients with dermatomyositis and polymyositis: A population based study. N Engl J Med 1992;326:363–367.

[30] Wagrowska-Danilewicz M, Danilewicz M. Glomerulonephritis associated with malignant diseases of non-renal origin. A report of three cases and a review of the literature.Pol J Pathol 1995;46(3):195-8.

[31] Zelen M. Keynote address on biostatistics and data retrieval. Cancer Chemother Rep 3 1973;4:31– 42.

[32] Stahel R, Ginsberg RJ, Havemann K, *et al.* Staging and prognostic factors in small cell lung cancer: a consensus report. Lung Cancer 1989;5:119 –126.

[33] Greene FL, Compton CC, Fritz AG, Shah JP, Winchester DP, (Eds.). American Joint Committee on Cancer Staging Atlas. Chicago, IL: Springer, 2006. Pp. 167–176.

[34] Sobin LH, Wittekind C, (Eds.). UICC: TNM Classification of Malignant Tumours, 6th Ed. New York, NY: Wiley, 2002.

[35] Valiieres E, Shephard FA, Crowley J, Van Houtte P, Postmus PE, Carney D, Chansky K, Shaikh Z, Goldstraw P on behalf of the International Association for the Study of Lung Cancer International Staging Committee and Participating Institutions.The IASLC proposals regarding the pathologic staging of small cell lung cancer in the forthcoming(seventh) edition of the tumour node, metastasis classification for lung cancer J Thorac Oncol 2009;4:1049-1059.

[36] Rusch V, Crowley JJ, Goldstraw P, *et al.* International Staging Com- mittee; Cancer Research and Biostatistics; Observers to the Committee; Participating Institutions. The IASLC Lung Cancer Staging Project: proposals for revision of the N descriptors in the forthcoming (7th) edition of the TNM classification for lung Cancer. J Thorac Oncol 2007;2:603– 612.

[37] Postmus PE, Brambilla E, Chansky K, *et al.* International Association for the Study of Lung Cancer International Staging Committee; Cancer Research and Biostatistics; Observers to the Committee; Participating Institutions. The IASLC lung cancer staging project: proposals for revision of the M descriptors in the forthcoming (7th) edition of the TNM classification of lung cancer. J Thorac Oncol 2007;2:686 – 693.

[38] Argiris A, Murren JR. Advances in chemotherapy for small cell lung cancer: single-agent activity of newer agents. Cancer J 2001;7:228–235.

[39] Jalal S, Ansari R, Govindan R, *et al.* Pemetrexed in second line and be-yond small cell lung cancer: a Hoosier Oncology Group phase II study. J Thorac Oncol 2009;4(1):93–96.

[40] Turrisi AT III, Kim K, Blum R, *et al.* Twice-daily compared with once-daily thoracic radiotherapy in limited small-cell lung cancer treated concurrently with cisplatin and etoposide. N Engl J Med 1999;340:265–271.

[41] Noda K, Nishiwaki Y, Kawahara M, *et al.* Irinotecan plus cisplatin compared with etoposide plus cisplatin for extensive small-cell lung cancer. N Engl J Med 2002;346:85–91.

[42] Hermes A, Bergman B, Bremnes R, *et al.* A randomized phase III trial of irinotecan plus carboplatin *versus* etoposide plus carboplatin in pa-tients with small cell lung cancer, extensive disease (SCLC-ED): IRIS-Study. J Clin Oncol 2007;25(390s): abstract 7523.

[43] Socinski MA, Smit EF, Lorigan P, *et al.* Phase III study of pemetrexed plus carboplatin compared with etoposide plus carboplatin in chemotherapy-naive patients with extensive-stage small-cell lung cancer.

[44] J Clin Oncol 2009;27(28):4787–4792.

[45] Hande KR, Oldham RK, Fer MF, *et al.* Randomized study of high-dose *versus* low-dose methotrexate in the treatment of extensive small cell lung cancer. Am J Med 1982;73:413–419.

[46] Bozcuk H, Artac M, Ozdogan M, *et al.* Does maintenance/consolidation chemotherapy have a role in the management of small cell lung cancer (SCLC)? A Metaanalysis of the published randomized con-trolled trials. Cancer 2005;104:2650–2657.

[47] Froeschl S, Nicholas G, Gallant V, *et al.* Outcomes of second-line chemotherapy in patients with relapsed extensive small cell lung cancer. J Thorac Oncol 2008;3:163–169.

[48] Hodkinson PS, MacKinnon A, Sethi T. Targeting growth factors in lung cancer. Chest 2008;133:1209–1216.

[49] Krystal GW, Honswek S, Litz J, *et al.* The selective tyrosine kinase inhibitor ST1571 inhibits small cell lung cancer growth. Clin Cancer Res 2000;6:3319–3326.

[50] Krystal GW, Honswek S, Litz J, *et al.* The selective tyrosine kinase inhibitor ST1571 inhibits small cell lung cancer growth. Clin Cancer Res 2000;6:3319–3326.

[51] Nelson AR, Fingleton B, Rothenberg ML, *et al.* Matrix metallo-proteinases: biologic activity and clinical implications. J Clin Oncol 2000;18:1135–1149.

[52] Michael M, Babic B, Khokha R, *et al.* Expression and prognostic sig-nificance of metalloproteinases and their tissue inhibitors in patients with small-cell lung cancer. J Clin Oncol 1999;17:1802–1808.

[53] Raymond E, Alexandre J, Depenbrock H, *et al.* CCI-779, a rapamy-cin analog with antitumour activity: A phase I study utilizing a weekly schedule. Proc Am Soc Clin Oncol 2000;19:187a. abstract 728.

[54] Pandya KJ, Dahlberg S, Hidalgo M, *et al.* A randomized, phase II trial of two dose levels of temsirolimus (CCI-779) in patients with extensive-stage small-cell lung cancer who have responding or stable disease after induction chemotherapy: a trial of the Eastern Cooperative Oncology Group (E1500). J Thorac Oncol 2007;2:1036–1041.

[55] Spigel DR, Greco FA, Zubkus JD, *et al.* Phase II trial of irinotecan, carboplatin, and bevacizumab in the treatment of patients with extensive-stage small-cell lung cancer. J Thorac Oncol 2009;4(12):1555–1560.

[56] Spigel DR, Hainsworth JD, Yardley DA, *et al.* Tracheoesophageal Fistula Formation in Patients With Lung Cancer Treated With Chemoradiation and Bevacizumab. J Clin Oncol 2010;28(1):43-8.

[57] Radiotherapy alone or with chemotherapy in the treatment of small-cell carcinoma of the lung. Medical Research Council Lung Cancer Working Party. Br J Cancer 1979;40(1):1–10.

[58] Petrovich Z, Ohanian M, Cox J. Clinical research on the treatment of locally advanced lung cancer: final report of VALG Protocol 13 Limited. Cancer 1978;42(3):1129–1134.

[59] Perez CA, Krauss S, Bartolucci AA, *et al.* Thoracic and elective brain ir-radiation with concomitant or delayed multiagent chemotherapy in the treatment of localized small cell carcinoma of the lung: a randomized prospective study by the Southeastern Cancer Study Group. Cancer 1981;47(10):2407–2413. 35. Seydel HG, Creech R, Pagano M, *et al.* Combined modality treatment of regional small cell undifferentiated carcinoma of the lung: a coop-erative study of the RTOG and ECOG. Int J Radiat Oncol Biol Phys 1983;9(8):1135–1141.

[60] Bunn PA Jr, Lichter AS, Makuch RW, *et al.* Chemotherapy alone or chemotherapy with chest radiation therapy in limited stage small cell lung cancer. A prospective, randomized trial. Ann Intern Med 1987;106(5):655–662.

[61] Perry MC, Eaton WL, Propert KJ, *et al.* Chemotherapy with or without radiation therapy in limited small-cell carcinoma of the lung. New Engl J Med 1987;316(15):912–918.

[62] De Ruysscher D, Pijls-Johannesma M, Vansteenkiste J, *et al.* Systematic review and meta-analysis of randomised, controlled trials of the timing of chest radiotherapy in patients with limited-stage, small-cell lung cancer. Ann Oncol 2006;17(4):543–552.

[63] Fried DB, Morris DE, Poole C, *et al.* Systematic Review Evaluating the Timing of Thoracic Radiation Therapy in Combined Modality Therapy for Limited-Stage Small-Cell Lung Cancer. J Clin Oncol 2004;22(23):4837–4845.

[64] Lee JS, Murphy WK, Glisson BS, *et al.* Primary chemotherapy che-motherapy of brain metastases in small-cell lung cancer. J Clin Oncol 1989;7:916–922.

[65] Kristensen CA, Kristjansen PE, Hansen HH. Systemic chemotherapy of brain metastases from small-cell lung cancer: a review. J Clin Oncol 1992;10:1498–1502.

[66] Pignon JP, Arriagada R, Ihde DC, *et al.* A meta-analysis of thoracic radiotherapy for small-cell lung cancer N Engl J Med 1992;327(23):1618–1624.

[67] Aupérin A, Arriagada R, Pignon JP, *et al.* Prophylactic cranial irradia-tion for patients with small cell lung cancer in complete remission. Cranial Iradiation Overview Collaborative Group. N Engl J Med 1999; 341: 476–484.

[68] Le Péchoux C, Senan S, Quoix E, *et al.* Initial results from an inter-group phase III trial evaluating two different doses of prophylactic cranial irradiation (PCI) in patients with limited small cell cancer (SCLC) in complete remission (PCI99-01, IFCT 99-01, EORTC 22003–08004, RTOG 0212). J Thorac Oncol 2007;2(suppl 4):S389–S390.

[69] Shepherd FA, Crowley J, Van Houtte P, *et al.* The International Asso- ciation for the Study of Lung Cancer lung cancer staging project: proposals regarding the clinical staging of small cell lung cancer in the forthcoming (seventh) edition of the tumour, node, metastasis classifica- tion for lung cancer. J Thorac Oncol 2007;2:1067–1077.

[70] Yu JB, Decker RH, Detterbeck F, *et al.* Surveillance epidemiology and end results evaluation of the role of surgery for stage I small cell lung cancer. J Thora Oncol 2010;5:215–219.

[71] Badzio A, Kurowski K, Karnicka-Mlodkowska H, *et al.* A retrospective comparative study of surgery followed by chemotherapy *vs.* non-surgical management in limited-disease small cell lung cancer. Eur J Car- diothorac Surg 2004;26:183–188.

[72] Lucchi M, Mussi A, Chella A, *et al.* Surgery in the management of small cell lung cancer. Eur J Cardiothorac Surg 1997;12:689 – 693.

[73] Shepherd FA, Ginsberg RJ, Feld R. Surgical treatment for limited small-cell lung cancer. The University of Toronto Lung Oncology Group experience. J Thorac Cardiovasc Surg 1991;101:385–393.

[74] Shields TW, Higgins GA Jr, Matthews MJ, *et al.* Surgical resection in the management of small cell carcinoma of the lung. J Thorac Cardio- vasc Surg 1982;84:481– 488.

[75] Eberhardt W, Stamatis G, Stuschke M, *et al.* Prognostically oriented multimodality treatment including surgery for selected patients of small- cell lung cancer patients stages IB to IIIB: long-term results of a phase II trial. Br J Cancer 1999;81:1206–1212.

[76] Suzuki R, Tsuchiya R, Ichinose Y. Phase II trial of postoperative adjuvant cisplatin/etoposide (PE) in patients with completely resected stage I-IIIA small cell lung cancer (SCLC) (abstract). Proc Am Soc Clin Oncol 2000;19(492a):abstract 1925.

[77] Brock MV, Hooker CM, Syphard JE, *et al.* Surgical resection of limited disease small cell lung cancer in the new era of platinum chemotherapy: its time has come. J Thorac Cardiovasc Surg 2005;129:64–72.

[78] Lad T, Piantadosi S, Thomas P, *et al.* A prospective randomized trial to determine the benefit of surgical resection of residual disease following the response of small cell lung cancer to combination chemotherapy. Chest 1994;106:320S–323S.

[79] Prager RL, Foster JM, Hainsworth JD, Hande KR, Johnson DH, Wolff SN, Greco FA, Bender HW. The feasibility of adjuvant surgery in limited-stage small cell carcinoma: a prospective evaluation. Ann Thorac Surg 1984;38(6):622-6.

[80] Williams CJ, McMillan I, Lea R, Mead G, Thompson J, Sweetenham J, Herbert A, Jefferys M, Buchanan R, Whitehouse JM. Surgery after initial chemotherapy for localized small-cell carcinoma of the lung. J Clin Oncol 1987;5(10):1579-88.

[81] Baker RR, Ettinger DS, Ruckdeschel JD, Eggleston JC, McKneally MF, Abeloff MD, Woll J, Adelstein DJ. The role of surgery in the management of selected patients with small cell carcinoma of the lung. J Clin Oncol 1987;5(5):697-702.

[82] Shepherd FA, Evans WK, Feld R, Young V, Patterson GA, Ginsberg R, Johansen E.Adjuvant chemotherapy following surgical resection for small cell carcinoma of the lung. J Clin Oncol 1988;6(5):832-8

[83] Brock MV, Hooker CM, Syphard JE, Westra W, Xu L, Alberg AJ, Mason D, Baylin SB, Herman JG, Yung RC, Brahmer J, Rudin CM, Ettinger DS, Yang SC. Surgical resection of limited disease small cell lung cancer in the new era of platinum chemotherapy:Its time has come. J Thorac Cardiovasc Surg 2005;129(1): 64-72.

Send Orders of Reprints at reprints@benthamscience.net

CHAPTER 15

Pain Treatment in Thorax Malignities

Selami Ateş Önal*

Department of Pain, Euphrates University, Elazig, Turkey

Abstract: Acute pain is a form of pain that starts suddenly. Chronic pain arises when pain continues after an acute disease or a reasonable recovery period. This period varies between 1 and 6 months. Visceral pain is an acute pain that develops depending on abnormal functioning or disorder of viscera or their membranes (parietal pleura, pericardia, peritonea). Lung cancer related pain depends on the location of the primary tumour, its regional invasion and metastatic spread. Pain may develop secondarily, depending on the peripheral growth of the primary tumour (spread to pleura or chest wall) or nerve invasion (pain which spreads to the arms or shoulders, known as Pancoast syndrome). While visceral pain is experienced slightly in the ipsilateral hemithorax independent of the regional spread, it may also cause non-specific chest pain symptoms. Pain may be located at the metastasis as with the bone metastases seen in one-third of patients and brain metastases, which progresses with headache and intracranial hypertension.

Keywords: Lung cancer, pain.

The term "pain" derives from the Latin word poena (punishment, torture). According to the definition made by the International Association for the Study of Pain (IASP) in 1976: Pain is an unpleasant sensory and emotional experience associated with actual or potential tissue damage, or described in terms of such damage. It is evident that the subjective, physiological and emotional sides of pain are closely linked. Therefore, a response to a painful stimulant varies between individuals and it may arise at different times in the same person [1].

1. PAIN CLASSIFICATION

1.1. According to Duration

1.1.1. Acute Pain

Acute pain is a form of pain that starts suddenly. In this pain, there is a close relationship between causing lesions and place, time and severity. It starts with

***Address correspondence to Selami Ateş Önal:** Department of Pain, Euphrates University, Elazig, Turkey; Tel: +90 424 2333555/3319; Fax: +90 424 2388096; E-mail: aonal@firat.edu.tr tissue damage and gradually alleviates during the recovery period and finally disappears. Acute pain is almost always nociceptive. It helps protect the organism and to localise and classify the damage. Some symptoms, like tachycardia and hypertension, might be observed, depending on the concomitant autonomic nervous system. Examples of acute pain include postoperative pain, renal colic, myocardial infarction and pancreatitis [1-3].

1.1.2. Chronic Pain

Chronic pain arises when pain continues after an acute disease or a reasonable recovery period. This period varies between 1 and 6 months. A continuous pain for six weeks could be considered as chronic in clinic. A chronic pain might be nociceptive, neuropathic or a mixture of both. There are no autonomic responses in many patients with chronic pain, as in acute pain. However, sleeping disorders and affective disorders are recorded at a considerable level. Many chronic pain types are commonly seen in cases such as musculoskeletal disorders, chronic visceral disorders, peripheral nervous, nerve roots or dorsal root ganglion lesions (causalgia, phantom extremity pain, postherpetic neuralgia), central nervous system (CNS) lesions (paralysis, spinal cord damage, multiple sclerosis) and cancer [1-3].

1.2. Pain Classification according to Anatomical Location

1.2.1. Somatic Pain

Somatic Pain can be classified as superficial and deep. Surface somatic pain develops with stimulants coming from the skin, subcutaneous tissues and mucous membranes. It has a sharp, stinging, shooting and burning quality, which is well localised. Deep somatic pain originates from muscles, tendons, joints or bones. It is obtuse and stinging, which cannot be well localised. [1-3].

1.2.2. Visceral Pain

Visceral pain is an acute pain that develops depending on abnormal functioning or disorder of viscera or their membranes (parietal pleura, pericardia, peritonea). It starts lightly but it is obtuse and stinging and difficult to localise. It may occur as another pain that is referred to other locations. The best known examples are cardiac pain referred to left arm and diaphragmatic pain referred to right arm [1, 2].

1.2.3. Sympathetic Pain

Vascular pain and reflex sympathetic dystrophy are examples of sympathetic pain, which occurs with the activation of the sympathetic nervous system. It is described as a burning pain. Patients complain of coldness and chill at the site of the pain. Dystrophic changes may occur over time [1, 2].

1.3. Pain Classification according to Mechanisms

1.3.1. Deafferentation Pain

These are the forms of pain that occur when the transmission between the peripheral sensorial stimuli or the sensorial stimuli connected to the lesions in CNS and the central nervous system is cut off (phantom pain, post amputation extremity pain) [1].

1.3.2. Reactive Pain

Reactive pain occurs when the nociceptors are stimulated as a result of the reflexive activation of motor or sympathetic afferents. Myofascial pain is an example of this type of pain [3].

1.3.3. Psychosomatic Pain

It is any somatisation or hypochondriasis case which is defined as "pain" arising when psychic and psychosocial problems increase [3]. Although there may exist a painful case, the main concern is psychological. Patients may become increasingly troubled by a trivial tissue problem as their neurophysiologic sensitivity increases.

1.3.4. Nociceptive Pain

Nociceptive pain can be defined as an appropriate physiological response to a painful stimulant. This kind of pain is felt as a physiological response to tissue damage. Pain and sensitivity occur in the damaged tissue and peripheral tissues and the pain lessens during the recovery period. The pain results from normal activation of peripheral nociceptors localised around the damaged tissue from where it is transmitted to the central nervous system *via* normal functioning sensorineural routes. It is transmitted *via* A-delta with myelin and C-fibres without myelin. It is generally believed that nociceptive pain is proportional to the predicted tissue damage. It occurs when physiopathological mechanisms stimulate the nociceptors, which are the pain sensors. Somatic and visceral pain are examples of these kinds of pain. The main difference between somatic and visceral pain is that somatic pain is transmitted *via* sensory fibres and visceral pain is transmitted *via* sympathetic fibres. Muscle and joint pain, cancer pain and tension type headaches are examples of nociceptive pain. Opioid analgesics, non steroidal anti-inflammatory drugs and peripheral nervous denervation are effective in the treatment of nociceptive pain [1, 3].

1.3.5. Neuropathic Pain

Neuropathic pain is defined as a pain that results from a primary lesion and dysfunction of peripheral or central nervous system. As a result of the dysfunction or primary lesion of the central nervous system, it generally arises a long time after the nerve damage, in contrast to inflammatory pain. In contrast to physiological pain, neuropathic pain is characterised by an increased spontaneous pain without any external stimulant and/or against a normally harmless stimulant. Somatosensory system may be stimulated abnormally. Neuropathic pain follows a normal nociceptive pathway and generally starts with direct tissue damage [1, 2, 4].

2. NEUROANATOMY AND NEUROPYHSIOLOGY OF PAIN

2.1. Locations and Systems Used in Pain Transmission

The Pain system should primarily be called the nociceptive system, as pain is a physiological result of nociception [5]. The transmission of a painful stimulant from the periphery to the centre occurs in four steps. These are transduction, transmission, modulation and perception. Recently, expression is addressed *via* the slogan "If you have a pain, make your voice heard". Transduction and transmission have a role in periphery; modulation in medulla spinalis and in periphery; and perception has a role in the supraspinal perception of the pain, in other words, in perception in cerebral cortex [5].

Transduction: It is a mechanism that converts primary afferent neurons in periphery and noxious stimulant in sensory nerve ends into an electrical activity.

Transmission: This is a mechanism that transmits pain information to top centres *via* nociceptors. A-delta with myelin and drC- fibres without myelin (dorsal root C) play an effective role in this transmission. A-beta fibres, which are mainly sensitive to touch sensation, play a role in pain transmission from time to time. Other nerve fibres participate in the transmission of a painful stimulant in various ways. Neural transmission is comprised of 3 components:

a) Primary sensorial afferent neurons transmitted to the spinal cord (neurons in the first place);

b) The brain stem, from the spinal cord and control system neurons, extending to thalamus (neurons in the second place);

c) Thalamocortical projection (neurons in the third place).

Modulation: Modulation occurs mainly in the spinal cord. It is the reduction of transmission *via* descending pain-inhibitory pathways. Various neurons and laminas take place in pain transmission and modulation in the spinal cord dorsal horn. Modulation also occurs in the periphery. This is demonstrated by the determination of endogenous opioids in the damaged tissue.

Perception: Pain is perceived when the stimulant passing through the spinal cord is transmitted, *via* ascending pathways, to the top centres.

Expression: The information assessed in the cerebral cortex is projected and expressed by the person at the injury site, and pain behaviour is exhibited as a result [6].

Based on these phases, the neuroanatomy of nociception can be analysed in 4 parts: the nociceptor and its periphery, spinal cord dorsal horn neurons, ascending nociceptive tracts and antinociceptive tracts.

2.1.1. Nociceptor and its Periphery

The origin of nociceptive processes is primary afferent nociceptors. Under normal conditions, the painful stimulant is transmitted to spinal cords *via* nociceptor fibres. The receptors, which respond to harmful (thermal, mechanic, chemical) stimulants, called nociceptors, have a role in the perception of pain. Afferent nociceptive messages are carried to the dorsal horn of the spinal cord by A-delta and C tendons. A-delta fibres are the thinnest neurons of the sensory afferent neurons containing myelin; their axon diameters range between 2 and 7 μm and transmission speed ranges between 10 and 30 m/sec. C tendons do not have myelin; their diameter ranges between 1 and 5 μm and their transmission speed is less than 2.5 m/sec. They are called mechanothermal nociceptors, as the nociceptors which are the tips of A-delta tendons are activated by thermal and mechanical stimulants; the nociceptors which are the tips of C fibres are called polymodal nociceptors, as they are activated by various stimulants such as mechanical, thermal, chemical, hot and cold stimulants. A stringing, sharp and well-localised pain generally occurs with the stimulation of thin A-delta tendons. The stimulation of drC fibres without myelin causes an obtuse and a non-localised pain. The stimulation of thin A-delta fibres due to tissue damage causes a short-term, localised and sharp pain. A less-localised and long lasting pain and hyperalgesia follow this process; this may last for minutes and hours and even days and months if the stimulant continues.

Bradykinin and serotonin (5-HT) are secreted due to the deformation of membrane permeability as a result of tissue damage. At the same time, the release of P substance and calcitonin-gene related peptide (CGRP) from the sensory tips of nociceptors helps efferent functions to recover in the tissue. Correspondingly, vasodilatation, extravasation from plasma, oedema and macrophage infiltration, which are the indicators of local tissue damage, appear. This course, consisting of nociceptors, is called neurogenic inflammation [1-4].

2.1.2. Spinal Cord Dorsal Horn Neurons

After afferent fibres enter the spinal cord, thick fibres move to the medial, while the thin fibres without myelin move to the lateral. These fibres form the Lissauer tract, which is a thin layer leading from the external surface of the spinal cord by moving a few segments before creating synapses with the neurons in the second row. Rexed defined some structural layers in the spinal cord grey matter in 1954. Dedicated in his name, 10 different Rexed laminas are known today. The first six laminas form the dorsal horn, lamina VII, VIII and IX ventral horn. Lamina X includes the cells encircling the periphery of the spinal cord. Lamina I is the outer layer and is called the marginal zone. Its main function is to receive pain impulses transmitted by A-delta and C fibres. Some neurons in lamina I are only stimulated by nociceptors and are called "nociceptor specific neurons". Nociceptive specific neurons only receive the noxious stimulus, are quiet under normal conditions and respond only to severe stimuli. Lamina II and III are called substantia gelatinosa. Many afferent tendons coming from the skin disappear in this location. There are many bindings between this region and the upper and lower layers. The marginal zone and substantia gelatinosa have important roles in pain transmission. Central terminals of the nociceptive nerve ending form synapses with neurons in these two laminates. Lamina IV receives thick cutaneous afferent tendons, which carry non-noxious impulses originating from small, localised skin areas. The neurons in lamina V receive stimuli from various sources; they appear as visceral and somatic nociception and mechanoreception, which is the predominant function. They are very sensitive to painful stimulants in particular. The neurons in this layer receive stimulus from both nociceptors and low threshold mechanoreceptors and are therefore called "Wide Dynamic Range" neurons. The sensitivity of WDR neurons increases with repeated stimulus and, after time, the same stimulus causes a more intensive reaction (wind-up phenomena). Lamina VI generally receives proprioceptive stimuli. The proprioceptive sense coming from muscles, tendons and joints is transmitted *via* these tendons. Movement activates these layer cells. Cutaneous stimulation is carried to this layer. The neurons in lamina VII and IX participate in ascending tracts, which ensure pain transmission. Lamina X cells are similar to the cells in lamina I and II. They respond to heavy stimulants [1, 2, 4, 5].

2.1.3. Ascending Nociceptive Tracts

Spinothalamic Tract: The spinothalamic tract originates from lamina I, V, VII and VIII neurons and is classically accepted as the most important tract for transmission of pain. The spinothalamic tract is responsible for autonomic responses that develop against painful stimuli and for unpleasant emotional perceptions.

Spinoreticular Tract: The neurons of this tract originate from lamina I, V and VII. This tract is thought to be responsible for autonomous responses against pain.

Spinomesencephalic Tract: This plays an important role in the activation of antinociceptive ascending tracts. The presence of the neurons which have an analgesic effect in periaqueductal grey matter binds the spinomesencephalic tract with this area important in terms of nociception.

Spino-ponto-amigdal System: This starts from lamina I and V in the dorsal root and ascends in the dorsolateral funiculus. It first links to the parabrachial area and then the amygdaloid complex. This system is usually associated with pain and fear memory, which include autonomic and behavioural reactions such as scream, escape, mydriatic and cardiovascular responses.

Postsynaptic Dorsal Colon: The collateral axons of thick afferent tendons ascend in the dorsal root and form a large part of this pathway; the axons of the nociceptive neurons in lamina V also participate and end at the nuclei cuneatus and in gracilis. This pathway is thought to be particularly important in the transmission of visceral pain.

2.1.4. Antinociceptive Tracts (Descending Control System)

An antinociceptive activity arises in the dorsal horn and brain stem against painful stimulants. The spinal cord is under the effect of the ascending tract, which reduces or facilitates the antinociceptive process. It is comprised of the paths originating from descending inhibition brain stem nucleus (periaqueductal field, nucleus raphe magnus) and spinal cord dorsolateral funiculus. This system may suppress the nociceptive information formed by spinal cord dorsal horn interneurons. The enkephalinergic cells in the mesencephalic periaqueductal grey matter are interacted with the cells in nucleus raphe magnus and nucleus reticularis in the medulla, including serotonin. These inhibitor transmitters are conveyed by the tendons of the descending dorsolateral funiculus. These tendons are associated with the interneurons, including enkephalin in gelatinosa. The antinociceptive effects of descending tracts are provided by α_2 adrenergic, serotoninergic and opioid receptor mechanisms. As a result of the stimulation of these receptors, K^+ channels are opened after the activation of intracellular second messengers and the intracellular Ca^{2+} concentration increase is inhibited. The inhibitor originates primarily from adrenergic paths and periaqueductal grey matter and reticular formation. The main neurotransmitter of this path is neuroadrenaline. The effect of this system on dorsal horn nociceptive neurons through dorsolateral funiculus is in the form of an inhibition. In the formation of this effect, α_2 adrenergic receptors have an intermediary role. Another analgesia group is segmental inhibition. In this system, attention is especially paid to spinal enkephalinergic neurons. Enkephalinergic neurons are especially by both C fibres and collaterals coming from A-delta fibres and they inhibit the projection neuron as pre and post synaptic. Glycine and gamma-aminobutyric acid (GABA), which are the inhibitor neurotransmitters, have an important role in segmental inhibition of pain in the spinal cord. Some peripheral and neuropeptides, such as somatostatin and bombesin, which emerge from intermediate neurons, are also thought to have inhibitory effects [1, 2, 4, 5].

2.2. Gate Control Theory

This theory was suggested by Wall and Melzack in 1965, to explain different pain phenomena. According to this theory, stimuli reaching the transmission cells in lamina V of the spinal cord *via* afferent tendons undergo a modulation by the activity of substantia gelatinosa cells in lamina II and III of the dorsal horn. Substantia gelatinosa cells affect the transmission of afferent stimuli to T cells. It blocks the stimulus in A-delta and C-tendon axons in presynaptic field or inhibits it from release of chemical neurotransmitters in presynaptic field and changes the level of perception of the incoming excitatory stimulants. These cells inhibit thick and thin nerve endings. The door mechanism is basically controlled by the activity of A-alpha and A-beta tendons. These stimulate the door cells and prevent the transmission to T cells (the door is closed). In contrast, small fibres enable the door to be open and increase the stimulant transmission, inhibiting door cells. When the stimulant lasts longer, large fibres adapt and small fibres predominate. Accordingly, the door in the spinal cord is opened and the painful stimulant is conveyed to the supraspinal centres through ascending paths [5].

2.3. Neurobiology

2.3.1. Chemical Mediators of Pain

Many neuropeptides and excitatory amino acids mediate the afferent neurons, which transmit pain as neurotransmitters. Many neurons include more than one neurotransmitter, which is secreted simultaneously. A neuron is stimulated by many neurotransmitters a number of times. The molecules that serve as neurotransmitters may show excitatory or inhibitory effects in the transmission and perception of pain [7].

Those which show an excitatory effect can be listed as P material, CGRP, glutamate, aspartate, adenosine triphosphate (ATP), cytokines [Interleukin-1β, Interleukin-6, Tumour Necrosis Factor (TNF)-α] and cholecystokinin (CCK). Glutamate is the most important excitatory amino acid [7, 8].

Those showing inhibitory effects are enkephalins, β-endorphin, norepinephrine (NE), 5-HT, adenosine, somatostatin, acetylcholine, GABA, glycine, galanin, neuropeptide Y, cytokines (interleukin-2) and nociceptive [7, 8].

In recent years, many channels, receptors and regulator proteins have been found in pain pathways. In this context, new pain mechanisms and paths were discovered in the periphery and at a spinal level. Researchers are gradually examining the molecular mechanism of pain. The main research foci can be listed as follows:

As a response to tissue damage, inflammatory mediators secreted from various cell types, including immune system;

The effect of these mediators on the specific receptors in the nociceptive sensory neurons;

The formation of second messengers with the activation of receptors and the activation of phospholipases with the protein kinases;

The role of second messengers in facilitating peripheral sensitisation regulating various receptors and ion channels;

Opening the ion channels as a response to noxious stimulants and start of action potentials in sensory neurons and ensuring their diffusion;

The release of neurotransmitters from central terminals in the spinal cord as a result of the excitation of nociceptive sensory neurons;

Start of central sensitisation with the binding of secreted neurotransmitters with postsynaptic receptors;

Occurrence of unbearable pain as a result of the exaggerated activation of ion channels, receptor and regulator proteins.

2.3.2. Main Molecules and Cascades

2.3.2.1.Bradykinin

Tissue damage and inflammation start the activation of proteolytic kallikreins. Kallikreins reveal the kinins, which include bradykinin among kininogen substrates. Bradykinin is the first inflammation mediator and initiates the pain. Bradykinin is also known as an effective endothelium-dependant vasodilator. The effectiveness of bradykinin is related to the activation of two types of B1 and B2 G-protein receptors. While the B2 receptor is structurally defined, the B1 receptor is defined by inflammation indicators such as tissue damage and nerve growth factor (NGF), cytokines, TNF α, interleukin-1β (IL-1 β). Bradykinin receptors activate phospholipase C β (PLC β) and phospholipase A2 (PLA2) over G-proteins. PLC β starts the activation of protein kinase C (PKC). PKCε, a PKC isozyme, is activated by nerve growth factor (NGF) and increases the tetrodotoxin- resistant (TTX-R) sodium current in sensory neurons as a response to inflammation indicators [9]. PKCε sensitises the capsaicin receptor TRPV1 (vanilloid receptor) with direct phosphorylation. On the other hand, it is ensured that arachidonic acid (AA) among the cell membrane phospholipids is formed with the PLA2 activation and later on the prostanoids such as prostaglandin E2 (PGE2) emerge with the help of cyclooxygenase (COX) [10].

2.3.2.2.COX-2 and Prostaglandins

As the non-steroid anti-inflammatory drugs such as aspirin and ibuprofen (NSAID) ensure COX inhibition, they can be used as painkillers and antipyretics. COX-1 is structural and effective in general in the body. It is also important in gastrointestinal protection. COX-2 is induced by pro-inflammatory cytokines (such as TNF α, IL-1 β) in the inflammation area. PGG2 and PGH2, which are the prostaglandin precursors are formed with the transformation of AA by COX. Subgroup isomerases and oxyreductases catalyse the formation of various prostaglandin isomers such as PGD2, PGE2 and PGI. Prostaglandins stimulate the second messengers such as protein kinase A (PKA) and PKC binding to the G-protein receptors and increase the intracellular Ca^{2+} level [11]. Hence, the sensory neuron excitability also increases. Prostaglandins are also effective on the pre and post-synaptic receptors in the central terminals of sensory neurons in the spinal cord dorsal root. Therefore, the membrane excitability of dorsal root neurons increases and central sensitisation starts.

2.3.2.3. Serotonin (5-HT)

5-HT affects at least 14 different receptors that appear heterogeneously in the tissue after getting released from thromboses. Only the 5-HT3 receptor does not bind to second messenger related G-protein. 5-HT3 receptor causes intracellular Na^{+} entry and neural excitation. While 5-HT3 receptor antagonists have anti-nociceptive effect both in periphery and in dorsal root ganglion (DRG), these antagonists are known to block induced analgesia and to have a moderated hyperanalgesic effect when given intrathecally [12].

The 5-HT1B receptor is found in sensory neurons, spiral cord and in various places within the central neuron system; it inhibits adenylyl cyclase and regulates the release of 5-HT and other transmitters.

2.3.2.4. Adenosine Triphosphate (ATP)

When ATP is injected into the skin as an infusion, it initiates pain over the ATP-sensitive ion channels of the P2X family. To date, 7 P2X subgroups have been identified. Each subgroup has two transmembrane segments, separated from each other by a large ectodomain. ATP is assumed to bind to ectodomain and to increase membrane Ca^{2+} permeability [13]. Among these subgroups, only the P2X3 subgroup is commonly found in the small-scale nociceptive sensory neurons.

Microglial ATP is effective on P2X4 in the dorsal root after tissue damage and stimulates the release of brain-derived neurotrophic factor (BDNF). BDNF affects the neurons and increases intracellular C1 concentration. As a result, GABA, which is an inhibitor transmitter, gains the characteristics of an excitatory transmitter and the normal pain inhibition is cut.

2.3.2.5. Transient Receptor Potential (TRP) Channel

TRP channels have 6 transmembrane areas, such as the voltage-sensitive K^+ channels. These combine as homo- or hetero-tetramers and form action channels. Vanilloid receptor TRPV1, known as a capsaicin receptor, shows increased permeability against Ca^{2+} as a response to the endogen lipids like anandamide. TRPV1 is activated in high temperatures (>43°C) and with a low pH [14]. TRPV1, which is sensitised with ATP and bradykinin can be activated at 30°C. The sensitisation of TRPV1 also occurs with partially PKCε-dependent phosphorylation. Many other TRP channels can be activated in different temperatures (TRPV2>53°C, TRPV3 34-38°C, TRPV4 27-35°C, TRPM8 <28°C, TRPA1<17°C).

2.3.2.6. Nerve Growth Factor (NGF)

Neurotrophins are a family of polypeptide-structured nerve growth factors, which are necessary for the development and maintenance of vertebrate nervous system. These are the first defined brain-derived neurotrophic factors after the NGFs in this family (BDNF). BDNF is basically found in the brain, its objectives are in the central and peripheral nervous system and more than 50% of its molecular structure is identical to that of NGF. The level of NGF in the tissues increases with inflammation, resulting in a hyperalgesic response. NGF can be derived from various places, including Schwann cells, mast cells and macrophages. NGF takes effect through two receptors as $p75^{NTR}$ and tyrosine kinase A (TrkA). The signalisation of these two receptors is known to be synergic, antagonist or independent from each other. Much of the biological activity of NGF is realised by the receptor TrkA. The binding of NGF with the TrkA receptor in the nociceptive sensory neurons activates a part of the tyrosine autophosphorylation and signal transduction channels. These cascades are mainly the paths of mitogen-activated protein kinase (Rap-MAPK, Ras-MAPK), extracellular signal controlled kinase (ERK), phospholipase Cγ (PLCγ) and phosphatidylinositol-3 Kinase (PI3K). The sensitisation of TRPV1 by NGF is explained by such transformations, *i.e.* by post-translational modifications [15].

2.3.2.7. Voltage-Sensitive Ion Channels

2.3.2.7.1. Ca^{2+} Channels

The activation of voltage-sensitive Ca^{2+} channels directly affects the membrane potential and the electrical excitability of the neuron. These channels have a critical role in neurotransmitter release from dorsal root presynaptic terminals. The voltage-sensitive Ca^{2+} channel (Cav2.2) plays a role in the excitability control of damaged sensory neurons [10].

2.3.2.7.2. Na^{+} Channels

Voltage-sensitive Na^{+} channels temporarily open the door for Na^{+} ions and initiate excitability, ensuring the membrane depolarisation of the neurons in pain paths. Nine different channels were determined within alpha sub groups, of which Nav1.3, Nav1.7, Nav1.8 and Nav1.9 have a main role in pain transmission. For example, TTX-R sodium channel, which has the most important role in starting and maintaining the action potential in damage-sensitive sensory neurons, is Nav1.9. Nav1.8 is modulated by many inflammatory mediators, such as PGE2, 5-HT and NGF. When Nav1.8 in sensory neurons is subjected to NGF for a long time, it goes through a functional upper regulation over its transcriptional and post-translational control mechanisms [16]. This is realised by p11, which is a partially new accessory protein. The upper regulation of p11 in sensory neurons is stimulated by NGF and p11 binds directly to the amino terminus of Nav1.8 and provides the translocation of the channel to the plasma membrane and opens new functional channels.

2.3.2.8. Glutamatergic Effect

Glutamate plays a key role in transmitting stimulating information from primary afferent sensory neurons in the synaptic area in the spinal cord to dorsal root neurons. The excitation resulting from tissue and nerve damage in nociceptive sensory neurons starts the continuous glutamate release from the central terminals of these neurons. This glutamate release shows similar effects on postsynaptic glutamate receptors and N-methyl-D-aspartic acid (NMDA) receptors and starts the central sensitisation. Glutamate receptors are also found in the central terminals of primary afferent sensory neurons and control the neurotransmitter release from the primary afferents. Homer1, which is a structural protein, forms an effective stimulation complex connecting to metabotropic glutamate receptors and inositol 1, 4, 5- triphosphate (IP3) receptors in the postsynaptic area and excretes intracellular Ca^{2+} stores, stimulating IP3'ü [17]. Thus, Homer1 is of importance in pain plasticity.

2.3.2.9. Other

In addition to these pain pathways, other mediators, receptors, channels, enzymes and transcription factors also play a role in pain transmission mechanisms. Glutamate, substance P and GCRP make excitatory effects on the central terminals of primary afferent sensory neurons; GABA and glycine are released from interneurons and, when pre- and post-synaptic, bind to their own receptors, and show an inhibitory effect. In addition, opioid receptors modulate Ca^{2+} channel activity and show inhibitory effect in the neuron excitability with the activation of endogen opioids such as β-endorphin and enkephalins. Fos, which is a transcription factor, appears in the nuclei of spinal dorsal root neurons with noxious stimulants. Some neurons respond to nociceptive stimulants, a characteristic which enables detection of these neurons.

Lysophosphatidic acid is known to start Rho-Rho kinase activation by affecting the LPA1 receptor and to be effective in the emergence of neuropathic pain [10].

2.4. Pain and Genetics:

2.4.1. The Effect of Genetics on Pain Sensitivity in Humans

The genetic similarity and psychosocial simplicity that are seen in animal families have facilitated identification of the genetic effects of pain in animals. The technology of mating animals from the same families helps to demonstrate the role of genetics in pain; however, this is not applicable to humans. Investigation of the pain sensitivity relationships based on common genetic variations in humans is very difficult to perform, due to the intra-species differences among humans. There are 7 million common mononucleotide polymorphisms (SNPs) where there is a minor allele frequency that emerges in at least 5% of all the human population; in addition, there are 4 million SNP where 1-5% of MAF coexists [18]. SNPs can be used as genetic factors in high-resolution maps, which help the phenotype related loci, due to their high frequency and vast distributions.

In clinical applications, it may be difficult to bring patient populations together in appropriate groups according to the phenotype characterisations, due to the variety of their etiologies, different clinical presentations and the insufficiency of objective methods used in pain assessment. Experimental pain stimulants created through different mechanisms are suggested as a means to determine pain-sensitivity or pain-insensitivity phenotypes [19].

Association studies of genetic markers such as SNPs and nociceptive functioning studies are the most frequent genetic studies on humans. The polymorphisms in TRPV1-defined genes, which provide nociceptive transduction, or in OPRD1-defined genes, which modulate pain processes, are used in predicting the variations in hot and cold pain sensitivity and in identifying the association differences between pain tolerance and pain perception depending on the species and the type of the stimulants applied [20-22].

Congenital pain insensitivity together with anhidrosis is called hereditary sensory and autonomic neuropathy (HSAN) type IV. HSAN type IV is an example of a mutational change that results in the formation of a group of neuropathies characterised by nociception loss and other sensorial and autonomic abnormalities [23]. Following the analysis of familial data, a new gene was recently defined which causes HSAN type II.

2.4.2. Analgesia Pharmacogenetics

Improving drug efficiency and reducing drug toxicity are the two main objectives of examining the role of genetics in clinical applications [24]. Pharmacogenetics includes the genetic component of individuals' differing responses to drug therapies. The genetic coding of CYP 2D6 is highly polymorphic and varies in many people. CYP is a multigenerational enzyme family that is responsible for the metabolisms of various drugs such as tricyclic antidepressant, codeine, tramadol and dextromethorphan. The desired analgesic effect cannot be obtained in people with a weak metabolism, which inactivates the mutations in the genes where specific CYP is coded. While 10-20 mg nortriptyline daily is enough for a person with a weak metabolism, a 500 mg dose may be required for a person with an ultra fast metabolism, in which this gene is multiple-inherited [25]. Identifying pain mechanisms is an objective for the development of new analgesics. The individual protein that generates and controls the pain focuses on the specific role of cytokines and neurotransmitters in a general approach. Alternative approaches use mRNA series and identify hundreds of genes that change their expressions in sensory neurons after the inflammation.

Optimal pain control will be accomplished by understanding the molecular genetic structures where the dose regimes are calculated and the analgesic medications individualised to suit the genetic characteristics of every person.

3. CHEST PAIN AND ITS CAUSES

The causes of chest pain include complaints related to the lungs, oesophagus and musculoskeletal system in addition to complaints that cause people to attend emergency units, such as acute myocardial infarction and panic attacks (Table **1**).

Table 1: Chest Pain Resulting From Neuropathic, Musculoskeletal Diseases and other Diseases

I.	Primarily neuropathic-origin pain		
	A.	Spinal cord disease (myelopathy)	
	B.	Thoracic spinal nerve root origins or nerve stems lesions (radiculopathy)	
	C.	Former spinal nerve lesions (neuropathy)	
	D.	Intercostal nerve lesions (intercostal neuropathy)	
	E.	Peripheral branch disorders of spinal nerves (peripheral neuropathy)	
II.	Primarily musculoskeletal-origin pain		
	A.	Bone diseases or lesions	
		1.	Thoracic vertebra disease or lesions
		2.	Costa's disease or lesions
		3.	Costal cartilage diseases or disorders
		4.	Sternum disease or disorders
		5.	Sternoclavicular joint disease
	B.	Muscle disorders	
		1.	Myophasial pain syndromes
		2.	Chest pain resulting from other muscle disorders
III.	Skin diseases		
	A.	Burns and other traumas	
	B.	Cicatrises	
	C.	Postoperative pain syndromes	
	D.	Mastodynia	
	E.	Deep axillary abscesses	
	F.	Adiposis dolorosa	
	G.	Anterolateral chest phlebitis	
	H.	Other painful dermatological diseases	
IV.	Chest pain resulting from non-thorax diseases		
	A.	Shoulder and cervical spine disorders	
		1.	Intervertebral disc diseases
		2.	Thoracic outlet syndromes
	B.	Abdominal diseases	

Table 1: contd….

		1.	Inability to defecate
		2.	Gastrointestinal tract disorders
		3.	Biliary tract disease
		4.	Pancreas disease
		5.	Another abdominal visceral disease
	C.	Diaphragm disorders	
		1.	Acute primer diaphragmatitis
		2.	Subphrenic abscess
		3.	Diaphragmatic flutter
V.	Primarily physiologic-origin chest pain		
	A.	Abnormal emotional reactions developing against visceral disease	
	B.	Anxiety syndrome	
	C.	Depression syndrome	
	D.	Conversion reaction	
	E.	Hypochondriasis	
VI.	Psychiatric syndromes		

3.1. The Types of Lung-Dependent Pain

Lung cancer is the most common form of cancer. It may develop with symptoms such as chronic cough, haemoptysis, chest pain, fever, repetitive pneumonia and /or bronchitis, weight loss and fatigue. Cancer-dependent pain may develop directly due to tumour invasion or may develop, secondarily to metastases or in response to pressure on the neural tissue. While a sudden and one-sided chest pain occurs in pneumothorax, there are pain and dyspnoea referred to the abdomen and shoulders.

3.2. The Types of Cardiovascular Pain

In angina pectoris, pain may be felt in the chest, arms, shoulder and back. This pain increases with exercise and decreases with resting. Pain in pericarditis is sharp and stinging and may extend to the shoulders and neck. Pain intensifies when the patient is lying and is alleviated in a sitting or standing position. Pain in dissecting aorta aneurism is sudden and severe. Dissection in ascending aorta causes anterior or posterior chest pain, while dissection in descending aorta mostly causes backache [26]. In addition, aortic stenosis, aortic regurgitation, mitral valve prolapse and hypertrophic cardiomyopathy are painful. Pulmonary emboli develop as a result of the embolisation of the pulmonary artery and its branches with a thrombus and chest pain occurring in more than 90% of the cases. Dyspnoea, tachypnea, haemoptysis, cyanosis, tachycardia, anxiety and syncope may also complete the clinical picture.

3.3. The Types of Gastrointestinal Pain

There is a retrosternal burning pain in esophagitis. Pain may arise due to dysphagia and swallowing. Peptic ulcer pain may spread to the front, lower and middle part of the chest, as in epigastrium. Acute pancreatitis causes the feeling of retrosternal uneasiness, together with a severe epigastric pain. Pain spreads to the left part of the chest and is not affected by effort. It may develop together with severe abdominal muscle spasms, hypotension and hypoventilation. Abdominal organ perforation may result in an inflammation and subfrenic abscess in the diaphragm; and may develop as a sharp and stinging pain in the lower part of the chest which often spreads to the shoulders [27].

3.4. The Types of Neuropathic Pain

Entrapment and damage in the nerves spreading to thorax generally result in neuropathic pain in the chest. In contrast to general opinion, diseases and disorders of the spinal cord may be causes of chest pain, an example of which is thoracic myelopathy. It may cause partial pain in segmental neuralgia in the cutaneous and subcutaneous tissue or sharp, stinging or astringent pain that is frequent and resembles stabbing, depending on the nerve affected. The severity of pain increases at night. The increased intraspinal pressure may intensify the pain during thoracic vertebra movement or coughing, sneezing and straining. Hyperalgesia, hyperaesthesia and hyperpathia may be seen in the affected dermatomes. One or more intercostal nerves may be affected in cases such as a trauma, surgical activity, infection or a compression. Stinging and burning pain occurs in post-thoracotomy and post-mastectomy syndromes. A sharp and burning pain arises in the innervation area of the nerve in intercostal neuralgia. Breathing and thorax movements are painful.

3.5. The Types of Musculoskeletal System Pain

Musculoskeletal pain is the most common form of non-cardiac chest pain (10%). This group includes costovertebral arthritis, rib trauma and its fractures, slippedrib syndrome, costochondritis (anterior chest wall syndrome), Tietze syndrome, costal cartilage tumours and costochondral dislocation.

3.6. Pain Based on Sternum and Its Joints

Partial manubriosternal joint subluxation may develop after an obtuse blow to the sternum. A sharp pain is felt following the trauma or after a long delay, and this pain may spread to a wider area. The trauma and arthritis of the sternoclavicular joint, sternoclavicular hyperostosis, manubriosternal arthritis and xiphoidalgia syndrome are all causes of chest pain.

3.7. Myofascial Pain Syndromes

Such syndromes generally emerge gradually and worsen over time. Definitive diagnosis becomes difficult in cases of sudden emergence. Pain in the left hemithorax may be confused with cardiac ischemia. The severity of pain may range from dull to severe and may cause the patient continual discomfort.

3.8. Muscle Disorders Related Pain

Myotonia, muscle sensitivity and trigger points may emerge in trauma related muscle ruptures. Pain may be dull or persistent. A sudden and short-term pain arises in the periapical area in precordial pain syndrome; no local sensitivity occurs and it does not increase depending on effort [28].

3.9. Pain Related to Mediastinum and Diaphragm Disorders

Chest pain occurs with mediastinal emphysema and mediastinitis. Acute primary diaphragmatitis (Heddron syndrome) causes pain in the lower chest, upper abdomen and shoulders from mild low severity to an unbearable level. Patients complain of pain that spreads from the pericardial area or from any part of the chest to the shoulders in a prolonged diaphragm spasm. This may progress to fainting, perspiration and hypotension and imitates the symptoms of myocardial infarction. In the course of diaphragmatic flutter, short breaths and palpitations develop. Pain starts from the epigastric area and may spread to the neck, shoulders and arms.

3.10. Breast Related Pain

Idiopathic chronic mastalgia may continue for many years without the cause being identified and pain may be cyclic. There is long-term pain in Adiposis dolorosa. The phlebitis that develops as a result of the thrombus of the surface vein in the antero-lateral wall of the thorax is called Mondor's Disease. The painful band in the skin is palpable. Diagnosis requires knowledge of the existence of such a disease in order.

3.11. Non-Thoracic Related Pain

In case of a posterolateral herniation in the cervical disc, pain is deep, stinging and constant in character. Its severity may increase from time to time and it may spread to the arms and shoulders. Coughing, sneezing, straining and lateral flexion may increase the pain. In thoracic outlet syndrome, pain may spread to the chest. In addition, the forms of pain occurring in the visceral organ disorders, which are described above, may also be referred to the thorax.

3.12. Pain Related to Psychological Factors

In the organic chest pain, psychological pain may primarily occur as well as the emotional reactions. When no pathological physical cause is found in chest pain, psychological causes should be considered. Examples include acute anxiety attacks and chronic anxiety [28].

4. CLINICAL ASSESSMENT OF CANCER RELATED PAIN

While the prevalence of pain observed in different cancer stages is approximately 50%, this rises to 74% in the terminal period. Two or more types of cancer related pain arise in the advanced stage in cancer patients; they generally depend on different aetiologies. The severity of pain ranges from mild to severe in 40-50% of patients in the advanced cancer period, and becomes severe or unbearable in 25-30% of patients [29]. The most fatal type of cancer is lung cancer, which is generally diagnosed in the advanced stage [30]. Lung cancer related pain depends on the location of the primary tumour, its regional invasion and metastatic spread. Pain may develop secondarily, depending on the peripheral growth of the primary tumour (spread to pleura or chest wall) or nerve invasion (pain which spreads to the arms or shoulders, known as Pancoast syndrome). While visceral pain is experienced slightly in the ipsilateral hemithorax independent of the regional spread, it may also cause non-specific chest pain symptoms. Pain may be located at the metastasis as with the bone metastases seen in one-third of patients and brain metastases, which progresses with headache and intracranial hypertension. Moreover, pain does not depend on the cancer itself; it may depend on an associated disease like osteoarthritis, as seen in elderly people. The findings of the disease directly affect the quality of life and functional status. Pain is thc primary factor in patient discomfort. In addition, psychological control and spiritual problems also determine quality of life. The World Health Organization (WHO) suggests that more than 80% of cancer related pain can be alleviated. However, relatively high proportions of patients who suffer from cancer pain are not diagnosed or are yet to receive treatment. Pain assessment is of critical importance in managing pain. There are many factors involved, such as the severity of nociceptive pain, the person's perception (analgesia, anxiety, somatisation, and depression), and cultural and personal beliefs.

4.1. Pain Characteristics

The location, extent, the trigger, duration (fixed or at intervals), quality (burning, dull, gnawing, stinging or paroxysmal), increasing factors (movement), decreasing factors (response to analgesics) and simultaneous neurologic changes determine the character of pain as perceived by patients. Pain physiopathology is revealed with the help of these assessments and, thus, the therapy becomes easier.

4.2. Determination of Severity of Pain

The structure of pain is subjective. In determining the severity of pain, patient self-assessment is essential. It is not possible to objectively measure pain. However, it is possible to make an appropriate assessment using esthesiometry and thermography tools. One-dimensional and multi-dimensional assessment scales were developed for this purpose. Within one-dimensional assessment tools, the visual analogue scale (VAS) or numerical rating scale was used (Fig. **1**) to determine pain characteristics. If patient can recognise the numbers or there is difficulty in communication due to language, age or another reason, the numerical rating scale would be more useful.

Visual Analogue Scale - VAS (10 cm)

No pain ---Worst Pain Imaginable

Numerical Rating Scale

No pain -- Worst Pain Imaginable

0	1	2	3	4	5	6	7	8	9	10

Verbal Descriptor Scales

None	No Pain
Mild	Mild
Moderate	Discomforting
Severe	Distressing
Horrible	
Excruciating	

Figure 1: Single Dimensional Assessment Scales for Determining the Severity of Pain.

4.2.1. Multi-Dimensional Assessment

Besides pain, cancer patients may also experience complex symptoms such as fatigue, anorexia, nausea, vomiting, dyspnoea, hypokinesia, depression, anxiety, somnipathy and feeling unwell. Therefore, pain may not be the important compliant of the patient at that time. On the other hand, pain treatment may reveal other symptoms such as nausea and vomiting. Therefore, multi-dimensional assessment methods are important for cancer patients [31]. The assessment method for prostrate patients should be fast, simple, valid, reliable, precise and clinic-related; the Edmonton Symptom Assessment System (ESAS) VAS is commonly used. Other multi-dimensional methods of symptom assessment include Functional Assessment of Cancer Therapy (FACT) and Memorial Symptom Assessment Scale (MSAS). Countries determine their own assessment scales according to specific criteria. The European Organization for Research and Treatment of Cancer (EORTC) core questionnaire (QLQ-C30) and specific module of lung cancer (QLQ-LC13) were developed to assess the specific symptoms of lung cancer and quality of life (QoL). Moreover, the Pain Management Index provides the opportunity to determine the pain level of the patient with the strongest analgesic in order to determine how much pain is controlled by the analgesic [32].

Personal beliefs, cultural background, and psychiatric factors (somatisation) also affect perception and the means of expression. Typically, a multidisciplinary pain treatment team includes a doctor, nurse, pharmacist, physiotherapist, speech therapist, occupational therapist, social trainer, religious functionary, nutritionist and a psychiatric nurse. Therefore, determining the personal assessment and treatment type becomes easier.

It should be noted that, in opioid application, tolerance and timidity against addiction (psychological addiction), fear of side effects, various beliefs and expectations could make the patient reluctant to provide information about his/her pain [6].

4.2.2. Serious Pain Syndromes and Weak Prognostic Factors

The risk factors that make pain treatment difficult in cancer patients include neuropathic pain, breakthrough pain, drug tolerance, psychological disorders, and alcohol and drug addiction. The response of neuropathic pain, which occurs as a result of compression, invasion, destruction and dysfunction of the central or peripheral nervous system to pharmacologic agents is weak. What is important here is to determine such phenomena and to optimise the analgesic requirements.

4.2.3. Breakthrough Pain (Incident Pain, Movement-Related Pain)

Pain inflammation is a temporary pain that is superimposed on the stable, basal pain pattern in patients treated with opioids. This type of pain, called episodic pain in some countries, is very severe, has very rapid onset and its time is non-stable (30 min on average). Pain inflammation is thought to be a negative prognostic factor [33, 34]. A study of 1095 cancer patients in twenty-four countries found that pain inflammation was associated with higher pain scores and hindered physical activity [35]. The untreated patients had lower physical activity, while anxiety and depression levels increased. Patients' satisfaction with opioid treatment was decreased, while unexpected visits to emergency service and clinics increased. In a study that directly and indirectly investigated the cost of pain treatment in cancer patients, pain inflammation was found to increase medical expenditure [36].

In routine applications, breakthrough pain is still not known and cannot be assessed and treated [37]. Pain inflammation is seen in 65% of cancer patients [35]. Its prevalence is higher in the patients staying in a hospital or a nursing home than among outpatients.

Pain inflammation arises due to a pre-known activity (such as walking, coughing and sitting), just prior to insufficient duration of the previous dose (in other words, before the next analgesic dose) or often due to unknown reasons. Incident pain is triggered by movement and often associated with bone metastases or fractures and it is a subtype of a well-defined breakthrough pain. A reversible type of pain inflammation may occur during the opioid titration, before reaching the correct and stable dose.

Pain inflammation may be triggered by various mechanisms:

a) Deglutition or mastication in patients with oral or oesophageal mucositis;

b) Touching the area of allodynia in patients with neuropathic pain;

c) Defecation, miction or tenesmus in patients with pelvic tumour;

d) Spasm, irritation or obstruction of hollow organs (oesophagus, intestines, gall bladder and ureter).

Breakthrough pain without an obvious cause may indicate insufficient opioid dose.

It can be difficult to assess pain inflammation, especially in patients who have incidental pain and who avoid specific movements that can trigger the pain. It is important to assess this pain as a different pattern from basal pain. In a detailed pain assessment, the frequency, duration of each episode, pain intensity, precipitating factors and the previous and current treatments and activities applied for basal pain (persistent) should be examined.

4.3. Physical Examination

4.3.1. Neurological Examination

The location of the pain is determined through neurological examination. The extent of pain in the spinal cord or nerve stem lesions or sensorial changes may have a dermatomal character [38]. Muscle weakness, poor reflexes and reflected visceral pain may be associated with spinal segments.

4.4. Examinations

A new pain or the recurrence of a previously controlled pain is an indication that the disease has progressed. Need may arise for diagnostic - tests or interventions. However, if the patient is at an advanced stage of an illness, the examinations should envisage treatments that may change the progress of the disease and change the algorithm of pain treatment. If not, it would be appropriate to apply a known pain treatment without causing further distress to the patient and without incurring additional expense. Another point in the assessment is to determine the expectations of the patient. How the patient defines the cause of the pain, how he/she feels about the effect of the pain, the importance of pain control for the patient and his/her expectations of the health team should be examined so that the team does not purse unrealistic objectives and understands the need for collaborative working with other disciplines.

5. LUNG CANCER PAIN

5.1. Factors Observed with Lung Cancer Related Pain

5.1.1. Histology

There is no common view on pain frequency on the basis of small-cell carcinoma (SCLC) or non small-cell carcinoma (NSCLC) [39].

5.1.2. Stage

Pain generally arises at advanced stages of lung cancer. In other words, the severity of pain increases incrementally at advanced stages. When the relationship between pain and survival is analysed, survival rates in painful squamous cell carcinoma are found to be 5 years less than those in painless cells; however, no such finding has been obtained in adenocarcinoma [40]. It is said that pain cannot be a determinant of survival in non small-cell lung cancers [41]. Lung cancer is diagnosed late and pain comes into prominence in the diagnosis [42].

5.1.3. Ages and Sexes of Patient

The average age is reported to be 63 (56-68), and the sex is reported to be 79% male (48-100%) in lung cancer. Pain does not often arise in patients of advanced ages (80 and over), while it arises at the age of 40 and below [39].

5.1.4. Aetiology

Pain is regarded as one of the causes of malignity in general; it develops multifactorily and is felt in different anatomical locations. When patients are directed to pain clinics, the pain prevalence rises to 100% [43]. That is to say, pain assessment is performed more precisely in these clinics. Many patients are receiving radiotherapy (59%), a surgical intervention (43%) and chemotherapy (20%) together. Pain may develop due to these treatments. Moreover, adjuvant and hormonal treatments may also cause pain.

5.2. The Characteristics of Lung Cancer Related Pain

5.2.1. Localisation of the Pain

In lung cancer patients, pain frequently arises in the chest (63%) and in the lumbar spine (32%). Pain complaints may come from two or more different locations (38%).

5.2.2. Progression of the Pain

The progression of pain varies according to the severity and its frequency, and is also dependent on psychosocial function and distress. Unbearable pain is seen in 28% of lung cancer cases. Patients' levels of pain within palliative care services are found to be two times more than that of patients in clinics that accept out-patients. The survival rate of the patients with unbearable pain is lower than patients with mild low pain [44]. Pain varies according to the daily activities and occupations of patients. The more they enjoy living, and the better or higher their spiritual conditions and occupational statuses, the lower the severity of pain. Distress and excessively dealing with oneself increase the severity of pain.

5.2.3. Duration of the Pain

More than 6 months of survival rate is reported in 20% of patients after diagnosis [39]. In ambulant lung cancer, it was found that this time ranged between 1 and 177 weeks and the average value was 4 weeks [45].

5.2.4. Pathophysiology

Nociceptive or somatic pain forms a significant subgroup of lung cancer within the scope of pain pathophysiology (73%). The rate of visceral or neuropathic pain subgroup is between 30 and 32%.

6. PAIN TREATMENT

In lung cancer related pain treatment, having a good command of pharmacology is of great importance. This includes drug mechanisms, undesired effects and possible drug interactions. Pain treatment can be classified as pharmacologic and non-pharmacologic. The pharmacologic group includes non-opioids, opioids and adjuvant analgesics; the non-pharmacologic group includes non-invasive and minimal invasive techniques and surgical invasive techniques.

6.1. Control of Cancer Pain

After careful examination of the patient, pain control should be ensured according to the suggestions of the WHO:

1- Careful recording of medical history and assessment;

2- Selection of appropriate drug;

3- Selection of appropriate dose;

4- Repeated assessment is required. These suggestions are never alternative suggestions to the strategies for cancer related pain relief. Treatment can involve a combination of radiotherapy, chemotherapy, surgical intervention, physiotherapy, anaesthetic block techniques, relaxation treatment, transcutaneous electrical nerve stimulation (TENS) and acupuncture, which should be applied on an individual basis.

Many researchers report that the WHO analgesic ladder method gives good results and more than 88% of patients no longer suffer from pain. Therefore, it is inevitable to use analgesics in a series of specific rules.

6.2. Principles of Use of Analgesics:

The rules suggested by the World Health Organisation are as follows:

a) The selection of analgesics is performed in line with the ladder principle, according to the severity of pain.

In the ladder principle, analgesics are classified into groups from the least effective to the most effective in terms of their strengths. The three main groups are: non-opioids (NSAİİ, antipyretics), weak opioids (codeine, tramadol), and strong opioids (morphine, fentanyl). Each group of analgesics forms a ladder system based on their efficacy combined within the framework of certain principles.

b) The cause and quality of pain are taken into consideration in the selection of analgesics.

Although non-opioids are less strong in theory than opioids, when they are selected and applied directed to the cause (in somatic visceral pain) of the pain, they give better results in many pain syndromes than opioids as they can affect and prevent the occurrence mechanism of pain, or they can increase their efficacy.

c) Oral ways are primarily preferred in the use of analgesics.

The simplest treatment method in chronic pain is the oral pathway. The slow release preparations of the oral forms of analgesics are preferred, as they minimise the frequency of using drugs. When the oral pathway is not applicable, rectal, transdermal, transmucosal, sublingual, intranasal and inhalation pathways are tried.

d) Analgesic dose is determined on an individual basis.

The analgesic need differs significantly between patients, even with similar problems. The appropriate dose is therefore different for each patient. In order to find an optimal dose, the lowest dose of analgesics should be applied at first and the dose should be titrated according to the effect. Attention should be paid to the fact that the duration of efficacy of the analgesic should not fall below pharmacologic standard duration of efficacy while deciding the dose.

e) Analgesics are taken at regular intervals.

Stable analgesia is only possible with the pharmacological efficacy level of the drug. The method of administration “in case of necessity-pro re nata" is inappropriate. A period of 24 hours of interrupted efficacy is of great importance in analgesia. The determined regular time intervals should be consistent with the known pharmacologic duration of the drug. The traditionally applied 3x1 programme is a deficient definition. On the other hand, the concept of administering analgesics with meals has been abandoned. The appropriate expression takes the form "at x hours intervals"

f) Side effect prophylaxis and its treatment are applied.

Analgesics have a range of side effects, and it is appropriate to inform patients of these issues. When necessary, an analgesic drug should be replaced with another one. Side effects such as constipation due to weak or strong opioids, nausea and vomiting are insufficient reasons for stopping the treatment.

g) Adjuvant drugs are used.

Adjuvants (secondary analgesics, off label drugs) are a different group of drugs, the main use of which is not pain management, but which can be effective in some pain types (antidepressants, anticonvulsants, *etc.*).

h) The patient and patient's relatives are assured.

Successful analgesia requires close cooperation between the doctor and the patient. A mutual environment of trust should be established. The side effect most feared by patients is tolerance and opioid addiction. Tolerance is that the patient experiences a gradual loss of efficacy of the determined dose of the drug. A rapid dose increase may be required in cancer patients, depending on the progress of the tumour, which does not imply the development of tolerance. Psychological and physical addiction should be distinguished in the concept of addiction [46].

6.3. Application of Analgesic Ladder Method

The WHO developed a three-step analgesia ladder system for analgesic medications used in the treatment of cancer pain:

1. Firstly, non-opioid analgesics are used for dull pain during stage I;

2. In the second stage, "mild" opioids are given to the patients with mild low pain to which a non-opioid analgesic can be added, if necessary;

3. In the third stage, "strong" opioids are given to the patients with severe pain, to which a non-opioid analgesic can be added, if necessary. If necessary, at each step, adjuvants can be added [47, 48]. The components that are effective in ascending or descending one step are pain severity, response to analgesic and side effects. And, one should wait for at least 24 hours before changing the step.

The three-step ladder system specifies treatment according to the intensity of pain. The WHO method has been of enormous benefit for the treatment of cancer pain worldwide. Cancer patients may need alternative methods of drug administration or strategies like invasive procedures. Despite its success, the WHO method should be carefully examined. It was found that effective analgesia could be provided in 70-90% of cancer patients suffering from pain, while no effective analgesia could be provided in 10-30% of patients [49]. Therefore, alternative methods of drug administration such as nerve blocks or other invasive procedures will be necessary as pain cannot be satisfactorily relieved in a significant proportion of cancer patients. Moreover, the WHO analgesia ladder system does not explain how these procedures should be ideally integrated with the medical cancer pain treatment. Secondly, the above mentioned series do not give any information on how fast and effective analgesia is provided for the patients who respond to the medications at different steps of the ladder. The aim of all the pain treatments is to receive a response as soon as possible, regardless of the aetiology and clinic. Finally, some data support the theory that more effective analgesia can be provided with fewer undesired effects by using earlier administration of invasive procedures; and, when compared to traditional analgesic treatment, the survival rate might be higher.

In order to climb a ladder, while we place one foot in a consistent and progressive way on the step, we move one step forward with the other foot without steering to any other shortcut. In the three-step ladder system developed by the WHO, the treatment starts with the first step and when no effective analgesia is provided with non-opioid drugs, it progresses to the second step. The same situation is valid for climbing from step two to step three. This approach may be appropriate in the treatment of progressively increasing pain; however, is it effective in the treatment of pain which is initially severe? If a patient coming to the first assessment has an initially unbearable pain, should we progress through the various steps, or start the treatment with strong opioids? The answer for the treatment of regular cancer pain is quite clear. Moreover, it may be difficult to choose the appropriate procedure for a less experienced clinician and this may delay the use of strong opioids by starting the treatment with steps one and two in order to follow the WHO guidelines. In order to avoid the misinterpretation of the ladder system, the expression that "opioids should be chosen depending on the intensity of pain at that time" should be emphasised. There are some discussions about the clinical benefits of weak opioids (or medications in Step two) in the treatment of cancer pain. A statistically significant difference was found between the outcomes for patients who started with "strong" opioids and those who were treated according to the WHO guidelines. The results in the first group were found to be much better than those of the second group.

Invasive procedures should be considered as adjuvant treatment, together with commonly used analgesic regimes at any stage, not as a "last resort".

A new algorithm suggests the following three treatment phases for cancer pain.

1) For dull pain, non-opioid analgesic treatment should be started. If the pain cannot be controlled in this way, then low dose "strong" opioids should be added and titrated according to the needs of the patient.

2) For moderate pain, low dose "strong" opioids should be applied and titrated; if necessary, non-opioids can be added.

3) For severe pain, "strong" opioids should be applied immediately; if necessary, non-opioids can be added.

For patients with moderate or severe cancer pain, invasive procedures like neurolytic blocks should be considered as an alternative or as an addition to pharmacology at any phase. Adjuvants should be used at all stages when indicated. As a rule, "weak" opioids should be omitted from cancer treatment, except in countries where "strong" opioids cannot be easily found or there are no well-trained doctors to use them. In such cases, clinicians should keep in mind that the efficacy of "weak" opioids is limited. Finally, although data from many controlled studies support the efficacy and reliability of this algorithm, it is suggested that further research is required, using prospective studies with large cancer patient populations [49].

In pain assessment, pain distress and pain severity should be distinguished. The treatment type varies according to the intensity, type and cause of pain. While the intensity of pain determines the level of analgesic requirement, its type and cause determine the adjuvant medications.

6.4. Intensity of Pain

Opioid analgesic response varies according to patient and pain. There is no pain that does not respond to opioids. However, there may be a partial response, as in neuropathic pain. Opioid analgesia is essential in all cancer pains, whether mild or severe. Cancer pain is persistent and it is necessary to maintain a constant plasma level of the analgesics. Therefore, the drug schedule should be determined according to the pharmacodynamic and pharmacokinetic characteristics of the drug. It would be very useful to familiarise the patient with these factors, and he/she should know that the optimal effect can only be provided by this way.

6.5. Selection of Analgesics

Paracetamol and non-steroid inflammatory medications are included in non-opioids and non-steroidal anti-inflammatory drugs (NSAID). Paracetamol is one of the most reliable agents used additionally in long-term management of mild low pain or in severe pain. However, especially in bone metastases, it is not preferred among non-opioids as its anti-inflammatory efficacy is limited. It would be reasonable to avoid its use or to use it in low doses in cases of renal and liver failure and more specifically with alcohol addictions. Paracetamol is generally available in combination with aspirin and caffeine, which increase its effectiveness. NSAIDs suppress prostaglandin biosynthesis and show their analgesic efficacies. The cascade of the inflammatory effects which initiate, increase or maintain the nociception is therefore inhibited. These types of drugs are effective on the central or peripheral nervous system independently of anti-inflammatory mechanism and also reduce the pain transmission. Even if the daily dose is increased, the analgesic efficacy will not increase as there is a ceiling effect.

6.5.1. Cyclooxygenases in Cancer

Upon the discovery of two different gene codes of cyclooxygenases in 1991, all of their characteristics were revealed (COX-1 and COX-2). Selective inhibitors were developed for both enzymes. These enzymes form hydrophobic troughs or channels that provide the transition from cell membrane. An arachidonic acid or an inhibitor binds to this trough. Interestingly, COX-2 protein forms a wider channel than COX-1 and the selective inhibitor of COX-2 binds here. COX-1 and COX-2 genes are on human chromosomes 9 and 1 respectively. While the COX-1 gene does not include any TATA box (transcription), COX-2 includes TATA box and has the capacity to fasten many transcription factors such as nuclear factor-κB (NF- κB), nuclear factor interleukin-6 (NF-IL-6) and the protein that binds to the response element (CAMP) of cyclic adenosine monophosphate. Therefore, COX-2 is regulated by various mediators included in the inflammation. While lipopolysaccharides, proinflammatory cytokines (interleukin-1β, tumour necrosis factor [TNF]) and growth factors induce COX-2, glucocorticoids, interleukin-4, interleukin-13 and interleukin-10, an anti-inflammatory cytokine inhibits it. Prostaglandin E2 is a major product of COX-2; it regulates COX-2 using a feedback mechanism with its cAMP increasing capacity in various cell types. COX-2 is also regulated at post-transcriptional level. Its level is greatly increased in colorectal, breast and prostate carcinogenesis. Its upper-regulation is reported in skin, lung, bladder and pancreatic cancers. When we consider the role of chronic inflammation in cancer occurrence and development, we can assume the NSAID may be an effective way of preventing cancer. However, it is reported that an ectopic increase in COX-2 level prevents cancer occurrence [50]. In addition, a high level of COX-2 in seminal vesicles reduced the risk of cancer occurrence.

6.5.2. Inhibition of COX-2 Activity by NSAID

The active part of COX is the last part of the hydrophobic channel. NSAIDs affect this active part in various ways. Aspirin irreversibly inactivates COX-1 and COX-

2 with acetylation in this active part, and thus inhibits the binding of arachidonic acid to this site. In contrast, the reversible competitive inhibitors compete with arachidonic acid in order to bind to the active part of COX. NSAIDs such as flurbiprofen and indomethacin inhibit COX-1 and COX-2 slowly, reversibly and time dependently.

6.5.3. Opioids

The analgesic plasma level of the blood varies according to the intensity of pain for every patient in opioid analgesia. For those who have skin pain, analgesic plasma level of the blood reaches a certain value, thus sufficient analgesia is provided and pain is relieved. This is called the "minimum effective analgesic blood concentration" (MEAC). Minor increases beyond this threshold result in a substantial increase in analgesia, which means no ceiling effect is observed.

6.5.3.1. Opioid Classification

The alkaloids obtained from opium are classified in two chemical groups as phenanthrene and benzylisoquinoline. The main phenanthrene alkaloids are morphine, codeine and thebaine. The main benzylisoquinoline alkaloids are papaverine (vasodilator) and noscapine; and they do not have morphine-like effects. Opioids can be divided into four main groups: Agonist, partial agonist, agonist-antagonist and antagonists (Table **2**).

Table 2: Intrinsic Activity (Drug-Receptor Complex) and Classification According to Synthetic Origin

	Agonists	**Partial agonist**	**Agonist-antagonists**	**Antagonists**
Natural opioids (Phenanthrene alkaloids)	Morphine Codeine Thebaine			Naloxone Naltrexone
Semi-synthetic opioids	Diacetylmorphine (heroin) Hydrocodone Hydromorphone Oxycodone Oxymorphone	Buprenorphine	Nalbuphin	
Artificial opioids	<u>Morphinan derivatives</u>: Levorphanol		<u>Benzomorphan derivatives</u>:	

Table 2: contd….

	Phenylpiperidine derivatives: Meperidine-Pethidine Fentanyl Sufentanyl Alfentanil Remifentanil Propionanilide derivatives: Methadone Propoxyphene		Pentazocine Morphinan derivatives: Butorphanol Dezocine	

6.5.3.2. Mechanism of Opioid Action

When the analgesia -induced by electrical brain stimulations- is reversed by naloxone, the endogenous opioid system comes to the agenda. Opioids show their effects by activating the endogenous opioid system. This system consists of the opioid receptors, neurotransmitters and endogenous opioid peptides widely spread throughout the central and peripheral nervous system. It is also included in the immune system and in the reproduction system. It activates in different ways:

a) The secretion of endogenous opioid peptides (electrical stimulation, placebo);

b) Increasing the endogenous opioid peptide concentration in receptor areas;

c) Pharmacological activation of opioid receptors, *i.e.* the release of opioid agonists.

Enkephalins, endorphins and dynorphins are genetically independent endogenous opioids. Recently, some endomorphines that show excessive affinity for mu receptors were detected as endomorphine 1 and endomorphine 2. There are 5 types of opioid receptors in general: mü (μ_1 and μ_2); κ - kappa; σ - sigma; δ-delta; ε-epsilon. Endogenous opioids are secreted depending on a stimulant or tonically in the nervous system.

Opioids show their antinociceptive effects over the opioid receptors located in supraspinal, spinal and peripheral areas. The receptors have similar effects, such as adenylyl cyclase inhibition, increasing the K^+ transmission and reducing Ca^{2+} channel activity.

With the developments in molecular biology, μ, κ and δ opioid receptors were found in humans. The pharmacological and functional features of the asexually reproduced (cloned) receptors, the development of "knockout" animals (which have no receptor or some receptors) and the manipulation and change of some amino acids included in various opioid receptors provide new information about receptor function and progress was made on opioid neurotransmission at the molecular level. Thus, perhaps it will be possible to control the factors that cause the development of tolerance to opioid drugs.

6.5.3.3. Opioid Metabolism

The liver is the first site of biotransformation for many drugs, including opioids. In the first contact place during absorption, the metabolism starts to function (First transition metabolism); in the gastrointestinal tract in oral intake and in the lungs in respiratory intake. The kidneys and brain also join the metabolism. However, the skin does not join the metabolism in the administration of transdermal fentanyl.

Although there are various classifications of drug metabolism in liver, one or two options can simply explain the metabolic reactions: Phase I and Phase II. While there are generally conjugation reactions with glucuronic acid in Phase I; in Phase II, both N and O- dealkylation are catalysed by 3A4 and 2D6, which are hepatic cytochrome P450 (CYP) isoforms. While many opioid drugs react in either Phase I or Phase II, some of them can react in both phase types. Some metabolites with positive effects (relieving pain) or negative effects (toxicity) arise.

Many opioids have high clearance; the liver blood stream determines the metabolic rate. Opioids can be classified into two groups as stream-limited and capacity-limited. Those that are stream-limited depend on liver perfusion. Pethidine clearance decreases in patients with cirrhosis. Methadone clearance is already very low and is therefore included in the capacity-limited opioids.

6.5.3.4. Undesirable Effects of Opioids

Some undesirable effects may occur, depending on systemic and administration factors. It depends on pharmacodynamic characteristics. The most feared effect is the respiratory depression, which occurs because the respiration system loses its carbon dioxide sensitivity. Xerostomia develops in 77% of patients receiving morphine. It may develop due to antidepressant and anticholinergic drugs. The mouth should be cleaned with sodium bicarbonate. Pilocarpine is also effective in overcoming xerostomia.

Nausea and vomiting may be observed initially or when the dose is increased. Moreover, nausea may develop, depending on the disease or chemo/radiotherapy, intestinal obstruction, ulcer and various metabolic disorders. Metoclopramide is effective and 5-HT3 antagonists (ondansetron, granisetron) can also be administered.

It is necessary to use prophylactics in the fight against constipation. Various laxatives such as intestine stimulants (senna) and stool softening (docusate sodium), actualise and fibrous foods are given. Sometimes an enema may even be required.

Sedation is usual in opioid-sensitive patients. Methylphenidate is treated with adjuvant drugs like modafinil.

Neurotoxicity may develop, depending on the opioid used [51]. Cognitive disorders, heavy sedation, hallucinations, delirium, myoclonus, contractions, hyperalgesia and allodynia are recognised as side effects. Such side effects typically occur with continuous high dose opioid usage or with shortage of liquid and in renal failure. These effects are treated using opioid rotation, hydration and dose restriction. The need to increase dose in order to achieve the same analgesic response is called "tolerance". Tolerance develops in all the opioid analgesics and when tolerance develops to one opioid, it develops to other opioids due to cross-tolerance, although to a lesser extent. Tolerance may develop without any physical dependence.

When opioids are used in repetitive doses, "physical dependence" may develop at different levels. Physical dependence does not mean addiction. When opioids are discontinued in physical dependence or an antagonist is administered, some deficiency symptoms such as rhinorrhea, yawning, hyperventilation, hyperthermia, mydriasis, muscle pain, vomiting and diarrhoea (abstinence or withdrawal syndrome) are observed. These symptoms reach the highest level at 72 hours. When deficiency symptoms appear, tolerance against opioids suddenly disappears.

6.5.4. Fundamental Principles in the Management of Cancer Pain

a. If possible, the use of oral or transdermal opioid, as specified in analgesics usage principles;

b. The use of long term effective opioids for persistent pain and the use of short term effective opioids in breakthrough pain;

c. Avoiding side effects by reducing the dose of opioids, using analgesic adjuvants such as NSAIDs, anticonvulsants;

d. Struggling with constipation, nausea and vomiting prophylactically;

e. Trying to increase the quality of life using parenteral infusion, intraspinal infusion and nerve blocks and palliative chemo/radiotherapy and surgical interventions.

6.5.5. The Use of Opioids in Cancer Pain

Almost 33% of patients who suffer from severe cancer pain are receiving active cancer treatment [52]. Despite developments in pain control methods, there are many people who suffer from cancer pain. One of the reasons for this is insufficient pain treatment and the other reason is inappropriate pain treatment. In terms of opioid treatment, the risk of addiction and avoiding undesirable effects causes physicians to adopt a position termed opiophobia, in which they are reluctant to prescribe the necessary drugs.

6.5.5.1. Opioids used in Dull and Moderate Pain:

6.5.5.1.1. Tramadol

Tramadol is a racemic mixture of two isomers and a synthetic analgesic that binds weakly to μ receptor. As tramadol is a selective noradrenalin and serotonin re-uptake inhibitor, it has also non-opioid central effects [51]. It has a weak affinity to M (mu) receptor, 6000 times less than morphine and 10 times less than codeine. It metabolises with CYP 2D6. Oral tramadol dose is 200-400 mg/day [53]. Its equivalent dose with morphine is around 5:1. It creates synergistic analgesia with paracetamol.

6.5.5.1.2. Codeine

Codeine, which is an opium alkaloid, is administered alone or in combination with other analgesics. It turns into morphine, which is an active metabolite, metabolising with CYP 2D6 [54]. The efficacy of codeine is one tenth that of the equivalent dose of morphine. If CYP 2D is at a low level, codeine does not show any analgesic effect. Codeine cannot relieve severe pain.

6.5.5.1.3. Hydrocodone

It is a ketone derivative of hydrogenised codeine. When administered in combination with paracetamol or aspirin, it is effective in treating cancer pain. Hydrocodone turns into a high affinity hydromorphone and into the active metabolite Mu receptor with CYP 2D6. While the equivalent analgesic rate to morphine is 1: 0.15, which rises to 1: 0.5.

6.5.5.2. Opioids used in Moderate and Severe Pain:

6.5.5.2.1. Morphine

Morphine is a major painkiller and commonly administered for cancer pain (WHO, 1986). It metabolises in liver. Its major metabolic enzyme is UDP-glucuronosyl- transferase (UGT) [55]. First passage reveals three metabolites in the metabolism: normorphine, morphine-3-glucuronide (M3G) and morphine-6-glucuronide (M6G). M3G does not have any analgesic activity; however, it is held responsible for some morphine-based neurotoxicity findings. M6G, on the other hand, is a hydrophilic metabolite, it rarely crosses into the central nervous system and it is more effective than morphine. It should be used carefully in cases with renal failure as metabolic products are removed from the kidneys and should be assessed in terms of neurotoxicity [56]. The half-life of morphine is 2-4 hours.

Administration routes for morphine may be oral, rectal, sublingual, IV, SC, topical and intraspinal (intrathecal/epidural). The oral route is preferred and it is available in Turkey. Intraspinal administration is much more effective than oral administration. First passage skips the metabolism; very few metabolites are encountered in CSF (Cerebrospinal Fluid). The metabolism of morphine is affected by the use of other drugs. Carbamazepine, phenobarbital, phenytoin and rifampin induce UGT enzyme and accelerate the morphine clearance. Phenothiazines, tricyclic antidepressants and cimetidine increase the effect of morphine. Benzodiazepines inhibit metabolism of morphine; therefore, sedation, hypertension and delirium may be observed.

Short and long-acting morphine preparations may be administered together *via* oral route. Short-acting preparations are preferred in episodic pain (breakthrough pain) and the first dose titration. Those can be administered at regular intervals or when necessary (pro re nata-PRN). The ceiling concentration occurs in 30-60 minutes. As there is no ceiling effect in morphine, insignificant dose increase causes a substantial increase in analgesia. When an optimal dose is reached with short-acting morphine, long-acting morphine preparation is administered for maintenance treatment. Long-acting preparations are in tablet or capsule form in continuous (modified) release formulation; they are also available in Turkey.

6.5.5.2.2. Hydromorphone

Hydromorphone is a semi artificial opioid and has been in clinic use since 1926. When administered orally, it undergoes the first passage metabolism and three metabolites are formed: hydromorphone-3-glucuronide (H3G), dihydromorphine and dihydroisomorphine. H3G is inactive and the others have more analgesic activity than H3G [57]. Hydromorphone has lower bioavailability than morphine, but it has greater dissolubility. Besides immediate release tablet, solution and suppository types, there are also continuous release tablets, which are not available in Turkey. Hydromorphone is effective on mu and delta receptors, but it is ineffective on kappa. Its metabolites are removed from the kidneys. Opioid toxicity may occur in renal failure and, in such cases; it is preferred over morphine [58]. It is more effective against chronic obtuse pain than episodic sharp pain. In renal and biliary colic pain, its analgesic efficacy is high when administered in high doses. It is most effective when administered *via* the intraspinal route, in combination with adrenaline. In sensitive cancer patients, opioids may be administered orally 1-3 mg at intervals of 3-4 hours. The dose titration must be performed afterwards.

6.5.5.2.3. Oxycodone

Oxycodone is a thebaine derivative and has been used for over 80 years. It is divided into active oxymorphone and inactive noroxycodone metabolites with CYP2D6 [59]. It shows antinociceptive effect over kappa receptors. It may be administered *via* oral, rectal, IM, IV, intranasal, sublingual or intraspinal routes. It has immediate release or extended release in oral forms. Oxycodone is removed from the kidneys. Its clearance decreases in renal failure. The equivalent analgesic rate between oxycodone and morphine is about 1:1.5. Extended-release oxycodone preparations are effective in moderate and severe pain and they are administered at intervals of 8-12 hours. Selective serotonin re-uptake inhibitors (SSRI) inhibit the oxycodone mechanism and toxicity findings occur. It interacts with cyclosporine and rifampicin. It is not available in Turkey.

6.5.5.2.4. Fentanyl

Fentanyl is a semi artificial opioid with high lipid dissolubility. It is 75-100 times stronger than fentanyl morphine. It turns into phenylacetic acid, norfentanyl and less active hydroxy fentanyl in the liver. It is administered *via* transdermal and transmucosal routes. Due to its low molecular weight and high lipophilicity, it is more practicable for transdermal administration (transdermal therapeutic system-TTS) [60]. Duragesic® preparates (12, 5; 25, 50, 75, 100 μg/hr) are adhered to bare and dry skin at 72 hours intervals (Table **3**). The sufficient concentration in plasma for analgesia is 1-2 nanogram/ml. Oral transmucosal fentanyl is sucked like a lollipop and passes through the mucosa. It is administered in episodic pain and in cases in which tolerance develops; there are Actiq® 200, 400, 800 μg preparates. It is not recommended in acute and postoperative pain. As there is no specified administration table, 200 μg of fentanyl is accepted to be equal to 2 mg IV morphine and 800 μg is accepted to be equal to 10 mg IV morphine.

6.5.5.2.5. Methadone

Methadone is a synthetic opioid. While previously used to treat addiction, it has begun to be used for its analgesic characteristics in recent years. Methadone affects mu, delta and NMDA receptors. Due to its NMDA receptor activity, it is of great importance in neuropathic pain treatment [61]. It may be administered *via* oral, rectal and parental routes. Oral methadone is in the form of 5-10 mg tablets, 40 mg/tablet liquid (10mg/ml) and powder for oral/rectal use; it is not available in Turkey. It is decomposed into its inactive metabolites with CYP 3A3/4 isoenzyme. As it affects NMDA receptors, it is more advantageous than other opioids. Its bioavailability is high, regardless of the administration route. As its metabolites are removed with the stool, it does not pose a risk for patients with renal problems. However, its half-life is very long (6-150 hours); respiratory depression is the most important side effect. Its administration interval may be 8-12 hours.

Table 3: Transdermal Fentanyl Comparative Dosage Guide

IV/SC Morphine (mg/day)	**Oral Morphine (mg/day)**	**Fentanyl TTS (µg/hour)**
20	60	25
40	120	50
60	180	75
80	240	100

6.5.5.3. Other Administration Routes

6.5.5.3.1. Spinal Administration

Opioid administration *via* intraspinal route (epidural or intrathecal) is preferred in cases when cancer pain cannot be controlled *via* oral route. This also became a commonly applied route for non-cancer chronic pain. This is because, it does not only provide good quality analgesia but it also produces the fewest side effects. The dosage considerably decreases: 1 mg intrathecal morphine is accepted to be equal to 10 mg epidural; 100 mg parenteral is accepted to be equal to 300 mg oral morphine. The blood concentration of opioid administered *via* intrathecal route is quite low, equal to sub-therapeutic doses. In contrast, when administered epidurally, it rapidly and significantly mixes with blood, thus analgesia is provided with both spinal and supraspinal effect. There are many catheter systems that can be implemented *via* intrathecal or epidural routes in clinic. The catheter end can be suitably placed in a desired dermatomal area.

6.5.5.3.2. Intranasal Administration

Intranasal administration with the opioid absorption from nasal mucosa is effective in pain which starts suddenly or in preoperative sedation. It is administered as a nasal spray. Fentanyl, oxycodone and sufentanyl may be administered *via* this route. The intranasal bioavailability of oxycodone is 45% and 78% for sufentanyl. Sufentanyl has the same effect in preoperative sedation whether in the form of drops or spray.

6.5.5.3.3. Inhalation Administration

Opioid drugs are absorbed rapidly but variably although their inhalation administration is found to be strange. Morphine and fentanyl can be inhaled as aerosols [62]. A similar average blood level is obtained in inhalation administration as in the intravenous route. Inhalation may be preferred in breakthrough pain, as it is a non-invasive route.

6.5.5.3.4. Rectal Administration

Rectal route is preferred for patients who cannot take drugs orally or who vomit. The rectal bioavailability of suppository opioids is higher than oral bioavailability. Special rectal preparates of methadone are successfully administered in cancer pain.

6.5.6. Response to Opioids

The terms of response to opioid and efficacy are often confused. Pharmacists use "intrinsic efficacy" to indicate the receptor rate that the drug affects; by "efficacy" they mean the maximal effect of the drug. For a clinician, this refers to the balance between analgesia and side effects or high pleasure of the patient. Potential responses to opioids include the possibility of achieving proper analgesia as a result of dose titration.

The response of a person to different opioids or the response of different people to the same opioid is quite variable. This is why different results are obtained in long-acting opioid treatment in cancer patients. The mechanism varies to a great extent due to various reasons related to both the type of pain and the individual patient. Two of these reasons are neuropathic mechanism and movement pain.

The patient-related factors include psychological factors, advanced age or major organ failure.

Giving weak response to various opioids is called "opioid resistance". The factors or factor groups in pain/patient variability, which may be resistant to opioids, could not be identified. While an opioid is effective against all forms of pain in people who have similar demographic characteristics, it may not be effective in neuropathic pain. It is not possible to make a generalisation, as there are many such cases.

On the other hand, when a resistance occurs to an opioid, this does not mean that the same resistance will occur to another opioid. In this case, it is necessary to change the opioid (opioid rotation).

6.5.6.1. Analgesia Strategies in Cases Generating Weak Responses

In order to determine the response to opioid administrations, it is necessary to record the analgesia and side effects throughout dose titration. A good balance can be developed in many patients and this balance may be maintained for a long time. An additional dose of opioid may be administered in movement pain, while gradual additional doses can be administered into the determined base dosage in ever-increasing pain [6].

In some cases, undesirable effects may occur and so sufficient analgesia is never provided. In such a case, a weak response occurs, depending on the method of administration and a certain drug. In such cases, it is necessary to apply new methods. Four main strategies are mentioned:

a. Opening the Therapeutic Window

If the undesirable effect occurring while determining the effective dose titration of opioid is significant and becomes prominent, more aggressive actions are taken and the opioid administration continues [63]. Therefore, the therapeutic window is opened, rising to therapeutic levels, while attempting to eliminate the limited undesirable effect(s). The occurrence of undesirable effects is inevitable in the use of opioids. Somnolence and mental confusion are the best examples; attempts are made to improve the situation by administering a psychostimulant. Methylphenidate, dextroamphetamine, amphetamine, pemoline and modafinil may be administered as a psychostimulant in cancer patients. When pemoline and modafinil are administered, insignificant sympathomimetic effects may occur; anxiety, insomnia and anorexia may occur in sensitive people. Fatal fulminant hepatitis may develop in pemoline administration.

b. Opioid Rotation

If a weak response develops against a μ-agonist opioid drug, proper analgesia may be achieved by trying another drug. The equivalent analgesic doses for this change are determined according to the methods of administration for each opioid.

c. Pharmacologic Methods that Reduce the Need for Systemic Opioid

It is thought to reduce the systemic opioid need, benefiting from some pharmacologic agents at the third stage in the phenomena generating weak response to opioid therapy. There are two pharmacological strategies for this: The first strategy is to administer non-opioids or adjuvant analgesics simultaneously; the second is to administer opioids *via* intraspinal route.

d. Non-Pharmacological Methods that Reduce the Need for Systemic Opioid

The fourth step aims to strengthen the weak response to opioids using non-pharmacological methods and to minimise the daily total opioid dosage. There are some minimal invasive interventions, such as surgical approaches and also non-invasive methods such as rehabilitation and psychological approaches.

6.5.6.2. Treatment of Breakthrough Pain

Patients or family doctors may contribute to the treatment of breakthrough pain by changing the position of the patient, applying cold or hot, massaging the painful area and using relaxation techniques until the positive effects of the medication are obtained. Beyond these simple, non-medicament methods, two major medical strategies are recommended for the treatment of episodic pain: opioid titration and auxiliary medication.

In order to develop the balance between analgesia and negative effects in the best way, it is necessary to optimise the timing of the analgesia with a proper opioid titration. Different opioid doses can be administered in optimisation processes and an analgesic support may be provided for the adjuvants. A careful opioid titration may increase the basal analgesia level while restricting negative effects. As a response to the breakthrough pain that may develop, depending on the insufficiency of last-dose efficacy duration, the basal medication dose may increase or the time between the doses may be reduced.

The physician should also prescribe an auxiliary medication, instructing the patient how and when to use it, in addition to the basal medication. The aim of pain treatment is to personalise the auxiliary medication according to the underlying mechanisms. The effect, onset time and the strength (potency) of the auxiliary medication used should be appropriate to the patient's needs and should be easily administered (or if possible, the person can administer it on his/her own). Administering rapid oral morphine, oxycodone, hydrocodone and transmucosal fentanyl citrate forms the basis of breakthrough pain pharmacotherapy treatment. If possible, it is necessary to administer the same opioid given for this basal pain to the patient with an auxiliary medication in order to identify some potential negative effects. The first dose to be administered is recommended to be as much as a fixed fraction of the daily total opioid dose of the patient. According to the European Association for Palliative Care (EAPC); one sixth of the daily morphine dose (17%) should be administered as a starting point and this dose can be increased or reduced according to the clinical effect [64].

The oral route is the most appropriate choice for patients for whom the IV route is not appropriate, or who are treated at home or outpatients. Moreover, while the peak concentration of episodic pain lasts 5-15 minutes, the activation of tablet or liquid oral opioid forms may take 45 minutes. In the United States of America, oral transmucosal fentanyl citrate (OTFC) received FDA approval for managing pain inflammation of cancer patients, which develops depending on the opioid tolerance. Little is known about the increasing plasma opioid concentrations and metabolites after the pharmacokinetics of the auxiliary doses, which are superimposed on regular opioid doses, or after the pain disappears.

6.5.7. Adjuvant Analgesics

Adjuvant analgesics are used as non-indicatory drugs in a very large painkiller group within the non-opioid drugs. They are called analgesic adjuvants or auxiliary analgesics. They show analgesic effect even when not administered alone. This group includes antidepressants, anticonvulsants, corticosteroids and antiarrhythmics.

In some lung cancer cases, bisphosphonates, radiotherapy and chemotherapy are used as painkillers.

6.5.7.1. Antidepressants

These types of drugs produce analgesic effect in lower doses than antidepressant doses. Both effects occur with the inhibition of presynaptic re-uptakes of serotonin, noradrenalin or both. The analgesic effects of the old tricyclic selective antidepressants are more effective than that of the selective serotonin re-uptake inhibitors. On the contrary, they have more effective SSRIs. They increase opioid efficacy and provide a regular sleep pattern. They have various side effects, including some antimuscarinic effects such as xerostomia, accommodation failure, urinary retention and constipation. Antihistaminic effects such as sedation and increase in acid concentration in stomach (H_1 and H2); alpha-adrenergic blockage which may result in orthostatic hypotension may reveal some effects similar to kinidin, as seen particularly in amitriptyline.

All of these drugs undergo the first pass metabolism of liver and bind to protein at a significantly high rate. Many of them have high lipophilicity value and a high distribution volume. Elimination half-lives range between 1 and 4 days and many of them have active metabolites.

6.5.7.2. Anticonvulsants

These drugs suppress neural discharge. They are commonly used in neuropathic pain. The most commonly used ones are phenytoin, carbamazepine, valproic acid, clonazepam and gabapentin. Lamotrigme and topiramate may also be effective. They all bind to protein at a high rate and their half-lives are long. It is necessary to follow the blood level to obtain an optimal effect, as carbamazepine has a slow and unpredictable absorption. Gabapentin is licensed for use in neuropathic pain. In long-term use, they might depress bone marrow function.

6.5.7.3. Neuroleptics

Some clinicians use neuroleptics in the patients with reflected neuropathic pain. Neuropathics are useful in patients with agitation and psychotic symptoms. The most commonly used are flufenazin, haloperidol, chlorpromazine and perphenazine. Their therapeutic effects occur when they block the dopaminergic receptors in mesolimbic areas. As the same effect occurs in nigrostriatal pathways, some extrapyramidal side effects such as mask face, horse walking, cogwheel rigidity and bradykinesia occur. Some patients may develop acute dystonic reactions such as oculogyric crisis and torticollis. Akathisia (extreme anxiety) and tardive dyskinesia (involuntary choreoathetoid movements of the tongue, pout and body imbalance) may be observed in neuroleptic areas for a long time.

In many of these drugs, there are antihistaminic, antimuscarinic and alpha-adrenergic blockage effects as in the antidepressants.

6.5.7.4. Corticosteroids

Corticosteroids inhibit the tissue inflammation and oedema, which have a great role in pain occurrence. Glucocorticoids, in particular, are frequently used. They inhibit the occurrence of cytokines (İL-6, İL-1, TNF), lymphokine (interferon-g), leukotrienes and prostaglandins, which cause tissue inflammation. Therefore, they inhibit both the occurrence of inflammation and the chemical activation of the nociceptive neuron *via* these mediators. Moreover, it is suggested that corticosteroids provide analgesia by decreasing the pathologic electrical activity in the damaged neuron. They are administered *via* topical, oral or parenteral (intravenous, subcutaneous, intrabursal, intra-articular, epidural). High doses or long-term usage may result in serious side effects. Hypertension, hyperglycaemia, increase in infection sensitivity, peptic ulcer, osteoporosis, femoral head necrosis, proximal myopathy, cataracts and, rarely, psychosis may occur due to excess glucocorticoidal activity. The symptoms of Cushing syndrome may occur in patients. Due to mineralocorticoid activity, the symptoms of sodium retention, hypokalemia and congestive heart failure may appear.

6.5.7.4.1. Dexamethasone

Dexamethasone may be administered as a single dose or 8-18 mg in total daily. If it is not effective in one week, it is discontinued. After the desired effect is achieved, the dose is reduced by 2-4 mg in each 3-5 days.

In some cases, the medication is not discontinued; it is administered in optimal dose. Courses lasting 3-5 days are administered in order to avoid side effects in pediatric oncology.

6.5.7.5. Antiaritmics

Antiaritmics are effective in neuropathic pain. In associated conditions, monitorization arises. Antiaritmics are used after antidepressants and anticonvulsants. There are proof-based studies on their uses in peripheral nerve injury and non-cancer neuropathic pain [65].

However, there is not much proof of their efficacy in cancer pain. Flecainide, mexiletine and lidocaine can be classified in this group. Local anaesthetics can be used in the treatment of neuropathic pain where the intensity is gradually increasing or is ineradicable due to its probable serious side effects. The undesirable effects of antiaritmics include arhythmy, lethargy, convulsion, hypertension and cardiovascular collapse.

6.5.7.6. Bisphosphonates

Bisphosphonates are inorganic pyrophosphate analogues which inhibit osteoclastic activity. Therefore, they reduce bone resorption in many diseases. They are important in malignity with bone metastasis, Paget disease in bone and bone pain treatment. The analgesic efficacy of these components, especially pamidronate, has been demonstrated. Their side effects are generally hypomagnesemia, hypocalcemia, hypokalemia, hypophosphatemia, nausea, diarrhoea and constipation. These side effects may arise as soon as they are administered. Fever, arthralgia and sudden increase in pain are commonly seen during the first days. It is contraindicated in renal failure. It has various occupancies. It can be administered as long as the metastatic bone disease continues.

6.5.8. Interventional Methods

Among the interventional methods in non-pharmacological pain treatment, opioids, local anaesthetics or clonidines are administered alone or together with neuropharmacological drug transmitter systems. Dosages are determined according to the administration route (epidural, intrathecal, intraventricular). Neurostimulators may provide analgesia with stimulation in the selected area with the help of electrodes implanted in the peripheral or central nervous system. Another method is neuroablative techniques such as cordotomy, rhizotomy, myelotomy and dorsal root entry zone lesions (DREZ). The success of spinal opioid administration among drug transmitter systems depends on the appropriate patient selection [66]. Therefore, it is necessary to take some principles into consideration:

a) If oral route or other simple routes have become ineffective;

b) If spinal route provides a more effective pain control and increases the quality of life;

c) If efficacy is proved in the testing period;

d) If the people around the patient can use these devices;

e) If the general and psychological situation of the patient is appropriate to use these devices;

f) As the drug to be administered requires a drug transmitter system, if it is not expensive, it can be administered.

Intraspinal drug transmitter systems are as follows:

a) Percutaneous epidural and intrathecal catheters;

b) Epidural and intrathecal catheters subcutaneously placed;

c) Epidural and intrathecal catheters bound to subcutaneously placed ports;

d) Subcutaneously placed mechanical pumps;

e) Subcutaneously placed infusion pumps;

f) External pumps.

Percutaneous catheters can be used temporarily during method assessment before applying more expensive systems. Port systems are permanently placed. However, there are some disadvantages, such as the risk of infection, injecting many times into a small part of the patient's skin, the need for a new surgical intervention in case of a blockage or dislocation.

It is possible to affect the bone metastases with percutaneous radiofrequency thermocoagulator ablation. Their combination with cementoplasty gives better results [67].

7. PALLIATIVE CARE

Palliative care is the name of an active treatment applied to patients who do not respond to curative treatment [68]. The aim of palliative care is to improve the quality of life of patients and their families as much as possible. Palliative care:

a. Affirms life and regards dying as a normal process;

b. Intends neither to hasten nor postpone death;

c. Provides relief from pain and other distressing symptoms;

d. Integrates the psychological and spiritual aspects of patient care;

e. Offers a support system to help patients live as actively as possible until death;

f. Offers a support system to help the family cope during the patient's illness and in their own bereavement.

The development of palliative care marks the establishment of hospices; palliative care was institutionalised and accepted as a field of expertise. A teamwork approach is required, within which all the health teams participate. The leader of the team may change depending on the problems of patients and local factors. Team members should give importance to patient confidentiality.

Well-trained health care personnels are required for professional inspection who could assess the wishes and complaints of patients and provide guidance for patients and their families; they should know the principles of administration of the drugs used in pain control and other symptoms very well and could provide psychological support to patients and their families.

The continuity between home and hospital care should be provided in ideal home care. Family members have a great role in the home care of advanced cancer patients. Therefore, they should be trained in preparing appropriate meals for patients, administering analgesics or other drugs and how to deal with some special medical problems such as paraplegia and incontinence.

ACKNOWLEDGEMENTS

Declared none.

CONFLICT OF INTEREST

The author confirms that this article content has no conflict of interest.

REFERENCES

[1] Önal A: Nöropatik Ağrı. In Önal A (ed): Algoloji. İstanbul: Nobel Tıp Kitabevleri, 2004, p.1.
[2] Ertekin C: Ağrının Nöroanatomi ve Nörofizyolojisi. In Yegül İ. (ed): Ağrı ve Tedavisi. İzmir: Yapım Matbaacılık, 1993, p.1.
[3] Raj P: Ağrı Taksonomisi. In Erdine S (ed): Ağrı. İstanbul: Nobel Tıp Kitabevleri, 2002, p.12.
[4] Erdine S: Ağrı Mekanizmaları. In Erdine S. (ed): Ağrı. İstanbul: Nobel Tıp Kitabevleri, 2002, p.20.
[5] Uçkunkaya N, Gurbet A: Ağrı Fizyolojisi. In Güldoğuş F, Güleç S, Uçkunkaya N (eds): Baş ve Yüz Ağrıları. Ankara: Öncü Basımevi, 2003, p.34.
[6] Bruera E: Assessment of cancer pain. In Giamberardino MA (ed): Pain 2002- An Updated Review. Seattle: IASP Press, 2002, p.15.
[7] Morgan GE, Mikhail MS, Murray MJ, Larson CP: Klinik Anesteziyoloji. Çeviri: Tulunay M, Cuhruk H. 3. Baskı, Ankara: Güneş Kitabevi 2004, p.310.
[8] Fürst S: Transmitter involved in antinociception in the spinal cord. Brain Res Bulletin 48:129, 1999.
[9] Khasar SG, Lin YH, Martin A, Dadgar J, McMahon T, Wang D, Hundle B, Aley KO, Isenberg W, McCarter G, Green PG, Hodge CW, Levine JD, messing RO. A novel nociceptor signaling pathway revealed in protein kinase C epsilon mutant mice. Neuron 24(1):253, 1999.

[10] Okuse K: Pain signalling pathways: From cytokines to ion channels. Int J Biochem Cell Biol 39:490, 2007.
[11] Baer AN, Green FA. Cyclooxygenase activity of cultured human mesothelial cells. Prostaglandins 46(1):37, 1993.
[12] Giordano J, Dyche J. Differential analgesic actions of serotonin 5-HT3 receptor antagonists in the mouse. Neuropharmacology 28(4):423, 1989.
[13] Bouvier MM, Evans ML, Benham CD. Calcium Influx Induced by Stimulation of ATP Receptors on Neurons Cultured from Rat Dorsal Root Ganglia. Eur J Neurosci 3(3):285, 1991.
[14] Caterina MJ, Schumacher MA, Tominaga M, Rosen TA, Levine JD, Julius D: The capsaicin receptor: A heat-activated ion channel in the pain pathway. Nature 389:816, 1997.
[15] Zhuang ZY, Xu H, Clapham DE, Ji RR: Phosphatidylinositol 3-kinase activates ERK in primary sensory neurons and mediates inflammatory heat hyperalgesia through TRPV1 sensitization. J Neurosci 24:8300, 2004.
[16] Okuse K, Chaplan SR, McMahon SB, Luo ZD, Calcutt NA, Scott PB et al: Regulation of expression of the sensory neuron-specific sodium channel SNS in inflammatory and neuropathic pain. Mol Cell Neurosci 10:196, 1997.
[17] Tappe A, Klugmann M, Luo C, Hirlinger D, Agarwal N, Benrath J et al: Synaptic scaffolding protein Homer1a protects against chronic inflammatory pain. Nat Med 12:677, 2006.
[18] Hinds DA, Stuve LL, Nilsen GB, Halperin E, Eskin E, Ballinger DG et al: Whole-genome patterns of common DNA variation in three human populations. Science 307:1072, 2005.
[19] Lariviere WR, Wilson SG, Laughlin TM, Kokayeff A, West EE, Adhikari SM et al: Heritability of nociception. III. Genetic relationships among commonly used assays of nociception and hypersensitivity. Pain 97:75, 2002.
[20] Mogil JS, Richards SP, O'Toole LA, Helms ML, Mitchell SR, Belknap JK: Genetic sensitivity to hot-plate nociception in DBA/2J and C57BL/6J inbred mouse strains: possible sex-specific mediation by delta2-opioid receptors. Pain 70:267, 1997.
[21] Zhu Y, King MA, Schuller AG, Nitsche JF, Reidl M, Elde RP et al: Retention of supraspinal delta-like analgesia and loss of morphine tolerance in delta opioid receptor knockout mice. Neuron 24:243, 1999.
[22] Kim H: Genetic influence on pain sensitivity in humans. In: Dostrovsky JO, Carr DB, Koltzenburg M (eds): Proceedings of the 10th World Congress on Pain. Seattle: IASP Press, 2003, p.513.
[23] Einarsdottir E, Carlsson A, Minde J, Toolanen G, Svensson O, Solders G, Holmgren G, Holmberg D, Holmberg M: A mutation in the nerve growth factor beta gene (NGFB) causes loss of pain perception. Hum Mol Genet 13:799, 2004.
[24] Bell J: Predicting disease using genomics. Nature 429:453, 2004.
[25] Wolf CR, Smith G, Smith RL: Science, medicine, and the future: Pharmacogenetics. Br Med J 320:987, 2000.
[26] Burma O: Vasküler Ağrı. In Önal SA (ed): Algoloji. İstanbul: Nobel Tıp Kitabevleri, 2004, p.281.
[27] Şahin A: Göğüs ağrısı. Doktor 36:74, 2007.
[28] Gavrin JR: Chest Pain from Other Disorders Including Cancer. In Loeser JD (ed): Bonica's Management of Pain. Philadelphia, PA, USA: Lippincott Williams & Wilkins, 2001, p.1210.

[29] Di Maio M, Gridelli C, Manzione L, Brancaccio L, ve ark: Prevalence and management of pain in Italian patients with advanced non-small-cell lung cancer. Br J Cancer 90:2288, 2004.
[30] Parkin DM: Global cancer statistics in the year 2000. Lancet Oncol 2:533, 2001.
[31] Önal A: Kanser Ağrısı. Erdine S. (ed): Ağrı. İstanbul: Nobel Tıp Kitabevleri, 2002. p.397.
[32] Cleeland CS, Gonin R, Hatfield AK, Edmonson JH, Blum RH, Stewart JA, Pandya KJ: Pain and its treatment in outpatients with metastatic cancer. N Engl J Med 330:592, 1994.
[33] Bruera E, Schoeller T, Wenk R, MacEachern T, Marcelino S, Hanson J, Suarez-Almazor M: A prospective multicenter assessment of the Edmonton staging system for cancer pain J Pain Symptom Manage 10:348, 1995.
[34] Mercadante S, Radbruch L, Caraceni A, Cherny N, Kaasa S, Nauck F et al; Steering Committee of the European Association for Palliative Care (EAPC) Research Network: Episodic (breakthrough) pain: consensus conference of an expert working group of the European Association for Palliative Care. Cancer 94:832, 2002.
[35] Caraceni A, Martini C, Zecca E, Portenoy RK, Ashby MA, Hawson G *et al.* Working Group of an IASP Task Force on Cancer Pain: Breakthrough pain characteristics and syndromes in patients with cancer pain. An international survey. Palliat Med 18:177, 2004.
[36] Fortner BV, Demarco G, Irving G, Ashley J, Keppler G, Chavez J, Munk J: Description and predictors of direct and indirect costs of pain reported by cancer patients. J Pain Symptom Manage 25:9, 2003.
[37] Mercadante S, Arcuri E. Breakthrough Pain in Cancer Patients. Pain Clinical Updates 16 (1), 2006.
[38] Woodruff R: Kanser Ağrısı. Çeviri: Babacan A, Akçalı DT. Victoria, Avustralya: Asperula Pty Ltd,1997.
[39] Potter J, Higginson IR: Pain experienced by lung cancer patients: A review of prevalence, causes and pathophysiology. Lung Cancer 43:247, 2004.
[40] Furuta M, Hayakawa K, Saito Y, Niibe H: Clinical implication of symptoms in patients with non-small cell lung cancer treated with definitive radiation therapy. Lung Cancer 13:275, 1995.
[41] Martins SJ, Pereira JR: Clinical factors and prognosis in non-small cell lung cancer. Am J Clin Oncol 22:453, 1999.
[42] Medina FM, Barrera RR, Morales JF, Echegoyen RC, Chavarria JGRFT: Primary lung cancer in Mexico city: A report of 1019 cases. Lung Cancer 14:185, 1996.
[43] Grond S, Zech D, Diefenbach C, Rdabruch L, Lehmann KA: Assessment of cancer pain: a porspective evaluation in 2266 cancer patients referred to a pain service. Pain 64:107-114, 1996.
[44] Schonwetter RS, Robinson BE, Ramirez G: Prognostic factors for survival in terminal lung cancer patients. J Gen Int Med 9:366, 1994.
[45] Portenoy RK, Miransky J, Thaler H, Hornung J, Bianchi C, Cibas-Kong I, et al: Pain in ambulatory patients with lung or colon cancer. Cancer 70:1616, 1992.
[46] Önal Ac: Analjezikler. In Önal A. (ed): Algoloji. İstanbul: Nobel Tıp Kitabevleri, 2004, p.47.
[47] WHO: Cancer Pain Relief. Geneva: World Health Organization, 1986.
[48] WHO: Cancer Pain Relief, 2nd ed. Geneva: World Health Organization, 1996.
[49] Eisenberg E, Marinangeli F, Birkhahn J, Paladini A, Varrassi G: Time to Modify the World Analgesic Ladder? Pain Clinical Updates 8(5), 2005.

[50] Zha S, Yegnasubramanian V, Nelson WG, Isaacs WB, De Marzo AM: Cyclooxygenases in cancer: progress and perspective. Cancer Letters 215:1, 2004.

[51] Bruera E, Kim HN: Cancer Pain. JAMA 290:2476, 2003.

[52] Fukshansky M, Are M, Burton AW: The role of opioids in cancer pain management. Pain Practice 1:43, 2005.

[53] Tawfik MO, Elborolossy K, Nasr F: Tramadol hydrochloride in the relief of cancer pain: a double blind comparison against sustained release morphine. Pain 5(suppl):337, 1990.

[54] Lurcott G: The effects of the genetic absence and inhibition of CYP2D6 on the metabolism of codeine and its derivatives, hydrocodone and oxycodone. Anesth Prog 45:154, 1999.

[55] Paul D, Standifer KM, Inturrisi CE, Pasternak GW: Pharmacological characterization of morphine 6-beta-glucuronide, a very potent morphine metabolite. J Pharmacol Exp Ther 215:477, 1989.

[56] Donnely S, Davis M, Walsh D, Naughton M: Morphine in cancer pain management: a practical guide. Support Care Cancer 10:13, 2002.

[57] Babul N, Drake AC, Hagen N: Hydromorphone metabolite accumulation in renal failure. J Pain Symptom Manage 10:184, 1995.

[58] Lee MA, Leng ME, Tiernan EJ: Retrospective study of the use of hydromorphone in palliative care patients with normal and abnormal urea and creatinine. Palliat Med 15:26-34, 2001.

[59] Heiskanen T, Olkkola KT, Kalso E: Effects of blocking CYP2D6 on the pharmacokinetics and pharmacodynamics oxycodone. Clin Pharmacol Ther 64:603, 1998.

[60] Gourlay GK: Treatment of cancer pain with transdermal fentanyl. Lancet Oncol 2:165, 2001.

[61] Egbert B, Andersen S, Krogsgaard-Larsen P: Ketobemidone, methadone and pethidine are noncompetitive N-methyl-D-aspartate (NMDA) antagonists in the rat cortex and spinal cord. Neurosci Lett 187:165, 1995.

[62] Onal SA, Keles E, Toprak GC, Demirel I, Alpay HC, Avci L: Preliminary findings for preemptive analgesia with inhaled morphine: efficacy in septoplasty and septorhinoplasty cases. Otolaryngol Head Neck Surg 135:85, 2006.

[63] Önal Ab: Kanser Hastalarında Ağrı. In Önal A (ed): Algoloji. İstanbul: Nobel Tıp Kitabevleri, 2004, p.73.

[64] Hanks GW, Conno F, Cherny N, Hanna M, Kalso E, McQuay HJ, *et al.* Expert Working Group of the Research Network of the European Association for Palliative Care: Morphine and alternative opioids in cancer pain: the EAPC recommendations. Br J Cancer 84:587, 2001.

[65] Lussier D, Portenoy RK: Adjuvant analgesics in pain management. In Doyle D, Hanks G, Chemy N, *et al.* (eds): Oxford Textbook of Palliative Medicine. Third Edition. Oxford, England: Oxford University Pres, 2003, p.349.

[66] Erdine Sb: İntraspinal Analjezikler. In Erdine S. (ed): Ağrı. İstanbul: Nobel Tıp Kitabevleri, 2002, p.627.

[67] Toyota N, Naito A, Kakizawa H, Hieda M, Hirai N, Tachikake T, Kimura T, Fukuda H, Ito K: Radiofrequency ablation therapy combined with cementoplasty for painful bone metastases: initial experience. Cardiovasc Intervent Radiol 28:578, 2005.

[68] WHO: Kanserde Ağrı Tedavisi ve Palyatif Bakım. Çeviri: Erdine S. Dünya Sağlık Örgütü Uzmanlık Komitesi Raporu. İstanbul: Cemturan Ofset Cağaloğlu, 1992.

CHAPTER 16

Palliative Care in Lung Cancer

Selçuk Dinçer* and Süleyman Özyalçin

Istanbul University, Istanbul Faculty of Medicine, Department of Algology, Monoblok, Capa, 34390 Istanbul, Turkey

Pre

Smoking is the most important factor of lung cancer etiology. 90% of lung cancer patients use cigarette. While smoke prevalence in developed countries is 40-60% in men and 20-40% in women, and that in developing countries respectively 40-60% and 2-10%.

The aim of the palliative care is to decrease the cough, sickness, dyspnea, pain, loss of weight because of diet problem, and also make them comfortable to decrease stress, anxiety and depression based on patients' physiology.

Most of the lung cancer patients have hope that they will become health. However, most of them have defeated their illness. According to lung cancer characteristic, the most important problem that patients have is dyspnea complain because of pain and air way obstruction. In addition to having care in hospital, home care condition for terminal term can be designed.

Selçuk Dinçer

Istanbul University

Abstract: Lung cancer rate in all cancer types is 21% in men and 5 % in women in European Union Countries. Smoking is the most important factor of lung cancer etiology [1]. The rate of Turkey is found 63% in men and 14% in women in 1988. 88.7% of the patients in Turkey have got smoking story. Lung cancer risk increases 3.5 times in passive smoking. Because there are carcinogens in air and they are not filtered; therefore, they are denser on air [2].

The primary care practitioner must maintain a close working relationship with medical and surgical oncologists to help guide patients and families through various treatment options.

***Address correspodence to Selçuk Dinçer:** Istanbul University, Istanbul Faculty of Medicine, Depratment of Algology, Monoblok, Capa, 34390 Istanbul, Turkey; Tel: (+90 212) 531 31 47; Fax: (+90 212) 631 0541; E-mail: selcukdincer@yahoo.com

Akın Eraslan Balcı (Ed)

In the lung cancer patients, the pain occurred based upon the oncologic period in 77 % percentage. Moreover, it depends on cancer treatment in 19 % percentage and the other effects which are not depending on cancer in 4 %. It is hard to join the analgesic aims if the innovations related to cancer pain control are not heard, the doctors and the other medicine workers are not trained well and if some legal problems exist while finding the drugs which are used in the pain control.

Keywords: Lung cancer, palliative care, pain treatment.

EPIDEMIOLOGY AND RISK FACTORS

Lung cancer is the most common seen cancer type. About one million people die because of lung cancer every year. The survey shows that 8 months between 5 years are the survival 15 % as an average percent. Incident rate is 71/100.000 in developed countries, is 14/100.000 in developing countries. It is also found that it is seen 52.5/100.000 in European countries [3]. There is no correct analysis related to incident rate in Turkey, but based on the known incidents, gathered from Health Ministry, it is 11.5/100.000, 9.9/100.000 in men, 1.0 in women. Lung cancer rate in all cancer types is 30 % in men, and 5% in women. Incidence rate increases with age [1]. Most of the lung cancer patients are between 50-70 ages. Average diagnosis is about at the age of 60. However, 3 % of patients are young-under 40. 58.4 % is the average age percent in Turkey. Lung cancer rate in all cancer types is 21% in men and 5 % in women in European Union Countries. This difference results from smoking habit. Lung cancer is the most common seen cancer type which is the result of death in men. It has gone ahead the breast cancer in recent years and has been at the fore front. Rate of men/women changes from 5 to 2 in various countries [4]. Rate of men/women in lung cancer events is 9.4 in Turkey. This rate increases more than in black race than white race.

Smoking is the most important factor of lung cancer etiology. 90% of lung cancer patients use cigarette. Smoking and the lung cancer relation was realised in 1950, and then it is confirmed in further studies. Risk of the lung cancer in patients who smoke 24-36 times is more [5]. Some usage increased between World War I and 1960s, but decreased from 1970s to today in USA. It is also same with the other countries. While smoke prevalence in developed countries is 40-60% in men and 20-40% in women, and that in developing countries respectively 40-60% and 2-10%. The rate of Turkey is found 63% in men, 14% in women in 1988. 88.7% of the patients in Turkey have got smoking story. There are 4000 chemical matters in smoke. More than 60 of them have carcinogenic characters. Some of them are radioactive including radon, lead, bismuth and polonium. Especially, polycyclic hydrocarbons and N-nitrosamine are defined as pro-carcinogenic. Cancer builds up changes with smoke usage period, number of used smoke, type of smoke, age of smoke, used unfiltered smoke and density of tar [2]. There are some results about mentholated cigarettes which are more carcinogenic. The reason for that they are more harmful as they lead to bad breath, with decreasing nicotine metabolism, with increasing permeability of toxic matters in cigarette, and with increasing diffusion of it.

Lung cancer risk increases 3.5 times in passive smoking. Because there are carcinogens in air and they are not filtered; therefore, they are denser in air. Air pollution is responsible for lung cancer 1% in mice which inhale matters such as benzopyrene and SO_2. Lung cancer results are more in place where there is dense hydrocarbon. People who live in urban areas have 1.2-2.3 times more risks. Cancer risks have been found 3 times more in sarcoidosis. Scar existence risk increases 8 times more with depending on tuberculosis. Risk is also more in systemic sclerosis. Especially, adenocarcinoma type increases the lung cancer which builds up scar area. In Turkey, it is found that cancer built up in idiopathic fibrosis area in 3% of lung cancer patients and in fibrosis area where develops secondary lung tuberculosis in 2.9 % of patients. Genetic factors are also analysed for lung cancer built up, and it is found that cancer risk is 2.4 times more increase in patients who have lung cancer in that first remove. Aryl hydrocarbon hydroxylase enzyme change the polycyclic hydrocarbons, which are dense in the smoke, to active carcinogen [5]. Risk may increase people who have high enzyme activity. Changes in "oncogene" occurrence are important in carcinogen in genes which have role cell development together with external influences such as radiation, chemical matters and viruses. The oncogene is the most important groups are "myc" (C-myc,L-myc,N-myc) and "ras" (K-ras,H-ras,N-ras) families. Polycyclic aromatic hydrocarbons harm the DNA bond, therefore, DNA repair, apoptosis and p53 gene, which adjust cell cycle, result in mutation. The p53 gene is found as defeated percent as 50-70% in lung cancer. Diet deficiencies affect the lung cancer development [2]. For example, in animal models, vitamin A and beta-carotene deficiencies increase the risk of lung cancer. In human experiment, beta-carotene retinol amount in diet decreases the risk of lung cancer in 40% percent. Beta-carotene is the primer of the vitamin A, and it is in the orange-gil, green-stuff and fish. Smoke addicted people who consume fatty foods have more risk of developing cancer. There are some results about that consumption of tea, especially green tea, is protective. Lung cancer risk is 2-6 times more in people who have low socioeconomic level. And it is probably related to the etiologic factors. The other treatments increase the lung cancer risk. The radiotherapy application increases the lung cancer rate 2 times more in women, and the risk starts 10 years after the therapy. At the same time, if the patient smoke, the risk increase about 40 times [6]. In the Non-Hodgkin's lymphoma patients, it starts 5 years later after the radiotherapy with increasing the risk 1.5 times more. In the studies which has observed the Hodgkin's lymphoma patients for 30 years, it is found that lung cancer risk increases 2.9 times more [7].

CLINICAL FINDINGS

In addition to breath findings such as cough, hemoptysis or shortness of breath, structural findings such as uncountable loss in weight can be seen in patients. In some cases a chest X-ray done for other reasons reveals a pulmonary nodule or mass lesion. In cases of metastatic pulmonary lesions, the symptoms of the primary cancer may be predominant or it may be completely occult.

Special Cases in Lung Cancer

Superior Sulcus Tumour and Pancoast Syndrome; Superior sulcus term is defined as anatomic case dependent on pres which occurrs by subcalvian artery passing in lung lobes apex. The tumour areas develop generally through the posterior and they are well localised. While it is generally adenocarcinoma, other primer or metastatic tumours in granulomatous infections and vascular anevrisma can be located to this special area of lung. "Pancoast tumour" which is defined by a radiologist Henry Pancoast in 1932 shows special findings. The findings arise with depending on upper part of brachial plexus and linkage between top of thoracic ribs and vertebrae matter, invasion of stellate ganglion and subclavian vessel. It occurs with findings like arm and shoulder pain characteristically, atrophy at the hand muscle. Horner syndrome and apical opacity at lung graphy, and it is named like "Pancoast syndrome". Depending on retention of medulla spinalis, paraplegia can develop in patients. Transthoracic thin needle aspiration biopsy has an important role in defining these tumours. Carcinoma with squamous cell is the most common seen pathologic type. Diagnosis and treatment plan are done with computerised tomography and magnetic resonance visualisation. In treatment, it is applied alone as a combination with radiotherapy, chemotherapy and surgery. Pancoast tumours are seen in lung tumours rarely (2-5%).

Superior Vena Cava Syndrome; Superior vena cava arises depending on cutting of blood stream. The most common reason is bronchogenic carcinoma in older patients. In young patients, the most common reason of super vena cava syndrome is non Hodgkin's lymphoma. Dyspnea, sensation of fullness in head, and/or light headedness may be seen in patients.

Sometimes, facial swelling, cough, pain and dysphagia can arise. Dilatation at neck veins, front of breast wall and venous collateral in stomach swelling on face, arms and shoulder, blue-purple colour changes on skin, depended on edema in vocal cords and tracheas can be seen. GIS bleeding depended on esophagus successor may also be seen in the patients who have suffered from vena cava superior syndrome for a long time. Diagnosis can also be confirmed with venography venous pressure measurement in the upper extremity. Chemotherapy, radiotherapy, or surgical techniques can be used for treatment.

Paraneoplastic Syndrome generally arises with indirect effects like hormones, neurologic, haematologic effects, without direct effects like metastatic, obstructive or invasion of tumour. Paraneoplastic syndrome is seen as a percent of 10%-20% in patients who have carcinoma. It is hard to evaluate paraneoplastic syndrome because of defining hardness and hided symptoms through the underlying illness. In addition to general symptoms like anorexia, loss of weight, electrolyte defects, fever, loss of weight, dysproteinemia and cachexy. Being together with the specific organs and systems, paraneoplastic syndromes like endocrine, nervous and muscle defects, haematopoietic, cardiovascular, gastrointestinal, immunopoietic, uropoietic dependence are also known [8].

The exact classification of paraneoplastic syndromes is hard because of variability of clinic results and complication of effects of mechanisms. Fever, high sedimentation, anemia, hypercalcemia, hypocalcemia, hypoglycemia through the way of hormone and tumours which generate hormone like matters, and also increase the level of ACTH, ADH, TSH, HCG hormones can be observed.

Diagnosis

Any pulmonary symptoms persisting beyond 3 weeks are an indication for a more extensive evaluation, and smokers and patients older than 40 years should receive a more aggressive workup. Diagnostic evaluation can begin with chest X-ray, but a negative X-ray does not rule out lung cancer, nor does it provide tissue diagnosis or staging. High-resolution CT scanning (HRCT) is a more sensitive test for identifying lung cancer even at asymptomatic stages. HRCT can also provide some anatomic detail for staging and determining operability of the cancer. Tissue diagnosis is essential not only for confirming the presence of malignancy but also for determining the histopathology. Fiberoptic bronchoscopy with biopsy, brushings, and washings is highly accurate for diagnosing centrally located bronchogenic carcinoma in the proximal bronchial tree. Transbronchial biopsy can reach deeper tissues for diagnosis of metastatic pulmonary nodules or even lymph node biopsy. Peripheral pulmonary lesions or pleural lesions can be reached by CT-guided needle biopsy or by surgical open lung biopsy [9]. The combination of tissue biopsy and imaging studies yields both the histopathologic type of cancer and the stage of cancer. The non–small cell lung cancer may be further classified into various histopathologic cell types, such as adenocarcinoma and squamous cell carcinoma.

Treatment

General treatment principles and guidelines provide a framework for the primary care practitioner. Histopathology and stage at diagnosis drive treatment options. For example, surgical resection is not generally effective in treating small cell carcinomas of the lung, which may respond better to chemotherapy. On the other hand, a stage I, non–small cell carcinoma might have as much as a 50% 5-year survival rate with appropriate surgical resection.

Treatment options in addition to surgery include radiation therapy and chemotherapy. Response to each of these forms of therapy differs by cell type (squamous cell *versus* adenocarcinoma, for example), by stage of disease, and by whether the tumour is primary or secondary. Metastatic pulmonary nodules from estrogen receptor–positive breast cancer may be treated quite differently from primary adenocarcinoma of the lung, for example, although both generally receive some form of chemotherapy. The primary care practitioner must maintain a close working relationship with medical and surgical oncologists to help guide patients and families through various treatment options [9].

One specific role for the family physician is to help the patient and family address psychosocial needs in a proactive manner. The family physician may facilitate the first conversation between the patient and the patient's family in which the word "cancer" is mentioned or an ongoing conversation in which issues of death and dying can be addressed. The family physician must find the balance in encouraging the family to maintain hope but also in helping the family to develop contingency plans for potential crises such as respiratory arrest or loss of function that leave the patient unable to live independently at home [10]. Health care power of attorney and advance-directive documents are a much needed complement to living wills, which cover only a narrow set of circumstances at the end of life [9]. The family physician can help ensure that pain and other forms of discomfort are managed appropriately and can work closely with patient, family, oncologist, nurses, hospice, and the patient's faith community to proactively manage the balance between preserving life and preventing suffering, especially in a patient with a terminal illness.

Prevention

Smoking causes lung cancer. Never smoking is the most important preventive measure available, but smoking cessation reduces the risk of all the major histologic types of lung cancer. β-carotene and vitamin-E do not prevent lung cancer, and in therapeutic doses β-carotene might be associated with a slight increase in cancer [3].

Regular chest X-ray screening with or without sputum cytology does not improve mortality rates. Recent studies suggest that routine screening of smokers with spiral CT every 6 months does increase detection of early stage cancer and might improve mortality by increasing the percentage of non–small cell cancers that are operable. Stage I non–small cell lung cancer has a 5-year survival rate of nearly 50%, but only 15% of lung cancer are found at this stage without routine screening [10].

Another aspect of preventing lung cancer deaths is the rates at which patients of different racial and ethnic groups receive potentially curative surgery in stage I disease. African American patients, for example, have significantly lower rates of surgery and significantly higher mortality rates. Causes of these racial disparities include patient factors (locus of control, acceptability of surgery, or health beliefs about the risks of opening such cancers to air during surgery), provider factors (biased treatment recommendations or assumptions about what patients might want), systemic or institutional factors (lack of insurance, poverty), and, perhaps most importantly, the patient-physician dyad around which issues of respect, trust, and effective communication influence the outcome of negotiating the treatment plan.

Neoplasms of the lung are most commonly either primary lung carcinomas or metastatic lesions that arise in other organs. Lung carcinomas may be further divided into small cell and non-small cell cancers. Overall, survival for patients with lung carcinoma is only 15%, in part because lung cancer is often diagnosed at inoperable stages.

The Characters of Palliative Care at Lung Cancer

The aim of the palliative care is to decrease the cough, sickness, dyspnea, pain, loss of weight because of diet problem, and also make them comfortable to decrease stress, anxiety and depression based on patients' physiology.

One of the most important patient problems is the limitations because of cancer. After the diagnosis of cancer, it is unreasonable that the limitations are increased by the patients' relatives. However, patients' consciousness is important. Therefore, the patients' relatives may get trained related to palliative care. For this training there should be a well developed organisation. Ideally, a doctor group who works cooperatively for the palliative care, and they should guide the relatives.

As mentioned before, in palliative care, life standard comes into prominence more than life long. Therefore, it is different from the other care principles. The aim is to find and get rid of the patients' discomforts. In order to do that, whatever the symptoms which give discomfort to patients should be analysed in detail. The symptoms may be seen because of the passivity of the patients, not only because of the cancer. The relatives' observations are important for the patients' home resting period. Therefore, the doctor should access their observations. While getting rid of symptoms, the side effects of the medicines should be analysed carefully in order not to be reason of a new symptom. Moreover, the palliative care is not only a symptom control. In the upper level of cancer, the needs are provided by palliative care. If the psychological supports to patients and their relatives are not provided, the pain and the symptom control become impossible. One of the most important works of palliative care group is to determine the level of disease and how it can be stopped. The work results in several argumentations. In developed countries, the patient and their relatives' life standards increase with putting into practice the experiences related to pain and other inconvenient symptoms.

Pain Treatment in Lung Cancer

In the lung cancer patients, the pain comes into existence based upon the oncologic period in 77 % percentage. Moreover, it depends on cancer treatment in 19 % percentage and the other effects not depending on cancer in 4 %. It is hard to join the analgesic aims if the innovations related to cancer pain control are not heard, the doctors and the other medicine workers are not trained well and if some legal problems exist while finding the drugs which are used in the pain control [11].

It a principle that the pain reasons which are pathologic occurrence are not analysed carefully in cancer pain treatment. Like all treatment techniques, the first step is getting rid of the pain reason. For this reason, some techniques such as surgery, chemotherapy and radiotherapy which are applied for cancer treatment should be applied firstly. The pain treatment in cancer patients is started when the other techniques are insufficient. In order to relax the patients while applying the techniques, such as radiotherapy and chemotherapy, and despite the pain, in order to accommodate treatment, it is the true way to control the pain.

Secondarily, the pain threshold should be increased. In order to increase pain threshold, the traditional techniques are given central and peripheral analgesic. Unfortunately, although it is a commonly used medicine both doctors and the patients do not have sufficient information related to analgesic usage. The irregular and unprincipled analgesic usage is the reason of drug addicts and intoxication. One of the upper levels of pain problems in cancer patients' basic reason is the wrong and unprincipled drug usage [11]. The basic principles which should have been carefully followed in analgesic usage, the dose should be arranged as to each patient, it should be given regularly, at the beginning of the pain and orally. Moreover, the analgesic usage principles which are arranged by World Health Organisation (WHO) should be applied.

Several therapeutic techniques are developed for cancer pain treatment. Antineoplastic treatments, analgesic pharmacotherapy, analgesic, neurosurgical, physiological techniques and rehabilitation techniques are used cancer pain treatments. The successful pain treatment is the choice of treatment which is the best therapeutic index. There should be a balance between symptomatic relaxation and the side effects. In 1988, World Health Organisation (WHO) advised the step treatment in cancer pain. Recently, European Association of Physicians has analysed the same principles again. According to that, it is suggested the regulation of analgesic treatment as to intensity of the pain which is evaluated in every step with Visual Analogue Scale (VAS). While evaluating as to 10 point, for between 1-3 point low intensity pain, the 1st level treatment, for between 4-6 point 2nd level of treatment, for between 7-10 point, the 3rd level of treatment can be applied. It is possible to get under control in 90 % percentage with this three step treatment. If the first three levels are not sufficient, as to 4th level of treatment, invasive or interventional pain treatment techniques have been applied [12]. It should be kept in mind that the steps can be applied in any steps of step treatment. The common applied interventional treatment in the pain treatment is the neurolytic nerve blocks and spinal opioid applications.

Neurolytic Nerve Blocks in peripheral or medulla spinalis level nerve fibers, neurologic areas such as alcohol, phenol and glycerol are the long term destruction provided processes [11].

The most commonly used nerve blocks in cancer pain include, gasser ganglion blockage for the cranial neuralgia especially trigeminal, glossopharingeal, vagus, geniculate and atypical facial neuralgies. Ophthalmic, maxillary and mandibular nerve parts are also blocked selectively. Generally, glycerol is chosen as a neurolytic agent.

Subarachnoid and Peridural Neurolytic Blocks are applied as common pains' control depending on lung cancer. Especially, subarachnoid neurolytic block is used commonly. However, the serious complications such as especially sphincter disorder and motor deficit, the techniques have recently almost abandoned.

Spinal Opioid Application provides an effective analgesia with applying opioid as a central way in lung cancer patients. In 1970s, after endogenous opioid peptides and opioid receptors came into existence, usage of that in a way of intrathecally and epidural way was effective and long term analgesia was also put forward. Therefore, when the opioid which is given orally is insufficient, epidural and intrathecal opioid usage comes into existence. When opioids are used epidural and intrathecal way, long term analgesia is provided in lower dosages instead of other ways. Opioid application in these ways is called spinal opioid application.

There are several different ways of spinal opioid application;

1. Percutaneous catheter.
2. Catheter which is put under skin.
3. Port systems.
4. Manual or programmed pump system.

Recently, in parallel with port and pump technological innovations, instead of percutaneous and under skin catheter, especially port and pump systems are chosen in intrathecal applications. For more than ten years, the disadvantage of epidural opioids exists, intrathecal way is being used. In epidural applications, combustion during the injection and fibrosis are the huge disadvantages. In intrathecal applications, subarachnoid fistula and infection are the most important side effects.

In spinal opioid application, morphine is the most commonly used agent. With morphine usage, long term analgesia with a limited dosage can be provided. Because of morphine, the side effects such as sickness, vomiting, and irritation can be seen. In both intrathecal and epidural applications, late breathing depression comes into existence in more rare than the other opioid usage ways. In spinal opioid applications, tolerance comes into existence later than the other ways. The advantages of spinal opioid applications are providing effective and long term analgesia by applying easily; rarely permanent disorders which are neurolytic blocks by decreasing opioid side effects in patients' daily activities.

It should be accepted that every cancer patient has the right to get rid of pain, and to do that, the pain treatment is necessary. In spite of that, the pain treatment should be applied without isolating the patient from the social environment [13]. For the most patients, pain complaints are not only because of the physiological reason and social reasons.

The active care which does not respond to curative treatment is called palliative care. Physiological and social problem control with pain and the other symptom control is very important. The aim of the palliative care is to provide the patients' and their patients' comfort. Palliative care can be applied with the anticancer treatment at the beginning of the disease [14].

Symptomatic Treatment in Lung Cancer

In most of the upper level of lung cancer patients, anorexia, cachexia and asthenia are seen. In some studies, it is more frequently seen than the symptoms such as pain and dyspnea. A direct relationship cannot be found between tumour amount and cachexia. These patients have short life, limited response to cytotoxic agent and high level of side effects of used treatment [15]. Powerlessness, fatigue and weakness are seen together in patients and their life qualities are low. These findings are also concerned with patients' relatives. Nutritional supports, enteral and parenteral support if necessary appetitives megestrol acetate and steroids should be applied. However, it is kept in mind that nutritional support cannot prolong life in terminal patients [16].

Psychiatric disorder is a frequently seen symptom in malignant patients in 50% percentage. If it is not treated, life quality degrades seriously and the conformity to the treatment can be harder. Depression and anxiety are more commonly seen in psychiatric disorders. Applied diagnosis and treatment techniques, the cancer in oneself (brain metastasis), electrolyte imbalances, hormonal imbalances, used drugs and insufficient pain control can be the reason of depression and anxiety [17]. It should be researched if there are the other background reasons, or not. Physiotherapy, antidepressant and anxiolytic drugs are the important parts of the treatment. Anxiety can be seen with not well treated pain. Suddenly cutting the corticosteroids, neuroleptics, bronchodilators, antihistaminics, digitalis preparations, in old patients benzodiazepines, alcohol, opioids, nicotine and benzodiazepines are the reason of the anxiety and the agitation. Moreover, hypoxia, pulmoner emboli, sepsis, hypoglisemi, thyroid abnormalities and the congestive heart failure are together with the anxiety.

Primer metastatic lung disorder and chronic cardiopulmonary disorders result in dyspnea and anxiety based on that, Lorazepam 0.5-2 mg. which has short term effect and lower side effects and can be given four times in a day or sublingually. Moreover, it can be applied parentally or with infusion in patient who has aglutition problem. Delirium is the most common symptom especially in the patients who have upper level of cancer. It appears generally because of indirect effects of cancer. Metabolic disorder, treatment side effects, infection, the deficiencies of nutrition are the reasons of delirium. In the treatment of delirium, insufficient medications, especially psychoactive drugs, should be cut and also background disorder should be corrected. Haloperidol is the most important drug in delirium treatment. 0.5-1 mg of that can be applied twice a day orally. Moreover, in addition to chlorpromazine, risperidone and olanzapine, non-pharmacologically breath taking and giving techniques and stargazing techniques can be tried.

Serious debilitating fatigue and weakness are common in cancer patients. While every modalite in cancer treatment can be the reason of fatigue and weakness, inflammatory cytokines, infections, malnutritions, hypothyroidism and anemia can contribute to same results. Depression and fatigue are seen in most patients. For this reason, the patients should be often examined. The sufficient examinations for depression should be done in order to return the results. In patients who did not have any reasons, exercises programs, patient trainings, energy conversation strategies and stimulation medications can be used [18]. Depression diagnosis is very hard at the terminal term. Fatigue, inappetence and sleeping disorder which are together with the cancer can be seen in patients independent of depression. The questions that "Are you sad?" or "Are you feeling depressed?" help to find the diagnosis. Serotonin specific feedback, inhibitors such as fluoxetine, paroxetine and sertraline can be tolerated well. However, the effect comes into existence in two or three weeks in upper level cancer patients or patients who have short life-long. In addition to fast effect term, the lower side effects are the reason in choosing new or atypical antidepressants such as mirtazapine venlafaxine and methylphenidate. For patients who have short life-long, stimulants such as methylphenidate and pemoline provide fast effects in hours and days.

Dyspnea is a symptom that has an increasing pace in lung cancer patients and especially in patients who are very close to dying. Its prevalence is known as between 29-74% in upper level lung cancer. Dyspnea treatment is one of the most difficult and most fearful symptoms. In addition to direct effect of cancer, indirect effects such as lymphagitis carcinomatosa or pleural infusion; cachexia, anemia, electrolyte disorder pneumonia and emboli also exist. It can develop depending on the toxicity of radiotherapy and chemotherapy which are applied for lung cancer treatment, background chronic obstructive lung disorder, congestive heart failure and asthma. In dyspnea treatment, it should be combined with antitumour and palliative treatments. Local effects of tumours should be get rid of with applied surgery, chemotherapy or radiotherapy. Pleurocenthesis and diuretic are the possible techniques in pleural infusion treatment. Bronchodilators, corticosteroids, inhale or intravenous morphine are effective in symptomatic wellbeing. Especially, low dosage morphine application provides sufficient sedation in terminal term patients. Short term effected anxiolytic can be used.

Sickness and vomiting symptoms may be seen as a percentage 62% of cancer patients who have terminal term. Physiological and physical factors should be considered in these symptom treatments.

The main strategies that should be applied are getting rid of vomiting expectancies and anxiety, giving meal as a small portion, decreasing gastric motilities, and arranging constipate, on and mechanic intestines obstruction. The over dose steroid may be effective at vomiting and sickness because of radiotherapy which is applied to brain and gastrointestinal system. The principal application for vomiting and sickness because of mouth and gastrointestinal system candidiasis is the antifungal treatment. The main reasons of vomiting and sickness are chemotherapy, antibiotics and opioids, and also metabolic problems such as uremia and hypercalcemi. For symptomatic treatment of sickness and vomiting, serotonin antagonist, lorazepam and haloperidol such as metoclopramide, steroids and granisetron can be used. In addition to problems which are mentioned above, cancer patients can experience a sleeping defect, paresis and plegia, incontinence, speaking defect, stubborn cough, pulmonary problems and edema.

To solve the problems of lung cancer patients, well palliative care is needed. Palliative care supports life as accepting the death result. Its aim is to get rid of pain and the other inconvenient symptoms without affecting the lifelong [19]. It provides the patients' integration as physically and socially. Moreover, it provides a supportive system for patients' active life till death. It supports the patients and their families during the disease and after that.

SUMMARY

The life quality of cancer patients has increased in the last 20 years. The main reason is that there is a consensus about necessities of construction of palliative care centres, the conscious usage of analgesic drugs, the symptom control of upper level of patients, and also providing quality life.

However, because of neglecting the palliative care, there are millions of people who complain about pain and other symptoms. The main obstacles about palliative care application are that there are no political applications and that there is deficient training of medicine workers, politicians, administration and public who have fear about possibility of increasing the drug addiction of morphine and the other drugs. Moreover, especially in developing countries, there are limitations about attainment and transporting the drugs which are used for pain and other symptoms, and deficiencies of professional medicine workers who give analgesic and other medicine sufficient doses, and also limitations about financial sources related to palliative care.

ACKNOWLEDGEMENTS

Declared none.

CONFLICT OF INTEREST

The authors confirm that this article content has no conflict of interest.

REFERENCES

[1] Rivera MP, Stover DE. Gender and lung cancer. Clin Chest Med 2004; 25: 391-400.
[2] Albert AJ, Samet JM. Epidemilogy of lung cancer. Chest 2003; 123:21-49.
[3] Simonato L, Agudo A, Ahrens W, *et al.* Lung cancer an, cigarette smoking in Europe: an update of risk estimatesandan assessment of inter-country heterogeneity. Int JCancer 2001;91:876-87.
[4] Jemal A, Tiwari RC, Murray T *et al.* Cancer statistics, 2004. CA Cancer J Clin 2004; 54: 8-29.
[5] Beckett WS. Epidemiology and etiology of lung cancer. Clin Chest Med. 1993; 14: 1-16.
[6] Hecht SS. Cigarette smoking and lung cancer: Chemical mechanism and approaches to prevention. Lancet Oncol 2002;3:461-9.
[7] Skuladottir H, Olsen JH. Epidemiology of lung cancer. Eur Respir Mon, 2001, 17, 1–12.
[8] Beckles MA, Spiro SG, Colice GL, Rudd RM. Initial evaluation of the patient with lung cancer. Symptoms, signs, laboratory tests, and paraneoplastic syndromes. Chest 2003; 123: 97-104.
[9] Collins LG, Haines C, Perkel R, Enck RE. Lung cancer: diagnosis and management. Am Fam Physician. 2007 Jan 1;75(1):56-63.
[10] Spiro SG, Douse J, Read C, Janes S. Complications of lung cancer treatment. Semin Respir Crit Care Med. 2008 Jun;29(3):302-17.
[11] Fine PG, Casaretti D. Pain management at the end of life. In Benzon HT, Rathmell JP, Wu CL, Turk DC, Argoff CE, Raj's practical management of pain. Philadelphia, Mosby-Elsevier, 2008; 1159-1177.
[12] Coyle N. Pain management in the home: Using cancer patients as a model. In Benzon HT, Rathmell JP, Wu CL, Turk DC, Argoff CE, Raj's practical management of pain. Philadelphia, Mosby-Elsevier, 2008; 1179-1186.
[13] Freedman OC, Zimmermann C. The role of palliative care in the lung cancer patient: can we improve quality while limiting futile care?. Curr Opin Pulm Med. 2009 Jul;15(4):321-6.
[14] Plunkett TA, Chrystal KF, Harper PG. Quality of life and the treatment of advanced lung cancer. Clin Lung Cancer. 2003 Jul;5(1):28-32.

[15] Gilbert CR, Smith CM. Advanced lung disease: quality of life and role of palliative care. Mt Sinai J Med. 2009 Feb;76(1):63-70.

[16] Borneman T, Koczywas M, Cristea M, Reckamp K, Sun V, Ferrell B. An interdisciplinary care approach for integration of palliative care in lung cancer. Clin Lung Cancer. 2008 Nov;9(6):352-60.

[17] De Leon Casasola O, Yarussi A. Cancer pain. In Benzon HT, Rathmell JP, Wu CL, Turk DC, Argoff CE, Raj's practical management of pain. Philadelphia, Mosby-Elsevier, 2008; 413-425.

[18] Cortazzo MH, Fishman SM. Major opioids and chronic opioid therapy. In Benzon HT, Rathmell JP, Wu CL, Turk DC, Argoff CE, Raj's practical management of pain. Philadelphia, Mosby-Elsevier, 2008; 597-611.

[19] Burton AW, Phan PC, Cousins MJ. Treatment of cancer pain: role of neural blockade and neuromodulation. In Cousins MJ, Carr DB, Horlocker TT, Bridenbaugh PO. Neural blockade in clinical anesthesia and pain medicine. Philadelphia, Lippincott Williams&Wilkins, a Wolters Kluwer business, 2009; 1111-1153.

INDEX

A

B

D

E

F

G

H

I

K

L

N

R

U

V

W

Y

Made in the USA
Las Vegas, NV
03 November 2026

57424107R00369